ER
A Ready Reckoner

for Emergency Room (ER)
Doctors and First Responders

ER
A Ready Reckoner
for Emergency Room (ER) Doctors and First Responders

Editors

Jamshed D Sunavala
MD FCCP FICP FICSE (Hon)
Director
Department of Critical Care and Emergency Services
Jaslok Hospital and Research Centre, Mumbai
Consultant Intensivist
Breach Candy Hospital and Research Centre and
BD Petit Parsee General Hospital
Mumbai, Maharashtra, India

Sachna P Shetty
MD (Emergency Medicine)
Consultant
Department of Emergency Medicine
Jaslok Hospital and Research Centre
Mumbai, Maharashtra, India

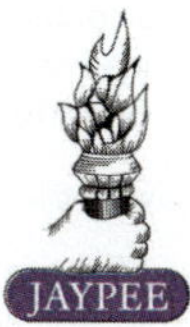

JAYPEE BROTHERS MEDICAL PUBLISHERS
The Health Sciences Publisher
New Delhi | London

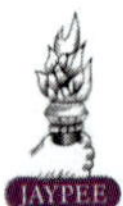

Jaypee Brothers Medical Publishers (P) Ltd

Headquarters
Jaypee Brothers Medical Publishers (P) Ltd
EMCA House, 23/23-B
Ansari Road, Daryaganj
New Delhi 110 002, India
Landline: +91-11-23272143, +91-11-23272703
+91-11-23282021, +91-11-23245672
Email: jaypee@jaypeebrothers.com

Corporate Office
Jaypee Brothers Medical Publishers (P) Ltd
4838/24, Ansari Road, Daryaganj
New Delhi 110 002, India
Phone: +91-11-43574357
Fax: +91-11-43574314
Email: jaypee@jaypeebrothers.com

Overseas Office
JP Medical Ltd.
83, Victoria Street, London
SW1H 0HW (UK)
Phone: +44 20 3170 8910
Fax: +44 (0)20 3008 6180
Email: info@jpmedpub.com

Website: www.jaypeebrothers.com
Website: www.jaypeedigital.com

Inquiries for bulk sales may be solicited at: jaypee@jaypeebrothers.com

ER A Ready Reckoner for Emergency Room (ER) Doctors and First Responders

First Edition: **2025**

ISBN: 978-93-5696-977-3

Printed in India

Dedication

To all nurses who are indeed the first responders and the heartbeat of emergency care!

Jamshed D Sunavala

To my wife who has embraced both motherhood and patient care wholeheartedly.

Sachna P Shetty

To my lifelines, my beloved parents, Usha and Pramod, whose unwavering faith and support have carried me through every stage of my life. Your belief in me has manifested the reality I live today.

And to my grandmother, Rama, who envisioned this journey long before it began—I am sure she is smiling from up there with pride, saying, "I told you so".

They say that finding a good mentor is a rare stroke of luck, but I have been fortunate to have many throughout my journey—from my postgraduate days at Dr DY Patil Medical College to my experiences at Jaslok Hospital and Research Centre to whom I am obliged. However, I want to give special recognition to Dr Jamshed D Sunavala, who has believed in me, challenged me, and inspired me to chase my dreams. His patient guidance and words of wisdom have not only shaped my professional life but also profoundly impacted me personally. I will forever cherish his support.

Lucky is the patient for whom the Bell Tinkles before it Tolls.

–Anonymous

For what are we born if not to Aid One Another.

–Ernest Hemingway

EM has no Rehearsals.

–Jamshed D Sunavala

Contributors

Aabha Nagral
MD DNB (Gastroenterology) CST (UK) Hepatology and Liver Transplantation FINASL Master-ISG
Director
Department of Gastroenterology
Jaslok Hospital and Research Centre
Mumbai, Maharashtra, India
President, Women's Wing South Asian Association for Study of Liver
Chairperson, Liver Committee ZTCC, Mumbai
Managing Trustee, Children's Liver Foundation
Past President/Secretary, Maharashtra Chapter of ISG

Ajay B Jhaveri
DNB (General Medicine) DNB (Gastroenterology)
Consultant Gastroenterologist
Department of Medical Gastroenterology
Jaslok Hospital and Research Centre
Mumbai, Maharashtra, India

Ajit Desai
MD DM (Cardiology) DNB (Cardiology) FACC
Interventional Cardiologist
Department of Cardiology
Jaslok Hospital and Research Centre
Mumbai, Maharashtra, India

Altaf Patel
MD FRCP (lon) FRCP (Edin) FCPS FCMT
Director (Medicine)
Jaslok Hospital and Research Centre
Mumbai, Maharashtra, India

Ameet P Pispati
MS (Orth, Mumbai) MMed Sc (Surgery of Trauma) (UK) DSports Med (UK) MCh Orth (Liverpool, UK) FRCS Trauma & Orth (UK)
Director of Orthopedic Surgery and Consultant Orthopedic Surgeon
Department of Trauma and Orthopedic Surgery
Jaslok Hospital and Research Centre
Mumbai, Maharashtra, India

Anand Bhabhor MD IDCCM
Additional Director and Consultant
Department of Critical Care
Jaslok Hospital and Research Centre
Mumbai, Maharashtra, India

Anjana Sainani MD
Consultant
Department of Medical Oncology
Jaslok Hospital and Research Centre
Mumbai, Maharashtra, India

Ashay Shingare MD DNB
Consultant Nephrologist
Department of Nephrology and Transplantation
Jaslok Hospital and Research Centre
Mumbai, Maharashtra, India

Ashitosh R Patil
DrNB (Nephrology)
Trainee
Department of Nephrology
Jaslok Hospital and Research Centre
Mumbai, Maharashtra, India

Ashwin B Mehta MD FACC FSCI
Director of Cardiology
Department of Cardiology
Jaslok Hospital and Research Centre
Mumbai, Maharashtra, India
Mentor
Sir HN Reliance Foundation Hospital and Research Centre
Mumbai, Maharashtra, India

Ashwin Patil MD DNB
Consultant Nephrologist
Department of Nephrology
Jaslok Hospital and Research Centre
Mumbai, Maharashtra, India

Ayesha J Sunavala
DNB (Gen Medicine) FNB (Infectious Diseases)
Consultant, Infectious Diseases
Division of Infectious Diseases
Department of General Medicine
PD Hinduja Hospital, Jaslok Hospital and Breach Candy Hospital
Mumbai, Maharashtra, India

Azad M Irani DNB (Neurology)
Consultant
Department of Neurology
Jaslok Hospital and Research Centre
Mumbai, Maharashtra, India

Balkrishna P Padate
MD (Med) MRCP (UK) FRCPATH (UK) CCST (UK)
Director and Head
Department of Hematology, Hemato-oncology, BMT
Nanavati Max Superspecialty Hospital
Mumbai, Maharashtra, India
Visiting Consultant
Jaslok Hospital and Research Centre
Mumbai, Maharashtra, India

Bharat Shivdasani
MD DNB (Cardiology) FCPS FESC
Interventional Cardiologist
Department of Cardiology
Jaslok Hospital and Research Centre
Mumbai, Maharashtra, India

Chintamani Godbole
MS DNB (Surgical Gastroenterology) FRCS (Ed)
Consultant Surgeon
Department of Surgical Gastroenterology
Jaslok Hospital and Research Centre
Mumbai, Maharashtra, India

Darius F Soonawalla
MS FRCS DNB DORTH
Consultant Orthopedic Surgeon
Jaslok Hospital and Research Centre
Mumbai, Maharashtra, India

Darshan Jhala
MD (Internal Medicine) DM (cardiology)
Consultant Cardiologist
Department of Cardiology
Lilavati Hospital
Mumbai, Maharashtra, India

Dhimant Goleria MS (Plastic Surgery)
Director
Department of Plastic and Reconstructive Surgery
Jaslok Hospital and Research Centre
Mumbai, Maharashtra, India

Divya A Samat MBBS
Resident
Department of Internal Medicine
Tower Health-Reading Hospital
Reading, Pennsylvania, USA

Divya Prabhat MS DOR DNB FICS
Head
Department of ENT
Wadia Children Hospital
Mumbai, Maharashtra, India
Jaslok Hospital and Research Centre
Mumbai, Maharashtra, India

Fali Poncha
MD (Med) DNB (Neurology) Fellowship in Cerebrovascular Diseases (Canada)
Consultant Neurologist
Department of Neurology
Jaslok Hospital and Research Centre
Mumbai, Maharashtra, India

Fazal Nabi DNB (Pediatrics)
Head
Department of Pediatrics and Neonatology
Jaslok Hospital and Research Centre
Mumbai, Maharashtra, India

Gautam Zaveri MS DORTH DNB
Director
Department of Spine Surgery
Jaslok Hospital and Research Centre
Mumbai, Maharashtra, India

GN Mansukhani
DGO DRCOG FRCOG (Lon)
Director
Department of Obstetrics and Gynecology
Jaslok Hospital and Research Centre
Mumbai, Maharashtra, India

Govind Purushothanam
DNB MCh GI Surgery
Consultant GI and HPB Surgeon
Department of Gastroenterology
Paalana Institute of Medical Sciences
Palakkad, Kerala, India

Hasnain Patel MD FCMT
Internist
Dr Patel's Clinic
Mumbai, Maharashtra, India

Heli S Shah
MD DM (Neurology) Post Doctorate (Movement Disorders)
Consultant Neurologist and Movement Disorder Specialist
Department of Neurology
Sterling Hospital, SVP Institute of Medical Science and Research
Ahmedabad, Gujarat, India
Former Post-doctoral Fellow
Jaslok Hospital and Research Centre
Mumbai, Maharashtra, India

Hemant P Thacker
MD (Bom) MRSH (London) FACP (USA) FACE (USA)
Head
Department of Medicine
Bhatia Hospital, Mumbai
Additional Director of Medicine
Jaslok Hospital and Research Centre, Mumbai
Consultant
Breach Candy Hospital
Mumbai, Maharashtra, India

Hemraj B Chandalia MD FACP
Director
Department of Endocrinology, Diabetes and Metabolism
Jaslok Hospital and Research Centre
Mumbai, Maharashtra, India

Indraneel P Raut
DNB (Medicine) IDCCM IFCCM EDIC
Additional Director
Department of Critical Care
Jaslok Hospital and Research Centre
Mumbai, Maharashtra, India

Jamshed D Sunavala
MD FCCP FICP FICSE (Hon)
Director
Department of Critical Care and Emergency Services
Jaslok Hospital and Research Centre, Mumbai
Consultant Intensivist
Breach Candy Hospital and Research Centre and BD Petit Parsee General Hospital
Mumbai, Maharashtra, India

Janhavi Gholap
MD (Anesthesia) DNB (Anesthesia) IDCCM
Junior Consultant and Intensivist
Department of Critical Care
Jaslok Hospital and Research Centre
Mumbai, Maharashtra, India

Janhvi Mehta DNB FRCS MAS
Consultant
Department of Ophthalmology
Jaslok Hospital and Research Centre
Mumbai, Maharashtra, India

Jeenam Shah MD DNB
Consultant
Department of Respiratory Medicine
Jaslok Hospital and Research Centre
Mumbai, Maharashtra, India

JK Maniar MD DVD DDV
Consultant
Department of Infectious Diseases
Jaslok Hospital and Research Centre
Mumbai, Maharashtra, India

Joy D Desai MD (Med) DNB (Neurology)
Director (Neurology)
Jaslok Hospital and Research Centre
Mumbai, Maharashtra, India

Judith Rebello
Fellow
Department Gastrointestinal Surgery
Jaslok Hospital and Research Centre
Mumbai, Maharashtra, India

Jyoti Narayan DNB (Radiology)
Clinical Associate
Department of Radiology
Jaslok Hospital and Research Centre
Mumbai, Maharashtra, India

Jyotiprakash Panda MD DNB
Consultant
Department of Microbiology
Apollo Hospital
Navi Mumbai, Maharashtra, India

Kaustubh Vaidya
MD (Internal Medicine) DM (Cardiology) Fellow of Indian Society of Electrocardiology
Consultant
Department of Cardiology
Jaslok Hospital and Research Centre
Mumbai, Maharashtra, India

Kayomars B Kapadia
MS FRCS (Eng) FRCS (Edin)
Consultant Surgeon
Department of Laparoscopic and Minimally Invasive Surgery
Jaslok Hospital, HN Reliance Hospital, Breach Candy Hospital
Mumbai, Maharashtra, India

Kiran M Ladkat
DNB (Orthopedics) MNAMS
Consultant Orthopedic Surgeon
Department of Orthopedics
Jaslok Hospital and Research Centre
Mumbai, Maharashtra, India

Kunal Dinesh Kale MD DrNB (Cardio)
Resident
Department of Cardiology
Jaslok Hospital and Research Centre
Mumbai, Maharashtra, India

Kunal Srivastava MBBS
Senior Manager
Medical Affairs
Wockhardt Ltd
Mumbai, Maharashtra, India

Madan M Bahadur MD DNB
Director
Department of Nephrology and Transplantation
Jaslok Hospital and Research Centre
Mumbai, Maharashtra, India

Mala Kaneria
MD (Internal Medicine) FICP Infectious Diseases Certificate Course (IDCC)
Professor and Unit Head
Department of Medicine
Topiwala National Medical College and BYL Nair Charitable Hospital
Professor and Unit Head
Department of Infectious Diseases
Kasturba Hospital for Infectious Diseases
Consultant, Infectious Diseases and HIV Medicine
Jaslok Hospital and Research Centre
Mumbai, Maharashtra, India

Malav Jhala
MD (Internal Medicine) DM (Cardiology)
Cardiologist
Lilavati Hospital and Research Centre
Mumbai, Maharashtra, India

Malavika Kohli MD DVD DNB
Founder and Director
Skin Secrets
Mumbai, Maharashtra, India
Consultant Dermatologist
Department of Dermatology
Jaslok Hospital and Research Centre,
Breach Candy Hospital Trust
Mumbai, Maharashtra, India

Manali Patel DA FCCCM C-IAPC
Former Consultant
Department of Critical Care and
Palliative Medicine
Jaslok Hospital, Mumbai
Consultant In-charge
High Dependency Unit and
Rehabilitation Medicine
Medanta Super Speciality Hospital
Lucknow, Uttar Pradesh, India

Manish Kothari
MS (Ortho AIIMS) FNB Spine, Spine Fellowship
RCS (Edin) UK
Consultant Spine Surgeon
Department of Spine Surgery
Jaslok Hospital and Research Centre
Mumbai, Maharashtra, India

Mehul S Bhansali MS DNB
Director
Department of Surgical Oncology
Jaslok Hospital and Research Centre
Mumbai, Maharashtra, India

Milind M Khadke
MD (Chest & TB) PGDGM (XLRI) PGDMLE
(National Law School)
Director (Medical Services)
Jaslok Hospital and Research Centre
Mumbai, Maharashtra, India

Natasha Tipnis
MD (Internal Medicine) DrNB (Neurology)
PDF (Epilepsy)
Consultant
Department of Neurology
Jaslok Hospital and Research Centre
Mumbai, Maharashtra, India

Nidhi Shah Gandhi
DGO DNB IFCPC IARC (Colposcopy)
Consultant Obstetrician and
Gynecologist, Colposcopist
Department of Obstetrics and
Gynecology
Jaslok Hospital and Research Centre,
Cama and Albless Hospital, Vora
Maternity and Nursing Home, Women's
Care Clinic
Mumbai, Maharashtra, India

Nihar Mehta
MD DNB (Medicine) DNB (Cardiology)
FRCP (London) FICP
Associate Director (TAVI and Structural
Heart Valve)
Department of Cardiology
Jaslok Hospital and Research Centre
Mumbai, Maharashtra, India

Nikesh Jain
DNB (Medicine) DNB (Cardiology)
Consultant
Department of Cardiology
Jaslok Hospital and Research Centre
Mumbai, Maharashtra, India

Nikhil S Chamankar
DNB (General Surgery) DrNB (Neurosurgery)
Consultant Neurosurgeon
Department of Neurosurgery
Sanjivani Hospital
Palghar, Maharashtra, India

Nilesh Doctor MS FRCS DNB
Consultant (Gastrointestinal and
Hepatopancreatobiliary)
Director
Department of Surgical
Gastroenterology
Jaslok Hospital and Research Center
Mumbai, Maharashtra, India

Nimish M Shah
MRCP (UK) MRCP (Respiratory Medicine) PG Cert Clin Ed (Kings College London)
Consultant (Pulmonary and Sleep Medicine)
Department of Respiratory Medicine
Jaslok Hospital and Research Centre
Mumbai, Maharashtra, India

Niraj Pawar MD (Med) DNB (Cardio)
Former Registrar
Department of Cardiology
Jaslok Hospital and Research Centre
Mumbai, Maharashtra, India

Nirmee N Shah
MRC Psych MSc (Clin Pharm)
Consultant Psychiatrist
Department of Psychiatry
Jaslok Hospital and Research Centre
Mumbai, Maharashtra, India

Parnasha Chemburkar
Fellow
Department of Gastrointestinal Surgery
Jaslok Hospital and Research Centre
Mumbai, Maharashtra, India

Percy J Chibber
MS FCPS FRCS MNAMS (Urology)
Senior Consultant
Department of Urology
Jaslok Hospital and Research Centre
Mumbai, Maharashtra, India

Pettarusp M Wadia
MD DNB (Med) DM DNB (Neurology)
Fellowship in Movement Disorders
Consultant Neurologist, Movement Disorder Specialist
Department of Neurology
Jaslok Hospital and Research Centre
Mumbai, Maharashtra, India

Phiroze Patel
MS FRCS (ED) FRC Ophth (UK)
Director and Head
Department of Ophthalmology
Jaslok Hospital and Research Center
Mumbai, Maharashtra, India

Pinank Pandya
MD (Anesthesia) FNB (Critical Care Medicine) EDIC (UK)
Consultant Intensivist
Department of Critical Care Medicine
Jaslok Hospital and Research Centre
Mumbai, Maharashtra, India

Pooja P Vyas
DMRE Fellowship in Fetal Medicine
Consultant Radiologist
Department of Ultrasound
Jaslok Hospital and Research Centre
Mumbai, Maharashtra, India

Preeti P Doshi MD FIPP FIAPM
Director and Consultant In-charge
Department of Pain Medicine
Jaslok Hospital and Research Centre,
Breach Candy Hospital
Mumbai, Maharashtra, India

Prerna Gomes
MD (Anesthesia) Executive Postgraduate Diploma in Hospital Administration
Head
Department of Anesthesia
Jaslok Hospital and Research Center
Mumbai, Maharashtra, India

Pushkar Mahajan DNB (Radiology)
Junior Resident
Department of Radio-diagnosis and Imaging
Jaslok Hospital and Research Centre
Mumbai, Maharashtra, India

Rafat Ali Khan
MNAMS DNB (General Surgery)
MCh (Plastic Surgery)
Honorary Consultant Plastic Surgeon
Department of Plastic and Reconstructive Surgery
Jaslok Hospital and Research Centre
Mumbai, Maharashtra, India

Rahul Chhabria DNB (Cardiology)
Associate Director (Emergency Cardiology)
Department of Cardiology
Jaslok Hospital and Research Centre
Mumbai, Maharashtra, India

Rajesh Sainani
MD DNB (Gastroenterology)
Consultant Gastroenterologist
Department of Medical Gastroenterology
Jaslok Hospital and Research Centre
Mumbai, Maharashtra, India

Rajiv S Mathur
MD (Gen Med) DNB (Resp Dis) Fellowship in Respiratory Medicine at Glenfield Hospital, Leicester, UK, Fellowship in Sleep Medicine from St Thomas Hospital, London, UK and Royal Prince Alfred Hospital, Sydney, Australia
Director
Department of Respiratory Medicine
Jaslok Hospital and Research Centre
Mumbai, Maharashtra, India

Ravi S Shah
MD DrNB (Gastroenterology)
Resident
Department of Medical Gastroenterology
Jaslok Hospital and Research Centre
Mumbai, Maharashtra, India

Resham Vasani
MD (Dermatology, Venereology & Leprosy) DDVL FCPS
Consultant Dermatologist
Bhojani Clinic
Mumbai, Maharashtra, India

Ritu Kashikar
DMRD DNB (Radiology)
Consultant
Department of Radiology
Jaslok Hospital and Research Centre
Mumbai, Maharashtra, India

Rushi V Deshpande
MD DM DNB (Nephrology)
Director of Academics
Department of Nephrology
Jaslok Hospital and Research Centre
Mumbai, Maharashtra, India

Sachna P Shetty
MD (Emergency Medicine)
Consultant
Department of Emergency Medicine
Jaslok Hospital and Research Centre
Mumbai, Maharashtra, India

Sadashiv Chaudhari
DNB (Gen Sur) FALS FMAS FIAGES
Consultant
Department of General Surgery
Jaslok Hospital and Research Centre
Mumbai, Maharashtra, India

Sana Aamir MBBS
Registrar in Orthopedic Surgery
Department of Trauma and Orthopedic Surgery
Jaslok Hospital and Research Centre
Mumbai, Maharashtra, India

Sandeep A Seth
DNB (Anes) IDCCM EDIC
Senior Consultant and Chief Intensivist
Department of Critical Care
Jaslok Hospital and Research Centre
Mumbai, Maharashtra, India

Sanjay Nagral MS FACS
Director
Department of Surgical Gastroenterology
Jaslok Hospital and Research Centre
Mumbai, Maharashtra, India

Santosh Gawali MS DNB (Urology)
Senior Consultant and PG Teacher
Department of Urology
Jaslok Hospital and Research Centre
Mumbai, Maharashtra, India

Sanyogita Warang DDVL DNB
Dermatologist
Department of Dermatology
Jaslok Hospital and Research Centre
Mumbai, Maharashtra, India

Savi J Kapila DNB (Anesthesiology)
Consultant Anesthesiology
Department of Anesthesiology
Jaslok Hospital and Research Centre
Mumbai, Maharashtra, India

Shailesh Raina
MS (Surg) D Urology (London)
Director
Department of Urology
Jaslok Hospital and Research Centre
Mumbai, Maharashtra, India

Shaival H Chandalia MD FRCP
Coordinator
Department of Endocrinology, Diabetes and Metabolism
Jaslok Hospital and Research Centre
Mumbai, Maharashtra, India

Shamsunder R Handa
MD (Medicine) DNB (Cardiology)
Cardiologist
Jaslok Hospital and Research Centre
Mumbai, Maharashtra, India

Shilpa P Agrawal
DGO DNB FCPS FNB (Fellowship in High-risk Pregnancy and Perinatology)
Consultant
Department of Obstetrics and Gynecology
Jaslok Hospital and Research Centre
Mumbai, Maharashtra, India

Shruti M Tandan-Pardasani
MD FNB
Consultant
Department of Critical Care
Jaslok Hospital and Research Centre
Mumbai, Maharashtra, India

Shweta Parekh
DrNB (Gastroeneterology)
Resident
Department of Medical Gastroenterology
Jaslok Hospital and Research Centre
Mumbai, Maharashtra, India

Siddharth Shah
MS (Ortho, Mumbai) FRCS (Glasgow)
Consultant Orthopedic Surgeon
Department of Orthopedics
Fortis SL Raheja Hospital
Mumbai, Maharashtra, India

SM Katrak
MD DM (Neurology) FRCP (Edinburgh)
Director Emeritus
Department of Neurology
Jaslok Hospital and Research Centre, Mumbai
Emeritus Professor
Grant Medical College and Sir JJ Group of Hospitals
Mumbai, Maharashtra, India

Snehal A Bhange
MS (General Surgery) MRCS (Eng)
Head
Department of General Surgery
Jaslok Hospital and Research Centre
Mumbai, Maharashtra, India

Sonar Narula MD (Microbiology)
Head
Department of Laboratory Medicine
Jaslok Hospital and Research Centre
Mumbai, Maharashtra, India

Sudeshna Ray
MD (Obs/Gyne) FRCOG (London)
Additional Director
Department of Obstetrics and Gynecology
Jaslok Hospital and Research Centre
Mumbai, Maharashtra, India

Sudheer Ambekar MCh IFAANS
Consultant Neurosurgeon
Department of Neurosurgery
Jaslok Hospital and Research Centre
Mumbai, Maharashtra, India

Sunil B Jain
MBBS PGCCAE PGCCCD PGDHHM MMED FACEE CCEBDM PGDCED CCCDM FDI FAIG
Head and Consultant Emergency
Department of Emergency Medicine
Jaslok Hospital and Research Centre
Mumbai, Maharashtra, India

Suresh V Joshi
MS (Gen Surg) MS (CVTS) FIACS FCCP FICS
Associate Director
Department of Cardiovascular and Thoracic Surgery
Jaslok Hospital and Research Centre
Mumbai, Maharashtra, India

Sushil C Munsi
MD DM (Cardiology) FRCP FACC
Emeritus Director (Cardiology)
Department of Cardiology
Jaslok Hospital and Research Centre
Mumbai, Maharashtra, India

Tulika Goleria
MS DOMS PGDML PGDHHM Fellowship in Cataract Surgery and Oculoplasty
Consultant
Department of Ophthalmology
Jaslok Hospital and Research Centre, Mumbai
Shushrusha Hospital, Mumbai
Conwest and Manjula S Badani Jain Hospital
Mumbai, Maharashtra, India

Upendra D Bhalerao
MS MCh (CVTS) DNB (CTS) FIACS
Senior Consultant, Cardiovascular Thoracic Surgery, Heart, and Lung Transplantation
Department of Cardiology and Thoracic Surgery
Jaslok Hospital and Research Centre
Mumbai, Maharashtra, India

Varshil Shah DNB (Pediatrics)
Clinical Associate
Department of Pediatrics and Neonatology
Jaslok Hospital and Research Centre
Mumbai, Maharashtra, India

Varun Deshmukh MD FNB EDIC FCCU
Consultant Intensivist
Department of Critical Care Medicine
Vishesh Jupiter Hospital
Indore, Madhya Pradesh, India

Vimesh Rajput MS (Gen Surg) DNB (Super-Specialty Thoracic Surgery)
Professor and Hon Senior Consultant
Department of Thoracic Surgery
Jaslok Hospital and Research Centre, Breach Candy Hospital, Mumbai
Professor
Sir JJ Hospital and Grant Medical College
Mumbai, Maharashtra, India

Vishal Gavali
MD (Gen Med) DrNB (Cardio)
Senior Registrar
Department of Cardiology
Jaslok Hospital and Research Centre
Mumbai, Maharashtra, India

Vismaya KB MBBS
Fellow
Department Gastrointestinal Surgery
Jaslok Hospital and Research Centre
Mumbai, Maharashtra, India

Vivek Shetty
MS DrNB (Surgical Gastroenterology)
Consultant Surgeon
Department of Gastrointestinal and Hepatopancreatobiliary Surgery
Jaslok Hospital and Research Centre
Mumbai, Maharashtra, India

Yash Gupte MD DrNB (Cardio)
Resident
Department of Cardiology
Jaslok Hospital and Research Centre
Mumbai, Maharashtra, India

Preface

Emergency medicine is now an established broad specialty dealing with patients suffering from acute and life-threatening illnesses arriving at the doorstep of the hospital.

In the emergency room (ER), patient situations can escalate rapidly, primarily because of the paucity of time for clinical assessment. The additional pressures of anxious relatives demanding attention and the inherent urgency of critical care make managing patients in this setting a formidable task.

Very often, the presenting diagnosis is not that simple to decipher, and it may be prudent to initiate therapy toward correcting the hemodynamic and respiratory derangement. This makes ER practice uniquely challenging compared to inpatient or ICU care.

This book is not intended to serve as a Comprehensive Textbook of Emergency Medicine. Instead, as the title suggests, it is a "Ready Reckoner" designed for quick bedside decision-making. However, we strongly recommend that readers familiarize themselves with its contents beforehand to maximize its utility during emergencies.

We have endeavored to make this book as concise as possible and easy for rapid reference.

It would benefit the reader to check the brief introduction on "*How to Use the Book*".

Structure of the Book

The book is organized into several parts:

1. *Fast Track to the Most Common Presentation in the ER:* The first part provides a fast-track approach to differential diagnosis, associated with presenting symptoms commonly encountered in the ER to facilitate rapid decision-making.
2. *Bedside Diagnosis and Management of Diseases Presented in the ER:* The second part delves into relevant differential diagnoses in greater detail, presented concisely in box formats to ensure clarity and ease of use. This avoids lengthy narratives, staying true to the purpose of a ready reckoner. Despite its brevity, the information provided is accurate and factual.

3&4. *Resuscitation in the ER and Emergency Support:* The third and fourth parts address supportive care, reflecting the evolving trends in modern emergency medicine, where longer ER stays are common. Supportive care initiated in the ER often continues seamlessly upon transfer to the ICU.

5. *Common Medical and Surgical Procedures:* The fifth part outlines common bedside medical and surgical procedures performed in the ER.

6&7. *Additional Resources:* Other parts provide insights into frequently used investigations, medicolegal queries, and broader perspectives on ER operations.

Final Thoughts

We hope this book serves as a valuable tool in enhancing the care of patients presenting to the ER with diverse and often devastating medical or surgical complications. It is our sincere effort to make a meaningful contribution to the field of emergency medicine and to the lives of those who practice it.

Jamshed D Sunavala
Sachna P Shetty

Acknowledgments

This book is indeed a Jaslok Hospital initiative and an acknowledgment of the encouragement and support, we always receive from the Jaslok Hospital trustees for all our academic pursuits.

The CEO of Jaslok Hospital and Research Centre, Mr Jitendra Haryan along with the Medical Director, Dr Milind M Khadke, were keen to have this book released simultaneously with the opening of the new emergency room (ER), and without their help and support this would not have been possible.

The main idea was to use the contribution from the consultants of various specialties attached to Jaslok Hospital and other leading hospitals. Their personal inputs regarding evidence and experience-based medicine were meticulously incorporated, to be followed in the emergency department, especially in their absence.

This was a monumental task for the Editors to follow-up, edit, maintain uniformity with timely submission, and most importantly to have a universal appeal of the subject matter. Hence, we are immensely grateful to our contributors for readily accepting to write their chapters despite their heavy schedule and pressing responsibilities.

We would like to express our gratitude to our part (sectional) editors: Drs Anand Bhabhor, Shruti M Tandan-Pardasani, and Indraneel P Raut for overseeing the Medicine and Surgery section; Dr Nimish M Shah for the Respiratory section; Drs Sanjay Nagral and Nilesh Doctor for the Gastrosurgery section; Dr Manali Patel for Part 1; and Dr Sandeep A Seth for the General Emergency section.

We would also like to thank M/s Jaypee Brothers Medical Publishers (P) Ltd, New Delhi, India and appreciate the constant support and encouragement of Shri Jitendra P Vij (Group Chairman) and Mr Ankit Vij (Managing Director) and their associate Ms Chetna Malhotra (Senior Director—Professional Publishing, Marketing, and Business Development). Special thanks go to the clinical assistants who helped to format the manuscript on the Internet and to Ms Kritika Dua (Senior Commissioning Editor) and Ms Somoshri Banerji (Development Editor) who have been prompt and efficient.

Contents

Section 2: Trauma

PART 3: RESUSCITATION IN EMERGENCY ROOM

PART 4: EMERGENCY SUPPORT

PART 5: PROCEDURES DONE IN THE EMERGENCY ROOM

Part 1

Fast Track to the Most Common Presentations in the Emergency Room

CHAPTER 1

Fast Track to the Most Common Presentations in the Emergency Room

1.1 FAST TRACK TO THE MOST COMMON PRESENTATIONS IN THE EMERGENCY ROOM

Sachna P Shetty, Jamshed D Sunavala

BOX 1: Presentation: Breathlessness/shortness of breath.

Pertinent bedside tests	***Differential diagnosis***	***Strong clinical indicators***
	Respiratory system	
SpO_2: Hypoxia Portable spirometry-FEV1, FVC CXR	Severe asthma (Page no. 35)	• Past history of asthma • Rhonchi or silent chest if severe
ABG: Type II respiratory failure CXR	COPD exacerbation (Page no. 42)	• Past history of COPD along with other relevant risk factor • Smoker • Drowsy • Diffuse crepitation or rhonchi
SpO_2: Hypoxia ECG CXR-WNL mostly, other signs in details in the chapter 2D echo-rv dilation and the other findings in respective chapter ABG: Type I respiratory failure, respiratory alkalosis might be noted, look for alveolar arterial oxygen gradient	Pulmonary embolism (Page no. 114)	**Risk factors:** Obesity/malignancy/bedridden/recent surgery/long flight/long bone fracture: • Sudden SOB • Unilateral leg swelling • Tachycardia • Tachypnea • Rule out other causes of SOB/chest pain
SpO_2: Hypoxia *CXR*: LRTI (usually bilateral/right dominant)	Aspiration	• Bedridden/decreased GCS/precise history of coughing or choking while eating/recent stroke • Decreased saturation • Crepitation right dominant • Fever

Contd...

Contd...

Pertinent bedside tests	*Differential diagnosis*	*Strong clinical indicators*
SpO_2: Hypoxia CBC Biomarkers (CRP/PCT) CXR	Pneumonia (Page no. 48)	• History of fever and cough, green/yellow phlegm • Focal crepitation/adventitious sounds
Mainly clinical and history	Anaphylaxis (Page no. 676)	• History of intake of new drug or food • Sudden breathless/wheeze/stridor • Itching/rash/diarrhea/abdomen pain • Edema face or oral • Chest discomfort • Shock in some cases
SpO_2: Hypoxia CXR	Airway obstruction	• History of foreign body ingestion/pediatric age group • Stridor • Ca larynx/radiation • Postprolonged intubation
CXR Bedside POCUS	Pneumothorax (Page no. 448)	• Trauma/TB/malignancy/iatrogenic • Desaturation • Reduced breath sound/movement unilaterally • Hemodynamic instability noted in moderate-to-severe cases
CXR USG chest	Pleural effusion	• Shortness of breath only with large amount of fluids • Pleuritic pain • Dullness in percussion • Classically reduced breath sounds on auscultation in the effected zone
Bedside CXR *ABG*: Hypoxia bedside POCUS 2D echo ECG	**Cardiovascular system** Acute heart failure (Page no. 101)	• History of cardiac ailment (ACS/arrhythmias/valvular heart disease/cardiomyopathy) • Desaturation/hypoxia • Chest discomfort • Basal crepitation • Pedal edema/raised JVP • Frothing/perspiration • Tachycardia • Tachypnea • Hypertension/hypotension
ECG: Electric alternans, low voltage ECG Bedside echo	Cardiac tamponade (Page no. 144)	• Trauma/iatrogenic • Triad of hypotension, raised JVP muffled heart sound

Contd...

Contd...

Pertinent bedside tests	*Differential diagnosis*	*Strong clinical indicators*
Beside USG	**Extrathoracic causes:** Raised intra-abdominal pressure (abdominal-ascites, obesity, pregnancy, tumor, obstruction, and paralytic ileus)	• Increased or normal respiratory rate • Pain/discomfort in the abdomen • Reduced breath sounds if pleural effusion secondary to ascites
	Metabolic acidosis (DKA and renal failure) (Page no. 845)	Details given in **Box 9**
ABG: Hypoxia or hypocarbia but very often normal	Neuromuscular [GBS, multiple sclerosis (MS)]	• Abnormal breathing pattern (SHALLOW)—GBS • Associated history • Ascending paralysis in GBS • Symptoms of limb weakens, loss of vision, tingling, and impaired coordination
	Toxicology: • Snake bite • Neuro toxins • Carbon monoxide poisoning • Methemoglobinemia • Organophosphate or salicylate poisoning (Page no. 525)	*History of bites/toxin administration:* Determine the appropriate toxidrome (anticholinergic, cholinergic, sympathetic, and opioid)
CBC: Neutrophilic leukocytosis or leukopenia ABG—elevated lactates (shock) Increased CRP/PCT cultures	Sepsis (Page no. 298)	• History of infection • Tachycardia • Tachypnea • Temperature • Organ dysfunction • Hypotension not responding to volume resuscitation (shock)
Most bedside tests are normal ABG: Low pCO_2 (hyperventilation)	Psychiatric	Diagnosis of exclusion normal lungs/saturation hyperventilation, anxiety

(ABG: arterial blood gas; ACS: acute coronary syndrome; BUN: blood urea nitrogen; CBC: complete blood count; CRP: C-reactive protein; COPD: chronic obstructive pulmonary disease; CVS: coronary artery vasospasm; CXR: chest X-ray; CXR-WNL: chest X-ray within normal limits; ECG: electrocardiography; FEV1: forced expiratory volume in the one second; FVC: forced vital capacity; GCS: Glasgow Coma Scale; JVP: jugular venous pressure; LRTI: lower respiratory tract infection; PCT: procalcitonin; POCUS: point-of-care ultrasound; SpO_2: arterial oxygen saturation; SOB: shortness of breath; USG: ultrasonography)

BOX 2: Presentation: Chest pain.

Pertinent bedside tests	*Differential diagnosis*	*Strong clinical indicators*
Bedside ECG Cardiac markers Echo	**Cardiovascular system** Angina (Page no. 71)	• Diffuse precordial or retrosternal chest pain can radiate (arms, neck, and jaw; epigastric), intermittently present, last few minutes can be associated with sweating, nausea, and giddiness • Usually on exertion • Inframammary an uncommon site of pain • Risk factors
Bedside ECG cardiac markers 2D echo	Acute myocardial infarction (Page no. 71)	• Acute severe chest pain at rest • Can present as heaviness/squeezing/pressing sensation of chest radiates mostly (arms/neck/jaw), associated with perspiration, nausea, discomfort, giddiness, and breathlessness • Unusual site is inframammary • Hypotension/hypertension • May mimic like acid reflux
Echo/POCUS/ 2D echo CXR	Aortic dissection (Page no. 130)	• Risk factors • Pain is acute sharp/stabbing/may or may not radiate to back • Most of the patients have severe-onset pain, maximal at beginning with radiation from anterior chest to the interscapular area; tearing quality; pain migrates • Neuro complications common—stroke, syncope, paresis, or paraplegia • Can mimic ACS, mesenteric ischemia, acute abdomen • Majority have **hypertension** or hemodynamic compromise, limb BP discrepancy
ECG Echo	Pericarditis myocarditis, stress cardiomyopathy (Page no. 144)	Postviral/infective
	Cardiac tamponade	Mentioned in **Box 1**
	Respiratory system • Pulmonary embolism • Pneumothorax	Mentioned in **Box 1**
	Pleuritic chest pain	Mentioned in **Box 1**
	Pneumonia	Discussed in **Box 1**

Contd...

Contd...

Pertinent bedside tests	***Differential diagnosis***	***Strong clinical indicators***
ECG and CXR (negative findings)	**Other causes** Chest wall pain	• Sharp/localized/positional/on inspiration or coughing • Can have tenderness—costochondritis • Can have xiphoid swelling—xiphodynia
UGI scopy	GI pain (Page no. 194)	• History/physical examination • Acid reflux-burning/burping/acid taste, relives with antacid • Peptic ulcer disease—postprandial dull aching • Esophageal spasm • Duodenal-relived pain on eating • Gastric ulcer increased pain on eating • Pancreatitis—mentioned • Biliary colic
CXR -mediastinal air/pleural effusion/widened mediastinum/ pneumothorax UGI scopy	Esophageal tear (Mallory Weiss or Boerhaave's) (Page no. 214)	• Risk factors—forceful vomiting, foreign body, caustic ingestion, trauma, alcoholism, esophageal disease • Pain is mostly retrosternal, persistent, precedes vomiting in most cases may be in shock might have signs of pleural effusion/pneumothorax/ consolidation
	Psychiatry	Hyperventilation, rule out other causes
	Shingles	Unilateral lesions/pain restricted to one dermatome for HZV
	Trauma (pneumothorax, cardiac tamponade, rib fracture/chest contusion)	History and examination mentioned in detail in the chapter

(HZV: Herpes zoster virus; GI: gastrointestinal; UGI: upper gastrointestinal)

BOX 3: Presentation: Headache.

Pertinent bedside tests	***Differential diagnosis***	***Strong clinical indicators***
Bedside LP-Xanthochromia	**CNS** Subacute arachnoid hemorrhage (Page no. 293)	• Worst headache ever • Hypertension • Other neurological signs and symptoms, check ottawa rule for SAH
LP: CSF examination	Meningitis/encephalitis/abscess (Page no. 361)	• Tachycardia/fever, seizure, and neck stiffness • History of sinus/ear infection or recent surgery • Impacted living conditions (e.g., military barracks and college dormitories)
CSF: Increased pressure Fundoscopy	Increased ICP	• History of prior benign intracranial hypertension • Presence of a CSF shunt-hypertension with normal HR or bradycardia
	Cluster headache (Page no. 248)	• Severe • Unilateral • Lasts 15–180 minutes (untreated) • Circadian/circannual pattern • Lacrimation/conjunctival injection • Nasal congestion or rhinorrhea Can have: • Ptosis and/or miosis • Edema of the eyelid and/or face • Sweating of the forehead and/or face
	Tension headache (Page no. 248)	• Tight, bandlike discomfort around the head that is nonpulsating and dull, may experience tightening of the neck muscles • Generally mild, self-resolving • Associated with anxiety/depression
	Migraine (Page no. 298)	• Classic—Aura-visual, sensory, speech, motor, brainstem, retinal, photophobia and phonophobia • Triggering factors, past history • Nonclassic—attack lasts 4–72 hours (untreated or unsuccessfully treated) – Unilateral location – Pulsating quality – Moderate-to-severe pain intensity – Aggravation by or causing avoidance of routine physical activity (e.g., walking or climbing stairs)

Contd...

Contd...

Pertinent bedside tests	***Differential diagnosis***	***Strong clinical indicators***
		– Nausea or vomiting – Not attributable to another disorder • In females, it is common to have migraines during menstruation
Important to refer for imaging as it is diagnostic	Cerebral venous thrombosis	• Generally severe, sudden, thunder-clap headache mostly in women of postpartum, peripartum, reproductive age/on oral contraceptive, prothrombotic • Near syncope such as features might be noted
Important to refer for imaging as it is diagnostic	Posterior reversible encephalopathy syndrome (PRES)	• Headache with visual loss, altered mental status, seizures • Patient has increased blood pressure mostly • Underlying associated conditions—autoimmune disorder, immunosuppression, chemotherapy, and preeclampsia hypertension
	Cervical dissection	• Sudden, thunderclap headache • Syncope
Important to refer for imaging as it is diagnostic	Stroke (ischemic/nonischemic) (Page no. 260)	• Focal neurological deficit • Hemiparesis • Speech impairment, gait impairment
	Others Sinusitis or infection (Page no. 625)	• Fulminant pain of the forehead and area of maxillary sinus • Nasal congestion, discharge
ESR Vascular work-up	Temporal arteritis (Page no. 248)	Headache with abrupt visual disturbance with tender temporal arteries more often in females
	Temporomandibular junction disease	• Clicking/snapping • Pain with jaw movement • Facial pain • History of trauma
ABG	Carbon monoxide Poisoning (Page no. 525)	• Breathing in enclosed/confined spaces with engine exhaust/CO producing equipment • Usually, gradual dull headache, drowsiness with no focal neurologic findings • After drowsiness or mild confusion depending on severity
	Hypertensive crisis (Page no. 124)	Markedly elevated BP

Contd...

Contd...

Pertinent bedside tests	***Differential diagnosis***	***Strong clinical indicators***
Tonometry	Glaucoma Sudden angle closure (Page no. 623)	• Past history • Eye pain, vision loss, and halos around lights • Age >30 years • History of pain increased in a dark environment • Tight pressure around eyeballs • Acute red eye (severe ciliary flushing) and poorly reactive, dilated pupils
	Postlumbar puncture/ spinal anesthesia	History of procedure, wrong posture postprocedure, inadequate hydration
Urine protein	Preeclampsia	Pregnancy >20 weeks
(CNS: central nervous system; CSF: cerebrospinal fluid; ESR: erythrocyte sedimentation rate; ICP: intracranial pressure; LP: lumbar puncture; SAH: subacute arachnoid hemorrhage)		

BOX 4: Presentation: Dizziness/giddiness.

Pertinent bedside tests	***Differential diagnosis***	***Clinical indicators***
HINTS	**VERTIGO** Peripheral (Page no. 251)	• Sudden, severe, lasts seconds to minutes mainly intermittent, one direction, worsened by position, no neurological signs, auditory signs-deafness/tinnitus may be present—ménière's • Walking preserved, unidirectional instability • Unidirectional-horizontal nystagmus • Spinning always indicates vestibular disease • History of drugs causing vestibulotoxicity, caffeine/nicotine • Post-trauma and whiplash • Head eye and ENT (HEENT) examination • HINTS TEST (mentioned in Chapter 6.2 Acute Giddiness)
	Central	• Gradual, mild intensity, weeks to months, multidirectional, no postural change • No auditory signs (deafness/tinnitus) • Neurological signs often present (Ataxia, diplopia, dysarthria, dysphagia, weakness etc.) • Check BP in both arms-subclavian steal neck bruits cranial nerves • Ophthalmoplegia fall while walking • Vertical/torsional nystagmus
Blood glucose, ECG, CBC, sepsis panel	**Non vertigo** Light-headedness/ Near syncope/ Disequilibrium	Look for signs and symptoms of anemia, hypoglycemia, dysrhythmias, myocardial infarction, dehydration, vasovagal, sepsis, drug side effect, peripheral neuropathy anxiety related

BOX 5: Presentation: Nausea/vomiting.

Pertinent bedside tests	*Differential diagnosis*	*Strong clinical indicators*
	CNS • Cerebellar infarct • Raised ICP (SOL, bleed, infarct, infection, and hydrocephalus) • Migraine • Seizure • CNS infection • CP tumor	• Central giddiness symptoms • Cerebellar signs • Papilledema • Nystagmus • (Details in Respective Boxes)
	GI Gastroenteritis (Page no. 306)	• Crampy abdomen • Might be associated with diarrhea, fever, and history of eating food outside
	Gastritis/peptic or duodenal ulcer disease	• Epigastric pain/tenderness • Belching • Regurgitation • Pain in relation to food
USG	Acute abdomen	See **Box 6**
HINTS (Refer Chapter 6.2: Acute Giddiness)	**Head, Eyes, Ears, Nose, Throat (HEENT)** Labyrinthitis, Ménière's disease, tumor, and iatrogenic	**Box 4** All signs and D/D of peripheral giddiness
UPT Pelvis USG	**Others** N/V of pregnancy	• UPT, pregnancy NVP typically starts in week 4–7 • Peaks in 12 weeks
ABG: Metabolic acidosis *Urine*: Ketones Blood sugar	DKA	Details given **(Box 6)**
	Uremia Alcohol/starvation	History
	Treatment related: • Drugs • Chemotherapy • Radiation	Get detail history
	Miscellaneous: • Emotional response • Psychiatric disorder	Anxiety

(CP: cerebellopontine; DKA: diabetic ketoacidosis; NVP: nausea and vomiting in pregnancy; SOL: space occupying lesion; UPT: urine pregnancy test)

BOX 6: Presentation: Abdomen pain.

Pertinent bedside tests	***Differential diagnosis***	***Strong clinical indicators***
USG-abdomen	**Abdomen** Ruptured or leaking abdominal aortic aneurysm (Page no. 130)	• Incidence increases with advancing age >60 • Risk factors—male sex, hypertension, family history, and peripheral vascular disease • Often asymptomatic until rupture • Acute epigastric and back pain + syncope or signs of shock • Pain may radiate to back, groin, or testes • Palpation of pulsatile mass usually possible in aneurysms >5 cm • Bruits or inequality of femoral pulses may be evident
	Descending aortic dissection (Page no. 130)	• *Risk factors:* Hypertension, connective tissue disorder, vasculitis, aortic surgery, aneurysm, family history, dissection, trauma, pregnancy • Other details mentioned in **Box 2**
USG abdomen X-ray abdomen erect	Perforated viscus (Page no. 188)	• Incidence increases with advancing age • Acute severe, mostly diffuse pain • Vomiting can cause peritonitis • Fever might be noted • Might result in shock • OE: guarding and rebound + "board-like" abdomen in later stages
Amylase—first 72 hours Lipase next 72 hours USG-abdomen	Pancreatitis (Page no. 183)	• Risk factors commonly noted are alcoholic/gall stones • Epigastric pain radiating to back in subscapular area, continuous (mainly upper abdomen section) • Vomiting/nausea • May worsen while lying flat, may improve on forward bending *Physical examination* not correlating to symptoms hypotensive or tachypneic if in shock, an alcoholic withdrawal patient can present with hypertension and tachycardia

Contd...

Contd...

Pertinent bedside tests	***Differential diagnosis***	***Strong clinical indicators***
USG/X-ray abdomen standing-air-fluid level	Intestinal obstruction Bowel strangulation ± gangrene (Page no. 188)	• Risk factors – History of previous abdominal surgery hence adhesions, hernia – Long-standing constipation, laxative abuse, drugs (sedatives, Parkinson medications, anticholinergics, etc.), malignancy, abscesses, ileus, volvulus, and infarction • Colicky diffuse abdominal pain associated with vomiting mostly bilious/feculent. Constipation or paradoxical loose stools. Vital signs usually normal unless dehydration or bowel strangulation has occurred. Abdominal distention, tenderness if peritonitis hyperactive bowel sounds distal to block and rectal examination might show impacted stools
	Diverticulitis	• Incidence with advancing age • Males > females • Recurrences are common • Fever usually low grade • Left lower quadrant pain without rebound is common • Rectal bleed
ABG—metabolic acidosis plus hyperlactatemia might show	Mesenteric ischemia	• *RF:* Elderly with cardiovascular dx, CHF, dysrhythmias, DM, sepsis and dehydration, atherosclerosis, low cardiac output, trauma, malignancy, and infection • Mesenteric venous thrombosis associated with hypercoagulable states, hematologic d/o, intraperitoneal inflammation, and trauma • Rapid, severe, disproportionate pain to physical finding (tenderness, peritoneal signs develops later) • Lactates can be normal initially • BS often still present • Rectal examination important because OB+ stools common. Metabolic acidosis of unknown etiology
USG-abdomen	*Biliary sepsis:* • Acute cholecystitis • Acute cholangitis	• RUQ—pain and tenderness • Fever, pain, jaundice (Charcot triad) • May lead to sepsis, shock, peritonitis, bowel obstruction

Contd...

Contd...

Pertinent bedside tests	***Differential diagnosis***	***Strong clinical indicators***
USG-abdomen	Liver abscess (Page no. 179)	• Amebic abscess-history of food intake from outside • RUQ pain and tenderness • Fever, diarrhea might be noted • In complicated cases shock may be noted
CBC POCUS	Splenic rupture	• LUQ pain • History of trauma—tachycardia, hypersplenism, and shock • Postsurgical/endoscopy
USG-abdomen	Spontaneous bacterial peritonitis in chronic liver disease	Diffuse pain with fever, altered mental status, and hypotension with ascites
	Gastritis/gastroenteritis	Clinical indicators see **Box 5** of Nausea
	Important extra-abdominal causes of abdominal pain	
	Toxicology: Toxic methanol poisoning heavy metal toxicity	History of consumption
	• Cardiac/pulmonary • Thoracic AMI/unstable angina • Pneumonia • Pulmonary embolism	Explained in **Box 2**
	Sickle cell disease, porphyria, SLE, and vasculitis DKA	Prior history of hematological and rheumatological disease
	Herniated thoracic disc	History of trauma or injury See details in back pain
	Abdominal wall muscle spasm/hematoma	Local findings
	Pelvic pain can also present as abdomen pain	
ECG	**Cardiac cause should be ruled out in an upper abdominal quadrant pain or epigastric pain**	Look for angina

(AMI: acute myocardial infarction; CLD: chronic liver disease; ECG: electrocardiography; DKA: diabetic ketoacidosis; POCUS: point-of-care ultrasound; SLE: systemic lupus erythematosus)

BOX 7: Presentation: Pelvic pain.

Pertinent bedside tests	***Differential diagnosis***	***Strong clinical indicators***
USG Abdomen/Pelvis	Appendicitis (Page no. 177)	• Generalized followed by localized RLQ pain with/without peritoneal sings • Low-grade fever, nausea, anorexia, and vomiting • RUQ pain in pregnant women or retrocecal appendicitis
USG-KUB	Renal/ureteral colic (Page no. 240)	• Pain is lateral usually moderate-to-severe. Often radiates into the groin (loin to groin) • Nausea and vomiting, prior history of stones • Hematuria might be present
USG-abdomen pelvis	Ovarian torsion (Page no. 471)	• Sudden onset of moderate-to-sever pain on the lateral side of the pelvis • Pain can be intermittent • Nausea and vomiting • Adnexal tenderness, possible peritonitis (+)
USG-abdomen pelvis **UPT** **Beta-hCG**	Ectopic pregnancy (Page no. 471)	• Classically severe sharp lateral pelvic pain, but both severity location and quality often variable, shoulder pain indicates hemorrhage • Vaginal bleeding • Patient might present to the ER in a complete hemodynamically collapsed state depending on the severity of bleeding • Delayed/scanty or missed period, history of previous ectopic, infertility, tubal ligation, or IUD use common
USG-abdomen pelvis	PID/tubo-ovarian abscess (TOA) (Page no. 471)	• Without TOA pain is usually bilateral. May present acutely within 48 hours or have more subacute presentation 1–2 week of pain • Fever, vaginal discharge, dyspareunia prior history of PID common pus from cervical os
USG-abdomen pelvis • Urine routine (bedside leukoesterase) • CBC/ biomarkers	UTI pain with urination (Page no. 235)	• Usually not severe unless has flank pain from associated pyelonephritis. • Urinary urgency and frequency, LUTS, fever, and vomiting, if has associated pyelonephritis
USG-abdomen pelvis	Endometriosis	• Unilateral or bilateral pelvic pain, often recurrent. Lower back pain • Dysmenorrhea and dyspareunia
USG-abdomen pelvis	Torsion testis (Page no. 245)	• Acute lower abdominal/inguinal/testicular pain not positional • Vomiting • Higher placed affected testis on physical examination
	Epididymitis (Page no. 245)	Gradual, lower abdomen/inguinal/scrotal/ testicular pain is positional, elevated scrotum relieves pain

(hCG: human chorionic gonadotropin; IUD: intrauterine device; LUTS: lower urinary tract symptoms; PID: pelvic inflammatory disease; UPT: urine pregnancy test)

BOX 8: Presenting symptoms: Bleeding from orifices.

Pertinent bedside tests	***Differential diagnosis***	***Strong clinical indicators***
	Vaginal bleed	
USG-abdomen pelvis or POCUS	**Vaginal bleed in pregnancy <20 weeks** Ectopic pregnancy	Discussed in **Box 7**
	Complication of termination (retained products)	History of pregnancy can be concealed by patient (illegal termination)
	(>20 weeks do not perform pelvic examination until placenta previa ruled out) Abruption placenta (Page no. 475)	• Mostly steady abdominal cramping pain • Dark vaginal bleeding • Hypotension, DIC, and shock can develop
	Placenta previa (Page no. 475)	• Usually very little pain, intermittent • Bright red vaginal bleeding, rarely severe • Incidence increased with multiparity and prior C-section
USG-abdomen pelvis or POCUS	Postpartum hemorrhage (first 24 hours postdelivery (Page no. 475)	• Pain often minimal, but can be severe with uterine inversion • Vaginal bleeding often brisk, but much blood loss can be hidden in uterus • Might be in shock • Tender abdomen with guarding (uterine rupture). Enlarged, doughy uterus (uterine atony) • Difficult, traumatic delivery (vaginal lacerations). Previous C-section although rare
USG-abdomen pelvis • Coagulation profile • Pelvic examination	**PV bleeding in nonpregnant** • Acute menorrhagia, endometriosis • Trauma, abuse, fibroid, and infection • Uterine AV malformation • Malignancy and coagulopathy	History and examination

Contd...

Contd...

Pertinent bedside tests	***Differential diagnosis***	***Strong clinical indicators***
	Oral bleed	
CBC, Coagulation profile BUN/ creatinine ratio >30 Ryle's tube insertion Endoscopy	Upper GI bleed (Page no. 205)	• Presents as Hematemesis/melena/ coffee ground emesis • Relevant drug history (blood thinners), NSAID abuse • History of peptic ulcer, alcohol history, liver disease, bleeding disorders • History of red colored food consumption
• CBC • Coagulation profile	Nasal bleed (Page no. 625)	• Bleeding nasally, fresh blood or clots orally to be confirmed with oral examination • History of trauma/hypertension, bleeding disorders • Past history of similar complaints • Ongoing upper respiratory tract illness
• CBC • Coagulation profile • CXR • Bronchoscopy	Hemoptysis (Page no. 54)	• Bleeding with sputum, cough is generally bright red or slightly dark with clots • PH testing is alkaline • Cough/SOB or signs of pulmonary involvement may be present, history of bleeding disorders • Rule out possibility of pulmonary embolism • New murmur can indicate mitral stenosis • Stable patient can deteriorate rapidly not due to bleeding but due to asphyxia
	PR Bleed	
• CBC • Coagulation profile • PR examination	Lower GI bleed	• Hematochezia or fresh blood per rectum • Could be due to anorectal/local reasons • PR examination will be helpful to differentiate from other sources of bleed • History of drug including blood thinner • History of constipation or straining • Bleeding disorders, malignancy

Contd...

Contd...

Pertinent bedside tests	*Differential diagnosis*	*Strong clinical indicators*
	Hematuria	
	UTI	Discussed in **Box 7**
	Bladder stones/renal colic	Pain
Serum PSA level	BPH	Dribbling of urine, frequency or urgency more at night, weak urinary stream, incomplete bladder emptying feeling, can have incontinence or sexual dysfunction
• Renal profile • Coagulation profile	• Systemic illness • Bleeding disorders, malignancy	Look for signs of kidney failure or LRTI
Urine routine: Red urine	• Drugs • Food dye • Metabolite	• Doxorubicin, rifampin, nitrofurantoin, chloroquine, brufen, iron, and deferoxamine • Beet blackberries, food color • Bile pigment, melanin, methemoglobin, porphyrin, and urate

(AV: arteriovenous; BPH: benign prostatic hyperplasia; DIC: disseminated intravascular coagulation; NSAID: nonsteroidal anti-inflammatory drug; PSA: prostate-specific antigen; PV: per vagina; UTI: urinary tract infection)

BOX 9: Presentation: Hyperglycemia.

Pertinent bedside tests	*Differential diagnosis*	*Strong clinical indicators*
• Bedside blood glucose • Ketones + • ABG: pH <7.35 HCO_3 <18	DKA (Page no. 377)	• Known or unknown diabetic • Generally younger individual • Generally backward social background • High sugars • History of fever/abdominal pain/vomiting/ischemia/infarct • Labored breathing (Kussmaul) • Can be altered mental sensorium
• Glucose >600 • Osmolality >320 • Serum bicarbonate >18 • pH >7.3 • Ketones small to negative	HHNK (Page no. 377)	• Severe hyperglycemia • Altered mental sensorium

(DKA: diabetic ketoacidosis; HHNK: hyperglycemic hyperosmolar non ketotic coma).

BOX 10: Presentation: Anuria.

Pertinent bedside tests	*Differential diagnosis*	*Strong clinical indicators*
USG-abdomen pelvis	Urinary retention (Page no. 238)	Palpable bladder
• USG • CT abdomen	Obstructive uropathy (Page no. 240)	Renal/ureteric calculi
• USG • Creatinine/BUN ratio • ABG: Metabolic acidosis • Urine proteins creatinine ratio	AKI on CKD (Page no. 220)	Signs of renal failure
(AKI: acute kidney injury; CKD: chronic kidney disease)		

BOX 11: Presenting complaints: Bowel disorders.

Pertinent bedside tests	*Differential diagnosis*	*Strong clinical indicators*
• Biofire [polymerase chain reaction (PCR)] • CBC • Electrolytes • Stool routine/culture/ hanging drop test	**Diarrhea** Noninfectious (toxins/ gastrointestinal/ systemic)	• History of drugs/toxins, travel history • Associated abdomen symptoms, comorbidities, epidemic
	Infectious (bacterial/ viral/amebic/hospital based)	• History of fever, blood in stools, travel history, comorbidities • Long stay in hospital or long duration of antibiotics, nursing home stay, epidemic
• PR examination • X-ray erect abdomen • USG	**Constipation** (Page no. 198) Acute	Change of daily routine, diet, psychological ailments, painful defecation secondary to local issues hypercalcemia or metabolic diseases, and drugs
	Chronic	IBS, neurogenic, DM-related autonomic neuropathy, bedridden limited mobility

BOX 12: Presenting complaints: Ophthalmology.

Pertinent bedside test	***Differential diagnosis***	***Strong clinical indicators***
Torch light, fundoscopy, SLIT lamp	Red eye (Page no. 623)	• History of foreign body • History of trauma • **Swelling of isolated structures more than lids**—orbital cellulitis, orbital compartment syndrome • **Swelling of lids**—hordeolum, blepharitis, chalazion • **Severe pain, FB sensation, or limbal injection**—acute angle closure glaucoma/ hyphema iritis/keratitis/ scleritis/anterior uveitis/ endophthalmitis/ keratoconjunctivitis/ episcleritis • Bulbar injection (not limbal)—bacterial conjunctivitis/chlamydia conjunctivitis/contact dermatoconjunctivitis/ allergic conjunctivitis/viral conjunctivitis
	D/D visual reduction loss	
Bedside-tonometry, fundoscopy slit lamp, fluorescein testing		
Clinical indicators	***Sudden***	***Gradual***
Painless	Central retinal artery occlusion central retinal vein occlusion, vitreous hemorrhage, amaurosis fugax, transient ischemic attack, cortical blindness, retinal detachment, CMV retinitis, functional	Macular degeneration, diabetic retinopathy, and cataract giant cell arteritis
Painful	Acute angle closure glaucoma corneal abrasion, keratitis, hyphema, and uveitis endophthalmitis	Optic neuritis

BOX 13: Presenting complaints: Back pain (Page no. 491).

Pertinent bedside tests	*Differential diagnosis*	*Strong clinical indicators*
Imaging	**Nonmechanical** Aortic dissection aneurysm	Mentioned above
	Spinal epidural abscess	Back pain with fever, focal neurological involvement
	Mechanical CAUDA equina syndrome	• History of back pain with urinary retention/fecal incontinence • Saddle anesthesia, bilateral leg pain. Lower extremity weakness with hyperreflexia
	Trauma	Acute onset, localized pain. Usually trauma history
	Disk herniation	A traumatic mechanism of lifting heavy weight, jerky twisting, stiffness, tenderness, decreased ROM, positive straight leg raise test are noted

BOX 14: Presenting complaints: Neck pain (Page no. 491).

Pertinent bedside tests	*Differential diagnosis*	*Strong clinical indicators*
X-ray	**Sprain/strain**	Trauma, whiplash, vertigo like symptoms might be associated
X-ray	**Disk herniation**	Trauma, nerve roots, and dermatomal involvement
X- ray	**Torticollis**	Mostly unilateral neck pain, acute

BOX 15: Presenting complaints: Shoulder pain (Page no. 500).

Pertinent bedside tests	*Differential diagnosis*	*Strong clinical indicators*
Imaging	Impingement	• Anterior/lateral shoulder or mid humerus • Pain at night or overhead movements
Imaging	Rotator cuff tears	• Trauma/hyperextension/hyperabduction • Chronic-gradual, persistent worsens at night • Diffuse or lateral arm • Limited motion • Palpation tenderness
Imaging	Adhesive capsulitis/ frozen shoulder	Limited shoulder movement

BOX 16: Presentation: Knee pain (Page no. 500).

Pertinent bedside tests	***Differential diagnosis [Location of pain/tenderness gives the clue]***	***Strong clinical indicators***
Imaging	Local knee injury	Give out
	Anterior knee pain	Quadriceps weakness
	Locking of knee	Meniscal injury
	Popping sensation	Ligamentous injury
	Pain at knee joint meniscal line	Knee effusion

BOX 17: Presentation: Confusion (Page no. 284).

Pertinent bedside tests	***Differential diagnosis***	***Strong clinical indicators***
Imaging EEG	Primary intracranial	Stroke (ischemic/nonischemic], trauma, tumor, and infection seizure (nonconvulsive)
• *Blood sugars* • *Lumbar puncture* • *Tox/alcohol screening* • *Arterial blood gases* • *S. electrolytes* • *Thyroid profile* • *POCUS for ICP*	Hypoglycemia, hypoxia, hypertension, and Wernicke's encephalopathy	• Check sugars/oxygenation/ventilation • Please check SpO_2 and HGT before proceeding further evaluation • IV thiamine push before dextrose drip
	Systemic disease affecting the CNS	Infectious encephalopathy, fever, signs of sepsis
	Exogenous toxins/sepsis Drug withdrawal/overdose	History
	Dyselectrolytemia	Mainly hyponatremia sometimes hypercalcemia
	Other	Psychiatry, dementia, and thyroid

BOX 18: Presentation for weakness.

Pertinent bedside tests	***Differential diagnosis***	***Strong clinical indicators***
	Non neuromuscular AMI, respiratory failure, sepsis, dehydration, fatigue, anxiety, depression, fibromyalgia, malignancy, sedatives, drug withdrawal [stimulant], toxins	Generalized weakness Along with clinical features of individual diagnosis mentioned in the respective sections
Imaging	**Neuromuscular** Ischemic stroke (Page no. 260)	• Unilateral limb weakness • Same side arms and legs • Look for facial involvement on the same side as the limb weakness for identifying the site of the lesion
	Brown-Séquard syndrome	• Ipsilateral position and vibration sense loss • Contralateral pain and temperature sensation loss • Motor loss ipsilateral to cord lesion
Imaging	Radiculopathy/ischemic stroke/neuropathy	• Unilateral limb weakness • Only one hand or leg • If only weakness and no loss of power consider AMI
Imaging	Complete cord transection [mainly trauma]	**Bilateral limb weakness**—Loss of sensation and motor function below level of cord injury. Sphincter control lost.
Imaging GBS-single breath tests, FVC, CSF analysis, EMG	• Anterior cord syndrome • Cauda equina syndrome • Guillain-Barré syndrome • Chronic polyneuropathy	**Bilateral limb weakness** • **Anterior cord**—Loss of pin and touch sensation. Motor loss or weakness below cord level. • **Cauda equina syndrome**—Saddle anesthesia may occur, with sensory loss varying from patchy distribution to a complete transverse pattern. • Weakness is typically of the lower motor neuron type. • Sphincter control is often compromised. • **Gullain-Barre syndrome**—Post 2 weeks of viral or acute gastroenteritis, presenting with progressive, symmetrical weakness that primarily affects the distal muscles.

Contd...

Contd...

Pertinent bedside tests	***Differential diagnosis***	***Strong clinical indicators***
		• The lower extremities are typically more affected, with reduced or absent deep tendon reflexes (DTRs), variable sensory changes, and preservation of anal sphincter function. Distal paresthesias further support a diagnosis. [Tongue weakness is a clue to need for mechanical ventilation]. • Common in LOWER extremities • Distal weakness
Imaging	Central cord syndrome	**Bilateral limb weakness** Common in UPPER extremities Distal>proximal
Imaging GBS-as above	Cervical anterior cord syndrome Guillain-Barré syndrome	**Bilateral limb weakness** All four limb weakness
EMG Rhabdomyolysis-myoglobins, CPK total, creatinine, urine testing	Myositis Rhabdomyolysis (Page no. 225) Neuromuscular junction disorder [tick paralysis, botulism]	**Bilateral limb weakness** • **Neuromuscular junction disorders**—mainly fatigue • **Botulism** presents as a descending, symmetrical, flaccid paralysis. It initially affects the cranial nerves and bulbar muscles, leading to symptoms such as diplopia, dysarthria, and dysphagia, followed by generalized weakness. Causes anticholinergic symptoms such as constipation, urinary retention, dry skin and eyes, elevated body temperature, and dilated, non-reactive pupils, which can help distinguish botulism from myasthenia gravis. Deep tendon reflexes are typically normal or reduced. • **Tick paralysis** causes an acute, ascending, flaccid motor paralysis • Ocular signs, such as fixed and dilated pupils, can help distinguish it from Guillain-Barré syndrome. • Commonly PROXIMAL

Contd...

Contd...

Pertinent bedside tests	***Differential diagnosis***	***Strong clinical indicators***
Myopathy-Inflammatory-EMG muscle biopsy	Myopathy inflammatory The most common are polymyositis and dermatomyositis.	**Polymyositis and dermatomyositis** • Proximal muscle weakness is predominant, often causing difficulties in rising from a seated position, climbing stairs, or lifting the arms overhead. This weakness is frequently accompanied by pain and tenderness in the affected muscles. • Reflexes are typically reduced, corresponding to the degree of muscle strength loss. • Dermatomyositis in addition is associated with skin symptoms.
Metabolic-serum electrolytes, thyroid function test, ECG changes for electrolytes	Metabolic-mainly potassium related or thyroid related periodic paralysis	Isolated or recurrent episodes of flaccid paralysis, more commonly affecting the lower limbs than the upper, though both may be involved. Bulbar, ocular, and respiratory muscles are typically spared. Can be triggered by high oral carbohydrate intake (leading to a subsequent insulin surge) and a period of rest
	Isolated CN VII • Mastoiditis • Parotitis • Idiopathic [BELLS PALSY] • Ramsay hunt • Lyme's disease **Not Isolated to CN VII** • Brainstem lesion • Neuromuscular junction disorder • Cranial polyneuropathy	• Facial muscle weakness only • For bells palsy -upper and lower face should be involved • Lid closing should be negative along with other symptoms • Lyme disease may present with systemic symptoms or bilateral facial paresis, particularly in regions where the disease is prevalent • Ramsay Hunt syndrome (herpes zoster oticus) is marked by unilateral facial paralysis, a vesicular rash resembling herpes, and vestibulocochlear impairment
Edrophonium testing and ice bag, both make ptosis go away. Serum Ach receptor antibodies	Myasthenia gravis	• Fluctuating weakness • Easy fatigue ability • Mainly diplopia, ptosis, neck and limb weakness may be present

BOX 19: Presentation: Jaundice.

Pertinent bedside tests	***Differential diagnosis***	***Strong clinical indicators***
• LFT, CBC, LDH, ALP, GGT • USG-abdomen	**Hepatic** Liver failure, alcohol, toxins with hepatotoxicity drugs, imaging, history of liver disease or drugs/toxins consumption (Page no. 205)	Signs of liver failure: Toxin/drug/alcohol ingestion
USG-abdomen	**Biliary** Cholangitis history of prior biliary/liver surgery	
• **ECHO** • **USG/POCUS** • Infective biomarkers	**Systemic** • Ischemic insult secondary to cardiac event • Sepsis • Heat stroke	• Cardiac event • Infections • History of heat exposure
• CBC, LFT, LDH, coagulation profile peripheral smear • Retic count	**Hematological** Transfusion reaction, hemolytic anemia by history	History
• CBC/LFT/LDH/ coagulation profile peripheral smear • Retic count	**Reproductive** HELLP (hemolysis, elevated liver enzymes—low platelet count) (Page no. 479)	• Can present antenatally or early postpartum • Usually presents in the late second and third trimester of pregnancy • Hypertension mostly noted • Nausea vomiting • Right upper quadrant pain • Headache • Blurring of vision
LFT/USG abdomen	Hepatitis (mainly HAV/HEV)	• History of eating outside food or contaminated water • Known case or exposure to HBsAg or HCV

(ALP: alkaline phosphatase; GGT: gamma-glutamyl transpeptidase; HAV: hepatitis A virus; HBsAg: hepatitis B surface antigen; HCV: hepatitis C virus; HEV: hepatitis E virus; LDH: lactate dehydrogenase; LFT: liver function test)

1.2 FAST TRACK TO FEVER IN EMERGENCY ROOM

Jamshed D Sunavala

APPROACH TO FEVER

BOX 1: Fast track—HISTORY (ICE PACK).

- **I**–Is the patient *I*mmunocompromised?
- **C**–Is the patient *C*ritically ill (shock or has organ dysfunction)?
- **E**–*E*nvironment, is it a community acquired or health care acquired infection?
- **P**–*P*rior history check the chronological history prior to the onset of fever (travel and exposure).
- **A**–*A*ssociated events (upper respiratory symptoms, localized pain, rash, dyspnea, burning micturition, neurological symptoms, hemoptysis, recent injuries, or insect bites)
- **C**–*C*omorbidities, ongoing comorbidities that may have influenced or may be the cause of fever (recent surgery, malignancy, diabetes, old age, or neurological cause for aspiration pneumonia, and medications for chronic illness like seizure)
- **K**–*K*ind of fever, intermittent, continuous, spiking with shivering and rigors, relapsing fever (borrelia infection), and primary adrenal lymphoma (PAL)—Ebstein (Hodgkin's lymphoma)

BOX 2: Fast track—PHYSICAL EXAMINATION.

- General and systemic examination
- Not to forget to check for hidden clues (*See* Figure 1 below)
  - Rash and skin lesions **(Box 3)**
  - Lymphadenopathy; cervical, axilla, inguinal region, and nape of the neck
  - Shallow respiration; often missed in GBS (breathless but may not be apparent)
  - Heart rate—temperature discrepancy, as seen in typhoid fever
  - Skin lesions—ulcers, wounds, and bed sores
  - Rub—pericardial or pleural often missed
  - Eye—particularly fundoscopy
  - Mouth for sores, ulcers, tonsils, and throat
  - Check for deep vein thrombosis (DVT)
  - Central lines, catheter
  - Gag reflex in elderly or neurologically compromised patients as they might have micro aspirations

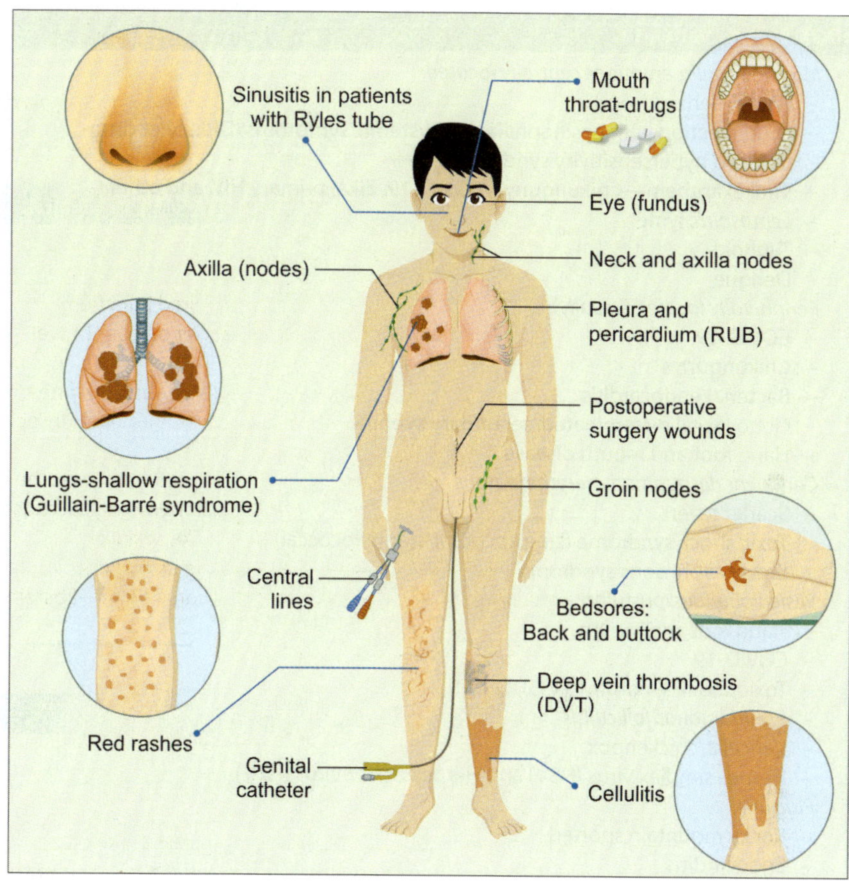

Fig. 1: Understanding fever; signs/symptoms/diagnosis.

BOX 3: Fever with rash.

- *Maculopapular eruptions centrally located:*
  - Acute meningococcus
  - Drug reaction with eosinophilia and systemic symptoms (DRESS) or drug-induced hypersensitivity syndrome
  - Viral exanthem—Chikungunya, COVID-19, Zika, primary HIV, and others
  - *Leptospira*, lyme
  - Typhoid
  - Dengue
- *Peripherally located (usually):*
  - COVID-19
  - Chikungunya
  - Bacterial endocarditis
  - Gonococcal disseminated, secondary syphilis
  - Hand foot and mouth disease
- *Confluent desquamative erythematous*
  - Scarlet fever
  - Toxic shock syndrome (streptococcal/staphylococcal)
  - Steven–Johnsons syndrome
- *Vesiculobullous/pustular:*
  - Hand foot and mouth
  - COVID-19
  - Toxic shock syndrome (TSS), DRESS
  - *Pseudomonas folliculitis*
  - Varicella/chickenpox
  - Herpes simplex virus (HSV) and Herpes zoster virus (HZV)
- *Purpuric:*
  - Rocky mountain spotted
  - Endocarditis
  - Dengue or viral hemorrhagic fever
  - COVID
  - Meningococcemia
  - Disseminated gonococcal infection
  - Purpura fulminans, thrombotic thrombocytopenic purpura/hemolytic uremic syndrome (TTP/HUS).
- *Eruptions with ulcers and /or eschars:* Scrub typhus rickettsia and anthrax

BOX 4: Fever with hematological abnormalities.

- ESR >100
  - Active Kochs
  - Giant cell (temporal) arteritis
  - Multiple myeloma
  - Pyogenic infections
  - Waldenstrom macroglobulinemia
  - Polymyalgia rheumatica and other collagen vascular diseases
  - Metastatic tumor
- *Increased WBC:*
  - Pyogenic infections
  - Patient on steroids
- *Normal WBC:*
  - Viral infections
  - Malaria
  - Typhoid

Increased procalcitonin: Bacterial infections

- *Decreased platelets:*
  - Dengue, malaria, and septicemia
  - Hematological causes, viral hepatitis, and HIV
- *Pancytopenia:* Hemato-oncology

BOX 5: Obligatory investigation in our country.

- ESR
- Blood for malarial parasite
- Dengue NS1/IgM
- Leptospira (during monsoon)
- Complete blood counts
- C-reactive protein
- Urine routine
- Chest X-ray
- Blood sugar
- AST/ALT
- LDH
- Renal functions
- Potentially diagnostic checks (PDCs) (all localizing signs and symptoms and abnormalities suggesting a certain diagnosis)

(AST: aspartate aminotransferase; ALT: alanine aminotransferase)

BOX 6: Guided diagnostic tests.

- *Increased WBC count*—blood cultures, and other appropriate cultures, PCT, and CRP imaging of suspected region
- *Fever with upper respiratory symptoms*—CBC/ESR/CRP, throat swab, or nasopharyngeal swab for viral infections, Biofire PCR
- *Fever with lower respiratory signs*—CXR/HRCT chest plus all obligatory tests
- *Neutropenic fever*—triple blood and urine cultures, HRCT chest, and USG abdomen
- *Immunocompromised patient*—imaging to rule out Kochs, fungal infections
- *Diabetic patient*—CXR/HRCT chest to rule out Kochs in our country
- *Very high ESR*—earlier mentioned diseases

(CRP: C-reactive protein; HRCT: high resolution computed tomography chest)

BOX 7: Therapeutic approach in ER.

First things first:

- Treat hemodynamics and/or respiratory failure/instability
- Treat hyperpyrexia with ice packs and intravenous paracetamol
- Check all vitals
- Blood and all other cultures before starting antibiotics
- *In suspected septic shock start* (see Chapter 7.1 on Sepsis):
  - Fluid resuscitation
  - Respiratory and inotropic support (refer Chapter 34.2)
  - Cultures followed by broad spectrum antibiotics with appropriate gram negative and positive cover
  - Treat severe hyperthermia (>103°F in axilla) *See Chapter 15.2.2 on heat stroke and heat emergencies*

SUGGESTED READING

1. Jameson JL, Kasper DL, Fauci AS, Hauser SL, Longo DL, Loscalzo J, et al. Harrison's principles of internal medicine. 20th ed. New York: McGraw-Hill Education; 2018.
2. Tintinalli JE, John Ma O, Yealy DM, Meckler GD, Stapczynski JS, Cline DM, et al. Tintinalli's Emergency Medicine: A Comprehensive Study Guide, 9th edition. McGraw Hill Professional; 2019.
3. Walls RM, Hockberger RS, Gausche-Hill M. Rosen's Emergency Medicine: Concepts and Clinical Practice. Philadelphia, PA: Elsevier; 2018.

Part 2

Bedside Diagnosis and Management of Diseases Presented in the Emergency Room

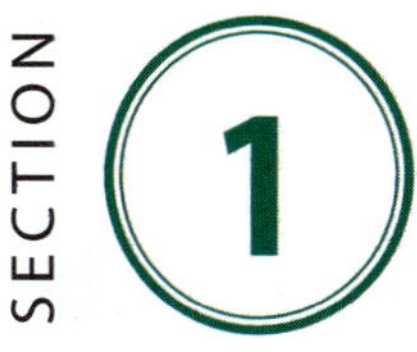

Medicine and Surgery

CHAPTER 2

Respiratory Emergencies

2.1 BRONCHIAL ASTHMA

Anand Bhabhor

BOX 1: Definition.

- Bronchial asthma is a chronic inflammatory disorder of the airway
- Bronchial asthma may have its onset in infancy through adulthood and the symptoms may be intermittent or persistent

BOX 2: History.

- Presence of cough, occasionally with yellow sputum and classically worse at night or early morning which may be perennial or seasonal
- Wheezing, continuous, or episodic
- Shortness of breath
- Chest tightness
- Nocturnal awakening
- Aggravating factors
- History of episodic symptoms
- History of allergy or atopic disease, family history, occupational history, and home pets
- History of hospitalization and intubation
- Use of corticosteroid or inhalers

BOX 3: Examination.

- Prolonged expiratory phase
- Wheezing
- Tachypnoea
- Use of accessory muscles if severe asthma

BOX 4: Differential diagnosis.

Diffuse airway obstruction	• COPD • Alpha-1 antitrypsin deficiency • Bronchiectasis • Cystic fibrosis • Bronchiolitis obliterans • Tracheobronchomalacia
Localized airway obstruction	• End bronchial tumor • Carcinoid tumor • Endobronchial foreign body • Extrinsic airway compression
Laryngeal obstruction	• Vocal cord dysfunction

BOX 5: Investigation.

- History and clinical
- *Objective pulmonary function test (PFT):*
  - *Spirometry:*
    - Reduced forced expiratory volume in one second/forced vital capacity (FEV1/FVC) ratio <70%
    - Reduction in FEV1 in associated with severity of asthma
    - Reversibility of bronchodilator if defined as FEV1/FVC increased by >12% or 200 mL from baseline
  - Peak expiratory flow rate (PEFR)
  - Chest X-ray
  - Complete blood count (CBC) and immunoglobulin E (IgE) level
  - Sinus CT scan
  - Allergy testing

BOX 6: Classification of acute asthma.

	Symptoms and signs	***Initial PEF (or REV1)***	***Clinical Course***
Mild or moderate	• Talks in phrases, not agitated, respiratory rate increased but no accessory muscle used • Pulse 100–120 bpm, oxygen saturation 90–95%	PEF ≥50	• Symptoms are relieved with inhaled SABA. Ipratropium might be required • Oral corticosteroids might be needed • Controlled O_2 to maintain 93–98%
Severe	• Breathlessness at rest; interferes with conversation • Respiratory rate >30 bpm • Pulse >120 bpm • Oxygen saturations <90% • Accessory muscle used • Agitated	PEF <50%	• Frequent inhaled SABA, ipratropium, ICS might be needed Needs longer duration of oral corticosteroids or IV corticosteroids • IV magnesium might be needed
Subset: Life threatening	Disoriented, drowsiness, silent chest	PEF <25% predicted or personal best	Minimal or no relief from frequent inhaled SABA; IV steroids; required; admission in intensive care unit

(ICS: inhaled corticosteroids; IV: intravenous; PEF: peak expiratory flow; SABA: short-acting β2-agonist)

BOX 7: Management of acute exacerbation.

	Mild to moderate	***Severe***	***Impending/acute respiratory arrest***
FEV or PEFR (percentage predicted/ personal best)	≥40%	Unable or <40%	
Oxygen therapy	Maintain SaO_2 ≥90%	Maintain SaO_2 ≥90%	
Initial therapy	• SABA by nebulizer or MDI up to three doses in first hour • Oral systemic corticosteroids if no immediate response or if patient recently took oral systemic corticosteroids	• SABA plus ipratropium by nebulization every 20 minutes or continuously for 1 hour • Oral systemic corticosteroids	• Needs urgent intubation and mechanical ventilation • Nebulized SABA and ipratropium • IV corticosteroids
Reassessment	*If moderate, exacerbation persists with the initial treatment:* • Continue to give inhaled SABA every 60 minutes • Add oral systemic corticosteroid • Continue treatment 1–3 hours, will need admission	*Severe exacerbation even after initial treatment:* • Oxygen nebulized SABA + ipratropium, hourly or continuous • Oral systemic corticosteroids • Consider adjunct therapies	
[Pharmacopoeia]			
Nebulized solution:			
Levosalbutamol	1.25 mg every 20 minutes for up to three doses	1.25 mg every 20 minutes for three doses continuous for 1 hour if severe	
Racemic salbutamol	2.5 mg every 20 minutes for up to three doses	5.0 mg every 20 minutes for three doses continuous for 1 hour if severe	

Contd...

Contd...

	Mild to moderate	***Severe***	***Impending/ acute respiratory arrest***
Salbutamol-metered-dose inhaler with valved holding chamber:			
Levosalbutamol (45 µg/puff)	6–12 puffs every 20 minutes for up to three doses with supervision	Same for three doses (if able to do) with supervision	
Racemic salbutamol (90 µg/puff)	6–12 puffs every 20 minutes for up to three doses with supervision	Same for three doses (if able to do) with supervision	
Ipratropium therapy:			
Nebulized solution	If previous response (same dose as for severe)	0.5 mg every 20 minutes for three doses (may mix with albuterol solution)	
MDI (18 µg/ puff) with VHC	If previous response (same dose as for severe)	8 puffs every 20 minutes for three doses	
Systemic corticosteroids:			
Oral (preferred)	• 40–80 mg of prednisone per day if no immediate response to albuterol • For outpatients: use 40–60 mg in one or two divided doses for 5–10 days	40–80 mg of prednisone per day	
IV (unable to take orally or absorb)	• Hydrocortisone 100–200 mg • Methylprednisolone 1 mg/kg every 4–6 hours • For outpatients, a single IM dose of 150 mg depot methylprednisolone may be used	• Hydrocortisone 100–200 mg • Methylprednisolone 1 mg/kg every 4–6 hours	
IV magnesium sulfate	Not indicated	2–3 g over 20 minutes (or at rates of up to 1 g/min) if FEV, ≤25% predicted	

(MDI: metered dose inhaler; PEFR: peak expiratory flow rate; SaO_2: oxygen saturation in arterial blood: VHC: valved holding chamber)

OTHER MANAGEMENT

- Intravenous/intramuscular epinephrine is an indication in anaphylaxis-induced asthma (Chapter 2.1)
- Noninvasive ventilation (NIV)—noninvasive positive pressure ventilation (NPPV) (details in Chapter 31):
  - Improves airflow and respirations compared with usual care.
  - It is commonly used in clinical practice for status asthmaticus but is quite controversial
- Ketamine demonstrates potent bronchodilator effect
- An IV bolus dose of 0.15, mg/kg followed by an infusion of 0.25 mg/kg/hour is sometimes used.
- Not used often in nonintubated patient
- Mechanical ventilation (details in Chapter 31)
  - Indications for intubation include coma, altered consciousness, cardiac or respiratory arrest, paradoxical breathing pattern, refractory hypoxemia, and failure of NPPV.
  - A ventilator strategy includes mainly avoiding barotrauma and assuring appropriate oxygenation and ventilation by target—low tidal volumes (6–8 mL/kg)
  - Low ventilation rates (below 10 breaths/min) and high inspiratory flow rates (above 60 L/min) provide prolonged time for expiration.
- *Caveat:* Methylxanthines aminophylline is no longer a first- or second-line treatment

BOX 8: Disposition.

The disposition of a patient—whether it involves a ward admission, ICU admission, or discharge—depends on the following criteria:

- *If there is a good response to the treatment:*
  - FEV1 or PEFR ≥70%
  - No distress
  - *Physical examination—normal:* Then discharge home:
    - To continue treatment with inhaled SABA
    - To continue course of oral systemic corticosteroid
  - *Patient education:*
    - On medicine use specially check inhaler usage knowledge
    - Recommend close medical follow-up
- *If there is an incomplete response to the treatment:*
  - FEV1 or PEFR 40–69%
  - *Mild-to-moderate symptoms:* Individualized decision can do the above or admit to the ward and do as per criteria for moderate asthma management
- *If there is a poor response to the treatment:*
  - FEV1 or PEFR <40%
  - PCO_2 ≥42 mm Hg
  - *Physical examination:* Symptoms severe, drowsiness, and confusion
  - Admit to ICU

FEV1: forced expiratory volume in one second; PEFR: peak expiratory flow rate; SABA: short-acting β2-agonist

SUGGESTED READING

1. Barnes PJ. Immunology of asthma and chronic obstructive pulmonary disease. Nat Rev Immunol. 2008;8(3):183-92.
2. Global Initiative for Asthma. (2021). Global strategy for asthma management and prevention. [online] Available from https://ginasthma.org/gina-reports/ [Last accessed September, 2024].
3. Holgate ST, Wenzel S, Postma DS, Weiss ST, Renz H, Sly PD. Asthma. Nat Rev Dis Primers. 2015;1(1):15025.
4. National Heart, Lung, and Blood Institute. (2007). Expert Panel Report 3: Guidelines for the Diagnosis and Management of Asthma. [online] Available from https://www.nhlbi.nih.gov/health-topics/guidelines-for-diagnosis-management-of-asthma [Last accessed September, 2024].
5. Walls RM, Hockberger RS, Gausche-Hill M. Rosen's Emergency Medicine: Concepts and Clinical Practice, 9th edition. Philadelphia: Elsevier: 2018.

2.2 CHRONIC OBSTRUCTIVE PULMONARY DISEASE

Nimish M Shah

BOX 1: Introduction/definition.

- Chronic obstructive pulmonary disease (COPD) is a heterogeneous lung condition characterized by chronic respiratory symptoms (dyspnea, cough, sputum production, and/or exacerbations) due to abnormalities of the airways (bronchitis and bronchiolitis) and/or alveoli (emphysema) that cause persistent, often progressive, and airflow obstruction
- An acute exacerbation of COPD (AECOPD) is defined as an event characterized by increased dyspnea and/or cough and sputum that worsens in <14 days which may be accompanied by tachypnea and/or tachycardia and is often associated with increased local and systemic inflammation caused by infection, pollution, or other insult to the airways

BOX 2: Etiopathogenesis.

Four biologic clusters (related to potential etiology and inflammation) have been identified in AECOPD—(1) bacterial, (2) viral or (3) eosinophilic-predominant, and (4) pauci-inflammatory—associated with limited changes in the inflammatory profile. Respiratory infections, both viral and bacterial and air pollution, are important triggers for AECOPD

BOX 3: Clinical features differentiating COPD and asthma.

	COPD	***Asthma***
Age of 35 years	Rare	Often
Symptoms	Persistent and progressive breathlessness, cough, and sputum production	Wheezing, variable breathlessness, chest tightness, and cough
Day-to-day symptom variability	Uncommon	Common
Risk factors	Smoking, occupational, and environmental exposures	Family history of asthma, history of allergic rhinitis or eczema, childhood respiratory infection, and exposure to irritants
Comorbidities	Cardiovascular disease, lung cancer, anxiety and depression, metabolic syndrome and diabetes, gastroesophageal reflux disease (GERD), bronchiectasis, obstructive sleep apnea, and cognitive impairment	Obesity, GERD, anxiety and depression, food allergy and anaphylaxis, rhinitis, sinusitis, and nasal polyps

BOX 4: Differential diagnosis.

Diagnosis	***Clinical condition***	***Clinical features***	***Diagnostic features***
Respiratory causes	Pulmonary embolism	History of deep vein thrombosis	Pulmonary angiography
	Pneumothorax		Chest X-ray, lung ultrasound
	Pleural effusion		Chest X-ray, lung ultrasound
	Chest trauma	History of trauma	Chest X-ray, CT scan chest
	Bronchiectasis	Purulent sputum	Chest X-ray—cystic changes, bronchial wall thickening
	Endobronchial tuberculosis	Hemoptysis, weight loss	Chest X-ray—upper lobe infiltrates
	Lung tumor	Hemoptysis, weight loss	Chest X-ray—lobar mass
Cardiac	Heart failure	History of ischemic heart disease	ECG, chest X-ray—cardiomegaly, and pulmonary edema
Other	Upper airway obstruction	History of foreign body inhalation	Chest X-ray—lobar collapse

BOX 5: Investigations.

The following three investigations are crucial in an emergency situation. The first two investigations help to diagnose concurrent conditions and complications:

1. Chest X-ray will diagnose pneumothorax, pneumonia, mucous plugging causing lung collapse, and pulmonary edema due to heart failure
2. *Lung ultrasound:* A-lines—lung sliding with horizontal repetitions of the pleural line indicative of normal lung. In pneumothorax, A-lines remain but there will be no lung sliding. They allow fast, accurate, and bedside examinations of most acute respiratory disorders
3. *Arterial blood gas (ABG):* To identify signs of type 2 respiratory failure. In patients with AECOPD, hypercapnia can be of recent onset, chronic or combination of acute chronic hypercarbia. Assessing serum bicarbonate levels helps to titrate therapy so as to bring patients back to baseline state prior to the episode of exacerbation

BOX 6: Management.

- Management of AECOPD should be directed to:
  - Correction of hypoxemia
  - Relieve obstructed airways
  - Reduce airway inflammation and treat infection
  - Prevent complications (e.g., air trapping, pneumothorax, and patient ventilator asynchrony)
  - Treat concurrent conditions

Oxygen therapy:
- Oxygen should be prescribed to prevent hypoxemia for all acutely ill patients to achieve a target saturation of 94–98%
- In patients with hypercapnic respiratory failure, oxygen therapy is titrated to achieve oxygen saturation of 88–92%, which can be delivered via low-flow nasal cannulae or via a Venturi mask to prevent untoward consequences of deteriorating hypercapnia
- Pulse oximetry is an invaluable tool to monitor in all patients and oxygen therapy should be titrated to it

Bronchodilators:
- Bronchodilators are the mainstay of treatment for immediate relief of symptoms
- Inhaled short-acting β2-agonists (salbutamol) are routinely administered to relieve dyspnea for AECOPD
- Addition of inhaled anticholinergics (ipratropium) has been found to have added benefit and is known to have fewer side effects than β2-agonists and tachyphylaxis is not exhibited
- In general, nebulizer therapy is the method of choice to deliver the drug, as it is convenient, easy to use especially in old frail and dyspneic patients, better aerosol particle size for deeper penetration and can be used continuously
- Metered-dose inhaler (MDI) administered using a spacer device is as effective as nebulizer, is cheaper to use, has less propensity for aerosolization of viral particles, can be administered directly into the ventilator circuit for intubated patients via an appropriate connection device

Corticosteroids:
- Corticosteroids are required to treat airway inflammation and mucus plugging and should be used in patients who fail to show a sustained clinical improvement in spite of initial inhaled bronchodilator therapy
- In AECOPD, short course of systemic corticosteroids has shown improvements on several in-hospital (symptoms, length of hospital stay, and treatment failure) and postdischarge (risk of relapse) outcomes
- Typically, a short course of oral prednisolone is used (40–50 mg/day for 5–7 days)
- Oral steroid is preferred due to the similar efficacy of intravenous and for the limitation of systemic effects
- Dose of intravenous steroid is solumedrol 80–160 mg, hydrocortisone 100–200 mg

Antimicrobial therapy:
- Antibiotic treatment is recommended for patients with AECOPD having clinical signs of a bacterial infection, e.g., increased sputum purulence and sputum volume
- The recommended length of antibiotic therapy is 5–7 days
- Initial choice of antibiotics should be guided by the local resistance pattern

Methylxanthines:
- In view of their poor clinical efficacy and significant side effects, methylxanthines are not recommended in the treatment of exacerbations. They should be considered only in subjects with severe exacerbation refractory to initial therapy

Details discussed in the pharmacopoeia section of asthma

BOX 7: Respiratory support therapy.

- The respiratory support therapy helps in:
  - Establishing adequate arterial oxygenation and removal of carbon dioxide
  - Reducing work of breathing, and
  - Resuming the power of normalized breathing
- Support in the form of high-flow nasal oxygen (HFNO) **(*see* Box 8)**
- Noninvasive ventilation (NIV) **(*see* Box 9)** or invasive mechanical ventilation (IMV) (*see* Chapter 31) may be required depending on the severity of the disease

BOX 8: High-flow nasal oxygen.

HFNO has multiple benefits: such as heated and humidified oxygen is delivered to the nose at high-flow rates (50–60 L/min), which may facilitate secretion removal, reduce airway inflammation and avoid epithelial injury, and generate low levels of positive pressure in the upper airways, which may counteract on the intrinsic positive end-expiratory pressure (iPEEP) and thus may decrease the work of breathing allow a known fraction of inspired oxygen (FiO_2) to be delivered, thereby reducing the dead space, patients are more compliant, able to communicate and permit oral intake. In spite of so many benefits, there is lack of evidence currently for the use of HFNO in AECOPD

BOX 9: Noninvasive ventilation.

- NIV has become benchmark in managing acute respiratory failure due to COPD exacerbations. NIV has several benefits:
  - Improves oxygenation and acute respiratory acidosis
  - Decreases the severity of breathlessness, respiratory rate, and work of breathing
  - Reduces intubation rates
  - Decreases complications such as ventilator-associated pneumonia
  - Reduces length of hospital stay and mortality. **Box 10** lists indications, contraindications and complications associated with NIV

BOX 10: Noninvasive ventilation—indications, contraindications, and complications.

Indications for NIV	*Contraindications to NIV*	*Complications of NIV*
Severe dyspnea	Cardiac or respiratory arrest	Pressure injury
Clinical signs of respiratory muscle fatigue	Obtunded or comatose patient	Gastric distension, aspiration
Respiratory acidosis (pH <7.3 and $PaCO_2$ >45 mm Hg)	Inability to clear secretions/ protect airway	Hypotension
Persistent hypoxemia despite adequate O_2 therapy	High risk for aspiration (vomiting)	Pneumothorax
Invasive mechanical ventilation is not appropriate	Upper airway obstruction	Claustrophobia
Postextubation of patients intubated for a COPD exacerbation	Facial surgery, trauma, or deformity, neck surgery	

- To initiate NIV, following settings are recommended:
  - Mode—spontaneous-timed (S/T)
  - A back-up respiratory rate of 10–15 breaths/minute
  - Expiratory positive airway pressure (EPAP) of 5 cmH_2O
  - An inspiratory positive airway pressure (IPAP) of 10 cmH_2O gradually titrated up
  - FiO_2 titrated to oxygen saturation of 88–92%
- The pressure support—difference of IPAP and EPAP will determine the tidal volume (target 6–8 mL/kg) delivered to the patient
- To get optimal benefit of NIV, following should be addressed before initiating NIV: adequate counseling as regards NIV, a cooperative patient, appropriate and comfortably fitting mask, gradual increments of IPAP for patient comfort
- Postinitiation of NIV, patient should be closely assessed for comfort, dyspnea, respiratory and heart rate, blood pressure, and oxygen saturation
- Patient should be closely monitored using ABG to monitor response
- Should a patient not improve with NIV, the critical care outreach team should be alerted, and a ceiling of care needs to established with the patient's next of kin to decide on the escalation of care plan

BOX 11: Disposition.

Following patients should be admitted to ICU:

- Inadequate response to initial therapy in emergency room
- Despite adequate oxygen therapy, there is worsening of hypoxemia or hypercapnia
- Altered level of consciousness
- Unstable hemodynamics
- Those who need ventilator support. The initial efforts should be directed in quick assessment and stabilization of airway, breathing, and circulation

SUGGESTED READING

1. Bafadhel M, McKenna S, Terry S, Mistry V, Reid C, Haldar P, et al. Acute exacerbations of chronic obstructive pulmonary disease: identification of biologic clusters and their biomarkers. Am J Respir Crit Care Med. 2011;184(6):662-71.
2. Chandra D, Stamm JA, Taylor B, Ramos RM, Satterwhite L, Krishnan JA, et al. Outcomes of noninvasive ventilation for acute exacerbations of chronic obstructive pulmonary disease in the United States, 1998–2008. Am J Respir Crit Care Med 2012;185:152-9.
3. Crisafulli E, Barbeta E, Ielpo A, Torres A. Management of severe acute exacerbations of COPD: An updated narrative review. Multidiscip Respir Med. 2018;13:36.
4. Dobler CC, Morrow AS, Beuschel B, Farah MH, Majzoub AM, Wilson ME, et al. Pharmacologic therapies in patients with exacerbation of chronic obstructive pulmonary disease: a systematic review with meta-analysis. Ann Intern Med. 2020;172:413-22.
5. Global Initiative for Chronic Obstructive Lung Disease. (2022). Global strategy for the diagnosis, management and prevention of chronic obstructive pulmonary disease. [online] Available from https://goldcopd/org [Last accessed September, 2024].
6. Johnston C, Nixon P. Asthma and chronic obstructive pulmonary disease in the intensive care unit. Anaesth Inten Care Med. 2022;23(10):628-34.
7. Lichtenstein DA. Lung ultrasound in the critically ill. Ann Intensive Care. 2014;4:1-12.
8. Lugogo NL, MacIntyre NR. Life-threatening asthma: pathophysiology and management. Respir Care. 2008;53(6):726-35.
9. McCory DC, Brown CD. Anti-cholinergic bronchodilators versus beta2-sympathomimetic agents for acute exacerbations of chronic obstructive pulmonary disease. Cochrane Database Syst Rev. 2002;4:CD003900.
10. O'Driscoll BR, Howard LS, Earis J, Mak V. British Thoracic Society Guideline for oxygen use in adults in healthcare and emergency settings. BMJ Open Resp Res. 2017;4:e000170.
11. Roman-Rodriguez M, Kaplan A. GOLD 2021 strategy report: Implications for asthma-COPD overlap. Int J Chron Obstruct Pulmon Dis. 2021;16:1709-15.
12. See KC, Ng J. Management of acute severe asthma and chronic obstructive pulmonary disease. Singapore Med J. 2022;63(9):535-41.
13. Torres-Sánchez I, Cruz-Ramírez R, Cabrera-Martos I, Díaz-Pelegrina A, Valenza MC. Results of physiotherapy treatments in exacerbations of chronic obstructive pulmonary disease: A systematic review. Physiother Can. 2017;69(2):122-132.
14. Veenstra P, Veeger NJGM, Koppers RJH, Duiverman ML, van Geffen WH. High-flow nasal cannula oxygen therapy for admitted COPD patients. A retrospective cohort study. PLoS ONE. 2022;17(10):e0272372.

2.3 PNEUMONIA

Rajiv S Mathur

BOX 1: Pneumonia.

- Pneumonia—infection of lung parenchyma
- *Classification of pneumonia:*
  - Community-acquired pneumonia (CAP)
  - Hospital-acquired pneumonia (HAP)
  - Ventilator-associated pneumonia (VAP)
  - Healthcare-associated pneumonia (HCAP)
- HCAP is cases of CAP caused by multidrug resistant (MDR) pathogens typically seen in HAP

BOX 2: Risk factors for infection with MDR organism in CAP.

- *MDR gram-negative bacteria:*
  - Hospitalization ≥2 days in previous 90 days
  - Use of antibiotics in previous 90 days
  - Immunosuppressed patients
  - Tube feeding
  - Severe COPD/bronchiectasis
  - Gastric acid suppression

BOX 3: Common microbial causes of CAP.

- *OPD setting:*
  - *Streptococcus pneumoniae*
  - *Mycoplasma pneumoniae*
  - *Haemophilus influenzae*
  - *Chlamydia pneumoniae*
  - *Respiratory viruses:*
    - Corona viruses
    - Influenza A and B viruses
    - Human metapneumovirus
    - Adenovirus
    - Respiratory syncytial virus
    - Parainfluenza virus
- *Hospital setting:*
  - Above +
  - *Staphylococcus aureus*
  - *Legionella pneumophila*
  - Gram-negative bacilli
  - Anaerobes

BOX 4: Risk factors for CAP.

- Alcoholism
- Asthma
- Immunosuppression
- Institutionalization
- Age ≥70 years

BOX 5: Risk factors for pneumococcal pneumonia.

- Dementia
- Seizure disorder
- Heart failure
- Cerebrovascular disease
- Alcoholism
- Smoking
- COPD
- Human immunodeficiency virus (HIV) infection

BOX 6: Risk factors.

- *CA-MRSA:*
  - Skin colonization with MRSA
  - Infection with CA-MRSA
- *Enterobacteria:*
  - Recent hospitalization with antibiotic therapy
  - Alcoholism
  - Heart failure
  - Renal failure
- *Pseudomonas aeruginosa:*
  - Bronchiectasis
  - Cystic fibrosis
  - Severe COPD
- *Legionella infection:*
  - Diabetes
  - Hematologic malignancies
  - Cancer
  - Severe renal disease
  - HIV
  - Smoking
  - Recent hotel stay
  - Ship cruise

BOX 7: Cardiac complications with pneumonia.

- Myocardial infarction (in first week of CAP)
- Congestive heart failure
- Arrhythmias

BOX 8: Diagnosis of CAP.

- Sputum gram stain, fungal stain, AFB smear, and gene Xpert
  - Sputum culture:
    - Aerobic/anaerobic/fungal/AFB cultures
    - Adequate sputum is >25 neutrophils and <10 squamous epithelial cells per low power filed
- Induced sputum analysis with hypertonic saline
- Deep suction aspirate in intubated patient
- Bronchoscopy with bronchoalveolar lavage
- *Blood cultures for high-risk patients:*
  - Neutropenia
  - Complement deficiency
  - Chronic liver disease
  - Severe CAP
  - At risk for MRSA/pseudomonas
    - Blood culture not recommended routinely due to low yield
- *Urinary antigen test:*
  - *Legionella pneumophila* serogroup 1
  - Pneumococcal urine antigen
    - Sensitivity 70%
    - Specificity >90%
- *PCR based test for:*
  - Viruses
  - Atypical organisms
  - Lower respiratory panel
- *Serology:*
  - Fourfold rise in specific IgM titer between acute convalescent serum samples
  - Not routinely done due to increased timeline
- *Biomarkers:*
  - C-reactive protein (CRP) useful in identification of worsening disease/treatment failure
  - Procalcitonin (PCT) distinguishes bacterial from viral infections

BOX 9: CURB-65 A Severity of illness score for hospitalization.

Detailed discussion in Chapter 44

BOX 10: Criteria for severe CAP.

- *Major criteria:*
  - Respiratory failure requiring invasive mechanical ventilation
  - Septic shock requiring vasopressors
- *Minor criteria:*
  - Respiratory rate ≥30 breaths/min
  - PaO_2/FiO_2 ratio ≤250
  - Multilobar lung infiltrate
  - Confusion/disorientation
  - Uremia (BUN ≥20 mg)
  - Leukopenia (TLC <4,000 cells/μL)
  - Thrombocytopenia (platelet <100,000 cells/μL)
  - Hypothermia (core temp <36°C)
  - Hypotension requiring fluid resuscitation

BOX 11: Risk factors for early deterioration in CAP.

- Multilobar infiltrates
- Severe hypoxemia SpO_2 <90%
- Severe acidosis pH <7.3
- Mental confusion
- Severe tachypnea RR >30 breaths/min

BOX 12: Empiric antibiotics for CAP in outpatients.

No comorbidities or no antibiotic in past 3 months and no contact with healthcare system:

- Amoxycillin (500 mg–1 g + tid) + either
- Clarithromycin 500 mg twice daily/azithromycin 500 mg once daily or
- Doxycycline 100 mg bid or
- Monotherapy with doxycycline 100 mg bid

BOX 13: Empiric antibiotics for CAP in outpatients.

With comorbidities + risk factors for antibiotic resistance:

- *Monotherapy with a respiratory fluoroquinolone:*
  - Moxifloxacin 400 mg once daily or levofloxacin 750 mg once daily or
- *A β-lactam:*
  - Amoxycillin or
  - Cefpodoxime 200 mg bid or
  - Cefuroxime 500 mg bid + plus a macrolide/doxycycline

BOX 14: Empiric antibiotic for cap in inpatients, non-ICU.

- Respiratory fluoroquinolones or
- IV β-lactam/carbapenem plus a macrolide

BOX 15: Empiric antibiotic inpatient ICU.

Inpatients ICU: β-lactam plus either macrolides or fluoroquinolones
If pseudomonas suspected:

- Antipseudomonal β-lactam
  - Piperacillin/tazobactam 4.5 g IV 6 hourly or
  - Cefepime 1–2 g IV 12 hourly or
  - Carbapenam + fluoroquinolones
- Above β-lactams + amikacin + azithromycin
- Above β-lactams + aminoglycoside + fluoroquinolones

If CA-MRSA suspected, add linezolid or vancomycin + clindamycin

BOX 16: Adjunctive measures.

- Routine use of steroids not recommended expect in patients with refractory septic shock
- Adequate hydration
- Oxygen
- Vasopressors
- Assisted ventilation

BOX 17: Failure to improve on treatment.

- *Conditions that mimic pneumonia:*
  - Pulmonary edema
  - Pulmonary embolism
  - Lung carcinoma
  - Radiation pneumonitis
  - Hypersensitivity pneumonitis
  - Connective tissue disease
- Resistant pathogen to the drugs selected
- Sequestered focus (lung abscess or empyema) blocking access of antibiotic to pathogen
- CAP due to fungus, CA-MRSA, or *M. tuberculosis*
- Nosocomial super infection

BOX 18: Complications of severe CAP.

- Respiratory failure
- Shock and multiple organ failure (MOF)
- Coagulopathy
- Exacerbation of comorbid illnesses
- Lung abscess
- Complicated pleural effusion
- Metastatic infection (rare)

BOX 19: Intercostal tube drainage in complicated pleural effusion.

- Fluid PH <7
- Glucose <40 mg%
- Lactate dehydrogenase (LDH) >1,000 U/L
- Bacteria are seen or cultured

BOX 20: Ventilator-associated pneumonia (VAP).

Common microbiologic causes:

- *Pseudomonas aeruginosa*
- MRSA
- *Acinetobacter* species
- Extended-spectrum beta-lactamase (ESBL) positive strains
- Carbapenem-resistant strains

BOX 21: Empiric antibiotic treatment for HAP and VAP.

Piperacillin-tazobactam or cefepime or carbapenem to be combined with aminoglycoside or colistin or polymyxin B.

BOX 22: Risk factors of MRSA.

- Add to above
- Linezolid 600 mg IV 12 hourly or
- Vancomycin IV

BOX 23: Standard recommendation for patient with risk factors for MDR infection in VAP.

Use three antibiotics: Two directed at *P. aeruginosa* + one at MRSA

BOX 24: Prevention of VAP.

- Use of NIV
- Minimize duration of ET tube ventilation
- Avoid heavy continuous sedation
- Elevating head end of bed by 45°
- Use of modified ET tube that allows removal of secretions above cuff
- Reduce transportation for diagnostic test outside the ICU
- Augment infection control practices, e.g., hand washing

SUGGESTED READING

1. Jameson JL, Kasper DL, Fauci AS, Hauser SL, Longo DL, Loscalzo J, et al. Harrison's principles of internal medicine. 20th ed. New York: McGraw-Hill Education; 2018.

2. Kalil AC, Metersky ML, Klompas M, Muscedere J, Sweeney DA, Palmer LB, et al. Management of Adults with Hospital-acquired and Ventilator-associated Pneumonia: 2016 Clinical Practice Guidelines by the Infectious Diseases Society of America and the American Thoracic Society. Clin Infect Dis. 2016;63(5):e61-e111.
3. Wunderink RG, Waterer GW. Community-acquired pneumonia. N Engl J Med. 2014;370(19):1861-3.

2.4 HEMOPTYSIS

Jeenam Shah

BOX 1: Definition.

Hemoptysis	Expectoration of blood originating from lower respiratory tract
Spurious hemoptysis	Hemoptysis present secondary to upper respiratory tract infection, above level of larynx, or from upper gastrointestinal (GI) tract mimicking hemoptysis
Massive hemoptysis	• Hemoptysis was initially defined based on the volume of blood expectorated within a specific time frame, but quantifying this volume accurately can be challenging. Additionally, blood present in the tracheobronchial tree is difficult to estimate. Generally, expectorating about 150 mL of blood over 24 hours or bleeding at a rate of 100 mL per hour is considered life-threatening • Currently, any level of hemoptysis that results in significant clinical issues, such as respiratory failure due to airway obstruction or hypotension, is regarded as life-threatening
Caveat: Criteria based solely on the volume of blood expectorated are imprecise because accurately quantifying the amount of blood can be challenging. Even small quantities of blood in patients with underlying cardiorespiratory conditions can pose a significant risk to life	

BOX 2: Etiology.

- Airway diseases—malignancy, foreign body, broncholith etc.
- Bleeding disorders—thrombocytopenia, platelet dysfunction, DIC etc.
- Trauma
- Infections—TB, NTM, Mycetoma etc.
- Rhematic diseases—SLE, GPA, Goodpasture etc.
- Drugs and toxins:
  - Cocaine use
  - Bevacizumab
  - Hydralazine
  - Riociguat
  - E-cigarettes/vaping
- Nitrogen dioxide toxicity
- Pulmonary vascular diseases—Pulmonary embolism, aneurysm, Heart failure etc.

BOX 3: Routine laboratory and bedside tests.

- Blood grouping and cross matching
- Complete blood count
- Prothrombin time (or international normalized ratio) and partial thromboplastin time
- Arterial blood gas
- Liver function test
- Serum electrolytes, creatinine, and blood urea nitrogen
- Urinalysis
- Sputum microscopy and culture (including *Mycobacterium tuberculosis*, bacteria, and fungi)
- Echocardiography

BOX 4: Selected laboratory testing (when selected conditions are suspected).

- Toxicity screen (e.g., cocaine and aspirin)
- Platelet function testing
- D-dimer
- Brain natriuretic peptide (BNP) or NT-proBNP
- Serologic tests—antinuclear antibody (ANA), antineutrophil cytoplasmic antibody (ANCA), double-stranded DNA antibodies, anti-glomerular basement membrane (GBM) antibodies, rheumatoid factor, and anticardiolipin antibodies
- Chest X-ray

BOX 5: Diagnostic modalities.

Chest X-ray	
CT chest with contrast	Superior to chest X-ray for pinpointing the site of bleeding, but it may not be practical for unstable patients or effective in identifying the source in those with pre-existing bilateral lung disease or blood aspiration in nonbleeding areas.
Bronchoscopy	Flexible bronchoscopy identifies the source of bleeding in 73–93% of cases of massive hemoptysis. It is the preferred initial investigation because it can be conducted at the bedside and is often effective in locating the bleeding site, especially when performed during active bleeding. Additionally, it can serve as a therapeutic tool to control the bleeding

Caveat: CT chest offers the highest diagnostic yield for identifying the source of bleeding. However, flexible bronchoscopy remains essential for patients requiring airway management or those with bilateral lung disease (post infective TB/bronchiectasis). In some situations, a combination of CT and bronchoscopy may be more effective than using either method alone.

BOX 6: Initial stabilization.

- Prioritize airway management, volume resuscitation, and correction of any coagulopathy
- If the bleeding site is identified, place the patient in a lateral decubitus position with the bleeding side down to reduce the risk of blood aspiration into the unaffected lung
- Intravenous tranexamic acid can be used for nonlife-threatening hemoptysis or as a temporary measure before definitive treatment in severe cases
- Use an endotracheal tube (ET tube) of size 8.0 mm or larger for endotracheal intubation to facilitate bronchoscopy if needed
- While unilateral intubation does not support bronchoscopic procedures, it can provide adequate ventilation and oxygenation while awaiting definitive treatment
- A double-lumen ET tube can enable single-lung ventilation and isolation of the bleeding site; however, routine use is not recommended due to the need for skilled personnel, difficulty in placement, and potential for obstruction by clots
- After initial stabilization and identification of the bleeding site, bronchial artery embolization (BAE) via the transfemoral approach is typically the first-line treatment for life-threatening hemoptysis
- *Bronchoscopy:*
  - Flexible bronchoscopy is the preferred initial diagnostic tool for most cases of life-threatening hemoptysis. It can be performed at the bedside and is effective in locating the bleeding site, particularly when done during active bleeding. It can also serve as a therapeutic measure to prevent recurrence
  - Advanced bronchoscopic techniques may be considered if flexible bronchoscopy alone is insufficient
- *Surgery:* With the advent of safe and effective endovascular embolization techniques, BAE has largely replaced emergency surgery for managing life-threatening hemoptysis. Emergent surgical intervention is reserved for:
  - Traumatic chest injury
  - Iatrogenic pulmonary artery rupture or hemorrhage associated with a resectable lung tumor
  - Failure of the BAE procedure, recurrent hemoptysis despite multiple BAE attempts, or maximum medical therapy
  - Life-threatening situations during hemoptysis that preclude safe interventional radiology
  - Definitive surgery may be crucial for patients with aspergillomas or those with tuberculosis who are at high risk for rebleeding after BAE

BOX 7: Management in nonlife threatening cases.

- Step 1: Ensure no life-threatening hemoptysis features such as below are present:
  - More than 150 and 100 mL in 24 hours
  - 100 mL/hour
  - Respiratory distress
  - Hypoxemia/hypercapnia
  - Hemodynamic instability
- Step 2: Obtain chest radiograph
  - If normal think of possibility of pseudohemoptysis secondary to nasal bleed or hemoptysis after vomiting or regurgitation and evaluate upper respiratory or GI sources
  - If not any of the above possibilities think of risk factors for lung malignancy or pulmonary embolism (Details given in respective chapters)
  - If above risk factors likely do the necessary investigation as per **Boxes 3 and 4**
  - But if above risk factor not likely consider acute bronchitis a likely possibility (if has concurrent Upper respiratory infections/productive cough mixed with mucous/quick resolution) then treat for same and observe for recurrence
  - If no recurrence no further work up needed
- Step 3: If there is recurrence work up as in **Boxes 3 and 4**
  - Or if as in step 2 if X-ray was abnormal do the initial work up and as per diagnosis manage the primary pathology
  - If no primary pathology has been incurred until now, do a flexible bronchoscopy, along with airway survey to identify source of bleeding, collect specimens for microbiological testing and if possible biopsy the lesion
  - Individualize further work up based on the results

Box 8: Management—life-threatening cases.

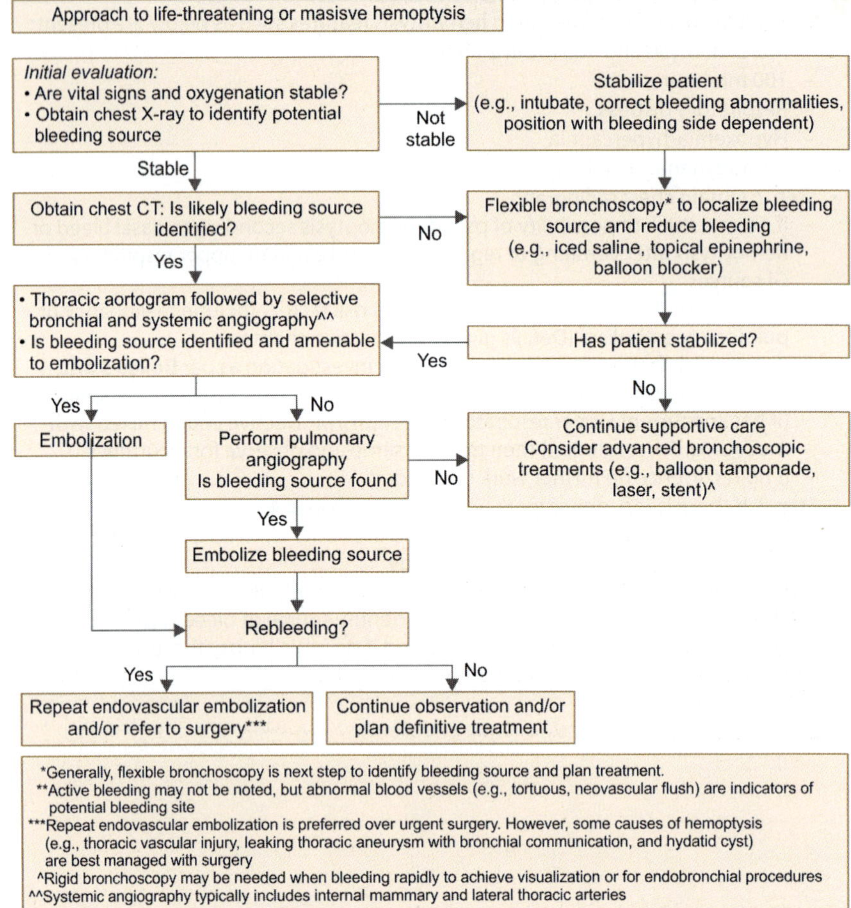

Source: Sakr L, Dutau H. Massive hemoptysis: an update on the role of bronchoscopy in diagnosis and management. Respiration. 2010;80:38.

SUGGESTED READING

1. Expert Panel on Thoracic Imaging, Olsen KM, Manouchehr-Pour S, Donnelly EF, Henry TS, Berry MF, Boiselle PM, et al. ACR Appropriateness Criteria® Hemoptysis. J Am Coll Radiol. 2020;17:S148.
2. Kathuria H, Hollingsworth HM, Vilvendhan R. Reardon C. Management of life-threatening hemoptysis. J Intensive Care. 2020;8:23.
3. Sakr L, Dutau H. Massive hemoptysis: an update on the role of bronchoscopy in diagnosis and management. Respiration. 2010;80:38.

2.5 ACUTE RESPIRATORY FAILURE

Jamshed D Sunavala

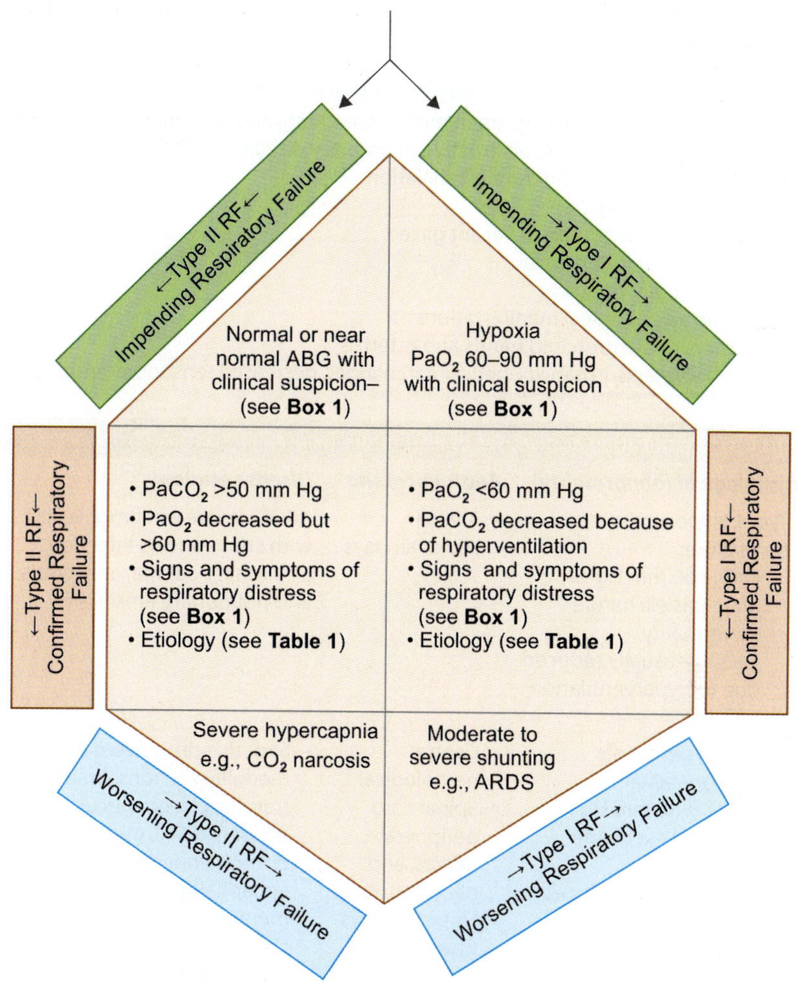

Fig. 1: Diagnosis of acute respiratory failure (ARF). (ABG: arterial blood gas; ARDS: acute respiratory distress syndrome; PaO_2: partial pressure of arterial oxygen; PiO_2: partial pressure of inspired oxygen; RF: respiratory failure)

BOX 1: Physical signs of acute respiratory distress.

- *Hypoxemic respiratory failure:*
  - Tachypnea, hypertension, and at times hypotension
  - Use of accessory muscles of respiration—intercostal, abdominal, and sternomastoid muscles
  - Tracheal tug
  - Exaggerated retraction of the intercostal space
  - Facial signs—nasal flaring, open mouth breathing, and pursed lips with labored breathing, as in chronic obstructive pulmonary disease (COPD)
  - Moaning and grunting during exhalation
  - Profuse sweating
  - Diminished mentation or vacant gaze
- *Hypercapnic respiratory failure:*
  - Mostly similar to above
  - Greater neurological manifestations
  - Tremors of outstretched hands and asterixis
  - Myoclonic jerks, irritability, behavioral changes, decreased sensorium, and seizures

TABLE 1: Classification and causes of respiratory failure.

Physiological (abnormality)	***Anatomical site***	***Disease etiology***
• *Type I:* Hypoxemic respiratory failure: – PaO_2 <60 mm Hg—main gas exchange abnormality – $PaCO_2$—usually reduced due to hyperventilation – V/Q <1	• Alveoli • Lower airways	ARDS, severe pneumonia, ILD with supra-added infection, pulmonary edema, atelectasis, and pulmonary embolism
• *Type II:* Hypercapnic respiratory failure: – $PaCO_2$ >50 mm Hg—main gas exchange abnormality – PaO_2—mildly reduced, appropriate to the $PaCO_2$ level – V/Q = 1 (normal)	• Central neurological • Spinal cord, peripheral nerves, and neuromuscular • Upper airways • Chest wall	• Sedative drug overdose, medullary lesions, brain trauma, cerebrovascular accident (CVA), metabolic encephalopathy, septic encephalopathy, and meningitis • Cervical cord injury, poliomyelitis, Guillan-Barre syndrome, myasthenia gravis, myopathies, and critical care neuropathy • Upper airways obstruction • Flail chest, pleural effusion, and increased intra-abdominal pressure
Combined respiratory failure: Hypercapnic and hypoxic: • $PaCO_2$ >50 mm Hg • PaO_2 <60 mm Hg	Airways	Acute exacerbation of COPD

Source: Sunavala JD. Acute Respiratory Failure. In: Sunavala JD (Ed). Essentials of Critical Care Medicine for the Physician. New Delhi: Jaypee Brothers Medical Publishers (P) Ltd.; 2022.

UNDERSTANDING HYPOXEMIA

BOX 2: Respiratory and nonrespiratory causes of hypoxemia.

Respiratory causes	***Nonrespiratory causes***
Decreased P_AO_2: Alveolar hypoventilation as in type II hypercapnic respiratory failure *Decreased transport of oxygen from alveoli to pulmonary capillaries:* • Diffusion impairment (ILD) • V/Q mismatch	*Decreased PiO_2:* Low barometric pressure at high altitude *Decreased FiO_2:* Anesthetic accident (very rare) Right-to-left intracardiac shunt

(FiO_2: fraction of inspired oxygen; ILD: interstitial lung disease; V/Q: ventilation to perfusion ratio; P_AO_2: partial pressure of alveolar oxygen; PiO_2: inspired oxygen partial pressure)

BOX 3: Alveolar arterial oxygen gradient [$P(A\text{-}a)O_2$] in clinical practice.

- Hypoxia with a normal $P(A\text{-}a)O_2$ suggests a type II RF, whereas an increased gradient confirms a lung parenchymal disease (type I RF)
- It is an essential calculation in clinical practice as PaO_2 alone has wide range of normality and is a function of three variables—ventilation, FiO_2, and respiratory quotient R
- Calculating $P(A\text{-}a)O_2$ can help to unravel subtle impairment of gas exchange which are otherwise not clinically apparent—Equation 1

EQUATION 1: Calculation for adequacy of O_2 transfer.

$$P_AO_2 = FiO_2\,(P_B - P_{H_2O}) - 1.2(PaCO_2)$$

$$P_AO_2 \text{ (at sea level)} = 0.21\,(760 - 47) - 1.2\,(40)$$

$$= 102 \text{ mm Hg}$$

P_AO_2 = Partial pressure of alveolar oxygen

P_B = Barometric pressure

P_{H_2O} = Water vapor pressure

$P(A\text{-}a)O_2$ = Alveolar arterial oxygen gradient; Gradient = 7–17 mm Hg in normal individuals. *Increased gradient suggests decreased oxygen transfer from alveoli to pulmonary capillaries as in type I respiratory failure.*

BOX 4: Pathophysiological causes of hypoxemia.

- Lung can either be poorly ventilated but well perfused (e.g., pneumonias, ARDS, etc.) or well-ventilated and poorly perfused (e.g., low cardiac output and pulmonary embolism)
- Diffusion defect is mainly manifest by a low PaO_2 worsening on exercise as in ILD
- Type II respiratory failure where main abnormality is an increase in $PaCO_2$ (>50 mm Hg) and a normal $P(A\text{-}a)O_2$
- For all above refer to **Flowcharts 1** and **Figure 2**

Flowchart 1: Physiological causes of hypoxemia.

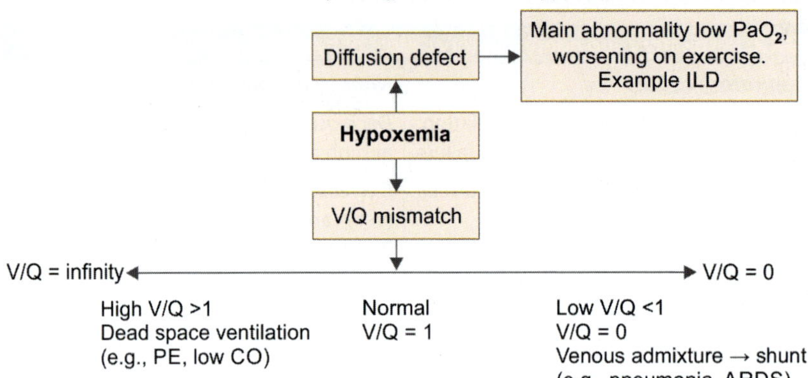

(CO: cardiac output; PE: pulmonary embolism)

Source: Sunavala JD. Acute Respiratory Failure. In: Sunavala JD (Ed). Essentials of Critical Care Medicine for the Physician. New Delhi: Jaypee Brothers Medical Publishers (P) Ltd.; 2022.

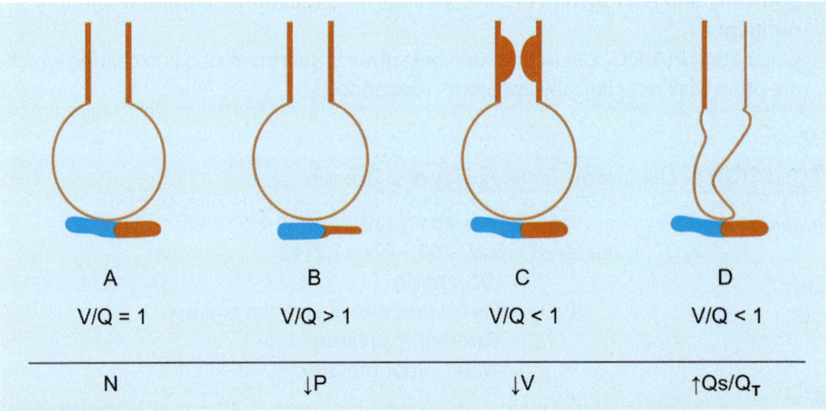

Fig. 2: V/Q mismatch and shunt. (N: normal; P: perfusion; Q_S/Q_T: total shunted blood flow/cardiac output; V: ventilation; V/Q: ventilation/perfusion)

Note:

A = Normal lung (uniform ventilation and perfusion)

B = Physiological dead space effect (uniform ventilation and nonuniform perfusion)

C = V/Q mismatch (nonuniform ventilation and uniform perfusion)

D = Shunt effect due to a collapse lung unit

Source: Sunavala JD. Acute Respiratory Failure. In: Sunavala JD (Ed). Essentials of Critical Care Medicine for the Physician. New Delhi: Jaypee Brothers Medical Publishers (P) Ltd.; 2022.

BOX 5: Differentiating shunt versus venous admixture **(Fig. 2)**.

Shunt	***Venous admixture***
Hypoxemia with totally unventilated alveoli	Hypoxemia with low V/Q mismatch of partially ventilated alveoli
Lung units where capillary blood receives no air from the totally unventilated alveoli	Lung units where alveolar air is less than the capillary perfusion
Delivery of 100% of oxygen will leave some degree of hypoxemia uncorrected. Hence supplemental oxygen will not significantly improve hypoxemia, e.g., ARDS	Delivery of 100% of oxygen will correct hypoxemia and eliminate venous admixture completely, e.g., lower respiratory tract infection (LRTI), mild-to-moderate pneumonia
Shunt equation (see Equation 2) helps to quantify the degree of shunt. However, at bedside the calculation of PaO_2/FiO_2 ratio gives a fairly good idea of the degree of shunting	

EQUATION 2: Quantifying shunt.

$$\frac{Q_S}{Q_T} = \frac{CcO_2 - CaO_2}{CcO_2 - CvO_2}$$

Where Q_T = Total cardiac output; Qs = Total shunted blood flow; Q_S/Q_T is the shunt fraction of the total cardiac output.

CaO_2, CvO_2, and CcO_2 are arterial, venous, and capillary O_2 contents respectively. Pulmonary catheterization is required to obtain CvO_2.

CcO_2 is assumed to be 100% on breathing 100% O_2 (as ventilated areas of lung are accepted to be perfused by ideal capillaries and the gas exchange is them is perfect).

UNDERSTANDING HYPERCAPNIA

EQUATION 3: Alveolar ventilation (V_A).

V_A is the volume of air that reaches the alveoli, and takes part in gas exchange between the alveoli and pulmonary capillaries. The portion of alveolar gas that is not involved in gas exchange because of dead space, is not considered a part of V_A.

$$\text{Hence } V_A = f \times (V_T - V_D)$$

where f = respiratory rate, V_T = tidal volume; V_D = dead space volume (physiological and anatomical).

BOX 6: Hypercapnia and PCO_2.

- CO_2 production (VCO_2) in the body is the by-product of food metabolism and needs to be continuously eliminated by the lungs. If for whatever reason VCO_2 increases (exercise) the excess load is eliminated by hyperventilation and does not result in hypercapnia.
- Hypercapnia would result if only the CO_2 excretion is impaired as in COPD, secondary to alveolar hypoventilation from central or peripheral neurological lesions (see **Table 1**) or from development of physiological dead space (see Equation 4)
- Hence as deduced from above, $PaCO_2$ is inversely proportional to V_A best expressed by the equation:

$$PaCO_2 = \frac{VCO_2}{V_A}$$

EQUATION 4: Dead space ventilation (V_D)

It is that portion of minute ventilation (V_E) that is not involved in gas exchange. V_D includes (1) anatomical V_D which remains in the airways and never reaches the alveoli and (2) physiological V_D that reaches the alveoli but for some reason does not take part in gas exchange.

$$\frac{V_D}{V_T} = \frac{PaCO_2 - PeCO_2}{PaCO_2}$$

$PeCO_2$ is the expired partial pressure of CO_2. Increased V_D/V_T >0.5 will result in hypercapnia and the most common cause is well ventilated but under perfused alveoli as in low cardiac output states or may occur transiently due to a passing pulmonary embolus.

BOX 7: Treatment of ARF.

- Correcting hypoxemia and ventilatory support (Details given in Chapters 2 and 31)
- Use and contraindication of NIV (Details given in Chapters 2 and 31)
- Oxygen delivery system (Details given in Chapter 31 Mechanical Ventilation)
- Treatment of the underlying causes of respiratory failure

SUGGESTED READING

1. Sunavala JD. Acute Respiratory Failure. In: Sunavala JD (Ed). Essentials of Critical Care Medicine for the Physician. New Delhi: Jaypee Brothers Medical Publishers (P) Ltd.; 2022.
2. Udwadia FE. Acute Respiratory Failure in Adults. In: Udwadia FE (Ed). Principles of Critical Care, 4th Edition. New Delhi: Jaypee Brothers Medical Publishers (P) Ltd.; 2024.

2.6 ACUTE RESPIRATORY DISTRESS SYNDROME

Jamshed D Sunavala

BOX 1: The Berlin definition of acute respiratory distress syndrome (ARDS).

Acute respiratory failure:

- Occurring within 1 week of a known clinical insult, or a new or worsening respiratory symptoms.
- Not explained by cardiac failure or fluid overload. May need objective assessment like 2D echo to rule out hydrostatic edema.
- Characterized by bilateral lung opacities which are not fully explained by effusions, consolidations, or collapse.

Severity of ARDS in relation to the degree of hypoxemia:

Mild	***Moderate***	***Severe***
Arterial oxygen partial pressure/fractional inspired oxygen (PaO_2/FiO_2) $\leq$300 but >200 on positive end-expiratory pressure (PEEP) 5 cmH_2O	PaO_2/FiO_2 $\leq$200 but >100 on PEEP 5 cmH_2O	PaO_2/FiO_2 $\leq$100 on PEEP 5 cmH_2O

BOX 2: Diagnosis.

- Sign and symptoms of pulmonary edema (PE) not explained by underlying cardiac failure or fluid overload
- X-ray chest showing characteristic bilateral lung opacities not fully explained by effusions, consolidations, or collapse. This is in contrast to peri hilar distribution seen in cardiogenic pulmonary edema
- Refractory hypoxia not responding to nasal or mask oxygen delivery
- These above features occur within 1 week of a known clinical insult or new or worsening respiratory symptoms
- 2D Echo may be useful in ruling out cardiogenic failure
- Presence of associated predisposing factors such as sepsis, pancreatitis, extensive burns, smoke inhalation, extensive trauma, severe bacterial, or viral pneumonia
- *Caveat:* Studies have shown that both cardiogenic PE and ARDS can coexist

BOX 3: Severity scoring.

- PaO_2/FiO_2 ratio in relation to the degree of hypoxemia **(Box 1)**
- High-resolution computed tomography (HRCT) picture may help in predicting severity of lung damage
- Knowing the severity or underlying predisposing factors or comorbidities **(Box 4)** associated with ARDS which can adversely influence the prognosis
- *Caveat:* Some large studies have found no clear association between degree of hypoxia to severity. However, bedside monitoring of the PaO_2/FiO_2 ratio is most convenient and a reasonably good measure of the extent of lung damage

BOX 4: Predisposing conditions for ARDS.

Major predisposing conditions:

Infection related:	*Noninfection related:*
• Septicemia • Septic shock • Pneumonia • Septic abdomen	• Gastric aspiration • Transfusion related acute lung injury (TRALI) • Pancreatitis • Shock (cardiogenic/hemorrhagic)
Postoperative: • Major abdominal surgery • Aortic surgery • Cardiac surgery • Thoracic surgery • Spine surgery	*Post-trauma:* • Polytrauma • Multiple fractures • Extensive burns • Lung contusion • Near drowning • Smoke inhalation

Risk modifiers:

(These are risk factors when combined with predisposing conditions are probably more prone to developing ARDS)

- Heavy smoking
- On chemotherapy
- Alcohol abuse
- Obesity
- Hypoalbuminemia
- High APACHE II score
- On high FiO_2
- Acidosis <7.35

MANAGEMENT

BOX 5: Immediate resuscitation and support.

Correcting hypoxia:

- Mode of oxygenation, type of mask, noninvasive ventilation (NIV), or mechanical ventilation (MV) depends of severity of ARDS
- High-flow nasal oxygen (HFNO) or NIV may be tried in less severe or uncomplicated cases. Also in some moderately severe and uncomplicated cases where the PE and the underlying pathology seems reversible within a short time
- *Intubation and MV:* All cases of severe ARDS (PaO_2/FiO_2 <100) plus those with life-threatening underlying disease or trauma or in cases of failed NIV or where NIV is contraindicated **(see Box 7)**
- *Immediate hemodynamic support:* This includes insertion of central line and arterial line, fluid management, and inotropic support

Note: Whenever there is delay in arterial blood gas (ABG), use O_2 at 8–10 L/min with face mask and if SpO_2 cannot be maintained >90% intubate.

BOX 6: Appropriate workup on admission.

- ABG, complete blood count (CBC), serum creatinine, serum electrolytes, blood sugar, liver function tests, prothrombin time and blood culture, and cultures from infected sites (aerobic, anaerobic, and fungus) when sepsis is suspected
- Urgent electrocardiography (ECG), X-ray chest, 2D echo, and appropriate biomarkers
- Appropriate empirical antibiotics when infection or sepsis is suspected (Details given in Chapter 7.1 Sepsis)

BOX 7: Contraindication for NIV.

- Unconscious or semiconscious patients
- Poor respiratory effort
- Uncontrolled seizures
- Life-threatening circulatory or respiratory failure or (PaO_2/FiO_2 <100)
- Copious tracheal secretions
- Vomiting/hemoptysis
- Serious injuries of the face and neck
- Laryngeal edema or obstruction

INVASIVE MECHANICAL VENTILATION: STEPWISE APPROACH

BOX 8A: Initiating MV in ARDS.

VT = 6–8 mL/kg
FiO_2 = 0.7–1.0 depending on PaO_2/FiO_2
Rate = 15–20 (increased if patient continues to fight the ventilator after sedation)
I:E = 1:2
PEEP = 5 cmH_2O
Mode = Volume-controlled ventilation or pressure-controlled ventilation or assist-control ventilation or pressure-regulated volume control (VCV or PCV or ACV or PRVC)

BOX 8B: Commonly used sedatives for patients on mechanical ventilator.

Drug	*Dosage*	*Comments*
Fentanyl	• *Bolus:* 0.35–0.5 µg/kg • *Infusion:* 0.7–10 µg/kg/h	• Short-acting opioid • No dose adjustment for renal failure • Less of adverse hemodynamic effects
Remifentanil	• *Loading:* 1.5 µg/kg • *Infusion:* 0.5–15µg/kg/h	• Ultrashort-acting opioid and effect is lost within 10 minutes of stopping infusion • No dose adjustment for renal failure
Midazolam	• *Loading:* 0.01–0.05 mg/kg • *Infusion:* 0.02–0.1 mg/kg/h	• Rapid acting benzodiazepine • Infusion to be limited to less than 48 hours
Lorazepam	• *Loading:* 0.02 – 0.04 mg/kg (not exceeding 2 mg as bolus dose) • *Infusion:* 0.01–0.1 mg/kg/h (not to exceed 8 mg/h)	• Longer acting benzodiazepine • Propylene glycol toxicity lasts up to 6 hours in high doses (lactic acidosis and delirium)
Dexmedetomidine	• *Loading:* 1 µg/kg over 10 minutes • *Infusion:* 0.2–0.7 µg/kg /h	• Cooperative sedation (like awakening from deep sleep and restoring back to sleep) • Sedation can be continued during spontaneous breathing trial (SBTs) during weaning • High loading and infusion rates can cause life-threatening bradycardia • Contraindicated in patients with heart blocks or cardiac failure

BOX 8C: PEEP settings.

- PEEP of 5–7 cmH_2O is used to prevent alveolar collapse in all patients. Hence, it should be a part of the initial setting
- Further increase in PEEP is required, if hypoxia is refractory to oxygen therapy; or to be more precise if FiO_2 of ≥0.6 is required to maintain a SaO_2 of ≥90%
- In patients with ARDS, a stepwise increase in PEEP levels (2–3 cmH_2O every 20 minutes) should be attempted, keeping VT, I:E ratio, and FiO_2 constant in order to obtain optimal lung recruitment. Achieving and maintaining SpO_2 of 90% or more reflects an optimal PEEP and recruitability
- Once the PEEP remains steady above 90% gradually decrease the FiO_2 to 0.6. Avoid increasing the PEEP levels above 20 cmH_2O
- Once the patient is recovering, weaning from PEEP is similarly done stepwise
- *Caveat:* PEEP trials based on SpO_2 titration may not give a correct idea of recruitability but is the most practical bedside method

BOX 8D: Management of refractory hypoxia.

- Subgroup of patients may require aggressive ventilator strategies as rescue therapy for refractive hypoxia
- These include prone positioning, inverse ratio ventilation and intermittent short recruitment trials, and airway pressure release mode (ARVA) (Details given in Chapter 31 Mechanical Ventilation)
- In worse scenarios, extracorporeal membrane oxygenation (ECMO) may have to be used (Details given in Chapter 34.1 ECMO)

BOX 8E: Weaning from MV.

- Most patient of ARDS take longer time to wean
- Weaning may be attempted once the lung pathology starts resolving and PaO_2/FiO_2 ratio >150 mm Hg
- Spontaneous breathing trial (SBT) is probably a good technique to weaning
- Check list for weaning failure (Details given in Chapter 31 Mechanical Ventilation) **(Box 7)**
- Weaning failure may manifest as sudden rise or fall in blood pressure (BP) or heart rate (HR), rising $PaCO_2$ or O_2 desaturation

Note: Weaning or weaning trials should be best attempted in the ICU after the transfer from ER.

BOX 8F: Prevention of ventilator-induced lung injury (VILI).

- There is a thin line between optimum recruitment using high level of PEEP and VILI
- Low V_T concept (using 4–6 mL/kg V_T) is now an accepted strategy, and is known as lung protective strategy (LPS)
- Avoid very high level of PEEP >20 cmH_2O
- Avoid FiO_2 levels above 0.6 and taper it slowly trying to maintain a SaO_2 >90% mm Hg by using optimum PEEP

BOX 9: Other strategies.

- *Steroids:* Use of steroids remains controversial. However, if used the Society of Critical Care Medicine (SCCM) and European Society of Intensive Care Medicine (ESCM) have suggested the use of methylprednisolone only in moderate-to-severe ARDS (PaO_2 <200 mm Hg) and to be started at a very early stage
- Prone position in severe ARDS is a strategy which should always be attempted to improve oxygenation in patient refractory to high FiO_2 and PEEP
- *ECMO:* Indicated in patients with refractory hypoxemia with failure of MV to achieve PaO_2/FiO_2 above 100. Also indicated in uncompromised hypercapnia with pH <7.2 not corrected by MV on high plateau pressure (Pplat) (Details given in Chapter 34.1 ECMO)

SUGGESTED READING

1. Acute Respiratory Distress Syndrome Network, Brower RG, Matthay MA, Morris A, Schoenfeld D, Thompson BT, Wheeler A. Ventilation with lower tidal volumes as compared with traditional tidal volumes for acute lung injury and the acute respiratory distress syndrome. N Engl J Med. 2000;342:1301-8.
2. ARDS Definition Task Force; Ranieri VM, Rubenfeld GD, Thompson BT, Ferguson ND, Caldwell E, Fan E, et al. Acute respiratory distress syndrome: The Berlin definition. JAMA. 2012;307(23):2526-33.
3. Bellani G, Laffey JG, Pham T, Madotto F, Fan E, Brochard L, et al. Noninvasive ventilation of patients with acute respiratory distress syndrome. Insights from the LUNG SAFE Study. Am J Respir Crit Care Med. 2017;195(1):67-77.

CHAPTER 3

Cardiovascular Emergencies

3.1 ACUTE MYOCARDIAL INFARCTION

Sushil C Munsi, Darshan Jhala, Malav Jhala

BOX 1: Initial evaluation.

1. *Typical symptoms of myocardial ischemia:*
   - Retrosternal/precordial chest discomfort/feeling of "pressure" radiating to left arm/jaws/epigastrium. In middle aged or elderly subjects associated with shortness of breath, diaphoresis, weakness, or fatigue strongly suggests myocardial ischemia
   - Diagnosis is further strengthened if diabetes, previous cardiac interventions on symptoms, and signs of heart failure are found
   - Women and elderly may present with atypical chest pain or with neurological symptoms.
2. Conduct a detailed history and physical examination to identify signs of hemodynamic instability and left heart failure
   - Assess baseline neurological function, especially important if considering fibrinolytic therapy
   - Obtain a 12-lead electrocardiogram (ECG) within 10 minutes of arrival; if the initial ECG is nondiagnostic but there is a high clinical suspicion, repeat it every 10–15 minutes
     - The initial ECG may not always provide a clear diagnosis.
       - *ST-elevation myocardial infarction (STEMI):* Look for ST-segment elevations >1 mm (0.1 mV) in at least two contiguous leads, or >2 mm (0.2 mV) in leads V2 and V3 **(Figs. 1A to C)**, or a new left bundle branch block (LBBB), combined with symptoms suggestive of acute coronary syndrome (ACS)

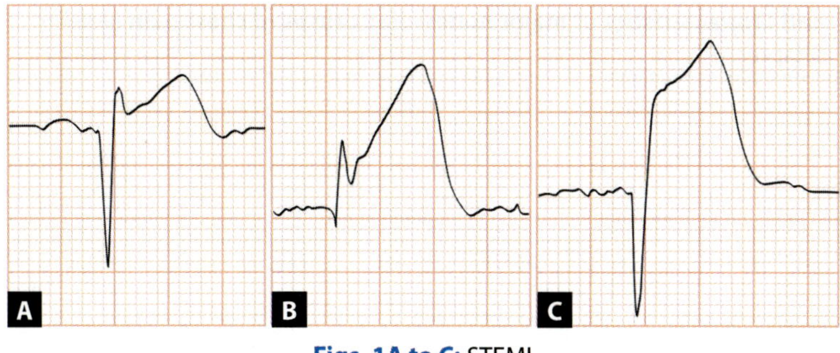

Figs. 1A to C: STEMI

Contd...

Contd...

- *Non-STEMI or unstable angina*: These conditions may present with ST-segment depressions or significant T-wave inversions without Q waves, or possibly no ECG changes at all **(Figs. 2 and 3)**

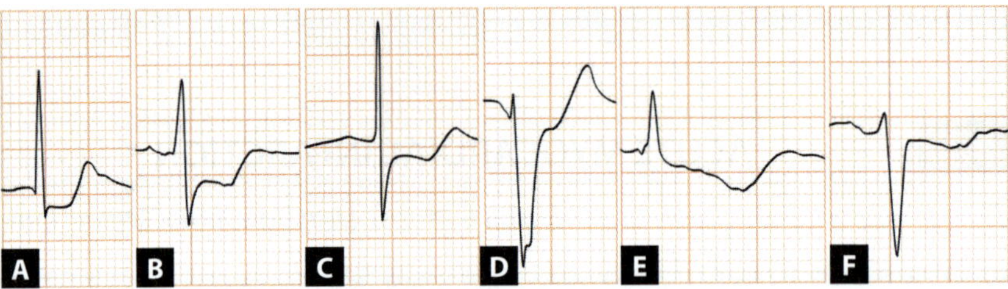

Figs. 2A to F: ST depression.

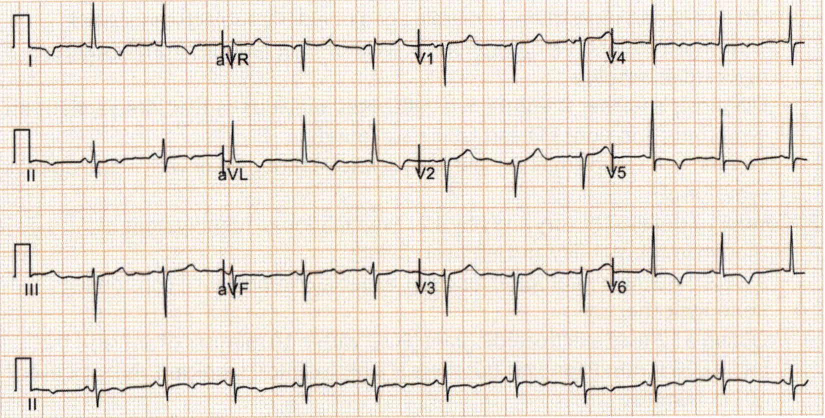

Fig. 3: T-wave inversion.

Manage on priority and immediately seek cardiology consultation for cases of ACS that are accompanied by cardiogenic shock, left heart failure, or sustained ventricular tachyarrhythmias.

Diagnoses other than cardiac ischemia for patients with chest pain and Characteristics of major noncardiac causes of chest pain (Refer to Chapter 1)

BOX 2: Differentiating myocardial infarction (MI) from pericarditis: How to distinguish Pericarditis from STEMI on ECG.

Three questions:

1. Is there ST depression in a lead other than aVR or V1? *If yes, it is an STEMI*
2. Is there convex up or horizontal ST elevation? *If yes, it is an STEMI*
3. Is the ST elevation in lead III greater than the ST elevation in lead II? *If yes, it is an STEMI*

If you are able to answer **NO to ALL** of the above then look for PR depression in multiple leads and a (usually transient) friction rub. PR depression is not specific for pericarditis **(Fig. 4)**.

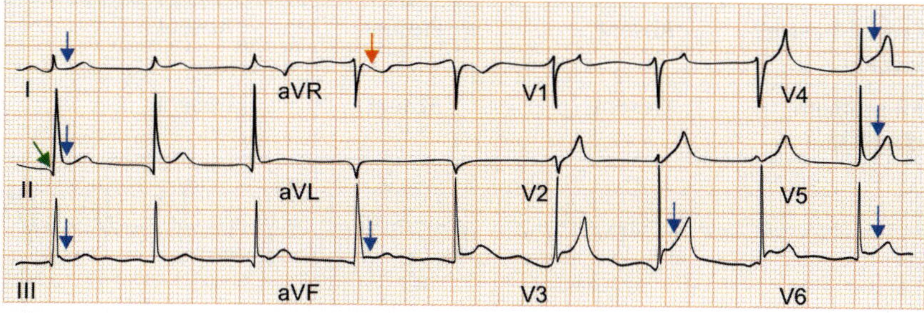

Fig. 4: ECG of acute pericarditis.

= ST-segment depression in aVR

= Diffuse concave upward ST-segment elevation

= PR-segment depression is best seen in leads II and V3

Lack of reciprocal ST-segment changes.

ST/T ratio is >0.25, a finding frequently indicative of acute pericarditis.

BOX 3: ECG characteristics in acute pericarditis and myocardial infarction (MI).

ECG finding	***Acute pericarditis***	***MI***	***Early repolarization (Fig. 5)***
ST-segment shape	Concave upward	Convex upward	Concave upward
Q waves	Absent	Present	Absent
Reciprocal ST-segment changes	Absent	Present	Absent
Location of ST-segment elevation	Limb and precordial leads	Area of involved artery	Precordial leads
ST/T ratio 1n lead V6	>0.25	NIA	<0.25
Loss of R-wave voltage	Absent	Present	Absent
PR-segment depression	Present	Absent	Absent

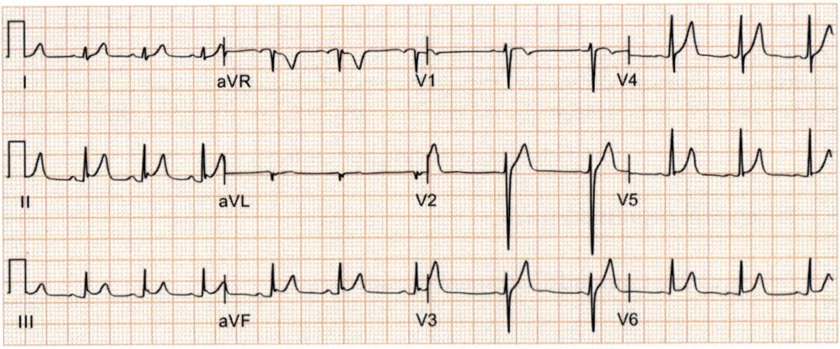

Fig. 5: Early repolarization.

BOX 4: Diagnosing MI in presence of bundle branch blocks.

In presence of right bundle branch block (RBBB), usual criteria of ST-segment elevation apply for anterior MI and MIs in other territories.

In presence of LBBB or paced rhythm (RV pacing), usual ST-elevation criteria cannot be used **(Box 5)**.

BOX 5: ST-elevation myocardial infarction (STEMI) diagnosis criteria in left bundle branch block (LBBB).

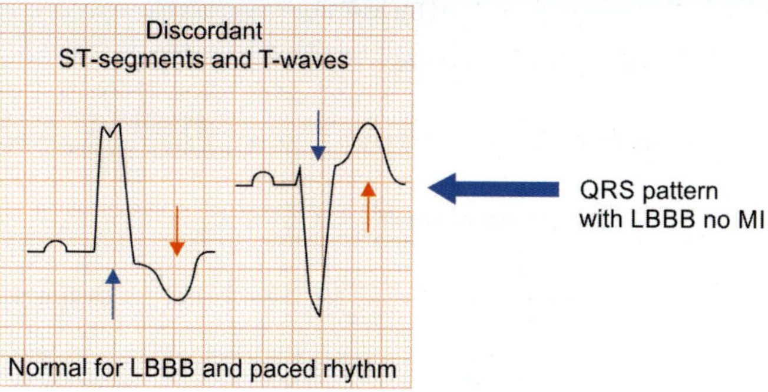

Fig. 6: QRS pattern with LBBB no MI.

Smith modified Sgarbossa criteria are used in of LBBB or RV paced rhythm **(Fig. 7)**:

- **Concordant ST elevation** ≥1 mm in ≥1 lead
- **Concordant ST depression** ≥1mm in ≥1 lead of V1V3
- **Proportionally excessive discordant ST elevation** in ≥1 lead anywhere with ≥1mm STE, as defined by ≥25% of the depth of the preceding S wave

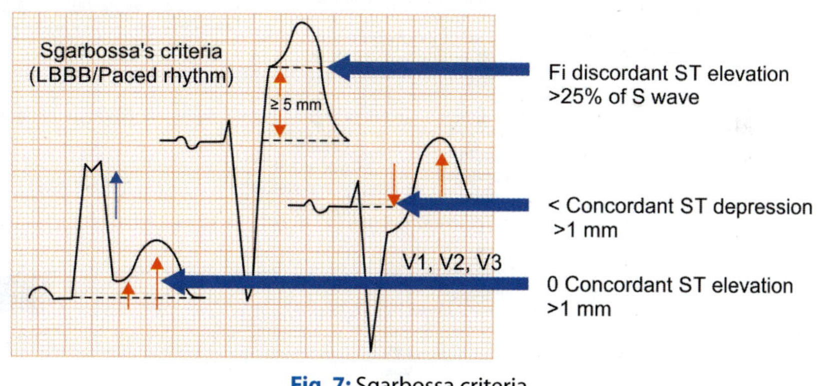

Fig. 7: Sgarbossa criteria.

BOX 6: Chest pain **(Flowchart 1).**

Flowchart 1: Chest pain training algorithm using high-sensitivity troponin I (TnI hs-TnI).

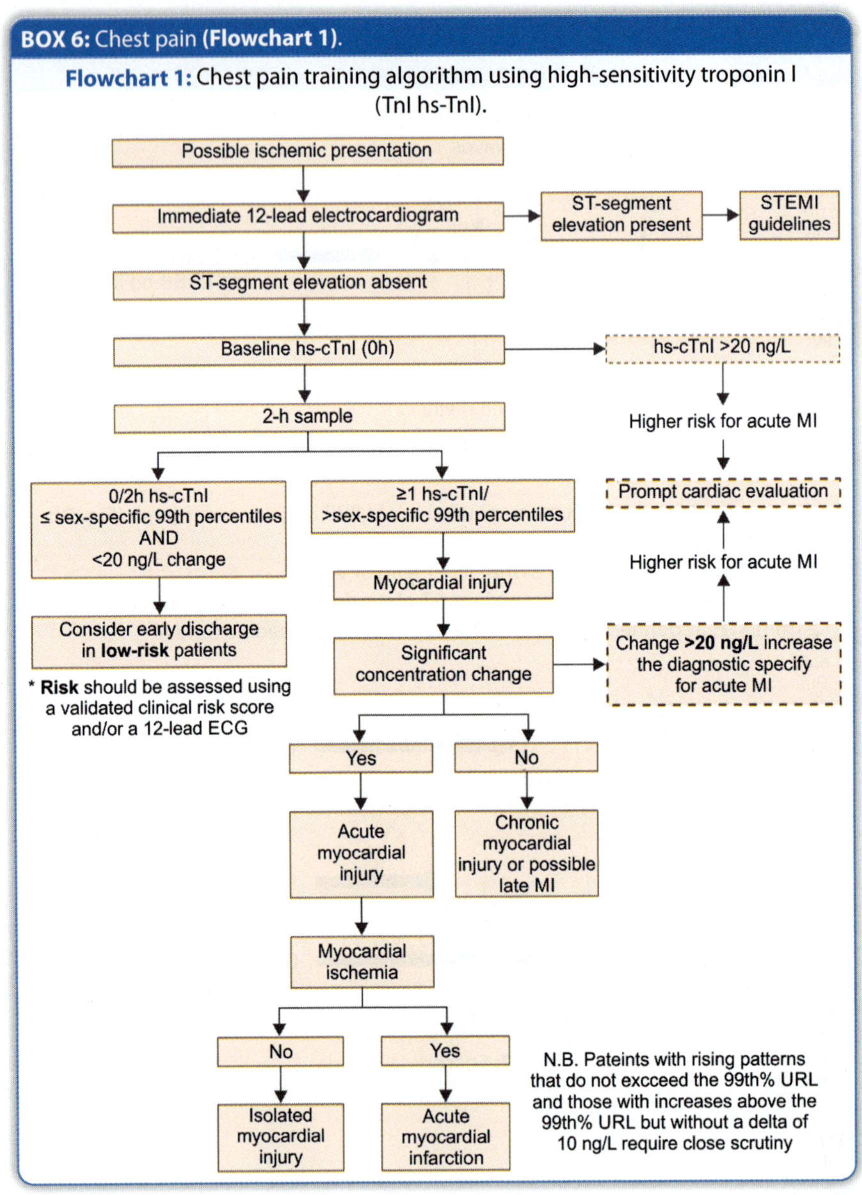

Contd...

Contd...

Flowchart 2: Chest pain pattern suggesting an acute coronary syndrome.

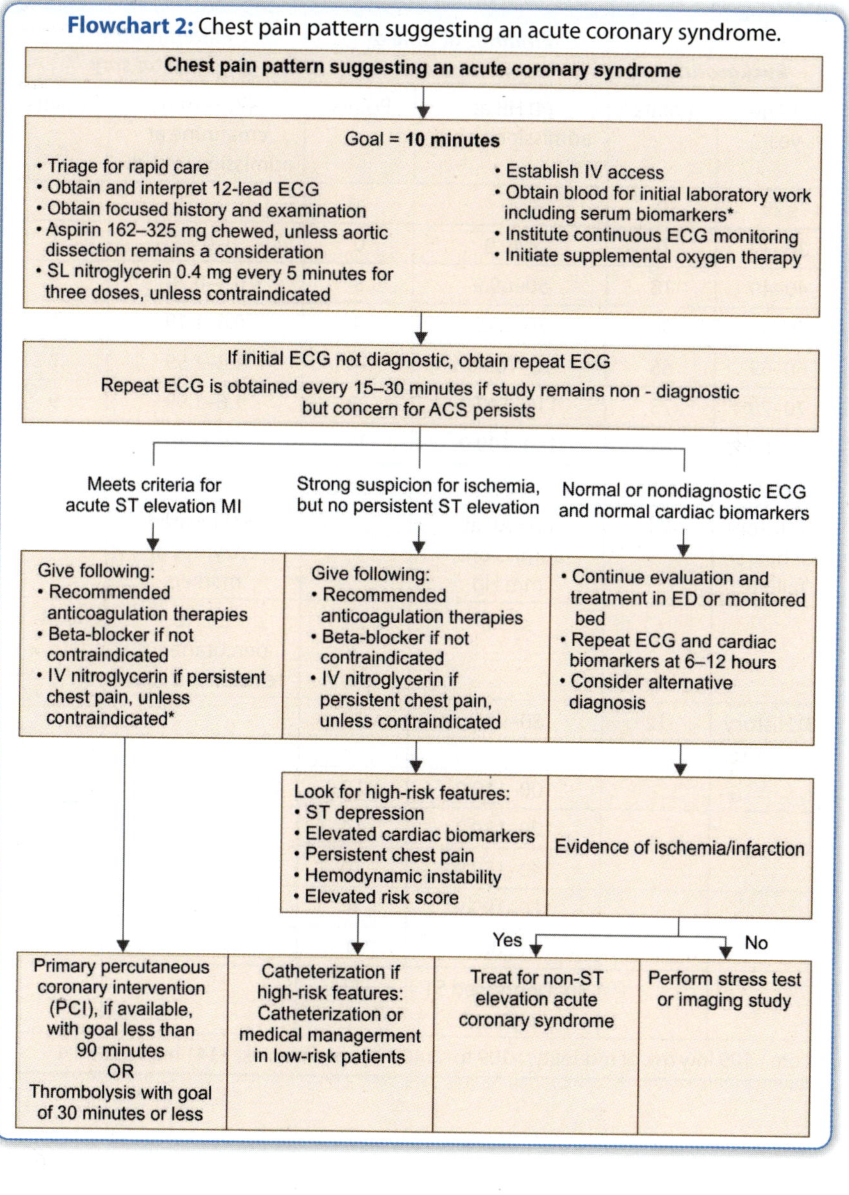

BOX 7: Grace score for ACS risk stratification.

Background		Findings at time of admission		Findings during hospital stay	
(1) Age, year	Points	(4) HR at admissions bpm	Points	(7) Serum creatinine at admission, mg/dL	Points
≤29	0				
30–39	0	≤49.9	0	0–0.36	1
40–49	18	50–69.9	3	0.4–0.79	3
50–59	36	70–89.9	9	0.8–1.19	5
60–69	55	90–109.9	14	1.2–1.59	7
70–79	73	110–149.9	23	1.6–1.99	9
80–89	91	150–199.9	35	2–3.99	15
≥90	100	≥200	43	≥4	20
(2) History of heart failure	24	(5) SAP at admissions, mm Hg		(8) Elevated enzymes or markers	15
		≤79.9	24	(9) No percutaneous revascularization	14
(3) History of AMI	12	80–99.9	22		
		100–119.9	18		
		120–139.9	14		
		140–159.9	10		
		160–199.9	4		
		≥200	0		
		(6) Depressed ST segment	11		
Score <109 low risk of mortality, >109 to <140 intermediate risk, >141 high risk					

BOX 8: Management of STEMI/non-STEMI.

Initial interventions:

- Assess and stabilize airway, breathing, and circulation
- Target SpO_2 >90%
- Establish IV access
- Obtain blood samples for Hs Trop to assess cardiac biomarkers, along with tests for electrolytes and hematocrit/hemoglobin levels. Conduct coagulation studies for patients currently on anticoagulants or if clinically indicated (e.g., known coagulopathy)
- Administer 325 mg of enteric coated aspirin to be chewed and swallowed unless there is a suspicion of aortic **dissection. If oral administration is not feasible, provide the aspirin as a rectal suppository**
- Administer three sublingual nitroglycerin tablets (0.4 mg) at 5 minute intervals, or use one aerosol spray under the tongue every 5 minutes for up to three doses if the patient continues to experience chest discomfort, hypertension, or signs of heart failure, provided there is no hemodynamic compromise (e.g., right ventricular infarction) and no recent use of phosphodiesterase inhibitors (such as those for erectile dysfunction). For persistent symptoms, consider intravenous nitroglycerin.
- Administer metoprolol tartrate 25 mg orally (beta-blocker) if there are no indications of heart failure, and the patient is not at high risk for heart failure, hemodynamic instability, bradycardia, or severe reactive airway disease. If the patient is hypertensive, initiate an intravenous metoprolol tartrate 5 mg IV (beta-blocker) every 5 minutes for up to three doses as tolerated.
  - *Treat left heart failure if present*: Administer an afterload-reducing agent (e.g., nitroglycerin sublingual tablet and/or IV drip at 40 µg/min), loop diuretic (e.g., IV furosemide), and noninvasive positive pressure ventilation [e.g., bilevel positive airway pressure (BIPAP)] to appropriate patients
  - *Treat sustained ventricular arrhythmia*: Follow ACLS protocols. Consider IV beta-blockers as above, or IV lidocaine (first bolus: 1.5 mg/kg, second and third bolus: 1 mg/kg, followed by infusion at 14 mg/min) or IV amiodarone (300 mg over 5 minutes via central line, followed by infusion of 900 mg in 24 hours)

BOX 9: Pain management.

- Administer morphine sulfate for chest discomfort that persists despite treatment with nitrates and other anti ischemic therapies. Administer 2–4 mg via slow IV push every 5–15 minutes as needed
- Statin therapy: Initiate atorvastatin 80 mg as soon as possible, ideally before PCI, in patients who are not currently on statin therapy, or even if they are on a low-to-moderate intensity statin

BOX 10: Acute management of STEMI.

Select Reperfusion Strategy:

Primary PCI is the preferred method, particularly for patients experiencing cardiogenic shock, heart failure, late presentation, or who have contraindications to fibrinolytic therapy. Activate the cardiac catheterization team as needed.

For patients with symptoms lasting >12 hours, fibrinolytic therapy is not recommended, but emergent PCI may be considered, especially in those with ongoing ischemia or at high risk of death.

If PCI is not available within 120 minutes of first medical contact, and symptoms have been present for <12 hours with no contraindications, administer fibrinolytic therapy.

Antiplatelet Therapy:

- *Patients treated with fibrinolytic therapy:* Clopidogrel loading dose 300 mg if age ≤75 years; if age >75 years, give a loading dose of 75 mg
- *Patients treated with no reperfusion therapy:* Ticagrelor loading dose 180 mg
- *Patients treated with primary PCI:* Ticagrelor loading dose 180 mg or prasugrel loading dose 60 mg (if no contraindications—prior stroke or TIA, or relative contraindications for prasugrel such as age ≥75 years, weight <60 kg). **For high bleeding risk or if prasugrel or ticagrelor cannot be used, give clopidogrel 600 mg**

Anticoagulant therapy:

- All patients with STEMI
- Patients treated with fibrinolysis enoxaparin for those not at high bleeding risk or fondaparinux for those at high bleeding risk

Dosing of enoxaparin:

- *Patients <75 years*:
  - Loading dose of 30 mg IV bolus followed by 1 mg/kg subcutaneously every 12 hours; maximum of 100 mg for the first two subcutaneous doses. The first subcutaneous dose should be administered with the IV bolus
  - Dose adjustment for renal impairment (CrCl <30 mL/min): Loading dose of 30 mg IV followed by 1 mg/kg subcutaneously every 24 hours. The first subcutaneous dose should be administered with the IV bolus
- *Patients >75 years:*
  - No IV loading dose. Administer 0.75 mg/kg subcutaneously every 12 hours; maximum of 75 mg for the first two doses
  - Dose adjustment for renal impairment (CrCl <30 mL/min): No IV loading dose. Administer 1 mg/kg subcutaneously every 24 hours
- *Dosing of Fondaparinux:*
  - 2.5 mg intravenously, followed by 2.5 mg subcutaneously every 24 hours. Avoid this drug in CrCl <30 mL/min
- *Patients not receiving reperfusion therapy:* Use enoxaparin or unfractionated heparin (UFH)
- *Dosing of UFH:* IV bolus of 50–70 units/kg to a maximum of 5,000 units, followed by an IV infusion of 12 U/kg/h adjusted to achieve a goal activated partial thromboplastin time (aPTT) of approximately 50–70 seconds (1.5–2 times control)

BOX 11: Acute management of unstable angina or Non-STEMI.

Antiplatelet therapy (in addition to aspirin in all non-STEMI patients):

1. *Patients not treated with an invasive approach:* Ticagrelor loading dose 180 mg. For very high-risk patients (e.g., recurrent ischemic discomfort, dynamic ECG changes, or hemodynamic instability), consider adding a GP IIb/IIIa inhibitor (e.g., eptifibatide or tirofiban)
2. *Patients managed with an invasive approach:* Ticagrelor loading dose 180 mg at presentation. Prasugrel loading dose 60 mg may be used as an alternative only after diagnostic coronary angiography

Anticoagulant therapy: For urgent catheterization (within 4 hours) or early invasive strategy (angiography within 4–48 hours), use UFH.

Dosing of UFH: IV bolus of 60–70 units/kg to a maximum of 5,000 units, followed by an IV infusion of 12 U/kg/h adjusted to achieve a goal aPTT of approximately 50–70 seconds (1.5–2 times control).

For noninvasive approach, use either fondaparinux or enoxaparin (see dosing above).

BOX 12: Other important considerations.

- *Cocaine-related ACS:* Administer benzodiazepines (e.g., lorazepam 2–4 mg IV every 15 minutes as needed) to alleviate symptoms. **Give standard therapies (e.g., aspirin and nitroglycerin) but avoid beta-blockers**
- Discontinue nonsteroidal anti-inflammatory drug (NSAID) therapy
- Correct electrolyte abnormalities, especially hypokalemia and hypomagnesemia, which often occur together

Dosing for fibrinolysis:

- *Fibrinolytic agents:*
  - *Streptokinase:* 1.5 million units over 60 minutes
  - *Alteplase:*
    - *Body weight >67 kg:* 15 mg initial IV bolus; 50 mg infused over the next 30 minutes; 35 mg infused over the next 60 minutes
    - *Body weight <67 kg:* 15 mg initial IV bolus; 0.75 mg/kg infused over the next 30 minutes; 0.5 mg/kg infused over the next 60 minutes
  - *Reteplase:* 10 units IV over 2 minutes followed by 10 units IV bolus 30 minutes later
  - *Tenecteplase:* Weight-based dosing (total dose not to exceed 50 mg):
    - <60 kg: 30 mg
    - 60–69 kg: 35 mg
    - 70–79 kg: 40 mg
    - 80–89 kg: 45 mg
    - ≥90 kg: 50 mg

BOX 13: Advanced cardiac life support **(Flowchart 3)**.

Flowchart 3: Advanced cardiac life support algorithm.

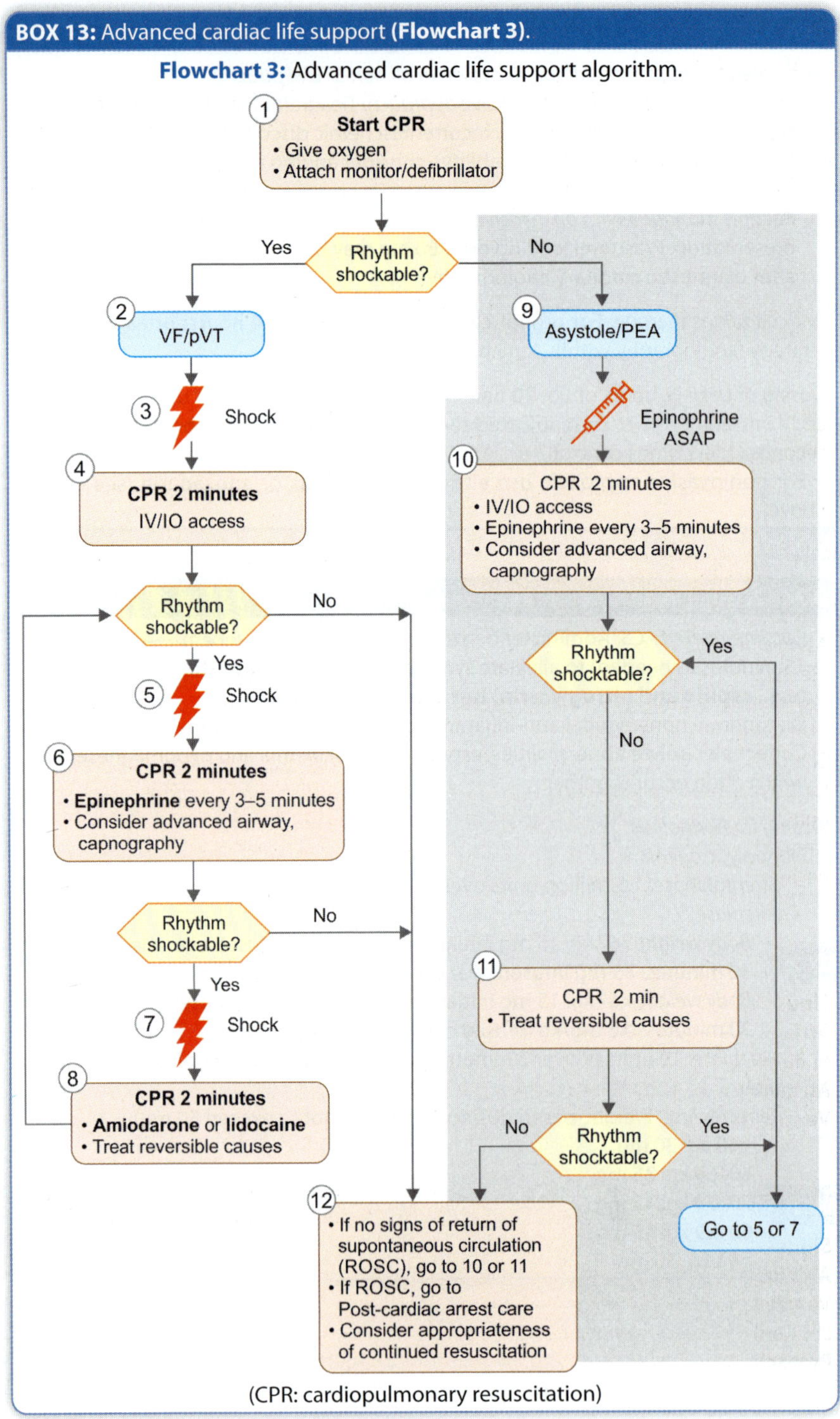

(CPR: cardiopulmonary resuscitation)

SUGGESTED READING

1. ACC/AHA Task Force on Clinical Practice Guidelines. (2022). Myocardial Infarction: Management Guidelines. [online] Available from https://www.jacc.org/doi/10.1016/j.jacc.2022.10.003 [Last accessed September, 2024].
2. "ESC Guidelines for the Management of Acute Coronary Syndromes"
3. "Clinical Practice Guidelines: Acute Coronary Syndrome" by NICE (National Institute for Health and Care Excellence)
4. "Acute Coronary Syndromes" by Adam Timmis
5. Journal of the American College of Cardiology (JACC)
6. Timmis A. Acute coronary syndromes. BMJ. 2015 Oct 30; doi:10.1136/bmj.h5849

3.2 CARDIAC RHYTHM DISORDERS

Shamsunder R Handa

BOX 1: Introduction.

- Cardiac rhythm and conduction disturbances can be
- Symptomatic (syncope, near syncope, dizziness, fatigue, or palpitations) or
- Asymptomatic
- Mechanistically, cardiac arrhythmias can be broadly classified into
  (a) Disorders of action potential formation or impulse formation
  (b) Disorders of impulse conduction
- Clinically, it is classified as bradycardia **(Box 2)** and tachycardia **(Box 3)**, with further categorization according to arrhythmia origin. This information is used to guide evaluation and management strategies **(Box 5)**
- Fatal arrhythmias are associated with reduced cardiac output causing decreased perfusion to myocardium and brain

BOX 2: Abnormalities of impulse formation.

- **Sinus node**—sinus arrythmia, sinus tachycardia, and sinus bradycardia
- **Atria**—supraventricular tachycardia (SVT), atrial tachycardia, atrial fibrillation (AF) or flutter, and ectopics
- **Atrioventricular (AV) node**—junctional rhythm and junctional tachycardia
- **Ventricles**—ventricular tachycardia, ventricular fibrillation, and ectopics

BOX 3: Abnormalities of impulse conduction.

- **Sinus**—sinoatrial block
- **AV block**—1, 2, and 3 types of block
- **Ventricles**—right bundle branch block/left bundle branch block (RBBB/LBBB)
- LEFT anterior and posterior fascicular hemiblock
- **Preexcitation syndrome**—Wolff–Parkinsons–White syndrome

BOX 4: Instability indicators in the patient with cardiac dysrhythmias.

- Low blood pressure
- Altered mental status
- Chest pain
- Dyspnea

BOX 5: Sinus arrythmia, bradycardia, and tachycardia.

- Sinus arrythmia is an irregular heart rate with variation in PP interval of >120 ms. It is mostly seen in young, healthy individuals
- Sinus bradycardia is defined as heart rate slower than 60 beats/min. It is due to enhanced vagal influence on the normal sinus node. In well-trained athletes, sinus bradycardia to rates of 50 beats/min may be a normal finding
- Sinus tachycardia defined as heart rate faster than 100 beats/minutes. It is a normal physiological adaptation to exercise or conditions with catecholamine release. "Inappropriate" sinus tachycardia is due to persistently elevated basal heart rate without any physiological demand **(Fig. 1)**
- Sick sinus syndrome includes patients with sinus arrest, sinoatrial exit block, or persistent sinus bradycardia. It can manifest as chronotropic incompetence which is defined as inappropriate heart rate response to exercise or stress

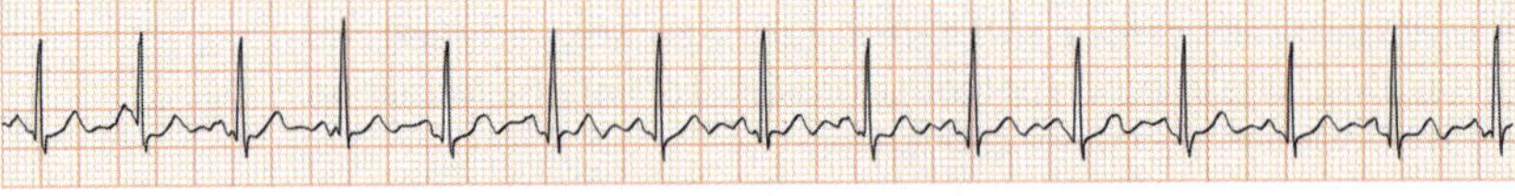

Fig. 1: Sinus tachycardia.

BOX 6: Paroxysmal supraventricular tachycardia (PSVT).

- Patients can present with palpitations of variable severity, hypotension, dizziness, or diaphoresis
- On **12-lead electrocardiogram (ECG), heart rate is regular varying between 160 and 220 beats/min, QRS duration will be narrow (<120 ms)**. P wave is often simultaneous with or just after QRS complex **(Fig. 2)**
- **Treatment:**
  - *Mechanical measures:*
    - Valsalva maneuver
    - Carotid sinus massage
    - Facial contact with cold water
  - *Medication therapy:*
    - *Intravenous adenosine:* It is a first-line agent due to its short duration of action and minimal negative inotropic activity. It is given rapidly as a 6 mg bolus followed by 20 mL of fluid
    - Intravenous calcium blockers
    - Intravenous beta-blockers
    - Intravenous amiodarone

Contd...

Contd...

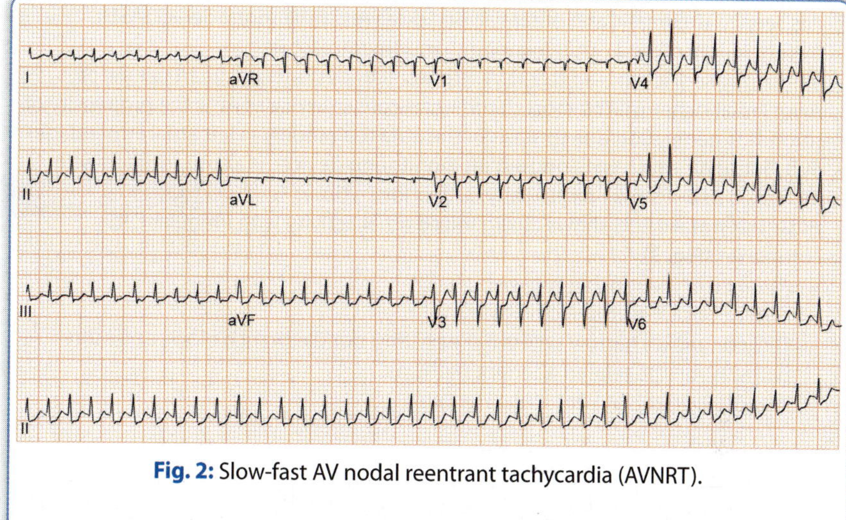

Fig. 2: Slow-fast AV nodal reentrant tachycardia (AVNRT).

- *Cardioversion:* If patient is hemodynamically unstable or if adenosine is ineffective or contraindicated, synchronized electrical cardioversion should be performed
- Radiofrequency ablation is the preferred approach to patients with recurrent symptomatic reentrant PSVT **(Flowchart 1)**

Flowchart 1: Acute therapy of narrow QRS tachycardia.

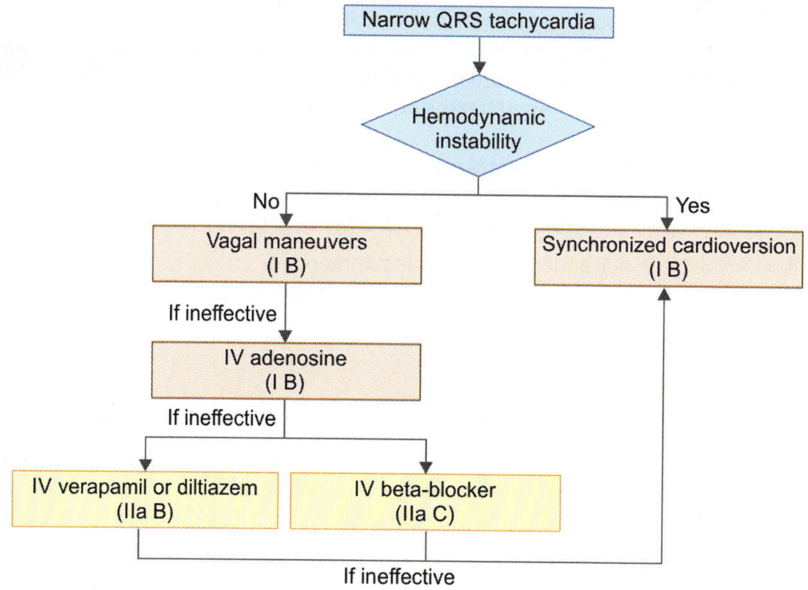

BOX 7: Atrial fibrillation.

- It is seen in rheumatic and other valvular diseases, atrial septal defect (ASD), hypertension, dilated cardiomyopathy, and thyrotoxicosis
- If uncontrolled, it can lead to left ventricular (LV) dysfunction, heart failure, or myocardial ischemia. The most detrimental consequence of AF is the propensity of thrombus generation due to stasis in the atria (commonly in left atrial appendage)
- Subclinical AF which is diagnosed on monitoring devices is also associated with increased risk of stroke particularly lasting for 24 hours
- **ECG:** The surface ECG shows disorganized atrial activity with irregular QRS complexes **(Fig. 3)**
  - Absence of identifiable P waves
  - Absent or chaotic isoelectric baseline
  - QRS complexes narrow unless a preexisting bundle branch block, accessory pathway, or rate related aberrant pathway
  - Irregularly irregular ventricular rhythm

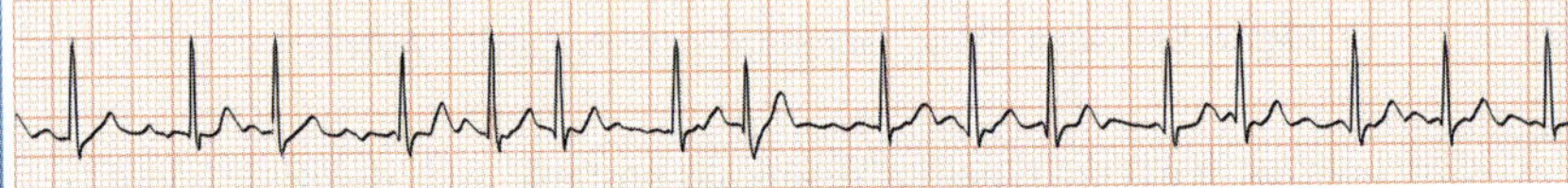

Fig. 3: Atrial fibrillation.

- **Echocardiography** gives information about LV function, associated valvular pathology and chamber volumes
- Transesophageal echocardiogram (TEE) may identify thrombi in left atrium or left atrial appendage
- **Treatment:**
  - Urgent electrical cardioversion is indicated in patients with shock or severe hypertension and ongoing MI or ischemia. An initial shock with 100–200 J is administered in a synchronized manner with R wave
  - In stable patients with AF, a strategy of rate control and anticoagulation is appropriate
- *Anticoagulation:* The need of anticoagulation should be assessed and offered to those without contraindication. The risk score most commonly used for assessing risk of stroke and antithrombotic therapy is CHA_2-DS_2-VASc (see Chapter 44)

  If the score is ≤2, oral anticoagulation is recommended

  Dabigatran, rivaroxaban, and apixaban have been shown be effective for stroke prevention in patients with AF

BOX 8: ECG features of atrial flutter.

- Identifiable P waves
- Single morphology
- Negative amplitude("flutter waves" in "sawtooth pattern") best seen in inferior ECG leads and V1
- Atrial rate is regular, usually at 300 beats/min (250–350 beats/min)
- QRS complexes narrow generally
- Ventricular rate regular, although occasional irregularity can be seen
- Ventricular rate often 150 beats/min due to 2:1 AV nodal block

ER management of AF/flutter in stable patients*

Given in the **(Box 17)**

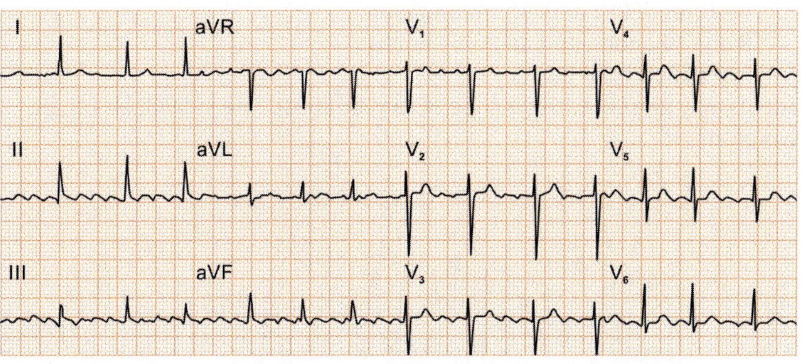

Fig. 4: Atrial flutter.

BOX 9: ECG features of multifocal atrial tachycardia.

- At least three distinct P-wave morphologies in a single ECG lead
- Varying P to P, PR, or R to R intervals
- Irregularly irregular rhythm with rates usually 100–180 beats/min
- Normal QRS complex unless preexisting bundle branch blocks
- Frequently confused with AF or flutter but isoelectric baseline between P waves

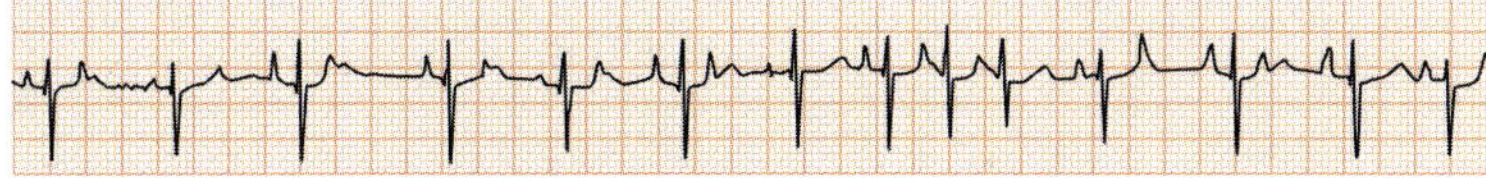

Fig. 5: Multifocal atrial tachycardia.

BOX 10: Ventricular tachycardia.

- Ventricular tachycardia is defined as three or more consecutive ventricular premature beats
- It is classified as either nonsustained (lasting <30 seconds and terminating spontaneously) or sustained with a heart rate >100 beats/min.
- It is frequently seen in acute myocardial infarction (MI) and dilated cardiomyopathy, hypertrophic cardiomyopathy (HCM), myocarditis, etc.
- **Torsades de pointes** is a form of ventricular tachycardia in which QRS morphology twists around the baseline and may occur in conditions causing hypokalemia, hypomagnesemia, or after taking medications that cause QT interval prolongation
  - **ECG shows:**
    - Features of PVT and QT prolongation
    - R on T phenomenon might be noted
    - Not sustained in bursts
- Patients may present with syncope or cardiac arrest. Few individuals can be asymptomatic

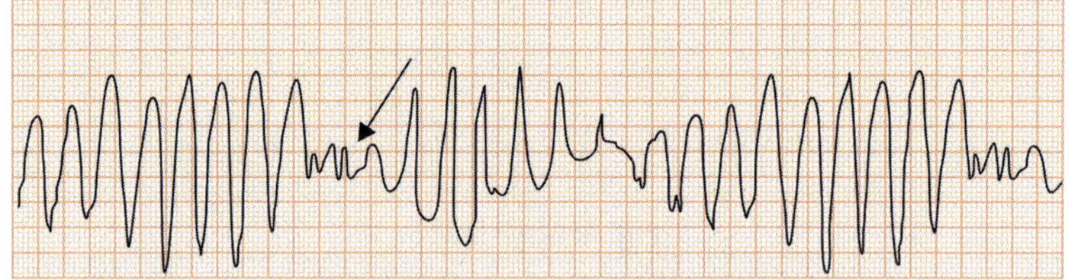

Fig. 6: Polymorphic ventricular tachycardia with torsades. (Torsades marked with the arrow)

BOX 11: Monomorphic ventricular tachycardia.

- No P waves-associated with QRS complex, occasional dissociated P wave **(Fig. 7)**
- Rapid and regular rhythm
- Rate usually 140–180 beats/min (range 120–300 beats/min)
- Widened QRS complex >160 ms but uniform
- Absence of typical bundle branch block
- Extreme axis deviation
- AV dissociation (P and QRS complexes at different rates) **(Fig. 8)**
- Capture beats (when sinoatrial node captures the ventricles transiently in the midst of AV dissociation, hence producing a normal complex QRS) **(Fig. 9)**
- Fusion beats—sinus and ventricular beats coincide resulting into a hybrid morphology
- Left axis deviation
- Monophasic (R) or biphasic (qR, QR, or RS) complexes in V1 and
- qR or QS complexes in V6
- **RSR' complexes with a taller "left rabbit ear". Very specific**
- *Caveat:* RBBB has taller right rabbit ear

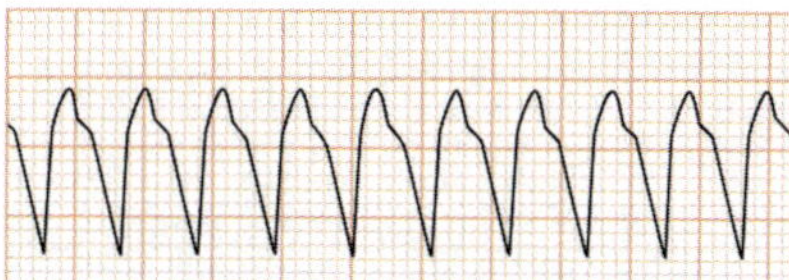

Fig. 7: Monomorphic VT.

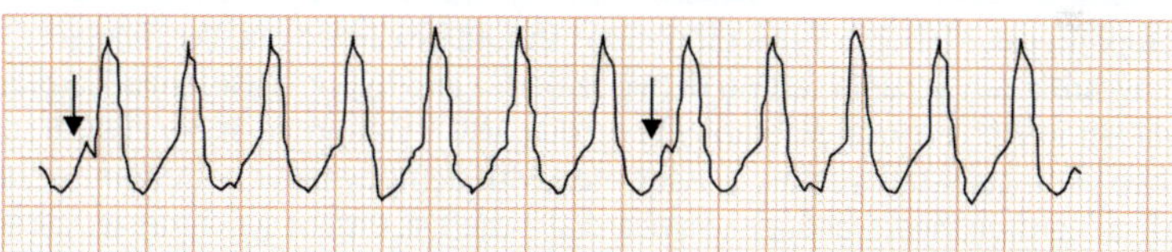

Fig. 8: AV dissociation in VT.

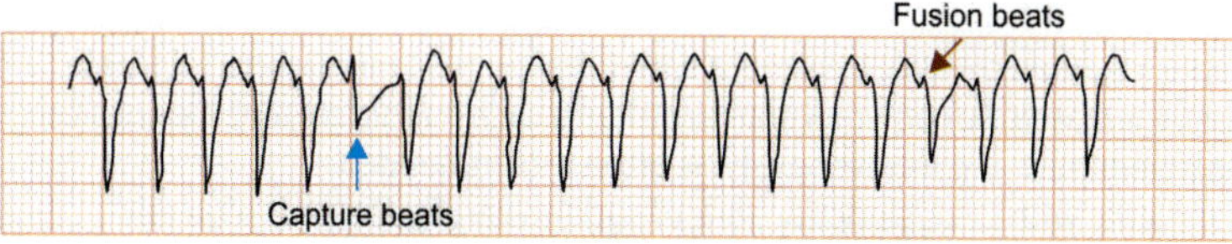

Fig. 9: Capture and fusion beats in VT.

BOX 12: Polymorphic ventricular tachycardia.

- *Polymorphic:*
  - No P waves-associated with QRS complex; may have occasional dissociated P wave
  - Rapid and irregular rhythm
  - Rate 140–180 beats/min (range 120–300 beats/min)
  - Widened QRS complex >100–120 ms with inconsistence beat-to-beat morphology **(Fig. 10)**.

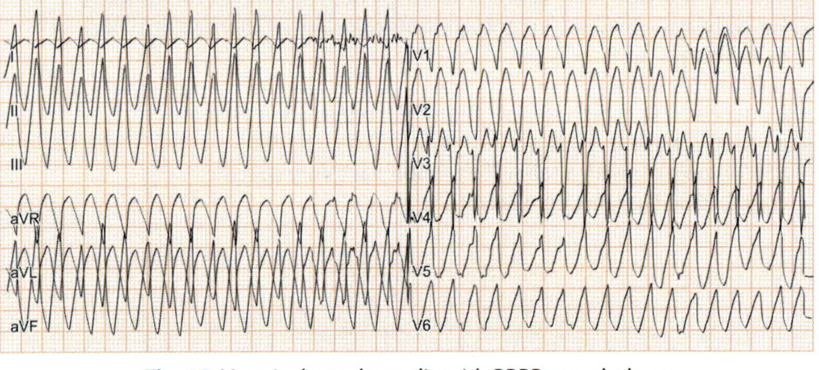

Fig. 10: Ventricular tachycardia with RBBB morphology.

BOX 13: Management of ventricular tachycardia.

- Comprehensive laboratory investigations should be carried out. Ventricular tachycardia can occur in setting of hypokalemia and hypomagnesemia. Cardiac evaluation with echocardiography or cardiac MRI is warranted as per clinical status
- When ventricular tachycardia is associated with hemodynamic compromise such as hypotension, heart failure or myocardial ischemia, urgent synchronized direct current cardioversion with 100–360 J should be performed
- Intravenous amiodarone (150 mg bolus followed by 1 mg/min infusion for 6 hours than 0.5 mg/min for 18 hours) should be administered
- In patients with sustained ventricular tachycardia who are hemodynamically stable, pharmacological treatment with intravenous amiodarone, lidocaine can be initiated. For polymorphic ventricular tachycardia empiric magnesium replacement (1–2 g intravenously) is often recommended
- In patients with LV dysfunction, risk of sudden cardiac death is high and Implantable cardioverter-defibrillator (ICD) implantation is recommended
- Beta-blockers remain the mainstay of the therapy in structural heart diseases
- Pulseless VTACH treatment is discussed in Chapter 26.

BOX 14: Ventricular fibrillation.

- Disorganized depolarization and chaotic contraction of small areas of ventricular myocardium complete absence of any mechanical cardiac activity and cardiac output
- **ECG changes** are a fine, irregular pattern without discernible P OR QRS WAVES **(Flowchart 2)**
- Catheter ablation can be a suitable option if tachycardia is recurrent and non-responsive to medical therapy

Flowchart 2: Acute therapy of wide complex tachycardia.

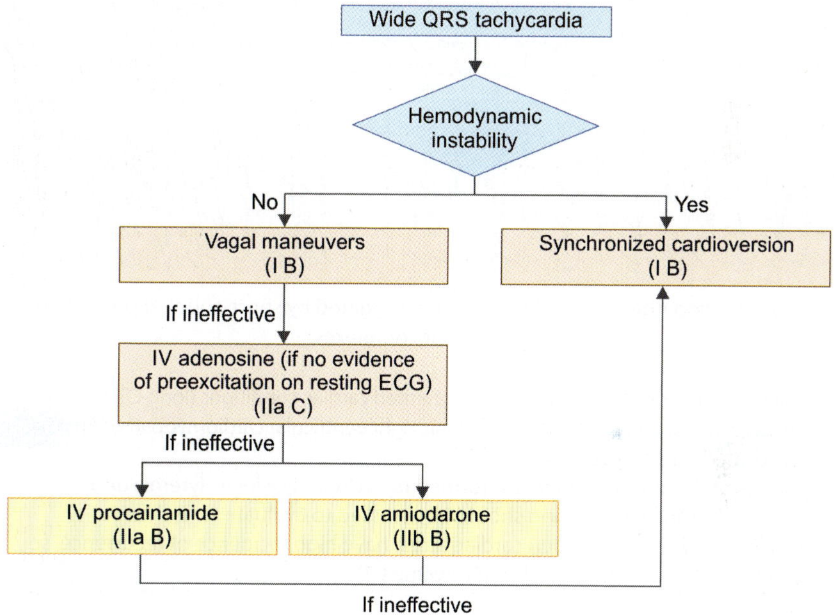

BOX 15: Sudden cardiac death.

- Sudden cardiac death is defined as unexpected nontraumatic death in clinically well or stable patients who die within 1 hour after onset of symptoms. It is most commonly caused by ventricular fibrillation
- In majority of the patients, cause attributable is underlying coronary artery disease **(Fig. 11)**

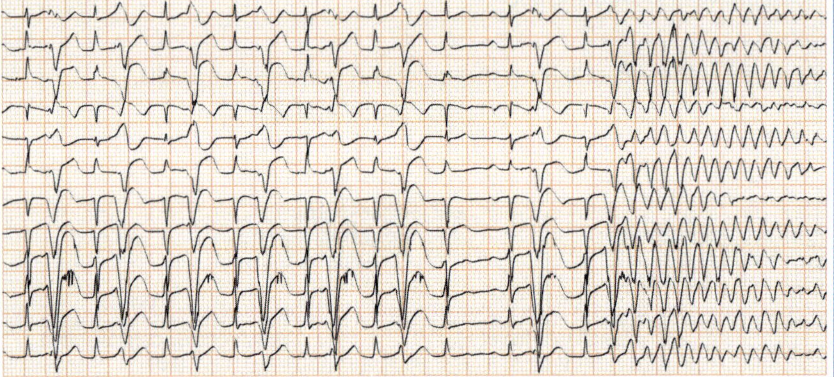

Fig. 11: Idiopathic ventricular fibrillation triggered by short-coupled premature ventricular complexes.

- In younger patients, SCD is caused by inherited cardiac conditions (long QT syndrome, Brugada syndrome, HCM arrhythmogenic right ventricular cardiomyopathy (ARVC), and dilated cardiomyopathy).
- Laboratory testing should be performed to exclude dyselectrolytemia and acidosis. Ventricular function should be assessed to evaluate for ischemia.
- Patients who survive sudden cardiac arrest have high incidence of recurrence, so an ICD implantation is indicated **(Flowchart 3)**.

Flowchart 3: Algorithm for evaluation of tachyarrhythmia.

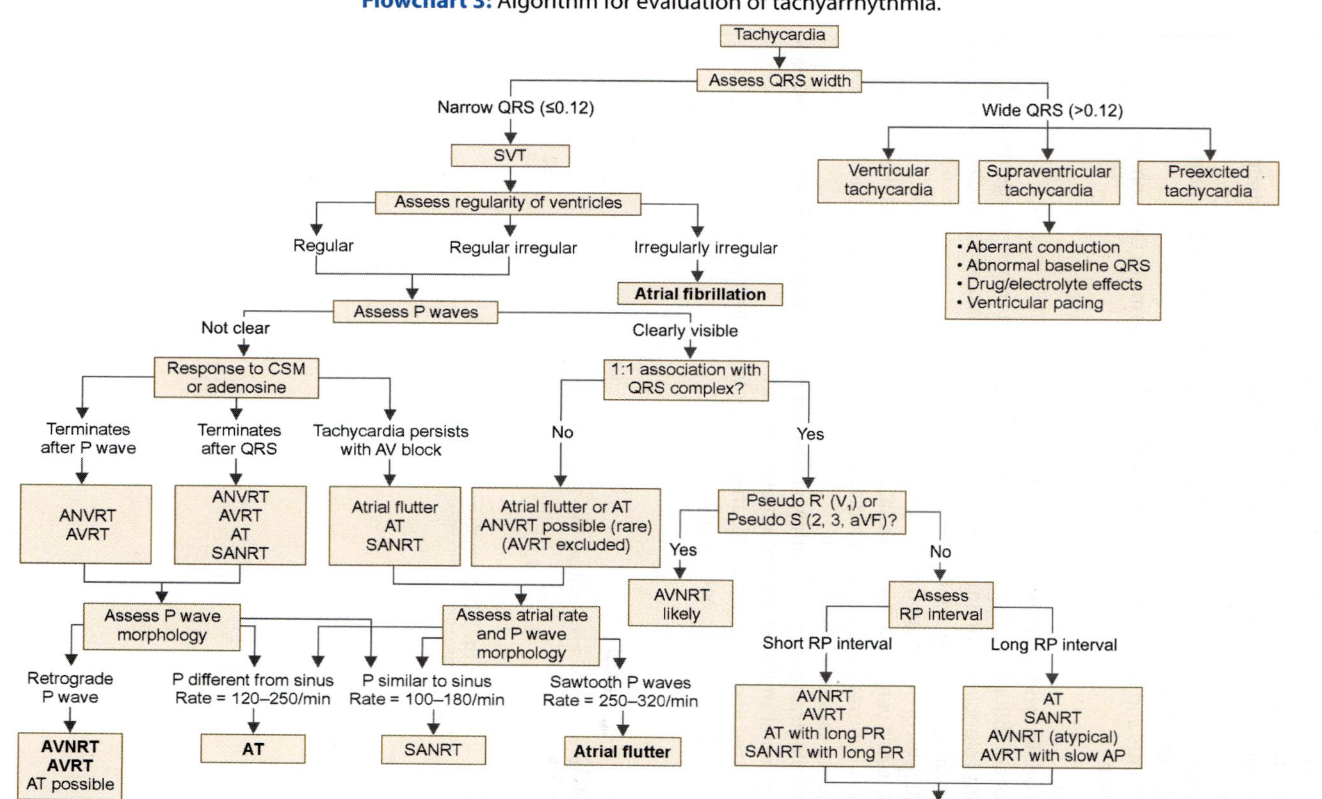

(CSM: carotid sinus massage; AVRT: AV reentry tachycardia)

Source: Brugada J, Katritsis DG, Arbelo E, Arribas F, Bax JJ, Blomström-Lundqvist C, et al. 2019 ESC Guidelines for the management of patients with supraventricular tachycardia, of the European Society of Cardiology (ESC). Eur Heart J. 2020;41(5):655-720.

BOX 16: ECG features of premature ventricular contractions (PVCs).

- Absence of P wave prior to the ectopic QRS complex
- Occasional retrograde P wave following QRS complex
- Widened QRS complex with different morphology from SA node–initiated QRS complex
- Commonly a compensatory postectopic pause following the PVC to next SA node–Initiated beat
- ST-segments and T waves that are directed opposite the major QRS complex deflection

Treatment:

- Mostly benign and might need intervention
- Look for conditions like that of ischemia or infarction, chamber enlargement, QT interval prolongation, or Brugada syndrome, hypoxia, drug effect, or electrolyte abnormalities and treat appropriately
- Patients with greater than three PVCs in a row are considered to have nonsustained ventricular tachycardia, which can be a marker for sustained tachydysrhythmias and sudden cardiac death. If this is a new dysrhythmia, initiate emergency cardiac investigation
- Pharmacological termination with IV antiarrhythmic is not generally advised, nor is long-term oral antiarrhythmic of a proven benefit
- ICDs are used in patients with PVCs that have potential to trigger malignant ventricular dysrhythmias or cardiac arrest

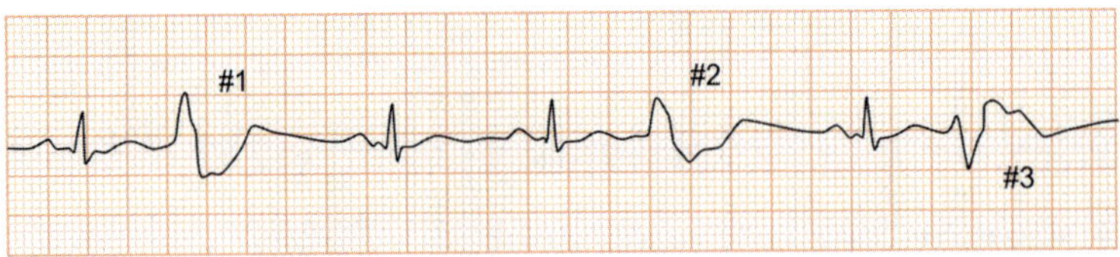

Fig. 12: Premature ventricular contraction.

BOX 17: ECG features of junctional rhythm.

- Absence of normal (sinus-mediated) P waves with normal PR interval
- Rare retrograde P wave (usually an inverted P wave and immediately adjacent to QRS complex, before or after)
- Narrow QRS complex AV dissociation might be present, with ventricular rate greater than atrial rate
- Ventricular rate:
  - Between 40 and 60 beats/min for junctional rhythm
  - Between 60 and 100 beats/min for accelerated junctional rhythm
  - >100 beats/min for junctional tachycardia

Treatment
- Isolated, infrequent junctional escape beats usually do not require specific treatment
- If sustained junctional escape rhythms are producing symptoms, the underlying cause should be treated. Atropine can be used to accelerate the SA node discharge rate and enhance AV nodal conduction
- Accelerated junctional rhythm and junctional tachycardia are managed by treating the underlying cause

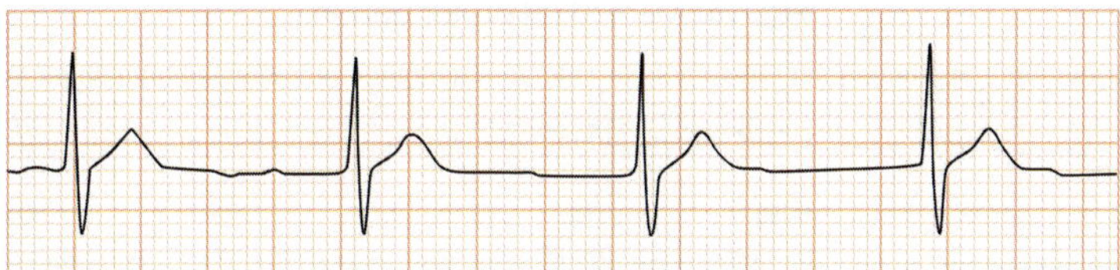

Fig. 13: Junctional rhythm.

BOX 18: ECG features of idioventricular rhythm.

- Widened QRS complex
- QRS complexes occurring regularly
- No evidence of atrial activity: no P waves
- Ventricular rate:
  - 30–50 beats/min for idioventricular rhythm
  - 50–110 beats/min for accelerated idioventricular rhythm
  - Fusion/capture beats might be noted

Treatment:
- With idioventricular rhythm producing hypoperfusion, drugs to increase the heart rate are appropriate.
- Atropine can be tried in some cases which might restore AV synchrony
- Cardiac pacing via the transcutaneous route might be superior
- In most cases of accelerated idioventricular rhythm, treatment is not necessary, suppression with antiarrhythmic agents may lead to asystole
- If sustained accelerated idioventricular rhythm produces symptoms secondary to a decrease in cardiac output, sequential AV pacing is recommended

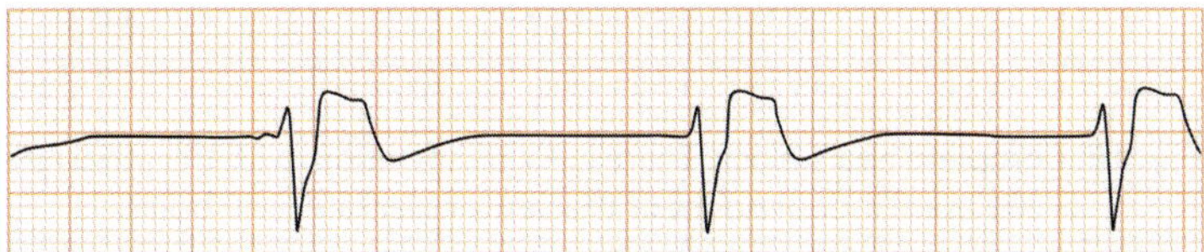

Fig. 14: Idioventricular rhythm with a ventricular rate of approximately 30 beates/min.

BOX 19: Atrioventricular block.

- AV block can be physiologic or pathologic due to various clinical conditions (ischemia, myocarditis, etc.)
- It is classified as *first degree* (PR interval greater than 200 ms with all P waves conducted), *second degree* (intermittent blocked impulses), or *third degree* (complete AV block, in which no P waves are conducted to ventricles) **(Fig. 15)**
- In second-degree *Mobitz type I (Wenckebach)*, the PR interval progressively lengthens before the blocked beat **(Fig. 16)**

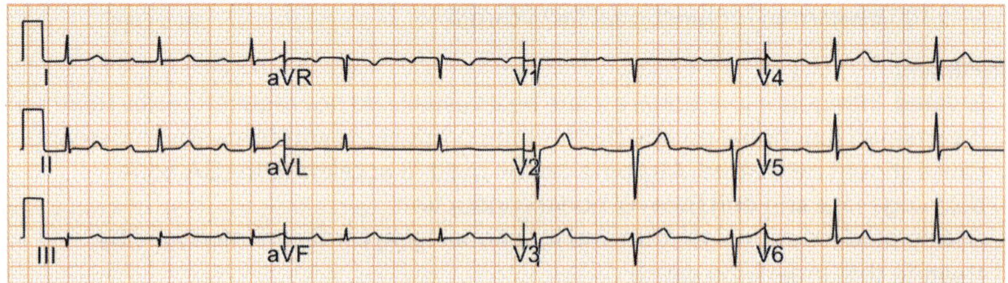

Fig. 15: Marked PR prolongation.

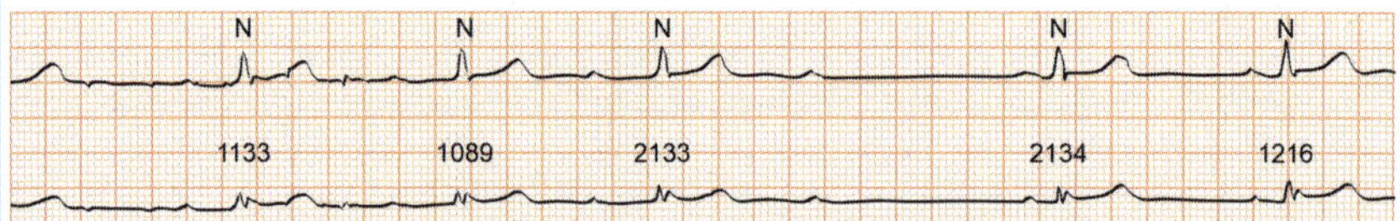

Fig. 16: Second-degree type 1 AV block (Mobitz I).

- In second-degree *Mobitz type II*, there are intermittently nonconducted P waves that are not preceded by AV conduction lengthening **(Fig. 17)**
- Symptomatic patients with any degree of heart block should be treated with atropine (0.5 mg given intravenously) or temporary pacing
- Indications for permanent pacing are symptomatic bradyarrhythmias with any degree of AV block **(Fig. 18)**

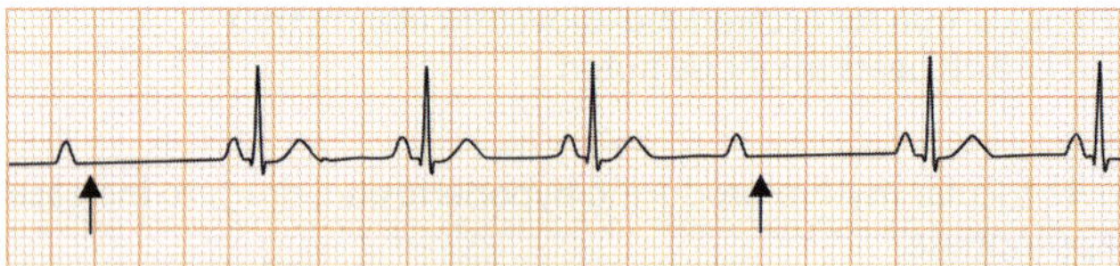

Fig. 17: Second-degree type 2 AV block (Mobitz II) with sinus rhythm and intermittent nonconducted P waves.

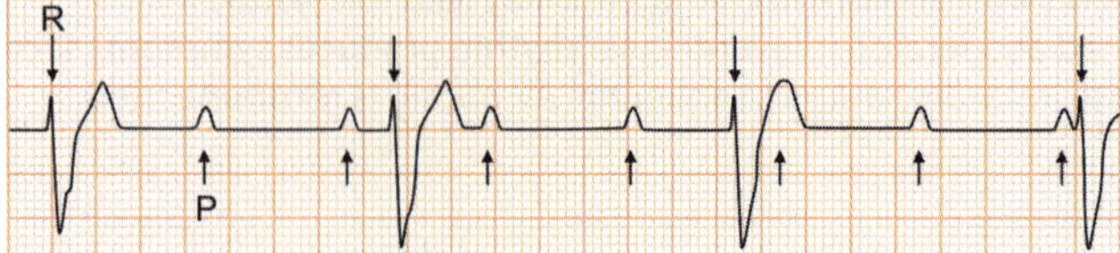

Fig. 18: Complete heart block: There is AV dissociation, with the atrial rate (~100 bpm) independent of the ventricular rate (~40 bpm).

BOX 20: Drug treatment for cardiac dysrhythmias in adults.			
Drugs for bradydysrhythmias	Atropine	0.5- to 1.0-mg IV push; may repeat every 3–5 minutes until desired heart rate is achieved or to total dose of 3 mg	
	Dopamine	IV infusion at rate 2–20 µg/kg/min; titrate to desired heart rate	
	Epinephrine	IV infusion at rate 2–10 µg/min; titrate to desired heart rate	
	Glucagon	3–10 mg IV infused over 1–2 minutes, followed by an IV continuous infusion of 1–5 mg/h	If beta-blocker overdose suspected
Drugs to block AV nodal conduction	Adenosine	6-mg rapid IV push; if after1–2 minutes the dysrhythmia persists, repeat rapid IV push with 12 mg; may repeat once more if dysrhythmia persists	Effective in terminating narrow QRS complex reentrant tachydysrhythmias involving the AV node
	Diltiazem	15–20 mg IV bolus over 2 minutes, followed by IV infusion at 5–10 mg/h; a repeat bolus of 20–30 mg may be given after 15 minutes if inadequate response to initial bolus	
	Verapamil	5–10 mg IV bolus over 2–3 min; if after 15 minutes the dysrhythmia persists, may repeat with dose of 10 mg	Effective in terminating narrow QRS complex, rate in AF or flutter
	Metoprolol	• 2.5–5 mg IV every 2–5 minutes; maximum total dose 15 mg • IV over 10–15 minutes	

Contd...

Contd...

Drugs to terminate tachydysrhythmias	Amiodarone	• Stable patient: 150 mg in 100 mL of D5W over 10 minutes, followed by infusion at 1 mg/min for 6 hours • If breakthrough arrhythmia occurs, may give repeat 150 mg boluses over 10 minutes • Maximum total daily dose is 2.2 g • Ventricular fibrillation or pulseless ventricular tachycardia: 300 mg • IV bolus; may repeat with additional dose of1 50 mg IV bolus	• Used in wide-complex tachydysrhythmias and new-onset AF • Preferred in setting of AMI or LV dysfunction • Contraindicated in pregnancy but can be used if benefits outweigh risk factors
	Lidocaine	• Loading dose: 50–100 mg over 2–3 minutes. May repeat in 5 min (up to 300 mg in any 1-hour period) • Maintenance: 1–4 mg/min	• (Start low in patients with liver dysfunction or CHF) • Not a first-line agent for ventricular tachycardia and ventricular fibrillation
	Magnesium sulfate	2 g IV over 2 minutes, followed by infusion of 1–2 g/h	Used in torsades de pointes with long QT interval
Conversion of new-onset AF or flutter	Ibutilide	• Weight <60 kg: 10 µg/kg IV over 10 minutes • Weight >60 kg: 1 mg IV over 10 minutes	
	Flecainide	• Weight <70 kg: 200 mg PO • Weight >70 kg: 300 mg PO • OR 2 mg/kg IV over 10 minutes	

Contd...

Contd...

	Digoxin	0.25 mg IV with repeat dosing to a maximum of 1.5 mg over 24 hours, followed by an oral maintenance regimen (0.125 to 0.25 mg once daily).	• Beneficial especially in CHF • Contraindicated mainly in patients with ventricular arrhythmias, but to avoid in patients with Wolff–Parkinson–White syndrome (increased risk of ventricular fibrillation), renal impairment, acute myocardial infarction, electrolyte imbalances, sinus node disease, and AV block

BOX 21: Vagal maneuvers.	
Carotid sinus massage	• Listen for bruit first • Do not massage an artery with a bruit • Massage only one side at a time • Massage for 20 seconds or less
Valsalva	• Patient lying flat or with head and chest elevated to 45° • Have patient hold breath and strain against closed glottis while tightening abdominal wall muscles • Hold for as long as practical, ideally >10–20 seconds • Increased vagal tone seen during release phase after breath hold
Modified Valsalva	• Patient lying on stretcher with head and chest elevated to 45° • Patient instructed to blow into 10-mL syringe with enough force to move plunger for 15 seconds • Patient then laid flat and legs passively elevated to 45° 15 seconds • Legs then lowered and patient lies flat for an additional 45 seconds • Diving reflex More effective in infants than adults

BOX 22: Peri cardioversion anticoagulation for unstable patients.

Nonvalvular AF:
- Onset >48 hours or unknown or
- Stroke or transient ischemic attack (TIA) <6 months or
- CHA2DS2-VASc scores ≥2
- Dabigatran 150 mg PO (75 mg if CrCl is 15–30 mL/min) or
- Rivaroxaban 20 milligrams PO (15 mg if CrCl is 15–50 mL/min) or
- Apixaban 5 mg PO (2.5 mg PO in patients with at least two of the following characteristics: age ≥80 years, body weight ≤60 kg, or serum creatinine ≥1.5 mg/dL)
- Mechanical prosthetic valve, rheumatic mitral stenosis, or CrCl <15 mL/min
- Enoxaparin 1 mg/kg SC

SUGGESTED READING

1. Brugada J, Katritsis DG, Arbelo E, Arribas F, Bax JJ, Blomström-Lundqvist C, et al. 2019 ESC Guidelines for the management of patients with supraventricular tachycardia, of the European Society of Cardiology (ESC). Eur Heart J. 2020;41(5):655-720.
2. Zeppenfeld K, Tfelt-Hansen J, de Riva M, Winkel BG, Behr ER, Blom NA, et al. 2022 ESC Guidelines for the management of patients with ventricular arrhythmias and the prevention of sudden cardiac death: Developed by the task force for the management of patients with ventricular arrhythmias and the prevention of sudden cardiac death. Eur Heart J. 2022;43(40):3997-4126.

3.3 HEART FAILURE

Bharat Shivdasani, Vishal Gavali

BOX 1: Introduction.

- Heart failure (HF) is a clinical syndrome characterized by structural and functional abnormalities displaying either reduced or preserved left ventricular ejection fraction (LVEF).
- Acute HF (AHF) is defined as new or worsening of symptoms and signs of HF. It is a common cause of unplanned hospital admission in patients of >65 years of age.
- *Etiology in India Trivandrum Heart Failure Registry:*

Ischemic heart disease	55%
Valvular heart disease	13%
Hypertensive	10%
Dilated cardiomyopathy	10%
Congenital heart disease	5%
Others (peripartum, infective, and infiltrative)	7%

- *Clinical stages of HF:*

Stage A	At risk for developing HF
Stage B	Structural heart disease but no symptoms of HF, e.g., left ventricular hypertrophy (LVH)
Stage C	Symptoms and signs of HF
Stage D	Advanced HF

- *Types of HF/Various terminology in heart failure:*
  - Acute versus chronic (pulmonary edema)
  - Systolic versus diastolic
  - Right versus left
  - High output versus low output
  - HFpEF: Heart failure with preserved ejection fraction
  - HFmrEF: Heart failure with mildly reduced ejection fraction
  - HFrEF: Heart failure with reduced ejection fraction

BOX 2: Clinical findings.

Clinical findings:

- Excessive salt or fluid intake, arrhythmias, and infection often cause exacerbation of the HF.

Signs and symptoms of HF	
Most common symptoms	***More specific signs***
1. Dyspnea	1. Tachycardia
2. Orthopnea	2. Elevated jugular venous pressure
3. Paroxysmal nocturnal dyspnea	3. Positive abdominojugular reflux
4. Fatigue	4. S3 (gallop rhythm)
5. Reduced exercise tolerance	5. Laterally displaced apical impulse
6. Ankle swelling, edema	

Less common symptoms	***Less specific signs***
1. Cough	1. Weight gain
2. Abdominal distension	2. Lung rales
3. Wheeze	3. Peripheral edema
4. Abdominal bloating	4. Ascites
5. Early satiety	5. Extremities that feel cool and/or appear mottled
6. Bendopnea	6. Narrow proportional pulse pressure (where the ratio of pulse pressure to systolic blood pressure is ≤0.25)
	7. Detection of murmurs indicative of valvular regurgitation or stenosis
	8. Presence of weight loss and cachexia, which are common in advanced HF

BOX 3: Investigations.

- Electrocardiogram (ECG): The ECG may reveal abnormalities such as atrial fibrillation (AF), Q waves, LVH, and a widened QRS complex—left bundle branch block (LBBB)
- Echocardiography for classification of HF:
  - Preserved EF >50%
  - Mildly reduced EF 40–49%
  - Reduced EF <40%
  - Severely reduced EF <25%
- Echocardiography offers comprehensive assessments including
  - Chamber dimensions
  - Presence of eccentric or concentric LVH
  - Regional wall motion abnormalities indicative of conditions such as coronary artery disease (CAD)
  - Takotsubo syndrome, or myocarditis
  - Right ventricular (RV) function
  - Pulmonary hypertension evaluation
  - Valvular function, and
  - Markers of diastolic function
- A chest X-ray is routinely recommended to explore potential causes of dyspnea, such as pulmonary diseases. It can also provide supportive evidence of HF, such as cardiomegaly or signs of pulmonary venous hypertension like Kerley lines
- Plasma concentrations of natriuretic peptides (NPs) serve as initial diagnostic tests in patients exhibiting symptoms suggestive of HF. Elevated levels support a diagnosis of HF, aiding in treatment, monitoring, and prognostication
- N-terminal prohormone of brain natriuretic peptide (proBNP):
  - Low cutoff point (rule out): 300 pg/mL
  - High cutoff points (high likelihood):
    - 450 pg/mL if under 50 years old
    - 900 pg/mL if between 50 and 75 years old
    - 1,800 pg/mL for >75 years old

BOX 4: Work-up for diagnosing HF.

Laboratory studies:
- BNP/NT-proBNP
- Complete blood count
- Basic metabolic panel
- Liver function tests
- Iron studies
- Thyroid function tests
- Lipid panel

Diagnostic imaging:
- ECG
- Chest X-ray
- Transthoracic echocardiography/transesophageal echocardiogram (TEE) (for vegetation, flail mitral leaflet, and dissection of aorta)
- Coronary angiography
- Consider cardiac imaging

Other:
- Right heart catheterization
- Endomyocardial biopsy

BOX 5: Emergent management of AHF **(Flowchart 1).**

Flowchart 1: Algorithm for management of AHF.

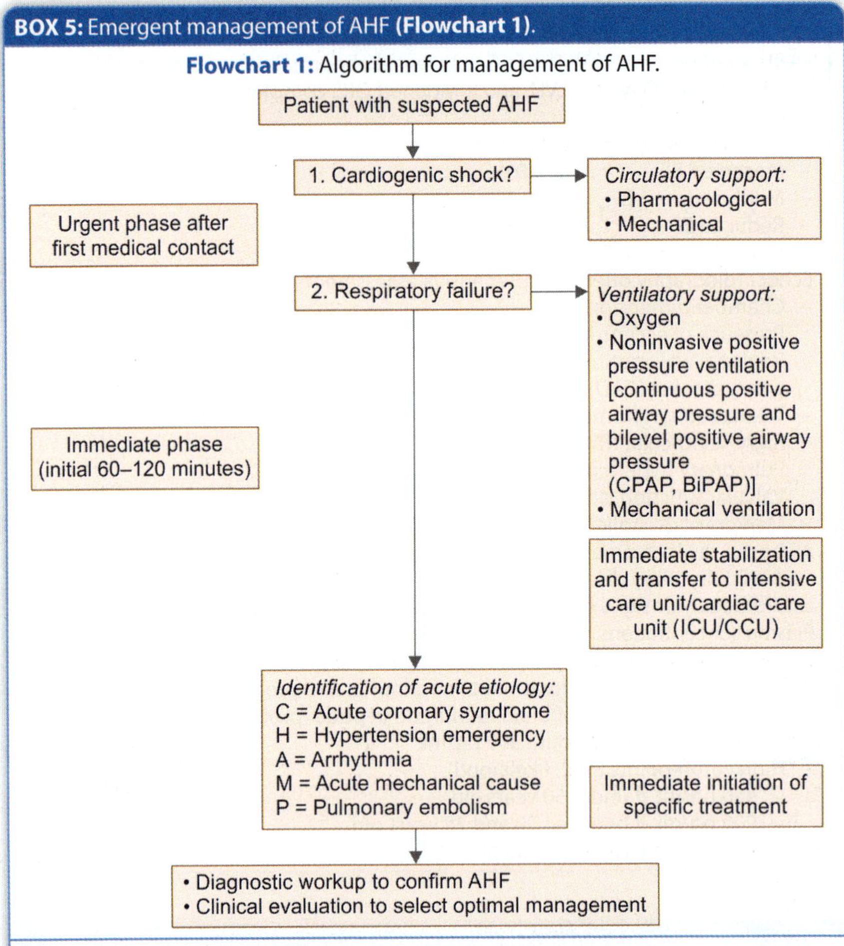

Emergent management of AHF

- Maintain oxygenation
- Supplement oxygen/ventilate to get PO_2 90%, escalating through the following as necessary:
  - Nasal cannula/face mask to begin with high-flow nasal oxygen (HFNO)—with (flow rates between 20 and 35 L/min) may be superior to standard oxygen delivered by nasal cannula and noninferior to noninvasive positive pressure ventilation in treatment of respiratory failure in patients presenting to the ER
  - High-velocity nasal insufflations are easier to use and better tolerated by many patients compared with noninvasive positive pressure ventilation
  - Noninvasive ventilation with combination of appropriate medical therapy can benefit a patient in AHF by preventing the need for endotracheal intubation
  - It also requires close monitoring, hemodynamic stability, facial anatomy allowing an adequate facemask seal, and patient cooperation

Contd...

Contd...

- Endotracheal intubation if none of the above works adequate perfusion
  - HF/hypertensive heart failure
    - Position sitting upright
    - Vasodilator agents
      - Nitroglycerin (NTG) (should be administered before diuretics in hypertensive HF for more benefits)
      - Loop diuretics (hypertension target—more details in Chapter 3.6)
  - Hypoperfusion-related HF (consider arterial catheter to monitor true blood pressure)
    - Consider careful crystalloid boluses (e.g., 250 cc NS)
    - Inotropic therapy (titrate to lowest adequate BP) (dose in **Box 7**)

Other considerations:

- *Correction of reversible causes:* These include myocardial ischemia, valvular heart diseases, hypothyroidism, infection, and high output states (anemia). Certain medication such as thiazolidinediones and nonsteroidal anti-inflammatory drugs (NSAIDs) are attributed to worsening of the HF.
  - Dialysis if severe renal failure
  - Blood transfusion if severe anemia (Hb <8 g/dL)
  - Rapid coronary revascularization if acute ST-elevation myocardial infarction (STEMI)
  - Rate/rhythm control if aberrant rhythm

BOX 6: Choice of vasoactive medications in HF.

- In patients with cardiogenic shock, vasopressors and inotropes should be initiated to mitigate hemodynamic instability and rapidly improve tissue perfusion
- Dobutamine and milrinone are common first choice agents in cardiogenic shock because of both inotropic and vasodilatory properties
- Norepinephrine is the first-line vasopressors of choice in HF and increases both systemic vascular resistance and cardiac output (CO)
- Epinephrine is associated with arrhythmia and compared to norepinephrine is less frequently used and reserved for refractory shock
- Dopamine improves renal perfusion and CO but repeated use may increase risk of death
- Vasopressin is often used in addition to norepinephrine and is particularly beneficial in RV failure due to increase in pulmonary vasodilation

BOX 7: Pharmacological therapy for HF.

- *Pharmacologic treatment:*
  - Nitrates/hydralazine:
    - Intravenous vasodilators, such as sodium nitroprusside or NTG, are particularly valuable in the context of acute, severely decompensated HF, especially when accompanied by hypertension or myocardial ischemia. However, side effects such as headache and hypotension may necessitate discontinuation. Oral hydralazine acts as an arterial dilator, enhancing symptoms, and exercise tolerance during maintenance therapy.
    - *Sublingual NTG:* 0.4 mg every 1–5 minutes
    - *IV NTG:* 0.5–0.7 µg/kg/min (starting dose if blood pressure is stable)
    - *Nitroprusside:* 0.3 µg/kg/min (initial dose), up to 10 µg/kg/min (maximum)
  - Diuretics for HF:
    - Diuretics offer symptomatic relief to patients experiencing dyspnea and systemic congestion. Common adverse effects include volume or electrolyte depletion, which can lead to hypotension and acute kidney injury.
    - Diuretic Dosage (IV) and Effects:
    - Furosemide:
      - First-time use: Administer 20–40 mg intravenous (IV), with diuretic effects starting within 15–20 minutes
      - Previous use: The total daily IV dose should be 1–2.5 times the patient's prior daily oral dose, divided in half, and given as an IV bolus every 12 hours
      - No effect observed: If there is no effect within 20–30 minutes, increase the subsequent dose
  - *Caveats*: Dosage Recommendations:
    - According to the DOSE trial, IV diuretic dosing should start at 1–2.5 times the patient's previous total daily oral dose, divided in half, and administered as an IV bolus every 12 hours. For example, a patient taking 80 mg of furosemide orally twice a day should receive an initial emergency room dose of 80–200 mg IV bolus
    - For patients who have not previously used loop diuretics, an appropriate starting dose is 40 mg of furosemide IV bolus
    - Sulfa allergies are generally not a concern with nonantibiotic drugs containing a sulfa group, such as diuretics
- *Nonpharmacologic treatment:*
  - *Implantable cardioverter defibrillators (ICDs):* It is recommended in patients with symptomatic or asymptomatic ventricular arrhythmias with LV systolic dysfunction
  - *Biventricular pacing:* Patients with wide QRS complexes LBBB morphology (>120 ms), reduced EFs (<35%) and moderate-to-severe symptoms have been shown to be responders to cardiac resynchronization therapy
  - *Coronary revascularization:* As CAD is the major cause of the HF, coronary revascularization has been thought to be able to improve symptoms, LVEF, and prevent progression
  - *Cardiac transplantation:* Transplantation can be a suitable option for patients with advanced refractory HF in expert center
  - *Device therapy:* Ventricular assist devices can be used in patients who require ventricular support either to recovery or bridge to transplantation

BOX 8: Disposition (HF ICU admission criteria).

- Patients with AHF requiring ICU support often present in cardiogenic shock, characterized by hypotension (systolic blood pressure <90 mm Hg or mean arterial blood pressure <60 mm Hg) (Chapter 29)
- Positive troponin or new Ischemic changes in ECG
- Signs of hypoperfusion such as cold extremities, low urine output, altered mental status, or elevated lactate are usually seen
- Many patients present with a "cold and wet" hemodynamic profile, although some with decompensated chronic HF may present without signs of overt congestion
- Creatinine >3.0 mg/dL, blood urea nitrogen (BUN) >40 mg/dL, and Sodium <135 mEq/L are some of the metabolic indicators
- New onset of AHF
- Significant comorbidities requiring acute interventions

SUGGESTED READING

1. Arrigo M, Jessup M, Mullens W, Reza N, Shah AM, Sliwa K, et al. Acute heart failure. Nat Rev Dis Primers. 2020;6(1):16.
2. McDonagh TA, Metra M, Adamo M, Gardner RS, Baumbach A, Böhm M, et al; ESC Scientific Document Group. 2021 ESC Guidelines for the diagnosis and treatment of acute and chronic heart failure. Eur Heart J. 2021;42(36):3599-726.
3. Murphy SP, Ibrahim NE, Januzzi JL Jr. Heart failure with reduced ejection fraction: A review. JAMA. 2020;324(5):488504.

3.4 CARDIOGENIC SHOCK

Ashwin B Mehta, Nikesh Jain

BOX 1: Introduction and definition of cardiogenic shock (CS).

Cardiogenic shock is a clinical state of impaired end-organ perfusion, due to reduced cardiac output.

BOX 2: Criteria for cardiogenic shock diagnosis.

Criteria for CS diagnosis are as follows:

- Systolic blood pressure (SBP) <90 mm Hg for over 30 minutes or the need for vasopressors to maintain SBP at or above 90 mm Hg
- Evidence of pulmonary congestion or increased left ventricular filling pressures [e.g., pulmonary capillary wedge pressure (PCWP) >18 mm Hg]
- Indications of impaired organ perfusion, with at least one of the following signs:
  - Altered mental status
  - Cold, clammy skin, and extremities
  - Oliguria with urine output <30 mL/h
  - Serum lactate levels higher than 2.0 mmol/L
- A reduced cardiac index (CI) (<1.8 L/min/m^2 without support and 2.0–2.2 L/min/m^2 with support)

BOX 3: Severity of cardiogenic shock can vary and can guide initial treatment modality.

	Pre/early shock	***Shock***	***Severe shock***
Severity of CS can be categorized as below:			
Clinical	• SBP <100 mm Hg • HR 70–100 bpm • Normal lactate • Normal mentation • Cool extremities	• SBP <90 mm Hg • HR >100 bpm • Lactate >2 mmol/L • Altered mentation • Cool extremities	• SBP <90 mm Hg • HR >120 bpm • Lactate >4 mmol/L • Obtunded • Cool extremities
Hemodynamics	• CI 2–2.2 • PCWP <20 • LVEDP <20	• CI 1.5–2.0 • PCWP >20 • LVEDP >20	• CI <1.5 • PCWP >30 • LVEDP >30
Vasoactive medicines	0 or 1 low dose	1 moderate to high dose	2 or more

(HR: heart rate; LVEDP: left ventricular end diastolic pressure)

BOX 4: Causes of cardiogenic shock.

The causes of CS can be categorized as follows:

- *Cardiomyopathic causes:*
  - Extensive myocardial infarction (MI) (involving >40% of the left ventricle or with widespread ischemia)
  - Severe right ventricular infarction
  - Acute exacerbation of severe heart failure due to dilated or ischemic cardiomyopathy
  - Stunned myocardium resulting from prolonged ischemia (e.g., cardiac arrest, hypotension, and cardiopulmonary bypass)
  - Myocarditis
  - Stress-induced cardiomyopathy
  - Myocardial contusion
  - Acute pulmonary embolism (PE)
- *Arrhythmogenic causes:*
  - Tachyarrhythmias: Atrial tachycardias (including fibrillation and flutter), ventricular tachycardia, and ventricular fibrillation
  - Bradyarrhythmias: Complete heart block, Mobitz type II second-degree heart block
- *Mechanical causes:*
  - Severe valvular insufficiency due to papillary muscle or chordae tendineae rupture, or infective endocarditis
  - Critical valvular stenosis
  - Ventricular septal rupture or ruptured ventricular wall aneurysm
  - Aortic dissection
  - Pericardial tamponade

BOX 5: Differential diagnosis of cardiogenic shock.

- The cardiogenic shock (CS) can be usually diagnosed easily by brief cardiac history, electrocardiography (ECG) and bedside two-dimensional (2D) echocardiography
- Other types of shock such as distributive shock or hypovolemic shock can be ruled out by brief history and physical findings
- Sometimes combined types of shock can coexist requiring multidisciplinary approach

BOX 6: Risk factors.

Risk factors for CS complicating acute coronary syndrome are as follows:

• Older age • Anterior MI • History of hypertension • Diabetes mellitus • Multivessel coronary artery disease	• Prior MI • SBP <120 mm Hg • HR >90 beats/minute • Diagnosis of heart failure on admission

BOX 7: Clinical presentation.

- The presenting symptoms of CS are variable
- The most common clinical manifestations of shock, such as hypotension, altered mental status, oliguria, and cold, clammy skin, can be seen in patients with CS
- *Importance of history:* A detailed patient history is crucial for identifying the underlying cause of CS, which in turn guides management. For example, angina may indicate MI, severe epigastric, or back pain and blurred vision with unequal peripheral pulses may suggest aortic dissection

BOX 8: Physical examination findings in cardiogenic shock.

- *General appearance:* Patients may exhibit altered mental status, cyanosis, cold and clammy skin, and mottled extremities
- *Peripheral pulses:* Pulses may be faint, rapid, and occasionally irregular if an arrhythmia is present
- *Jugular venous distension:* This may be observed
- *Heart sounds:* Diminished heart sounds may be noted. S3 or S4 gallops might be present, and murmurs may indicate valvular disorders such as mitral regurgitation or aortic stenosis
- *Pulmonary examination:* Pulmonary vascular congestion can present with rales
- *Peripheral edema:* This may be seen in cases of fluid overload

BOX 9: Initial evaluation and management.

Rapid diagnosis with prompt supportive therapy plays a vital role in achieving good outcomes in patients with CS. Irrespective of etiology immediate attention to ABC—airway, breathing, and circulation should be made.

Diagnostic evaluation of CS includes the following:

- Complete blood picture, comprehensive metabolic panel, magnesium, phosphorous, coagulation profile, thyroid-stimulating hormone
- Arterial blood gas
- Lactate
- Brain Natriuretic peptide
- Cardiac enzyme test
- Chest X-ray
- Electrocardiogram
- 2D echocardiography
- Ultrasonography to guide fluid management
- Coronary angiography

BOX 10: Hemodynamic support in cardiogenic shock.

- Most important is to ensure adequate volume status of patient. If hemodynamics do not improve in spite of adequate volume status, inotropes, and advanced hemodynamic support devices should be initiated
- Arterial line, Swan–Ganz catheter should be inserted to measure PCWP and to guide choice of hemodynamic support devices
- *Use of inotropes:*
  - Norepinephrine is preferred over dopamine in patients with CS. Dopamine can be added as second line, but has been associated with higher incidence of arrhythmias. However, inotropes should be used with caution as it can cause tachycardia and increased myocardial oxygen demand in patients with recent MI
  - Dobutamine is widely used, has beta1- and beta2-agonist properties, which can improve myocardial contractility, lower left ventricular end-diastolic pressure, and increased cardiac output. It should be used in patients with low cardiac output and maintained blood pressure. It is a good addon to norepinephrine
  - Milrinone, also a widely used inotrope, has been shown to increase cardiac contractility and reduces left ventricular filling pressures. It can cause peripheral vasodilatation, hypotension, and arrhythmias
  - Vasopressin can be used as addon or to reduce dose of norepinephrine requirement. Since it is a pure vasoconstrictor, it may reduce stroke volume and cardiac output, or precipitate ischemia
- *Mechanical circulatory support (MCS) devices:* Due to the poor prognosis associated with CS, medical therapy is often inadequate, and MCS therapy to improve end-organ perfusion is often required. Threshold should be low to initiate MCS devices. Team approach is required to select and rapidly initiate MCS

Various short-term MCS in CS are as follows:

- Intra-aortic balloon pump (IABP)
- Percutaneous transvalvular left ventricular assist device (LVAD) (Impella)
- Extracorporeal membrane oxygenator (ECMO)
- Percutaneous left atrial to femoral arterial ventricular assist device (TandemHeart)
- LVAD

These devices are used depending on severity of shock as categorized earlier. Comparison of commonly available MCS devices are described in **Table 2**.

TABLE 2: Comparison of commonly available mechanical circulatory support devices.

Device	***IABP***	***Impella 2.5, CP, RP***	***Tandem heart***	***Venoarterial (VA)-ECMO***
Flow, L/min	0.51	2.55	46	46
Cannula size, Fr	78	1,223	• Inflow 21 • Outflow 1,519	• Inflow 1,823 • Outflow 1,529
Duration of support, FDA approved	9 days	414 days	21 days	6 hours (limited by oxygenator durability)
Ventricle supported	LV	LV or RV	LV or RV	LV and RV
Additional requirements	–	Surgical cutdown for Impella 5	Transseptal puncture	LV venting or IABP or Impella
Advantages	Easy to place, widely available, fewer complications especially vascular	Multiple device options	Highest cardiac output (CO) comparable to VA-ECMO. No LV distension	• Highest CO • Complete cardiopulmonary support including oxygenation and CO_2 removal
Disadvantages	Limited hemodynamic support. Contraindicated in severe aortic regurgitation (AR)	More invasive. Position of catheter should be accurate. Hemolysis, vascular complications. Contraindicated in severe AR	• Needs tertiary care setup • Atrial transseptal puncture needed • Vascular complications. Retrograde blood flow	• Needs Tertiary care setup • Increases LV afterload, LV dilatation. Vascular complications, thrombocytopenia

BOX 11: Specific therapy for cardiogenic shock.

MI	• MI is the most common cause of CS. Window period for revascularization in CS is extended up to 24 hours. Fibrinolysis is not indicated in CS, and it may have more complications if done. Patient should be shifted for emergent coronary angiography and angioplasty. Though in CULPRIT SHOCK trial only culprit vessel revascularization was preferred, if feasible complete revascularization should be the goal • Mechanical complications of MI like ventricular septal rupture, severe MR warrants urgent surgery
Aortic dissection	• After stabilizing patient, urgent CT aortogram is required to delineate extent of dissection and urgent surgery is recommended. Mortality increases with each hour of delay in surgery
Pericardial tamponade	• Urgent pericardial tapping will immediately improve hemodynamics. Specific treatment for the cause should be done based on clinical evaluation and pericardial fluid analysis
Acute massive PE	• Thrombolysis is indicated in acute massive PE complicated by CS. Catheter-directed therapy is indicated in patient with contraindicated to thrombolysis or patient having huge thrombus load

BOX 12: Conclusion.

- CS is a life-threatening disorder and is the main cause of death after an acute MI. Even in the best of hands and the latest treatment, the condition carries a mortality rate in excess of 50%. Team approach is the key
- Initial resuscitation and determining hemodynamics most important—fluids and Swan–Ganz catheter
- Low threshold for MCS
- Specific therapy depending on cause of CS
- Percutaneous coronary intervention (PCI) strategy as per clinical condition and anatomy—complete revascularization should be the goal
- Judicious use of Inotropes

SUGGESTED READING

1. Nakata J, Yamamoto T, Saku K, Ikeda Y, Unoki T, Asai K. Mechanical Circulatory Support in Cardiogenic Shock. J Intensive Care. 2023;11(1):64.
2. Tehrani BN, Truesdell AG, Psotka MA, Rosner C, Singh R, Sinha SS, et al. A standardized and comprehensive approach to the management of cardiogenic shock. JACC Heart Fail. 2020;8(11):879-91.
3. Vahdatpour C, Collins D, Goldberg S. Cardiogenic shock. J Am Heart Assoc. 2019;8(8):e011991.

3.5 PULMONARY EMBOLISM

Vishal Gavali, Ajit Desai

BOX 1: Introduction.

- Acute pulmonary embolism (PE) represents the sudden obstruction of part of the pulmonary arterial vasculature, which is usually caused by thrombus embolization from the deep veins.
- *Predisposing factors:*
  - **Patient-related factors** include advanced age, obesity, previous venous thromboembolism, active cancer (mainly solid or hematological cancers or adenocarcinoma and metastasis, acute leukemia, and myeloma), underlying coagulopathy (including factor V Leiden and prothrombin mutations), smoking, hormone replacement therapy, and oral contraceptive pills.
  - Certain medical conditions elevate the risk of developing PE. These include heart failure, stroke, respiratory failure, sepsis, and inflammatory bowel disease.
  - Various situational factors also increase the risk of PE. These include extended periods of immobility following major general or orthopedic surgeries, significant fractures, long duration air travel, pregnancy, chemotherapy, or having a central venous line in place.

BOX 2: Hemodynamic instability in pulmonary embolism.

Cardiac arrest	***Obstructive shock***	***Persistent hypotension***
Need for cardiopulmonary resuscitation	Systolic blood pressure (BP) <90 mm Hg or vasopressors required to achieve a BP ≥90 mm Hg	Systolic BP <90 mm Hg or systolic BP drop ≥40 mm Hg, lasting longer than 15 minutes

BOX 3: Signs and symptoms of pulmonary embolism.

Symptoms
- Dyspnea
- Chest pain pleuritic/focal/substernal
- Wheezing or cough
- Calf or thigh pain in some cases
- Calf or thigh swelling
- Stroke
- Syncope
- Hemoptysis

Signs
- Hypoxia
- Reduced saturation on pulse oximeter
- Tachypnea (20/min)
- Tachycardia (>100/min)
- Hypotension if cardiovascular collapse
- Decreased breath sounds
- Rales (crackles) very rarely noted
- Increased P2 heart sound
- Jugular venous distension

Caveat:
- Dyspnea, no auscultatory findings tachypnea, and tachycardia could be the most important presentation.
- Arterial blood gas (ABG) might show hypoxia with increased alveolar gradient or respiratory alkalosis.
- The most common rhythm in a cardiac arrest secondary to PE is pulseless electrical activity (PEA).

BOX 4: Diagnosis of pulmonary embolism flowchart.

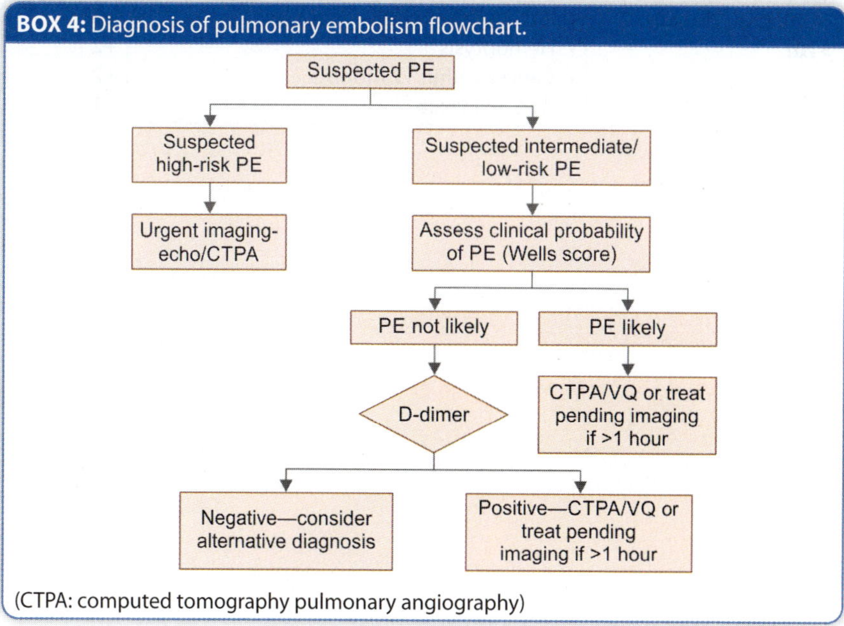

(CTPA: computed tomography pulmonary angiography)

BOX 5: Clinical prediction rules for the diagnosis of pulmonary embolism.

	Patient characteristic	*Score*
PERC system (score range 0–6 has low probability of PE) should be done after initial wells/Geneva or risk of most cases being false negative	• Unilateral leg swelling	+1
	• Heart rate >99 beats/min	+1
	• Immobilization or surgery in the previous 4 weeks	+1
	• Previous deep vein thrombosis (DVT) or PE	+1
	• Hemoptysis	+1
	• Age >49 years	+1
	• Oxygen saturation on room air <95% by pulse oximetry	+1
	• Estrogen use	+1
Wells system (Clinical probability of PE low: If score <4.5; intermediate if score 5/6; high if score >6)	• Clinically suspected DVT	+3
	• Heart rate >100 beats/min	+1.5
	• Immobilization or surgery in the previous 4 weeks	+1.5
	• Previous DVT or PE	+1.5
	• Hemoptysis	+1
	• Cancer within 6 months	+1
	• Alternative diagnosis is less likely than PE	+3
Revised Geneva system (preferred more in UK/USA as less subjective) **(clinical probability of PE low: If score <4; intermediate if score 5–10; high if score >10)**	• Unilateral lower limb pain	+3
	• Pain on lower limb palpation and unilateral edema	+4
	• Heart rate 75–94 beats/min	+3
	• Heart rate >94 beats/min	+5
	• Surgery or lower limb fracture within the previous 4 weeks	+2
	• Previous DVT or PE	+3
	• Hemoptysis	+2
	• Cancer within 12 months	+2
	• Age >65 years	+1

BOX 6: Laboratory investigations and imaging modalities in pulmonary embolism.

- D-dimer: If low or intermediate risk consider sending a quantitative D-dimer, if negative can easily rule out PE, but if positive consider associated factors and scoring method to come to a diagnosis.
  - Age-related cut off values is age × 10 nano/mL
  - *Caveat:*
    - False negative in warfarin treatment, symptoms over 5 days, small clots isolated palm, calf infarct/thrombosis
    - False positive in age >70 years, pregnancy, malignancy, liver disease, rheumatoid arthritis, infection, trauma, and recent surgical procedure (within a week)
- *CTPA*: A negative CTPA in a low-risk and intermediate-risk patient essentially rules out PE while a negative CTPA in patient with high pretest probability or high clinical suspicion may warrant additional evaluation.
- Ventilation/perfusion lung scintigraphy assesses ventilation and perfusion mismatch, which gives evidence of pulmonary artery obstruction.
- Magnetic resonance angiography (MRA) may be less effective at evaluating for distal PE.
  - *Caveat:* V/P scan as per some new articles has equal sensitivity as that of CTPA, less harm of radiation to breast but equal dose of radiation to a pregnant female, safe in kidney diseases. But the patient needs to be able to relatively stable.
- Venous US—rule out DVT.

BOX 7: Electrocardiogram in pulmonary embolism.

Electrocardiogram (ECG) findings that have been associated with PE include sinus tachycardia being the most common finding

- Tachyarrhythmias (sinus tachycardia and atrial fibrillation)
- Right bundle branch block (RBBB)
- Right-sided axis deviation
- Nonspecific ST changes
- T-wave inversions (in particular in early precordial or less commonly inferior leads)
- The S1Q3T3 seen in about 67% cases **(Figs. 1 and 2)**.

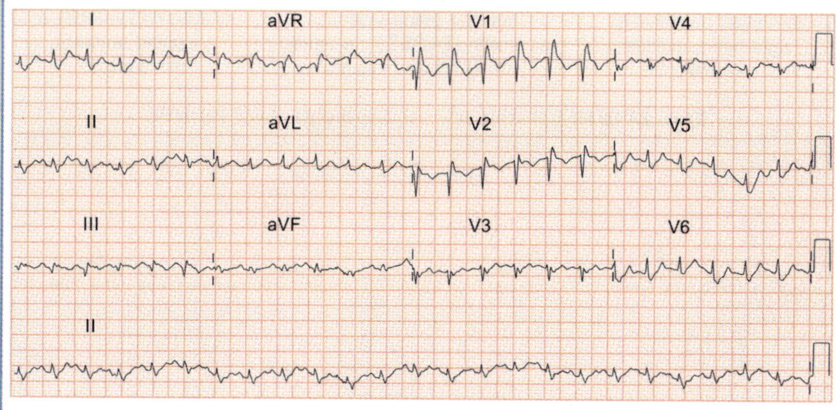

Fig. 1: ECG in PE with sinus tachycardia, RBBB and T-wave inversions in precordial leads.

Contd...

Contd...

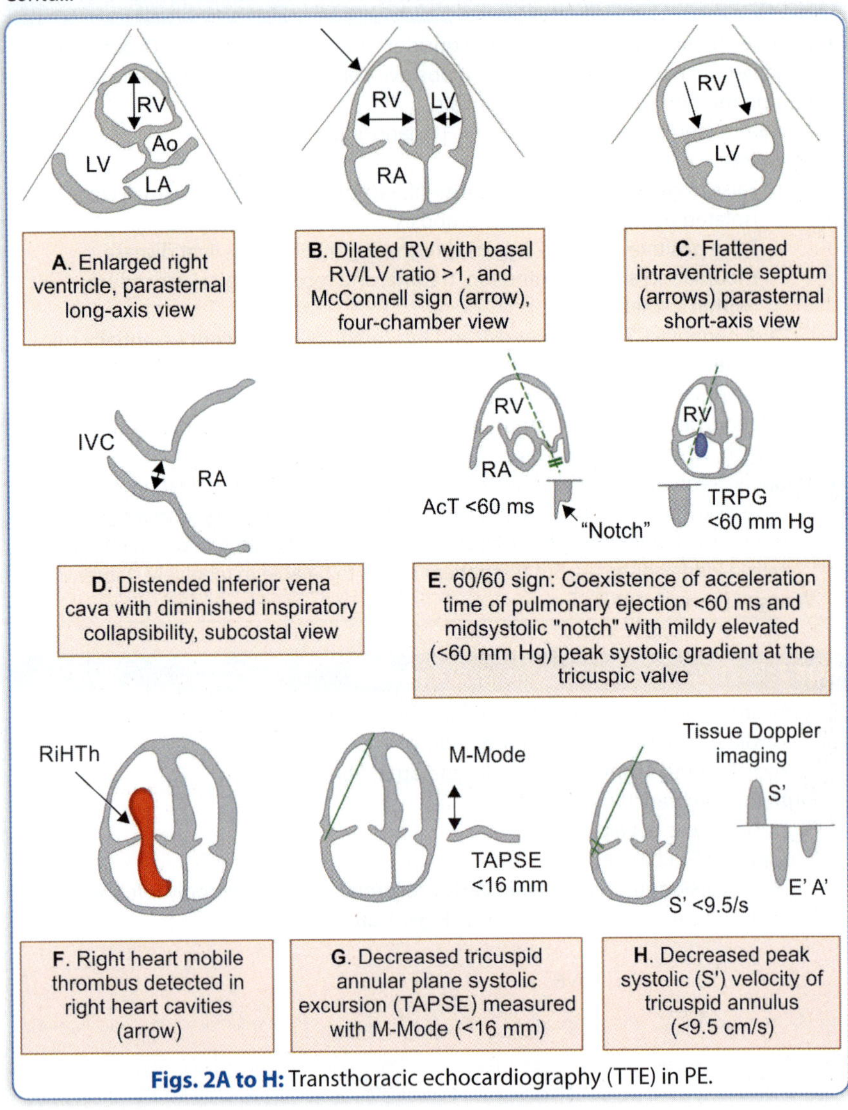

Figs. 2A to H: Transthoracic echocardiography (TTE) in PE.

BOX 8: Simplified pulmonary embolism severity index (PESI).

- Patient characteristics
- Age >80 years
- *Medical history:*
  - Cancer
  - Chronic cardiopulmonary disease
- Heart rate >109 beats/min
- Systolic BP <100 mm Hg
- Oxygen saturation by pulse oximetry on room air <90%
- *Interpretation:*
  - Each item is indicated as score 1
  - Score range: 0 (indicates low risk with a risk of 1.5% recurrent venous thromboembolism and a 1.1% risk of death at 30 days)–6 (score >0 indicates intermediate or high risk with a 10% risk of death at 30 days)

BOX 9: Classification of pulmonary embolism severity.

Indicators of risk				
Early mortality risk	**Hemodynamic** instability	**Clinically severe PE, PESI class IIIV or sPESI ≥1**	**RV dysfunction on TTE or CTPA**	**Elevated** cardiac **Troponin** levels
High	(+)	(+)	(+)	(+)
Intermediate				
Intermediate high	-	+	+	+
Intermediate low	-	+	One (none) positive	
Low	-	-	-	-

BOX 10: Treatment of pulmonary embolism.

- *Respiratory and hemodynamic support:*
  - PE leads to right ventricular (RV) obstruction, increased pulmonary vascular resistance (PVR), ventilation perfusion mismatch, and right-to-left shunting. It is crucial to address hypoxemia and maintain oxygen saturation above 90%
  - Supplemental oxygen can be provided through nasal cannula, simple face mask, or nonrebreather face mask. High-flow nasal cannula is generally favored over positive pressure ventilation methods such as continuous positive airway pressure (CPAP) or biphasic positive airway pressure (BiPAP)
  - Mechanical ventilation's positive intrathoracic pressure can reduce venous return and worsen low cardiac output (CO) caused by RV failure in patients with high-risk PE. Consequently, positive end-expiratory pressure should be used with caution.
  - Tidal volumes of about 6 mL/kg of lean body weight should be used to maintain end-inspiratory plateau pressure below 30 cmH_2O
  - Acute RV failure, leading to low systemic output, is the primary cause of death in high-risk PE patients.
  - If central venous pressure is low, a modest fluid challenge (≤500 mL) can be considered to increase the cardiac index in acute PE patients. However, volume loading may cause RV overdistension and ultimately reduce systemic CO

Management of RV failure in acute high-risk PE		
Volume optimization	**Vasopressors and inotropes**	**Mechanical circulatory support**
Volume challenge	• Norepinephrine (0.21 µg/kg/min) to raise RV inotropy and systemic BP • Dobutamine (220 µg/kg/min)	Venoarterial extracorporeal membrane oxygenation (VA-ECMO)

- *Initial anticoagulation:*
  - In patients with high or intermediate clinical probability of PE anticoagulation should be initiated as early as possible. Intravenous (IV) unfractionated heparin (UFH) is the recommended form of initial anticoagulation is recommended if systemic thrombolysis is planned
  - If IV UFH is chosen, an initial bolus of 80 U/kg or 5,000 U followed by an infusion of 18 U/kg/h or 1,300 U/h should be given, with the goal of rapidly achieving and maintaining the activated partial thromboplastin time (aPTT) at levels that correspond to therapeutic heparin levels
  - Low-molecular-weight heparin (LMWH) and fondaparinux are preferred over UFH for initial anticoagulation in PE, as they carry a lower risk of inducing major bleeding and heparin-induced thrombocytopenia LMWH is currently the preferred anticoagulant for active malignancy and pregnancy
  - A nonoral anticoagulant (NOAC) is recommended in preference to a vitamin K antagonist (VKA), however, they are not recommended with severe renal impairment
- *Reperfusion treatment:*
  - *Systemic thrombolysis:*
    - Thrombolytic therapy leads to faster improvements in pulmonary obstruction, pulmonary artery pressure (PAP), and PVR in patients with PE, compared with UFH alone

Contd...

Contd...

- It is recommended if patients with high-risk or intermediate high-risk PE progress to hemodynamic instability
- The ESC guideline recommended regimens for systemic thrombolysis include recombinant tissue type plasminogen activator (rtPA)

Thrombolytic agents, regimen, and contraindications		
Agent	***Regimen***	***Contraindication to thrombolysis***
rtPA	• 100 mg over 2 hours • 0.6 mg/kg over 15 minutes (maximum dose 50 mg)	• ***Absolute*** *contraindications:* – **History of hemorrhagic stroke or stroke of unknown origin** – **Ischemic stroke within the past 6 months** – **Central nervous system neoplasm** – **Major trauma, surgery, or head injury within the past 3 weeks** – **Bleeding diathesis** – **Active bleeding** • ***Relative*** *contraindications:* – **Transient ischemic attack within the past 6 months** – **Use of oral anticoagulants** – **Pregnancy or within the first postpartum week** – **Noncompressible puncture sites** – **Traumatic resuscitation** – **Refractory hypertension (systolic BP >180 mm Hg)** – **Advanced liver disease** – **Infective endocarditis** – **Active peptic**
Streptokinase	• 250,000 IU as a loading dose over 30 minutes, followed by 100,000 IU/h over 12–24 hours • Accelerated regimen: 1.5 million IU over 2 hours	
Tenecteplase	Tiered dose as per weight to be given single IV bolus: • <60 kg: 30 mg • ≥60–<70 kg: 35 mg • ≥70–<80 kg: 40 mg • ≥80–<90 kg: 45 mg • ≥90 kg: 50 mg	

– *Catheter-based therapies:*
  - Mechanical reperfusion involves inserting a catheter into the pulmonary arteries through the femoral route to perform mechanical fragmentation, thrombus aspiration, or a combination of both
  - A pharmacomechanical approach combines mechanical or ultrasound fragmentation of the thrombus with in situ reduced dose thrombolysis
– *Surgical embolectomy:*
  - Typically performed with cardiopulmonary bypass, this procedure avoids aortic cross clamping and cardioplegic cardiac arrest. It involves incising the two main pulmonary arteries to remove or suction fresh clots
    Recent reports have indicated favorable surgical results in high-risk PE, with or without cardiac arrest, and in selected cases of intermediate-risk PE

BOX 11: Management of intermediate-risk PE.

- Anticoagulation
- If there is no improvement in 24–48 hours of therapeutic anticoagulation then IV thrombolysis is performed
- If IV thrombolysis is contraindicated then catheter-based treatment (CBT) is offered.
- Even after IV thrombolysis or CBT, there is no improvement and patient remains critically Il, mechanical circulatory supports (VA ECMO/Impella RP) are utilized

BOX 12: Management of high-risk PE.

- It begins by categorizing patients into two groups—(1) Stable and (2) catastrophic.
- For stable patients, bleeding risk is assessed.
  - If bleeding risk is present, CBT is recommended. If there is ongoing shock after CBT, RV mechanical circulatory support (RV MCS) or VA-ECMO is suggested
  - If bleeding risk is absent, systemic thrombolysis versus CBT is considered
- In case of ongoing shock, RV MCS or VA-ECMO is advised, followed by right heart catheterization (RHC) and pulmonary angiography
- If the patient is a candidate for reperfusion, systemic thrombolysis is performed
- If there is a residual proximal clot burden, further intervention includes Impella RP versus ProtekDuo or VA-ECMO, CBT, or surgical embolectomy
- For catastrophic patients, the focus is on thrombolysis
- If the patient is an ECMO candidate, VA-ECMO is the primary treatment. If the patient is not an ECMO candidate, systemic thrombolysis is performed
- In the presence of ongoing shock, CBT or VA-ECMO is recommended, followed by anticoagulation
- If there is still ongoing shock, medical management or Impella RP versus ProtekDuo is advised

BOX 13: Definitive management.

- Systemic thrombolysis in ER is the main stay of treatment in a high risk and an intermediate risk unstable patients
- Interventional therapies are decided alongside multidisciplinary committees post the thrombolysis in such patients
- In other intermediate stable patients, the choice of treatment is anticoagulants followed by intervention as per the decision of a multidisciplinary committee

BOX 14: Disposition.

- High/intermediate high-risk patients need an intensive care unit (ICU) admission
- Intermediate-risk patients for initial few hours will require monitoring hence ICU admission
- While a low risk will suffice with a ward admission

PE in a pregnant female

- In a symptomatic patient do a venous US, if DVT present and suggestive of PE do a CT PA with a lead apron
- But if venous US is negative for DVT risk stratify with PERC rule and do the needful imaging if positive.
- If PERC is negative do a D-dimer as per the trimester cut off criteria (first trimester <750, second trimester <1,000, and third trimester <1,250)
- Can be thrombolyzed in a high risk or intermediate high risk but in presence of a multidisciplinary committee, which will involve an obstetrician

SUGGESTED READING

1. Khandait H, Harkut P, Khandait V, Bang V. Acute pulmonary embolism: Diagnosis and management. Indian Heart J. 2023;75(5):335-42.
2. Konstantinides SV, Meyer G, Becattini C, Bueno H, Geersing GJ, Harjola VP; ESC Scientific Document Group. 2019 ESC Guidelines for the diagnosis and management of acute pulmonary embolism developed in collaboration with the European Respiratory Society (ERS). Eur Heart J. 2020;41(4):543-603.

3.6 HYPERTENSIVE EMERGENCIES

Kaustubh Vaidya, Rahul Chhabria

BOX 1: Introduction.

- Severe hypertension in adults (often defined as a systolic pressure ≥180 mm Hg and/or diastolic blood pressure (BP) ≥120 mm Hg) can be associated with variety of acute, life-threatening complications, any one of which is considered as a hypertensive emergency
- If no signs of emergency, rapid drop in BP should not be the target hence oral antihypertensives instead of parenteral should be preferred

BOX 2: Causes of hypertensive emergencies.

- Noncompliance with antihypertensive medications
- Renal artery stenosis
- Adrenal disorders (such as pheochromocytoma)
- Acute glomerulonephritis
- Preeclampsia/eclampsia in pregnant women
- Drug-induced hypertension (e.g., cocaine use)
- *Neurologic disorders (e.g., intracranial hemorrhage and stroke)*
- Acute aortic dissection
- Acute hypertensive retinopathy
- Acute heart failure/coronary syndrome
- Hypertensive encephalopathy

BOX 3: Symptoms of hypertensive emergencies.

Variable

Common symptoms include:

- Severe headache
- Visual disturbances
- Chest pain
- Nausea and vomiting
- Seizures
- Altered mental status
- Focal neurologic deficits
- Signs of end-organ damage such as pulmonary edema, acute kidney injury, or hypertensive encephalopathy

BOX 4: Diagnosis of hypertensive emergencies.

Diagnosing a hypertensive emergency involves assessing BP levels and identifying signs of target organ damage.

Diagnostic tests may include:
- *BP measurement:* Persistent systolic BP (SBP) above 180 mm Hg or diastolic BP above 120 mm Hg indicates a hypertensive emergency
- *Laboratory tests:* Complete blood count, renal function tests, electrolyte levels, and urinalysis can help to evaluate organ damage
- *Imaging studies:* Brain imaging (CT or MRI) may be necessary to assess for intracranial hemorrhage or ischemic stroke
- *Electrocardiogram (ECG)*: ECG findings can reveal signs of cardiac ischemia or left ventricular hypertrophy

BOX 5: Management of hypertensive emergencies.

- Initial stabilization by managing the airway, breathing, and circulation (ABC)
- Achieve BP target according to emergencies or the target organ involved **(Box 6)** The primary goal of managing hypertensive emergencies is to lower BP gradually while avoiding complications such as cerebral hypoperfusion
- Use parenteral antihypertensive agents to reduce SBP no >25% in the first hour; if stable, then reduce to 160/100 mm Hg over the next 2–6 hours and then to normal over the following 24–48 hours

Treatment strategies may include:
- *Intravenous antihypertensive agents:* Drugs such as nitroglycerine, nitroprusside, and labetalol are commonly used to lower BP gradually.
- While using intravenous antihypertensive agents, arterial BP monitoring is ideal

Drug	***Dose range***	***Adverse effects***	***Role***
Nitroglycerine (NTG/glyceryl trinitrate)	5–100 µg/min as IV infusion	Reflex tachycardia, headache, flushing, and tachyphylaxis	Additional benefit in patients with angina, pulmonary edema
Nitroprusside	0.25–10 µg/kg per minute as IV infusion	Cyanide toxicity if excess dose. Elevated IC pressure, decreased cerebral blood flow, flushing, and sweating	Preferred in resistant cases only
Labetalol	Initial bolus of 20 mg IV followed by 20–80 mg IV bolus every 10 minutes (max 300 mg)	Nausea, vomiting, paresthesia, bronchospasm, dizziness, and heart block	Can be used in most hypertensive emergencies including with myocardial ischemia, hypertensive encephalopathy, preeclampsia, and postoperative hypertension

Contd...

Contd...

Drug	Dose range	Adverse effects	Role
Metoprolol	Initially, 1.25–5 mg IV followed by 2.5–15 mg IV every 3–6 hours	• Nausea, vomiting, paresthesia, bronchospasm, dizziness, and heart block • Avoid in acute decompensated heart failure	Myocardial ischemia, perioperative hypertension
Source: Walls RM, Hockberger RS, Gausche-Hill M. Rosen's Emergency Medicine: Concepts and Clinical Practice. Philadelphia, PA: Elsevier; 2018.			

BOX 6: Treatment and BP target according to hypertensive emergencies.

Diagnosis	Therapy goals	Agents
Intracerebral hemorrhage	If SBP >220 mm Hg, consider aggressive BP management. If SBP 150–220 mm Hg, use IV boluses of antihypertensive medications to acutely lower SBP to 140 mm Hg	Labetalol-Nicardipine-esmolol Initial IV bolus followed by infusion if needed
Acute ischemic stroke, recombinant tissue plasminogen activator (rtPA) candidate (BP ≤185/110 mm Hg)	If BP >185/110 mm Hg after three measurements: Treat before fibrinolytic therapy	Labetalol-nicardipine-nitroprusside last choice
Acute ischemic stroke, hypertension excludes reperfusion therapy	Treat if ≥220/120 mm Hg on the third of three measurements, spaced 15 minutes apart; BP should be reduced by ~15% in the first 24 hours	Same agents and doses as above acute ischemic stroke rtPA candidate
Aortic dissection	Lower SBP to 100–120 mm Hg ↓ PR ≤60 beats/min	Esmolol OR labetalol-nicardipine-nitroprusside continuous infusion
Acute hypertensive pulmonary edema	Reduce BP by 20–30%	A nitroglycerin push dose of 600-1000 mcg administered over 2-3 minutes has been practiced in Sympathetic Crashing Acute Pulmonary Edema (SCAPE) patients following a 2021 prospective study on the same
Acute myocardial infarction	Upto approx ≤25% reduction of MAP	Nitroglycerin-labetalol or metoprolol IV

Contd...

Contd...

Diagnosis	***Therapy goals***	***Agents***
Acute sympathetic crisis (cocaine, amphetamines, and MAOI toxicity)	Aim for SBP <140 mm Hg in the first hour	Benzodiazepine-nitroglycerin-phentolamine-nicardipine
Eclampsia and preeclampsia	Aim for SBP <140 mm Hg in the first hour	• Hydralazine • Labetalol • ACE/ARB inhibitors nitroprusides
Hypertensive encephalopathy	Decrease MAP 20–25% in the first hour of presentation	• Labetalol • Nicardipine
Subarachnoid hemorrhage	• Aim for SBP <160 mm Hg to prevent rebleeding	• Nicardipine • Labetalol • Esmolol

Source: Walls RM, Hockberger RS, Gausche-Hill M. Rosen's Emergency Medicine: Concepts and Clinical Practice. Philadelphia, PA: Elsevier; 2018.

BOX 7: Treatment caveats.

- Oral drugs are simultaneously started and titrated according to the need and underlying comorbidities
- Sublingual nifedipine should be avoided as it causes rapid fall in pressure which may lead to neurological complications as in most patients' cerebral autoregulation is altered
- *Close monitoring:* Continuous BP monitoring and frequent assessment of organ function are essential to gauge treatment response and detect complications
- *Targeted therapy:* Treatment should address underlying causes such as renal artery stenosis or pheochromocytoma if present
- *Neurologic support:* Patients with hypertensive encephalopathy may require sedation, mechanical ventilation, and neuroprotective measures.
- *Cardiac support:* Management of acute coronary syndromes or heart failure may be necessary in patients with cardiac complications.
- *Renal support:* Dialysis may be indicated in cases of acute kidney injury secondary to hypertensive crisis.

BOX 8: Prognosis and complications.

The prognosis of hypertensive emergencies depends on various factors, including the severity of target organ damage, the promptness of treatment, and the patient's overall health status. Delayed intervention can lead to life-threatening complications such as:

- Cerebral hemorrhage or ischemia
- Acute kidney injury requiring dialysis
- Myocardial infarction or heart failure
- Pulmonary edema
- Vision loss due to hypertensive retinopathy

BOX 9: Oral antihypertensive for urgency [noninvasive BP (NIBP) is sufficient for monitoring].

Agent	***Dosage***	***Contraindications***	***Adverse effects***
Labetalol	200–400 mg PO, repeat every 2–3 hours	Asthma, chronic obstructive pulmonary disease, bradycardia, heart block, and heart failure	Bronchoconstriction, bradycardia, and hyperkalemia
Metoprolol	50 mg PO	Relatively contraindication Asthma, chronic obstructive pulmonary disease, as cardioselective (bradycardia, heart block and heart failure)	Bronchoconstriction, bradycardia, heart block, and hyperglycemia
Losartan	50 mg PO	Second and third trimesters of pregnancy	Allergic reaction (rare)
Hydrochlorothiazide ideal first choice medication in most patients, but onset of action is delayed	25 mg PO	Renal insufficiency, pregnancy. Caution in diabetics; may raise glucose levels	Electrolyte imbalance dehydration, increased uric acid levels (may precipitate gout attacks)
Nifedipine (extended release) indicated for preeclampsia only	10 mg PO, may repeat every 30–60 minutes	Angina, acute hypertension	Myocardial infarction, cerebrovascular accident, syncope, heart block, and CHF
Amlodipine	2.5 mg starting dose, up to 10 mg can be given *Caveat:* Onset is slow up to 10 hours		Peripheral edema

(CHF: congestive heart failure; IR: immediate release)

Source: Walls RM, Hockberger RS, Gausche-Hill M. Rosen's Emergency Medicine: Concepts and Clinical Practice. Philadelphia, PA: Elsevier; 2018.

BOX 10: Management.

- For hypertensive urgency/severe hypertension, target should be gradual reduction of BP, hence parenteral antihypertensive should be avoided and oral hypertensive should be given (see in **Box 11**)
- Also newly diagnosed or incidental hypertensives should be managed as below in the ER.

BOX 11: Treatment protocol.

Recommended treatment protocol for ER patients with increased BP

SBP (mm Hg)		*DBP (mm Hg)*	*Follow-up/treatment*
130–139	or	80–89 and ASCVD risk <10%	Lifestyle modification and outpatient follow-up
130–139	or	80–89 and ASCVD risk ≥10%	Lifestyle modification; initiate antihypertensive; follow-up in <1 month
140–179	or	>90–109	Lifestyle modification; initiate antihypertensive therapy (ideally 2 agents); follow-up in <1 month
≥180	or	≥110	Evaluation for target organ damage; initiate lifestyle modification and antihypertensive therapy (ideally 2 agents); prompt outpatient follow-up (within a week)

(ASCVD: atherosclerotic cardiovascular disease; DPB: diastolic PB)

Source: Data adopted from Whelton PK, Carey RM, Aronow WS, Casey DE Jr, Collins KJ, Himmelfarb CD, et al. 2017 ACC/AHA/AAPA/ABC/ACPM/AGS/APhA/ASH/ASPC/NMA/PCNA Guideline for the Prevention, Detection, Evaluation, and Management of High Blood Pressure in Adults: Executive Summary: A Report of the American College of Cardiology/American Heart Association Task Force on Clinical Practice Guidelines. Hypertension. 2018;71(6):1269-324.

SUGGESTED READING

1. Bakris GL, Sorrentino M. Hypertension: A Companion to Braunwald's Heart Disease, 3rd edition. India: Elsevier; 2017.
2. Black HR, Elliott WJ. Hypertension: Principles and Practice. Philadelphia: Elsevier Health Sciences; 2006.
3. Camm AJ, Lüscher TF, Serruys PW. The ESC Textbook of Cardiovascular Medicine. India: Wiley-Blackwell; 2006.
4. Izzo Jr JL, Sica DA, Black HR. Hypertension Primer: The Essentials of High Blood Pressure, 4th edition. Philadelphia: Lippincott Williams and Wilkins; 2007.
5. Kaplan NM, Victor RG. Kaplan's Clinical Hypertension, 11th edition. Netherlands: LWW 50; 2015.
6. Mancia G, Grassi G, Agabiti-Rosei E. Hypertension: New Frontiers: From Past to Future, 3rd edition. Boca Raton: CRC Press; 2019.
7. Turner N, Lameire N, Goldsmith D, Winearls C, Himmelfarb J, Remuzzi G. Oxford Textbook of Clinical Nephrology, 4th edition. India: OUP Oxford; 2015.
8. Mathew R, Kumar A, Sahu A, Wali S, Aggarwal P. High-dose nitroglycerin bolus for sympathetic crashing acute pulmonary edema: a prospective observational pilot study. J Emerg Med. 2021;61(3):271-7.

3.7 ANEURYSMAL DISEASE RELATED EMERGENCIES

Suresh V Joshi, Upendra D Bhalerao

BOX 1: Introduction.

- Aortic aneurysm is pathologic dilatation of aorta that can lead to expansion in its size and rupture
- Aortic aneurysm can slowly increase in size causing compression of surrounding structures and can lead to acute aortic dissection
- Aortic dissection is life-threatening emergency, in which there is a split between the tunica intima and the tunica media of the aortic wall creating true and false lumens for blood flow
- *Risk factors,* development of aortic dissections, are hypertension, connective tissue disorders, Marfan syndrome, Turners and Ehler–Danlos syndrome, aortitis, preexisting thoracic aortic aneurysms, and bicuspid aortic valve disease with aortopathy and pregnancy

BOX 2: Classification.

Aortic dissection is classified as:
- *DeBakey classification by the site of origin:*
  - Type 1 starts in the ascending aorta and extends to the aortic arch
  - Type 2 starts in and is limited to the ascending aorta
  - Type 3 starts in the descending aorta and extends distally above or below the diaphragm
- *Stanford classification:*
  - Type A involves the ascending aorta (DeBakey types I and II)
  - Type B does not involve the ascending aorta (DeBakey type III) **(Figs. 1A and B)**

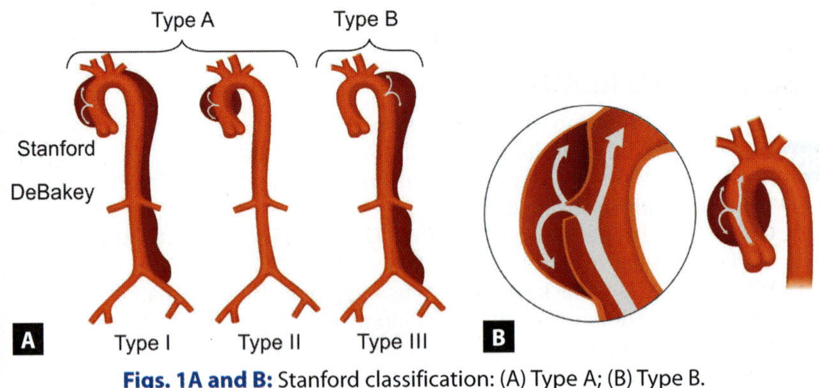

Figs. 1A and B: Stanford classification: (A) Type A; (B) Type B.

BOX 3: Clinical features.

- Acute onset and severe sharp stabbing chest pain, which can also involve neck and back pain
- Neurological symptoms due to malperfusion syncope attacks, stroke (hemiparesis/hemiplegia), and altered mental status
- Abdominal pain (with gut ischemia)
- Acute limb ischemia
- In severe cases, patient can present with features of cardiac tamponed following aortic rupture or sudden death **(Figs. 2A and B).**

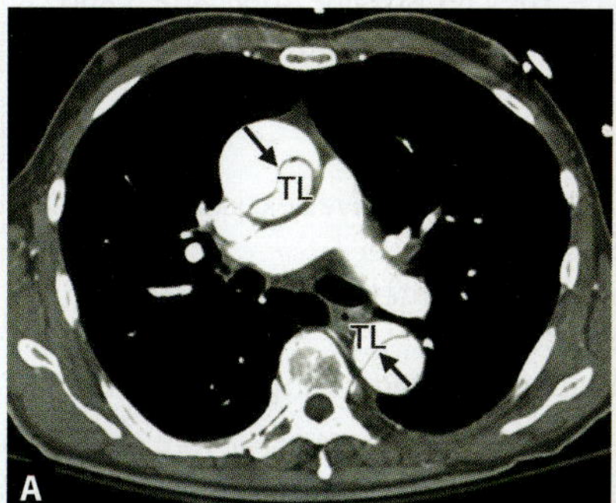

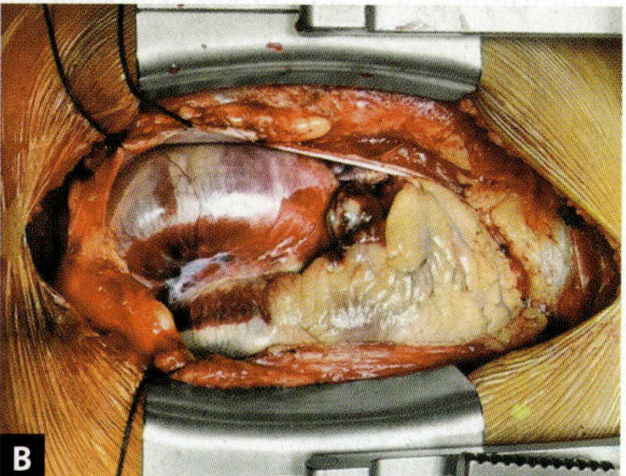

Figs. 2A and B: (A) Computed tomography (CT) scan showing dissection in the ascending aorta with true and false lumens; (B) Intraoperative photo showing dissection involving ascending aorta.

BOX 4: Signs.

- Acute aortic dissection presents with systemic hypertension. Hypotension can be present if there is pericardial collection
- Features of acute aortic regurgitation due to involvement of aortic root and valve, e.g., early diastolic murmur and wide pulse pressure
- Signs of cardiac tamponade such as pulsus paradoxus, muffled heart sounds, increase jugular venous pressure (JVP), and Kussmaul's sign
- Signs of malperfusion renal dysfunction, coronary ischemia, gut, or cerebral ischemia

BOX 5: Investigations.

- *Computed tomography (CT) with contrast:*
  - Definitive diagnostic test in cases suspicion of aortic dissection
  - It can reveal the origin, extent, and vessel involvement—coronary arteries, arch vessels, renal arteries, coeliac/superior mesenteric artery/inferior mesenteric artery (SMA/IMA), and iliac arteries
  - It identifies true and false lumens and the origin of different vessels from true/false lumens
  - It can diagnose pericardial collection and hemothorax
  - CT aortography helps in operative planning
- *Echocardiography:*
  - It can identify the dissecting flap in aorta, true lumen, and false lumen
  - Doppler evaluation can be a reliable tool to quantify the aortic regurgitation
- Transesophageal echocardiography helps in more detailed evaluation and intraoperative assistance

BOX 6: Management of acute aortic dissection.

Type A dissection involving ascending aorta needs immediate surgical intervention to prevent cardiac tamponade, correct acute aortic regurgitation, and prevent sudden death. Uncomplicated Type B dissection are treated with medical treatment antihypertensive and closely followed up with imaging.

Initial emergency room treatment:

- Lower systolic blood pressure (SBP) to 110–120 mm Hg (lowest tolerated without compromising mentation or urine output)
- Intravenous (IV) beta-blockers are first choice. They reduce SBP, shear stress and also prevent extension of tear (e.g., esmolol, labetalol, and propranolol)
- Analgesia IV opioids

Surgical treatment:

- The purpose of surgical treatment in type A dissection involves excision of intimal tear and obliterates the false lumen proximally
- This is done by replacing the ascending aorta with an interposition prosthetic graft which restores blood flow to the true lumen
- If the aortic valve is involved it can be repaired or replaced during the surgery

Commonly done procedure is replacement of aortic valve and aortic root (Bentall procedure) using the suitable valve as per patient's age (mechanical/tissue prosthesis). The ascending aorta is replaced with prosthetic graft. The replacement of aortic arch is done either partially (Hemiarch) or completely (total arch replacement and reimplantation of neck vessels) depending on pathology extent and technical expertise **(Figs. 3A to C)**.

Complicated type B dissections need emergency interventions, e.g., in presence of aortic rupture, visceral, or branch vessel ischemia. Endovascular grafts can be alternative to surgery in such cases of type B dissections with lesser short-term morbidity and mortality.

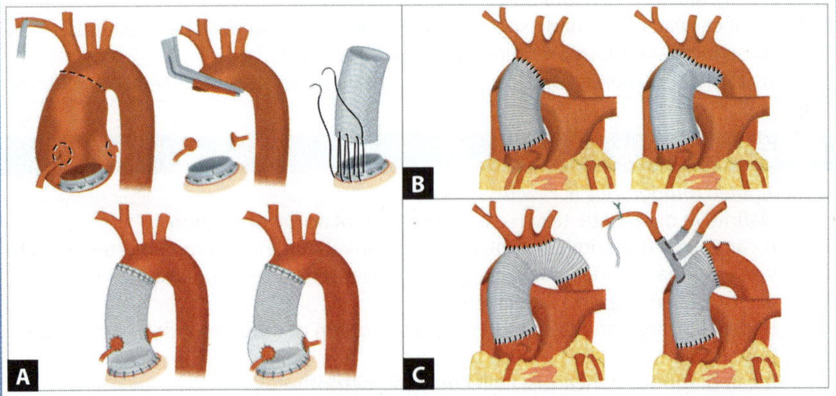

Figs. 3A to C: (A) Bentall surgery; (B) Ascending aorta and hemiarch replacement; (C) Total arch replacement.

BOX 7: Survival.

- Untreated type A acute aortic dissection has high mortality with >60% dying within 24 hours of developing symptoms
- Hence type A aortic dissection should be suspected in patients with chest pain, diagnosed early, and promptly referred for surgical treatment
- Overall in hospital mortality is 4–11% for stable patients with type A dissections and 15–18% in patients who are unstable at initial presentation
- Survival is better in high-volume aortic surgery centers with technical expertise of aortic surgical team

SUGGESTED READING

1. Baker JL, Kelly DT. Prognosis of acute aortic dissection: Impact of surgical intervention. Ann Thorac Surg. 2022;113(2):342-9. (This article examines the impact of surgical intervention on the prognosis of acute aortic dissection).
2. Evangelista A, Isselbacher EM. Aortic dissection: Diagnosis and management. J Am Coll Cardiol. 2021;78(5):527-36. (This review article discusses the clinical features, classifications, and management of aortic dissection).
3. Grassi V, Melissano G. Risk factors and management of aortic dissection. J Cardiovasc Surg. 2022;63(3):167-76. (This article discusses the risk factors and management strategies for aortic dissection).
4. Hiratzka LF, Bakris GL. Management of acute aortic dissection. Circulation. 2020;141(3):580-7.
5. Miller C, Cheng S. Role of CT and echocardiography in aortic dissection. J Cardiovasc Imaging. 2021;7(1):40-9. (This publication details the roles of CT and echocardiography in the evaluation and management of aortic dissection).
6. Nienaber CA, Clough RE. Aortic dissection: Clinical features and risk factors. N Engl J Med. 2021;385(4):337-48. (This paper outlines the clinical presentation and risk factors associated with aortic dissection).
7. Safi HJ, Miller CC. Outcomes of aortic dissection: Survival rates and prognostic factors. J Vasc Surg. 2021;73(4):1406-15. (This study analyzes survival rates and prognostic factors in patients with aortic dissection).
8. Stanford WS, Kirkland MA. Stanford classification of aortic dissection. Circulation. 2018;138(12):1237-45. (This article provides insights into the Stanford classification system and its clinical relevance).

3.8 PERIPHERAL ARTERIAL OCCLUSION

Nikesh Jain

BOX 1: Introduction.

Introduction and definition:
- Acute arterial occlusion also known as acute limb ischemia (ALI) is defined as sudden loss of limb perfusion for up to 2 weeks after the initiating event
- It can occur in any peripheral artery of upper or lower limb
- If not intervened in time, it can lead to limb infarction and loss of limb and even life.
- Lower limb is more commonly involved than upper limb

BOX 2: Etiology and risk factors.

- Conventional risk factors include age, smoking, hypertension, dyslipidemia, diabetes, obesity, sedentary lifestyle, preexisting coronary artery disease, family history of vascular disease, and chronic kidney disease
- Most common etiology is acute thrombosis of a native peripheral artery at the site of preexisting atherosclerosis. Various causes of ALI are as follows:
  - Atherosclerosis
  - Aneurysm
  - Dissection
  - Hypercoagulable states
  - Vessel injury
  - Embolism
  - Thrombosis following intervention

BOX 3: Clinical presentation.

- Clinical severity of ALI depends upon the time course of vessel occlusion; the location of the affected vessels, underlying cause; and the ability to recruit collateral channels to provide flow around the occlusion. Symptoms can develop over a period of hours to days and can range from new or worsening claudication to relatively sudden paralysis of the affected limb
- The classic presentation of acute arterial occlusion involves the "six Ps"—(1) pallor, (2) pain, (3) paresthesia, (4) paralysis, (5) pulselessness, and (6) poikilothermia. It can rapidly progress to gangrene if not intervened early and can result in loss of limb
- A careful examination of both lower extremities is necessary to detect signs of ischemia. The level of arterial obstruction is usually one joint above the line of demarcation between the normal and ischemic tissue. A handheld Doppler can be used to detect peripheral pulses. Ankle brachial index (ABI) can be measured and if <0.4 indicates severe ischemia

BOX 4: Evaluation.

- A clinical diagnosis can be quickly made based on history and examination of limb and comparing it opposite normal limb. Diagnostic evaluation and treatment strategy should be made in parallel to reduce ischemic time
- ALI can be classified clinically as below to guide our management strategy

	Viable (I)	***Marginally threatened (IIa)***	***Immediately threatened (IIb)***	***Nonviable (III)***
Pain	Mild	Moderate	Severe	Variable
Capillary refill	Intact	Delayed	Delayed	Absent
Motor deficit	None	None	Partial	Complete, paralysis (rigor)
Sensory deficit	None	None or minimal (toes)	More than toes	Complete, anesthetic
Arterial Doppler	Audible	Inaudible	Inaudible	Inaudible
Venous Doppler	Audible	Audible	Audible	Inaudible
Treatment	Urgent evaluation	Urgent revasculariza-tion	Emergent revasculariza-tion	Amputation

- Following imaging modalities are used to delineate site of obstruction. It is used depending on availability and underlying clinical urgency.
  - **Arterial Doppler:** Quick and widely available, no contrast required
  - **CT angiography:** It can exactly determine the extent of disease, but requires dye and imaging processing, and result may take some time
  - **MR angiography:** Used in CKD patients but has limited availability and time consuming
  - **Catheter-directed angiography:** In severe limb ischemia—grade II-a/II-b patient can be directly shifted to catheterization laboratory for limb angiography. Treatment can be done immediately and angiography. Brief and quick Doppler examination can guide procedure
- Routine blood tests—complete blood count, renal and liver function tests, coagulation parameters, electrocardiography (ECG), and chest X-ray (CXR) should be done at the time of presentation
- Blood creatinine kinase, lactate dehydrogenase (LDH), lactic acid, and acidosis should be done at baseline and repeated at regular intervals to monitor for myonecrosis, reperfusion injury

BOX 5: Management.

Initial stabilization:

- Antiplatelets and unfractionated heparin bolus followed by infusion should be administered immediately to prevent thrombus progression.
  - Antiplatelets—loading dose of 300 mg ecosprin and 300 mg of clopidogrel followed by 75 mg of each daily as maintenance dose
  - Unfractionated heparin—100 U/kg as bolus followed by 500–1,000 U/h. Partial thromboplastin time (PTT) should be maintained between 45 and 60.
- IV fluids should be started to maintain hydration and prevent kidney injury due to toxins of ischemia
- Pain management should be given liberally to alleviate pain and it allows imaging evaluation without discomfort
- *Specific treatment—options are as below:*
  - Surgical treatment—thrombectomy and bypass grafting. Usually preferred with extensive thrombus and when larger vessels are involved. It gives more rapid result
  - Endovascular treatment—catheter-directed thrombolysis, percutaneous thrombus aspiration followed by balloon angioplasty or stenting. It is more commonly used now. It is more suitable for grade I, II-a ischemia and occlusion at level of femoral and below
- In some cases, hybrid modality with combined endovascular and surgical treatment may be required. Endovascular treatment may be associated with more bleeding and stroke rates compared to surgical treatment as shown in few studies. In severe ischemia II-b, surgical modality may be preferred to relieve ischemia immediately. In grade III ischemia and in patients with extensive grade II-b ischemia of long duration, amputation is required, required in latter to prevent severe reperfusion injury.

BOX 6: Myonephropathic metabolic syndrome (MNMS).

- It is also called ischemia-reperfusion injury
- It is caused of perfusion of metabolites released through muscle liquefactive necrosis such as lactates, potassium, creatinine kinase, and superoxide throughout the body
- Preceded by prolonged ischemia, revascularization causes these metabolites to cause kidney injury, myoglobinuria, pulmonary edema, hyperkalemia, arrhythmias, and cardiac arrest
- It is life threatening with adequate hydration, forced alkaline diuresis, and dialysis (CRRT—continuous renal replacement therapy) being used with varying success

BOX 7: Compartment syndrome.

- It is another form of reperfusion injury, caused by increased capillary permeability following revascularization
- High suspicion should be made once there is appearance of pain, swelling, and discoloration of limb following revascularization
- Urgent fasciotomy is indicated to relieve pressure in muscle compartments

BOX 8: Summary.

- Acute limb ischemia should be diagnosed at earliest clinical presentation
- Delay in diagnosis and management can lead to limb or even loss of life
- Revascularization following prolonged ischemia can cause MNMS or compartment syndrome, necessitating early treatment as soon as diagnosis is made
- Management is usually a team approach between intensivists, interventional radiologist, imaging, and vascular surgeons

SUGGESTED READING

1. Berridge DC, Kessel DO, Robertson I. Surgery versus thrombolysis for initial management of acute limb ischaemia. Cochrane Database Syst Rev. 2013;6:CD002784.
2. Creager MA, Kaufman JA, Conte MS. Clinical practice. Acute limb ischemia. N Engl J Med. 2012;366:2198-206.
3. Fukuda I, Chiyoya M, Taniguchi S, Fukuda Wl. Acute limb ischemia: contemporary approach. Gen Thorac Cardiovasc Surg. 201563:540-8.
4. Olinic DM, Stanek A, Tătaru DA, Homorodean C, Olinic M. Acute limb ischemia: an update on diagnosis and management. J Clin Med. 2019;8(8):1215.
5. Sedghi Y, Collins TJ, White CJ. Endovascular management of acute limb ischemia. Vasc Med. 2013;18(5):307-13.

3.9 VALVULAR EMERGENCIES

Nihar Mehta, Divya A Samat

BOX 1: Introduction.

- Acute valvular emergencies account for around 8% of coronary care unit admissions
- However, their diagnosis can be challenging due to nonspecific clinical presentations and subtle examination findings
- Prompt identification and timely surgical or percutaneous intervention are crucial for a favorable prognosis
- This chapter will focus on the diagnosis and management of native left-sided valvular emergencies—regurgitation and stenosis—as these are the most common causes of hemodynamic decompensation

ACUTE VALVULAR REGURGITATION

Acute Mitral Regurgitation (MR)

BOX 2: Etiology.

- Acute MR can be caused by ischemic and nonischemic factors:
  - *Ischemic MR:* It occurs due to papillary muscle rupture or dysfunction following an acute myocardial infarction (MI) or trauma
  - *Nonischemic MR:* It arises from ruptured mitral chordae tendineae, which can be caused by mitral valve prolapse, infective endocarditis, blunt chest trauma, rheumatic heart disease, spontaneous rupture, or Takotsubo cardiomyopathy
- *Iatrogenic MR:* Occasionally, it happens during procedures such as transcatheter aortic valve implantation (TAVI) or removal of a transaortic left ventricular (LV) assist device

BOX 3: Clinical presentation.

- Acute MR often presents as a cardiac emergency with sudden-onset dyspnea and signs of cardiogenic shock due to rapid elevation in left ventricular end-diastolic pressure (LVEDP)
- It can be challenging to recognize because it mimics acute pulmonary conditions such as infection or acute respiratory distress syndrome (ARDS), and physical examination findings are often subtle
- In less dramatic cases, especially if acute MR is superimposed on chronic MR, patients might present with subacute symptoms such as increasing shortness of breath, fatigue, and weakness

Physical examination findings:

- Tachypnea
- Tachycardia
- Inspiratory crackles
- Hypoxemia
- Altered mental status
- Hypotension
- Narrow pulse pressure
- Pale, cool extremities
- Thready, rapid pulse
- Hyperdynamic apical impulse

Auscultatory findings:

- Soft, systolic, and decrescendo murmur best heard at left sternal border
- S3 commonly heard
- *Silent MR:* In moderate-to-severe acute ischemic MR, there may be no audible murmur, mostly seen in acute ischemic MR

Other clinical symptoms may be present owing to the etiology of regurgitation (e.g., fever or peripheral emboli in endocarditis, or chest pain secondary to ischemia or aortic dissection).

BOX 4: Diagnostic evaluation.

- *Transthoracic echocardiography (TTE):* First-line modality for evaluating valvular regurgitation. Color Doppler is crucial for identifying acute valvular regurgitation. Severe MR is indicated by flow reversal in the pulmonary veins. LV and left atrium (LA) sizes are often normal, and systolic function is normal or hyperdynamic
- *Transesophageal echocardiography (TEE):* Used when TTE is nondiagnostic. Essential for evaluating prosthetic mitral valves
- *Electrocardiogram (ECG):* No specific MR-related findings. However, ECG can provide clues to the etiology, such as ST-segment elevation and Q waves in ischemic MR
- *Chest X-ray:* Typically, it shows pulmonary edema with a normal cardiac silhouette

BOX 5: Treatment.

Acute MR is a medical and surgical emergency. Definitive treatment usually involves prompt surgical intervention, but medical therapy may be necessary to stabilize the patient until surgery can be performed.

Medical management:

- It focuses on *diuresis and afterload reduction*. Intravenous nitroprusside can reduce MR severity by decreasing systemic vascular resistance (SVR), which increases forward cardiac output and reduces pulmonary congestion
- *Inotropes* may be considered for patients with persistent hypotension. Norepinephrine is often used as a first-line pressor in cardiogenic shock due to its lower arrhythmia risk
- *Mechanical circulatory support (MCS)*, such as intra-aortic balloon counterpulsation (IABP), percutaneous transaortic LV assist devices (e.g., Impella and TandemHeart), venoarterial extracorporeal membrane oxygenation (VA-ECMO), or left atrial venoarterial extracorporeal membrane oxygenation (LAVA-ECMO), can be used as temporizing measures before emergency valve surgery

Interventional treatment:

- *Myocardial ischemia:* Percutaneous revascularization may resolve MR. Medical therapy and IABP may be used during the acute episode, with subsequent weaning
- *Transcatheter techniques* include transcatheter edge to edge repair (TEER) using MitraClip or Pascal Device and transcatheter mitral valve repair (TMVR), but appropriate patient selection is crucial

Surgery:

- *Chordal rupture/Papillary muscle rupture:* Early mitral valve repair is often necessary. Mitral valve repair is preferred over replacement.
- *Infective endocarditis:*
  - *Ischemic MR:* Surgical mitral valve repair or replacement with coronary artery bypass grafting (CABG) is indicated in patients with triple vessel disease and ischemic MR, although it carries a higher surgical risk

Acute Aortic Regurgitation

BOX 6: Etiology.

The two most common causes of acute AR of a native aortic valve are endocarditis and aortic dissection, others being:

- **Rupture of** sinus **of Valsalva aneurysm**
- **Traumatic rupture** of the valve leaflets (after deceleration injury or blunt trauma to the chest)
- **Iatrogenic**—complication of procedures such as aortic balloon valvotomy or TAVI

BOX 7: Clinical presentation.

Severe acute AR commonly presents with sudden cardiovascular collapse and pulmonary edema.

Other presenting symptoms are related to the cause of acute AR (refer Chapter 3.7)

Physical examination:

- Manifestations of cardiogenic shock usually dominate in patients with severe acute AR:
  - Profound hypotension
  - Pallor
  - Diaphoresis
  - Occasional cyanosis
  - Pulse is usually low amplitude and rapid
  - Pulse pressure is normal or may be reduced
  - If aortic dissection is the cause (refer the Chapter 3.7 for signs)

Auscultation findings:

- **Soft or absent S1** (due to early closure of the mitral valve)
- An **S3 is often heard**
- The murmur is a **low-pitched early diastolic murmur** beginning after S2
- A soft systolic murmur might be heard
- The combination of a soft systolic and a low-pitched diastolic murmur often produces a **"to and fro" murmur at the cardiac base** in acute AR

BOX 8: Diagnostic evaluation.

- *Electrocardiogram:* Nonspecific ST- and T-wave abnormalities are typical. If due to aortic dissection, right coronary artery involvement can show acute MI signs
- *Chest radiograph:* Cardiac silhouette size is usually normal but may show slight LV enlargement or signs of heart failure
- *Echocardiography:* Confirms AR, assesses severity, and identifies causes (e.g., aortic dilatation, dissection, and valvular vegetations). Transesophageal imaging is more precise than transthoracic. Color Doppler shows diastolic blood backflow across the aortic valve
- *CT or TEE:*
  - *Cardiac catheterization:* Rarely performed due to the urgency of the condition; coronary angiography is only considered if the patient is stable
  - *Aortography:* Used when noninvasive imaging fails to diagnose. It can confirm AR and identify dissection and aortic root widening, though it may underestimate AR severity

BOX 9: Treatment.

Emergency aortic valve replacement or repair is necessary for acute severe AR.

Initial management:
- Stabilize patients temporarily with **intravenous vasodilators (e.g., nitroprusside)** and possibly inotropic agents (e.g., dobutamine).
- Intra-aortic balloon pumps and LV assist devices are contraindicated due to worsening AR.
- **Aortic** dissection (refer Chapter 3.7)

Definitive management:
- **Endocarditis**
- **Aortic dissection** (refer Chapter 3.7)

ACUTE VALVULAR STENOSIS

BOX 10: Introduction.

Acute presentations of native mitral and aortic valve stenosis, typically chronic conditions, can occur during **acute decompensated heart failure or cardiogenic shock due to precipitating events,** resulting in acute elevations of LA and pulmonary venous pressures, and potentially a decrease in LV ejection fraction (LVEF) or cardiac output.

Causes of acute deterioration in severe valvular stenosis:
- Atrial fibrillation
- Fever/infection/sepsis
- Hypertensive urgency/emergency
- Ischemia
- Pregnancy
- Pulmonary embolism
- Emotional stress

BOX 11: Clinical presentation.

- Dyspnea
- Cardiogenic shock tachycardia, altered mental status, hypotension, cool extremities, and a narrow pulse pressure
- Hypoxemia
- Tachypnea
- Scattered inspiratory crackles
- Auscultatory findings are consistent with that of severe valvular stenosis

BOX 12: Diagnostic evaluation.

Mitral valve	***Aortic valve***
TTE	
• Rheumatic changes of the mitral valve will demonstrate the classic "hockey stick" appearance and may have associated leaflet thickening, calcification, or thickening of the subvalvular apparatus • LA enlargement	• Thickened/calcified valve leaflets • Decreased leaflet motion • Annular calcification • LA enlargement • LV hypertrophy
Color Doppler	
Turbulent flow (at the stenotic orifice)	
Multidetector CT (MDCT)	

BOX 13: Management of acute mitral stenosis.

- After initial stabilization of heart failure, the patient should be offered definitive treatment with balloon mitral valvuloplasty (BMV) or surgical mitral valve replacement based on the valve anatomy
- There is a greater role for percutaneous interventions (i.e., BMV) in patients with profound instability or metabolic disarray as long as the valve is pliable for BMV.
- For those who do not qualify for valvuloplasty, medical therapy combined with MCS may also be used as a "bridge" to eventual surgical intervention
- Transcatheter mitral valve replacement (TMVR) also represents a potential treatment option in the future
- **Contraindications to BMV:**
  - Calcific MS
  - Patients with an established LA appendage thrombus
  - More than mild MR or
  - Unfavorable valve morphology

Traditional medical therapy and MCS:

- Medical therapy for acutely decompensated valvular stenosis is limited. For patients with **pulmonary edema, diuresis** is a mainstay of therapy
- **To maximize LV filling** in patients with severe MS, heart rate should be lowered and restoring normal sinus rhythm using medications such as β-blockade (e.g., esmolol and metoprolol) amiodarone or digoxin
- As such, prioritizing the use of pressors that avoid chronotropy (e.g., vasopressin or phenylephrine) is preferred

Surgery:

As such, while surgical evaluation should be prompt, surgical replacement may not need to occur emergently.

BOX 14: Management of acute aortic stenosis.

Traditional medical therapy and MCS:

- **Afterload reduction**
- **Nitroprusside**
- Somewhat counterintuitively, **phenylephrine** has classically been recommended as the *pressor of choice* for AS with cardiogenic shock with the three primary reasons being:
  1. LV afterload is relatively "fixed" by the stenotic valve (and therefore increasing SVR will have a smaller effect on myocardial work)
  2. Higher diastolic blood pressure will translate to increased coronary perfusion pressure
  3. Reflex bradycardia will decrease overall myocardial work
- MCS can be used to support patients with severe valvular stenosis

Surgery:

Surgery is the definite management, but unstable patients can temporarily be managed with percutaneous coronary intervention (PCI)

Percutaneous intervention:

- **Balloon aortic valvuloplasty (BAV):**
  - BAV can be used in patients with severe AS but should only be considered as a *bridge* given its generally modest efficacy and suboptimal hemodynamic effects.
  - Contraindications:
    - Moderate or greater AR
    - Infectious endocarditis or
    - Patients with poor vascular access
    - For both procedures, patients can develop severe regurgitant lesions with the progression of hemodynamic instability
- **Transcatheter aortic valve replacement (TAVR):**
  - Good option for patients with cardiogenic shock and critical AS
  - While there are multiple important limitations to urgent TAVR (most notably the inability to obtain a gated MDCT for assessment of annular size and iliofemoral access) and mortality remains high, it is nonetheless feasible

BOX 15: Take away points.

- Physicians should include acute valvular regurgitation in the differential diagnosis of any patient presenting with pulmonary decompensation and consider echocardiography early in the disease course to exclude or confirm this possibility
- Even before the diagnosis of an acute valvular emergency is established, patients often will (or should) receive diuretics for the management of pulmonary edema and volume overload
- Once the diagnosis is made, the patient's hemodynamic and metabolic status, medical comorbidities, and goals of care should be considered when making a decision should be made regarding continuation of medical management alone, initiation of MCS, emergent surgery, or emergent PCI
- Notably, acute valvular regurgitation often requires emergent surgery given the highly unstable nature of the lesions and poor response to medical therapy, whereas acute valvular stenoses are more amenable to percutaneous interventions and medical temporization prior to surgery

SUGGESTED READING

1. Chiappini B, Schepens M, Tan E, Dell'Amore A, Morshuis W, Dossche K, et al. Early and late outcomes of acute type A aortic dissection: analysis of risk factors in 487 consecutive patients. Eur Heart J. 2005;26:180-6.
2. Iung B. Management of ischaemic mitral regurgitation. Heart (British Cardiac Society). 2003;89(4):459-64.
3. Mokadam NA, Stout KK, Verrier ED. Management of acute regurgitation in left-sided cardiac valves. Tex Heart Inst J. 2011;38:9.
4. Otto CM, Nishimura RA, Bonow RO, Carabello BA, Erwin JP 3rd, Gentile F, et al. 2020 ACC/AHA guideline for the management of patients with valvular heart disease: A report of the American College of Cardiology/American Heart Association Joint Committee on Clinical Practice Guidelines. Circulation. 2021;143:e72-e227.
5. Stout KK, Verrier ED. Acute valvular regurgitation. Circulation. 2009;119:3232-41.
6. Watanabe N. Acute mitral regurgitation. Heart (British Cardiac Society). 2019;105(9):671-7.

3.10 PERICARDIAL DISEASES RELATED EMERGENCIES

Rahul Chhabria, Yash Gupte

BOX 1: Types of pericarditis.

Pericarditis	*Definition and diagnosis*
Acute	*Should include two of the four criteria:* 1. Pericardial chest pain, which is usually pleuritic and postural (relieved by sitting). The pain is substernal but may radiate to the neck, shoulders, back, or epigastrium 2. Pericardial rub 3. Widespread ST-elevation or PR depression 4. Pericardial effusion (new or worsening)
	Additional suppurative findings: 1. Elevated inflammatory markers (ESR, WBC, and CRP) 2. Evidence of pericardial inflammation (CT/MRI)
Incessant	Pericarditis lasting longer than longer than 4–6 weeks but <3 months without remission
Recurrent	Recurrence after a documented first episode and a symptom free interval of 4–6 weeks or longer
Chronic	Pericarditis lasting longer than 3 months

(CRP: C-reactive protein; CT: computed tomography; ESR: erythrocyte sedimentation rate; MRI: magnetic resonance imaging; WBC: white blood cell)

BOX 2: Acute pericarditis.

- The most prevalent cause of acute pericarditis is viral infections
- Although it is uncommon in affluent nations, tuberculous pericarditis is nevertheless prevalent in some regions of the world
- Bacterial pericarditis is extremely uncommon and typically arises from the direct extension of lung infections. Nonetheless, a primary pericardial infection might be brought on by pneumococci. The Lyme disease-causing bacteria, *Borrelia burgdorferi*, can also induce myopericarditis (and sometimes heart block)
- One frequent side effect of chronic renal disease is uremic pericarditis
- In many nations, pericardial tamponade is most caused by lymphomas and Hodgkin disease
- An inflammatory response to transmural myocardial necrosis can cause pericarditis, which can manifest 2–4 days after myocardial infarction (MI) (also known as post-MI or postcardiotomy pericarditis, or Dressler syndrome)
- Radiation can cause a fibrinous and fibrotic process in the pericardium, which might manifest as constriction or subacute pericarditis. Treatments with >4,000 cGy delivered to ports encompassing >30% of the heart typically result in radiation pericarditis

Treatment:

- Experts advise limiting activities until symptoms of acute pericarditis resolve. Exercise limitation for athletes should last until all laboratory tests return to normal and symptoms have resolved, which is usually 3 months
- The 2015 ESC guidelines recommend aspirin 750–1,000 mg every 8 hours for 1–2 weeks with a taper by decreasing the dose 250–500 mg every 1–2 weeks or ibuprofen 600 mg every 8 hours for 1–2 weeks with a taper by decreasing the dose by 200–400 mg every 1–2 weeks. Gastroprotection should be included
- Research indicates that administering colchicine at the outset of an acute episode can help avoid its recurrence. For a minimum of 3 months, 0.5–0.6 mg of colchicine should be given to the nonsteroidal anti-inflammatory drug (NSAID) once day for patients under 70 kg or twice daily for patients above 70 kg
- When treating post-MI pericarditis (Dressler syndrome), aspirin and colchicine should be used in place of NSAIDs because corticosteroids and NSAIDs may impede the healing process of the heart
- The standard treatment for Dressler syndrome consists of 3 months of colchicine plus aspirin at doses of 750–1,000 mg three times a day for 1–2 weeks. About 30% of patients have recurred after receiving first treatment
- When treating recurrent pericarditis, indomethacin (25–50 mg every 8 hours) may be used instead of ibuprofen
- Patients with immune-mediated etiologies, severe symptoms, or refractory instances may benefit from the addition of systemic corticosteroids; however, this may come with an increased risk of recurrence and even lengthen the illness
- Oral prednisone dosages of 0.25–0.5 mg/kg/day are often advised, with a 4- to 6-week tapering phase

BOX 3: Cardiac Tamponade.

Cardiac tamponade is caused by a build-up of fluid in the pericardial area that is significant enough to seriously restrict blood flow into the ventricles.

The most frequent causes of tamponade include idiopathic pericarditis, pericarditis attributable to tuberculosis, neoplastic illness, or bleeding into the pericardial space following aortic dissection, heart surgery, trauma, or anticoagulant therapy.

Tamponade, often known as Beck's triad, is characterized by three main features:

1. Hypotension
2. Soft or missing heart sounds
3. Distention of the jugular vein with an early diastolic (early systolic) descent that is missing but pronounced in the x direction.

Lower cardiac output and arterial pressure are caused by restrictions on ventricular filling.

When an effusion develops slowly and the pericardium has had time to stretch and adjust to an increasing volume, the amount of fluid required to cause cardiac tamponade may be as little as 200 mL or as much as >2,000 mL.

Since there is frequently no clear explanation for pericardial illness, a high index of suspicion for cardiac tamponade is necessary.

Any patient who exhibits the following symptoms—acute, inexplicable enlargement of the cardiac silhouette, hypotension, and elevated jugular venous pressure—should be evaluated for this diagnosis.

Electrical alternans of the P, QRS, or T waves as well as decrease in the amplitude of the QRS complexes should further raise the possibility of cardiac tamponade.

BOX 4: Diagnosis.

Since cardiac tamponade might potentially be life-saving, it is imperative to establish the diagnosis as soon as possible, typically using echocardiography (ECHO).

Clinical appearance:

- Common symptoms include weakness, exhaustion, weight gain, increased belly circumference, discomfort in the abdomen, and edema
- The patient frequently presents as chronically sick, and in more severe cases, there may be anasarca, cachexia, and skeletal muscular wasting
- Both orthopnea and exertional dyspnea are prevalent, though the latter is rarely severe
- The venous pressure may not decrease after inhalation, and the neck veins may continue to swell even after receiving strong diuretic therapy (Kussmaul's sign).
- The pulse pressure is either lowered or normal. In around one-third of cases, a paradoxical pulse is detectable
- Profound congestive hepatomegaly can lead to jaundice and compromise hepatic function; ascites is frequently seen and typically more noticeable than dependent edema
- There may also be splenomegaly and pleural effusions
- In systole, the apical pulse is diminished and may retract (Broadbent's sign)

Contd...

Contd...

- **The paradoxical pulse** is a crucial indicator of cardiac tamponade, characterized by a systolic arterial pressure fall that is larger than normal (10 mm Hg) after inspiration. When severe, the arterial pulse may palpate weaken or even stop during inhalation; nonetheless, sphygmomanometric measurement of the systolic pressure during slow respiration is usually necessary
- **The electrocardiography (ECG)** typically shows diffuse flattening or inversion of the T waves together with low voltage of the QRS complexes. About one-third of patients have atrial fibrillation
- The chest radiograph reveals a heart that is either normal or somewhat enlarged. The most common cause of pericardial calcification is tuberculous pericarditis

Two-dimensional (2D) ECHO:

- The right atrium (RA) and right ventricle (RV) exhibit late diastolic inward motion, or collapse
- Early diastolic collapse of the RV
- Late diastolic collapse of the RA
- Septal bounce
- "Swinging" anteroposteriorly
- According to Doppler ultrasound, during inspiration, the tricuspid and pulmonic valve flow velocities significantly rise, whereas the aortic, mitral, and pulmonic vein flow velocities drop

Tamponade can be rapidly lethal if left untreated, hence pericardiocentesis utilizing an apical, parasternal, or most commonly, subxiphoid technique must be performed as soon as symptoms occur.

BOX 5: Pericardiocentesis.

Refer Chapter 34.4.

BOX 6: Conclusion.

- Large effusions that do not result to tamponade can be treated first with NSAIDS, colchicine, and/or corticosteroids
- Small to moderate effusions should be treated cautiously
- A low threshold should be maintained for pericardiocentesis if there is imminent tamponade or if the patient has a big effusion that is starting to cause symptoms

SUGGESTED READING

1. Adler Y, Charron P, Imazio M, Badano L, Barón-Esquivias G, Bogaert J, et al. 2015 ESC Guidelines for the diagnosis and management of pericardial diseases. Euro Heart J. 2015;36(42):2921-64.
2. Imazio M, Adler Y. Management of pericardial diseases. Euro Heart J. 2013;34(46):3753-63.
3. Imazio M, Trinchero R. Management of acute and recurrent pericarditis. Expert Rev Cardiovasc Ther. 2007;5(5):793-803.
4. Ristic AD, Imazio M, Adler Y, Anastasakis A, Badano LP, Brucato A, et al. Triage strategy for patients with pericardial effusion: a consensus statement of the European Society of Cardiology. Euro Heart J. 2014;35(1):16-27.
5. Spodick DH. (2003). Acute pericarditis: current concepts and practice. J Am Med Assoc. 2003;289(9):1150-3.
6. Spodick DH. Acute cardiac tamponade. N Engl J Med. 2003;349(7):684-90.

3.11 CARDIOMYOPATHY DISEASE-RELATED EMERGENCIES

Rahul Chhabria, Niraj Pawar

BOX 1: Introduction.

Cardiomyopathy: A primary myocardial disease, characterized by structural and functional abnormalities

Morphologically, the myocardium may be dilated, hypertrophied, or scarred.

Functionally, diastolic (restrictive) and/or systolic dysfunction (global/regional) may manifest.

Phenotypes:
- Dilated cardiomyopathy (DCM)
- Hypertrophic cardiomyopathy (HCM)
- Nondilated left ventricular cardiomyopathy (NDLVC)
- Arrhythmogenic cardiomyopathy
- Restrictive cardiomyopathy (RCM)

BOX 2: ECG in different cardiomyopathies **(Fig. 1)**.

DCM	AV block
	Low P-wave amplitude
	Low QRS amplitude
	Posterolateral infarction pattern
RCM	AV block
	Biatrial enlargement
	Atrial arrhythmias
ARVC	*TWI in V1-V3*: RV terminal conduction delay
	Atypical RBBB
	Epsilon waves in V1-V4
HCM is discussed separately	

(ARVC: arrhythmogenic right ventricular cardiomyopathy; AV: atrioventricular; ECG: electrocardiography; RBBB: right bundle branch block; TWI: T-wave inversion)

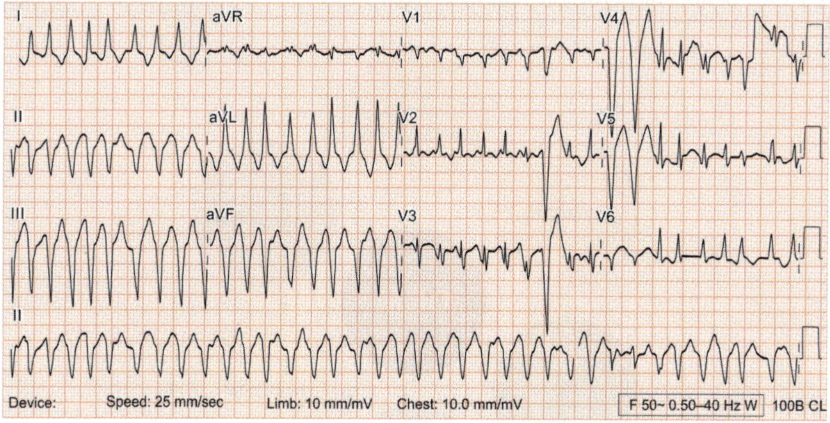

Fig. 1: 12-lead ECG of a cardiac sarcoidosis patient who presented with monomorphic ventricular tachycardia (VT).
Source: Department of Cardiology, JHRC Mumbai.

BOX 3: Dilated cardiomyopathy.

Left ventricular (LV) dilatation and systolic dysfunction [LV ejection fraction (LVEF) <50%], not explained solely by abnormal loading conditions or coronary artery disease (CAD) **(Fig. 2)**.

- Two-dimensional echocardiography (2D ECHO) in DCM—Checklist:
  - LV systolic function—global and regional
  - Diastolic function (LV filling pressures)
  - Right heart function
  - Valvular regurgitation
  - Pulmonary artery (PA) pressure
- Intracardiac thrombi, LV trabeculation (contrast ECHO)*
- Left atrial (LA) volume index, LV end-diastolic volume (LVEDV), LV end-systolic volume (LVESV)*
- Speckle tracking assessment*

Treatment principles:

- Urgent/emergent care
- Assess hemodynamic stability and congestion profile ("wet" or "dry")
- Assess peripheral perfusion ("warm" or "cold")

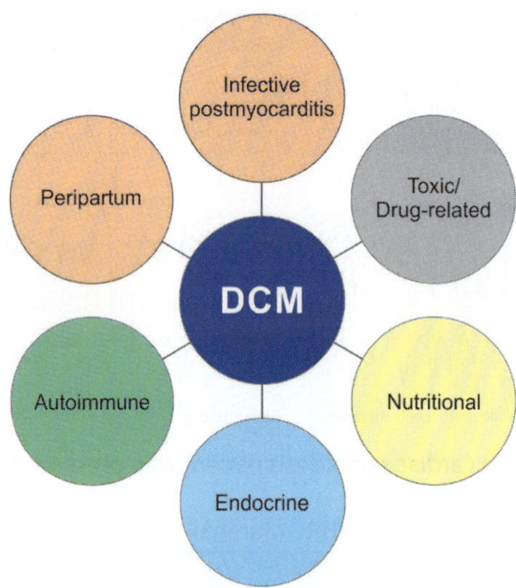

Fig. 2: Etiology of dilated cardiomyopathy (DCM).
Source: Department of Cardiology, JHRC Mumbai.

- *Treatment:*
  - *"Wet and warm:"* Blood pressure (BP) normal/↑- vasodilators, intravenous (IV) diuretics, ultrafiltration (if diuretic resistance)
  - *"Wet and cold:"*
    - Systolic BP (SBP) <90 mm Hg—inotropes, vasopressors, and mechanical circulatory support (MCS) if refractory
    - SBP >90 mm Hg—vasodilators, diuretics, and inotropes if refractory

Contd...

Contd...

- "*Dry and warm:*" Adequately perfused. Adjust guideline-directed medical therapy (GDMT)
- "*Dry and cold:*" Hypoperfused and hypovolemic. IV fluid challenge → inotropes
- Assess need for O_2 therapy (SaO_2 <90%), noninvasive ventilation (NIV) [continuous positive airway pressure/noninvasive positive pressure ventilation (CPAP/NIPPV)]

- *Specific challenges*:
  - *Atrial fibrillation (AF)*: IV beta-blocker/amiodarone, electrical cardioversion if unstable
  - *RV heart failure (HF)*: IV diuretics, inotropes, and PA vasodilators [target central venous pressure (CVP) 10–12 mm Hg]
  - Acute coronary syndrome (ACS)
  - *Cardiogenic shock*: SBP < 90 mm Hg, cardiac index (CI) <1.8 L/min/m^2, PCWP >18 mm Hg. Inotropes, vasoconstrictors, and early MCS—intra-aortic balloon pump (IABP) and extracorporeal membrane oxygenation (ECMO)

*Advanced techniques

BOX 4: Laboratory tests.

Routine	CBC, BUN, creatinine, serum electrolytes, LFT, HbA1c, fasting thyroid function, and lipid profile
Cardiac	Cardiac troponin-T (cTnT), NT-proBNP
Specific	• *Serum ACE:* Sarcoidosis • *CK-MB:* Myopathies, neuromuscular disorders • *CRP:* ARVC, NDLVC • *Serum iron, ferritin:* Hemochromatosis • *Lactic acidosis:* Mitochondrial diseases
Genetic testing	

(ACE: angiotensin-converting enzyme; BUN: blood urea nitrogen; CBC: complete blood count; CK-MB: creatine kinase-MB; HbA1c: glycated hemoglobin; LFT: liver function test; NT-proBNP: N-terminal prohormone of brain natriuretic peptide)

BOX 5: Restrictive cardiomyopathy.

Restrictive ventricular physiology, with normal/decreased systolic and diastolic volumes, presenting as HF with preserved EF (HFpEF) (LVEF ≥50%)

Etiology: Amyloidosis, sarcoidosis, hemochromatosis, Fabry disease, postradiation, metastatic, and idiopathic

Symptoms: Dyspnea (50%), orthopnea (20–30%), pedal edema (50%), fatigue, and palpitations

Signs: Advanced stages—↑ heart rate (HR), ↓ pulse volume, atrial arrhythmia ±, ↑ respiratory rate (RR), ↑ jugular venous pressure (JVP), hepatomegaly, ascites, and pedal edema. CVS: 3rd heart sound, mitral regurgitation/tricuspid regurgitation (MR/TR) murmurs

2D ECHO:
- Normal/near—normal LVEF and right ventricular EF (RVEF)
- Biatrial enlargement
- Restrictive diastolic filling
- ↑ LV wall thickness
- Tissue Doppler imaging (TDI)—↓ E', ↑ E/E' (LVEDP ↑) ↑ PASP
- Hepatic vein pulse—wave Doppler—inspiratory diastolic flow reversal
- *Sarcoidosis:* ↑ echogenicity of basal interventricular septum (IVS), inferior, anteroseptal, and RV free walls
- *Amyloidosis:* Granular/"sparkling" appearance of LV wall, IAS and valve thickening, small pericardial effusion, and thrombi

Treatment:
- *Acute HF:*
  - Loop diuretics, mineralocorticoid receptor antagonist (MRA), sodium-glucose co-transporter-2 inhibitor (SGLT2i) (dapagliflozin and empagliflozin)
  - Cautious use of ACE inhibitor/angiotensin receptor blocker (ARB)/beta-blockers may worsen hypotension
  - Avoid nondihydropyridine (DHP) calcium channel blockers (CCBs) (↓ BP, AV block)
  - Avoid excessive negative chronotropy; maintain adequate stroke volume
  - Maintain euvolemia
  - *Orthostatic hypotension:* Midodrine
  - *Advanced therapies:* MCS, referral for cardiac resynchronization therapy (CRT)
  - *Refractory HF, NYHA III-IV on maximal drug therapy:* Referral for cardiac transplantation
- *Arrhythmia:*
  - *Supraventricular:* Beta-blockers, amiodarone, digoxin (IV → PO), and sotalol
  - *Ventricular:*
    - Correct electrolytes, acidosis, ischemia, and hypoxemia
    - Antiarrhythmic drug (AAD) therapy—IV beta-blockers, amiodarone, and lidocaine
    - Electrical cardioversion
    - Overdrive pacing
  - *Refractory VT/electrical storm:* Epicardial ablation and cardiac sympathetic denervation

Contd...

Contd...

- *Atrial flutter/fibrillation—anticoagulation:* Direct oral anticoagulant (DOAC) > vitamin K antagonist (VKA), irrespective of CHA_2DS_2VASc score (cardioembolic CVA risk ↑)
- *Symptomatic persistent AF:* AV node ablation + CRT
- AV block—permanent pacemaker (PPM) implantation
- VT/resuscitated cardiac arrest; LVEF <35%, syncope—implantable cardioverter defibrillator

• *Etiology-directed therapy:*
  - *Amyloidosis:* Gene stabilizers (tafamidis), gene silencers (patisiran and inotersen)
  - *Sarcoidosis:* Immunosuppression—prednisolone, methotrexate, azathioprine, and cyclosporine
  - *Hemochromatosis:* Phlebotomy

BOX 6: Arrhythmogenic cardiomyopathy.

- Genetically determined cardiomyopathy characterized by fibrofatty replacement of the RV myocardium
- Up to 50% of patients may have LV involvement
- It presents most commonly in the second to fourth decade of life, as palpitations, syncope, HF, and sudden cardiac arrest/sudden cardiac death (SCA/SCD)
- Echo may show RV wall motion akinesia/dyskinesia, dilatation, and dysfunction **(Fig. 3)**
- Genetic assessment (PKP2, DSG2, and DSP), cardiac magnetic resonance (CMR) are central to confirming the diagnosis by the Padua international diagnostic criteria (2020)
- The cornerstone of treatment is antiarrhythmic drugs (beta-blockers, amiodarone, and flecainide)
- Electrophysiologist SCD prevention, to decide the need for invasive catheter ablation and/or implantable cardioverter-defibrillator (ICD) implantation

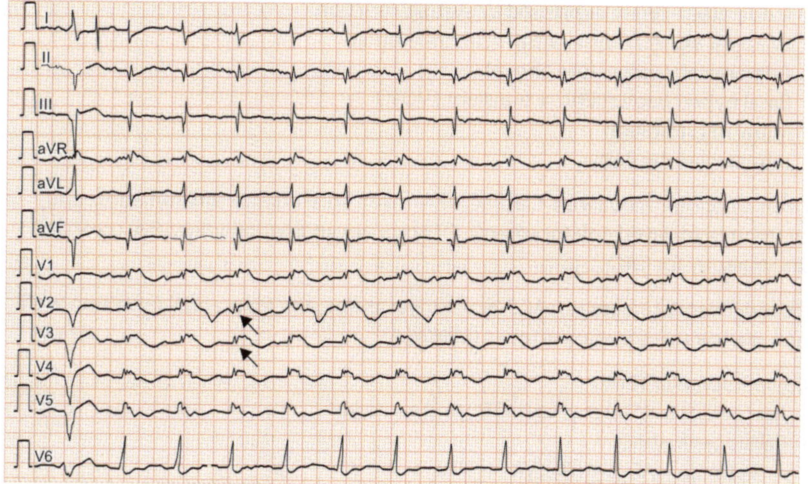

Fig. 3: 12-lead ECG of a 26-year-old male patient diagnosed with ARVC, showing prolonged PR-interval, indeterminate axis, wide QRS and epsilon waves (arrows) with TWI in V1-V4.

Source: Department of Cardiology, JHRC Mumbai.

BOX 7: Stress/takotsubo cardiomyopathy (TCM)/apical-ballooning syndrome.

Introduction:
- Acute coronary syndrome, with acute HF and normal epicardial coronaries/ nonobstructive CAD
- *Important risk factors*: Postmenopausal women, significant emotional and/or physical stress, subarachnoid hemorrhage, cannabis use, pheochromocytoma, and serotonin syndrome. However, 30% of patients do not have any identifiable triggering factors
- TCM is not benign as previously believed; the in-hospital mortality rate is 4–5%. The recurrence rate is 2–4%/year. Recovery of LV function is observed within 1–2 weeks of onset
- *Anatomical variants:* Apical (typical; 70–80%), midventricular (10–20%), basal/ inverted (5%), and biventricular (<0.5%). RV and focal varieties—very rare

Clinical features:
- Chest pain (75%)
- Dyspnea (50%) → pulmonary edema
- Syncope (5–10%)
- Palpitations—arrhythmia
- Tachycardia, tachypnea, and signs of shock and HF (S3, basal crepitations) may be detected.
- Systolic ejection murmur, if LV outflow tract obstruction (LVOTO) +

Diagnosis:
- *ECG*: 24–48 hours after symptom onset. Ischemic ST-T changes, deep and wide TWIs, and arrhythmias
- *Cardiac biomarkers*: ↑ cardiac troponin-i (>90% of cases), ↑ CK-MB, ↑ NT-proBNP (peaks at 48 hours)

2D ECHO:
- Moderate-severely depressed LV systolic function
- LV apical akinesia/dyskinesia—circumferential
- Anatomical variants (see above)
- Basal hypercontractility → transient LVOTO
- Mitral regurgitation
- Intracardiac thrombi

Other diagnostic modalities: Cardiac MR—myocardial edema, inflammation, and LV thrombi (delayed enhancement). CT coronary angiography/invasive coronary angiography for CAD

Close differential diagnoses: ACS, acute myocarditis, and myocardial infarction with non-obstructive coronary arteries (MINOCA)

Complications of TCM:
- Acute HF (12–45%) due to LVOTO and acute MR
- Cardiogenic shock
- Arrhythmia—AF (5–15%), VA (4–9%)
- LV thrombi → cardioembolic stroke
- Intramyocardial hemorrhage → rupture (very rare)

Contd...

Contd...

Management principles of TCM:

- *Pulmonary and systemic decongestion:*
  - Loop diuretics
  - *Arteriodilators:* ARB/angiotensin receptor-neprilysin inhibitor (ARNI), isosorbide dinitrate, and hydralazine
  - *Venodilators:* IV nitroglycerin and Na nitroprusside
- *Antiarrhythmics—Beta-blockers:* Metoprolol, and esmolol
- Anticoagulation, if LV thrombi—NOAC/VKA for 3 months
- *Cardiogenic shock:*
  - LVOTO + → IV fluids, vasopressin, and phenylephrine
  - LVOTO – → dobutamine, dopamine, and milrinone (+ve inotropy)
  - *Refractory cases—consider early MCS:* IABP, ECMO, and Impella

BOX 8: Hypertrophic cardiomyopathy.

Introduction: HCM may present at **any age** but it presents most commonly in the second decade of life. Pertinently, it is the most common cause of **sudden cardiac death (SCD) in young athletes**.

Clinical presentations:

- Dyspnea—diastolic dysfunction (↑ LVEDP, ↑ PCWP) → advanced stages—systolic dysfunction
- Chest pain—angina, due to subendocardial ischemia
- Fatigue
- Syncope-postexertional—Mechanisms:
  - Baroreceptor activation → reflex vasodilation
  - Dehydration → hypovolemia and ↓ preload → ↓ LV cavity size → ↑ LVOTO
  - Arrhythmogenic
- Palpitations—supraventricular arrhythmia SVA/VA, apical aneurysms
- Sudden cardiac death

One must keep in mind the possibility of valvular aortic stenosis, ischemic heart disease, and pulmonary hypertension as close differentials of HCM, especially in elder individuals.

BOX 9: ECG diagnosis of HCM.

- Classical asymmetric septal hypertrophy—**deep and narrow septal Q-waves <40 ms** in lead I, aVL, V5, and V6 ("dagger-like") **(Figs. 4 and 5)**
- *LV hypertrophy (LVH)* by voltage criteria, left atrial enlargement (LAE)
- Giant precordial **TWIs**—Yamaguchi disease (apical HCM)
- **Preexcitation** seen in 2–5%, may present with **atrioventricular nodal reentry tachycardia/AF (AVNRT/AF)**
- AF is seen in 20–25%.
- AV block

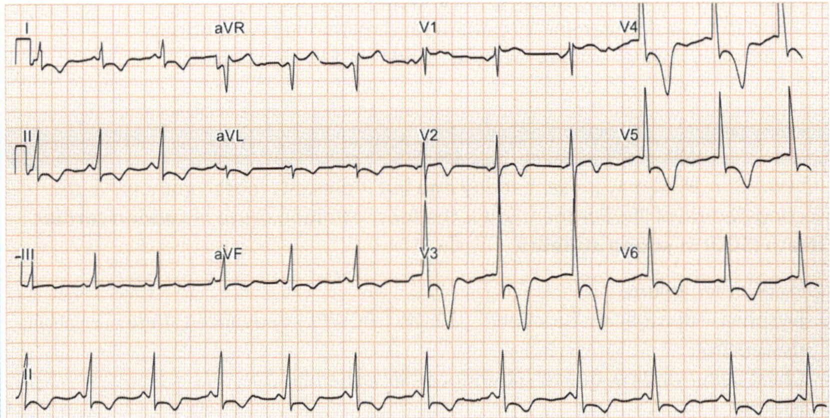

Fig. 4: 12-lead ECG of an apical HCM patient, showing deep precordial TWIs, inferolateral ST depressions and shortened PR-interval, s/o preexcitation.
Source: Department of Cardiology, JHRC Mumbai.

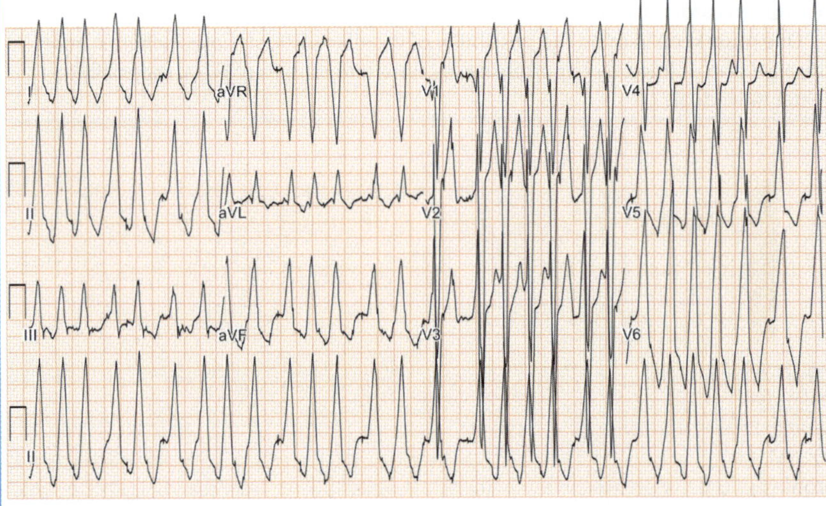

Fig. 5: 12-lead ECG, irregular wide-complex tachycardia—atrial fibrillation with HCM.

BOX 10: 2D echocardiography checklist **(Figs. 6 to 8).**

- *PLAX view:*
  - LV cavity—small, hypercontractile
  - LVOT—↑ flow velocity; resting LVOT gradient >30 mm Hg,* Valsalva maneuver
  - IVS—thickened; >30 mm at any site*
  - MR jet—posterolaterally directed, systolic anterior motion (SAM) +
- *PSAX view:*
  - Systolic function
  - LV dimensions (≥15 mm; ≥13 mm if family history +ve)
- *A4C view:*
  - *Morphology:* Asymmetric/basal/concentric/apical
  - LV systolic and diastolic function—LVEF ≤50%*
  - Continuous wave Doppler—dagger-shaped peak systolic gradient
  - LV aneurysms*, LA/LV thrombi
  - RV function [tricuspid annular plane systolic excursion (TAPSE)]
  - PA pressure

*Denotes ↑ SCD risk

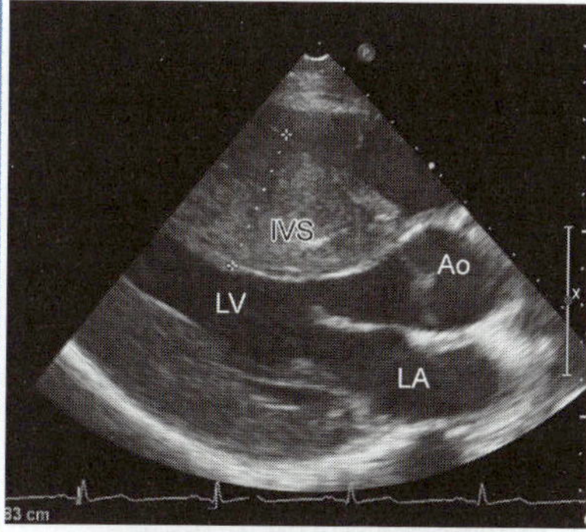

Fig. 6: PLAX view: Concentric variety of HCM.
Source: Pandian NG, Rowin EJ, Gonzalez AM, Maron MS. Echocardiographic profiles in hypertrophic cardiomyopathy: imaging beyond the septum and systolic anterior motion. Echo Res Pract. 2015;2(1):E1-7.

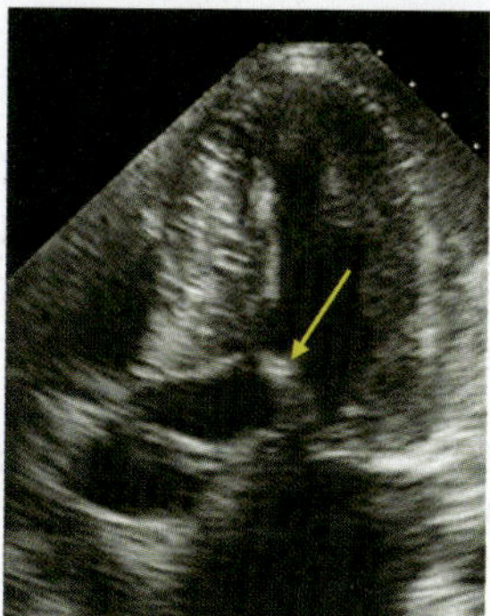

Fig. 7: A4C view: SAM of anterior mitral leaflet (yellow arrow).
Source: Pandian NG, Rowin EJ, Gonzalez AM, Maron MS. Echocardiographic profiles in hypertrophic cardiomyopathy: imaging beyond the septum and systolic anterior motion. Echo Res Pract. 2015;2(1):E1-7.

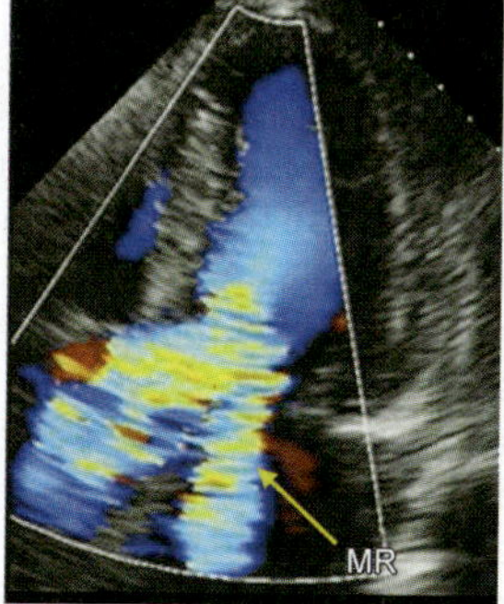

Fig. 8: A4C color Doppler: Posteriorly directed jet of MR.
Source: Pandian NG, Rowin EJ, Gonzalez AM, Maron MS. Echocardiographic profiles in hypertrophic cardiomyopathy: imaging beyond the septum and systolic anterior motion. Echo Res Pract. 2015;2(1):E1-7.

BOX 11: Treatment.

Asymptomatic obstructive/nonobstructive HCM—Close medical follow-up:

- *Heart failure:*
  - *Beta-blockers:* Carvedilol, bisoprolol, nebivolol, and metoprolol
    - **Negative inotropy**; ↑ LV diastolic time and ↓ myocardial O_2 consumption
    - Titrate dose as per **symptoms**, and not the LVOT gradient
  - *Non-DHP CCBs:* Verapamil 120–480 mg/day as add-on/substitute therapy
  - *Disopyramide (Class IA) dose:* 100–150 mg QID. ↓ basal LVOT gradient, ↑ exercise tolerance. Add-on if persistent symptoms/gradients with beta-blocker/CCB. Avoid in elderly (urinary retention, glaucoma). Monitor QTc.
  - *Loop diuretics:* If pulmonary congestion
  - *LVEF ≤50%:* B-b, ACE inhibitor/ARB/ARNI, MRA, SGLT2i, diuretics, and fluid restriction
- *Acute LVOT obstruction with hypotension:*
  - *IV fluid resuscitation:* Normovolemia
  - *IV Phenylephrine* (↑ systemic vascular resistance) + IV beta-blockers
- *AF:*
  - *Rate control strategy:* IV beta-blockers, verapamil
  - *Rhythm control strategy:* IV amiodarone, sotalol, and dofetilide
  - Anticoagulation warranted irrespective of CHA_2DS_2VASc score. NOAC > VKA
  - *Pregnancy:* LMWH/VKA; beta-blockers with fetal growth monitoring
  - *If AF + preexcitation [Wolff-Parkinson-White (WPW)]:* Avoid AV nodal blocking agents such as IV adenosine → ↑ conduction via AP → precipitates VT/VF
  - Frequent paroxysmal episodes/persistent AF → EP referral for catheter ablation
- *Sudden cardiac death prevention:* 1–3 yearly assessment of SCD risk should be performed with the ESC risk calculator:
  - *Primary prevention:* If ≥1 risk factor—refer for ICD
  - *Secondary prevention:* ICD therapy in patients with cardiac arrest/sustained VT

Avoid: **Digoxin**, nitrates, amlodipine, nifedipine, **ACE inhibitor/ARB. PDE5-i**, dobutamine, and dopamine

Advanced therapies:

- *Indications:* **Obstructive HCM** with NYHA-III/IV symptoms on maximal medical therapy; exertional syncope; LVOT gradient ≥50 mm Hg
- *Mavacamten:* Allosteric inhibitor of cardiac myosin ATPase improves myocardial energetics
- *Septal reduction therapy (SRT):* Younger patients and adults. Postprocedure PPM rate: 2–10%
- *Alcohol septal ablation (ASA):* Elderly patients with major comorbidities. Postprocedure PPM: 10%. Complications: ACS, VF, AV blocks, LAD perforation, tamponade, and VSD
- *Heart transplantation:* End-stage nonobstructive HCM

BOX 12: Myocarditis **(Figs. 9 and 10).**

- Inflammatory involvement of the myocardium, due to discrete external antigens (infections, toxins, and drugs), or internal triggers (autoimmune)
- The inciting cardiac injury triggers an immunological response in the host, leading to inflammation. If the immune response persists, cardiac remodeling leads to DCM and HF
- Classically, a bimodal incidence is seen, in infancy and adolescence (fulminant course) and >40 years (subtle, insidious clinical course). The mortality rate is 1–7%

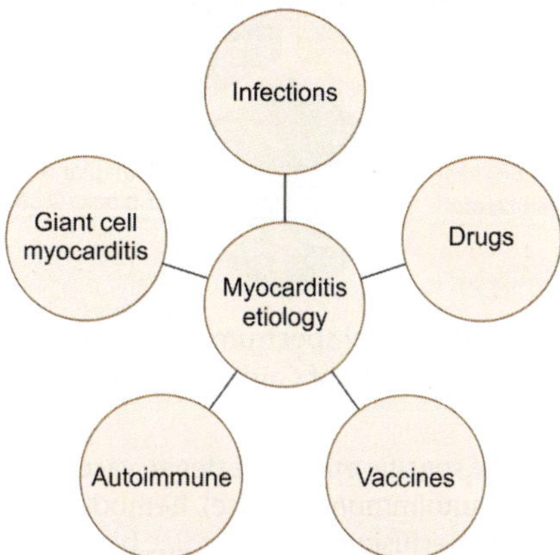

Fig. 9: Myocarditis etiology.
Source: Department of Cardiology, JHRC Mumbai.

Viral etiologies predominate, including influenza, adenovirus (2–23%), parvovirus B19 (11–56%), and enterovirus (15–30%). The SARS-CoV-2 (coronavirus) has globally prevailed since December, 2019. Bacterial causes include *Group A Streptococcus*, *Staphylococcus*, TB, Lyme disease, and diphtheria (50% mortality rate). In developing countries, Dengue fever and Chagas disease must be considered.

Autoimmune: Systemic lupus erythematosus (SLE), rheumatoid arthritis (RA), giant cell arteritis (GCA), eosinophilic myocarditis, and sarcoidosis

Rare but important vaccine-related causes include the tetanus toxoid and COVID vaccines.

Cancer chemotherapy, notably immune checkpoint inhibitors (ICI), trastuzumab (Herceptin), and anthracyclines (doxorubicin) are known to cause myocardial dysfunction.

Diagnosis of myocarditis:

- *Laboratory tests*: cTnT ↑, CK-MB ↑, NT-proBNP ↑, leukocytosis, ESR, CRP, and IL-10
- *ECG:* Sinus tachycardia; LBBB, **if myopericarditis: PR ↓, diffuse ST ↑. Ventricular arrhythmia*; QRS >120 ms*** AV block*: Giant cell myocarditis (GCM), Lyme disease
- *2D ECHO:* **LV dysfunction (LVEF < 50%)* and dilatation, segmental RWMA, and pericardial effusion**
- *Cardiac MRI:* Lake–Louise criteria (2018)—myocardial edema and nonischemic patterns of myocardial injury. Late gadolinium enhancement (LGE)
- *Endomyocardial biopsy:* Dallas criteria. If suspecting GCM, fulminant/refractory myocarditis

Contd...

Contd...

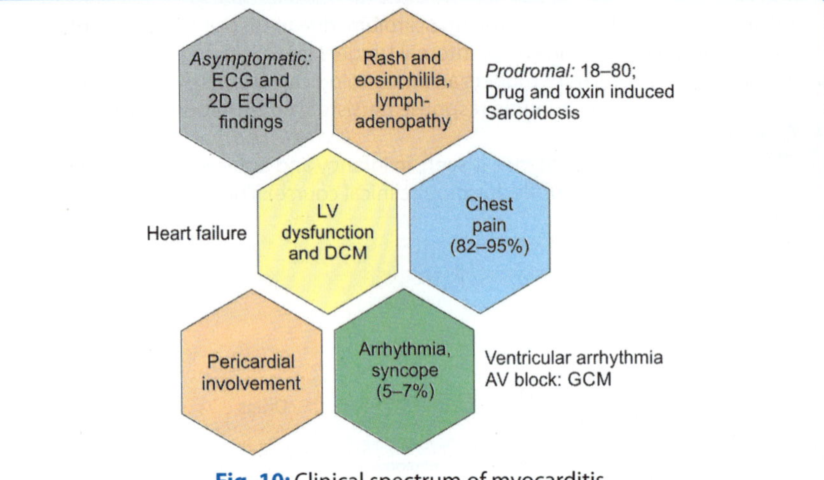

Fig. 10: Clinical spectrum of myocarditis.
Source: Department of Cardiology, JHRC Mumbai.

Treatment aspects:
Risk assessment: Presence of specific etiologies (fever, vaccines, allergies, asthma, chemotherapy, drugs, and autoimmune disease), hemodynamic stability and presence of congestion and perfusion status, cardiac biomarkers, ECG, and 2D ECHO.
- Hemodynamic support—vasopressors (noradrenaline and milrinone), MCS: IABP/VA-ECMO/Impella; consider LVAD if >2 weeks of MCS or early HT if refractory.
- *Mild-moderate cases:* ARB/ARN and beta-blockers
- *Immunosuppression*: Autoimmune, sarcoidosis—Corticosteroids, azathioprine, and mycophenolate mofetil (MMF). GCM—IV MPS, antithymocyte globulin (ATG), and cyclosporine.
- *Viral etiologies:* Interferon-β and antiviral
- *Arrhythmia:* Antiarrhythmics, beta-blockers, consider temporary external pacing and early ICD implantation.
- *Pericardial involvement:* Colchicine and NSAIDs

*↑ SCD risk.

SUGGESTED READING

1. Ammirati E, Moslehi JJ. Diagnosis and treatment of acute myocarditis: a review. JAMA. 2023;329(13):1098-113
2. Arbelo E, Protonotarios A, Gimeno JR, Arbustini E, Barriales-Villa R, Basso C, et al. 2023 ESC Guidelines for the management of cardiomyopathies: Developed by the task force on the management of cardiomyopathies of the European Society of Cardiology (ESC). Euro Heart J. 2023;44(37):3503-626.
3. Maron BJ, Desai MY, Nishimura RA, Spirito P, Rakowski H, Towbin JA, et al. Management of hypertrophic cardiomyopathy: JACC state-of-the-art review. J Am Coll Cardiol. 2022;79(4):390-414.
4. Ommen SR, Mital S, Burke MA, Day SM, Deswal A, Elliott P, et al. 2020 AHA/ACC guideline for the diagnosis and treatment of patients with hypertrophic cardiomyopathy: a report of the American College of Cardiology/American Heart Association Joint Committee on Clinical Practice Guidelines. J Am Coll Cardiol. 2020;76(25):e159-240.

3.12 SYNCOPE

Shruti M Tandan-Pardasani

One-third of individuals will experience syncope at least once.

BOX 1: Recognition.

- **Sudden** loss of consciousness that is often **complete**
- Lasts a few seconds to a few minutes (2–3 minutes) with **spontaneous and complete** neurological recovery
- Patient is often limp during the episode—has a **loss of tone**
- **Myoclonic jerks/other motor movements may occur in 90%**
- **Premonition**—blackout sensation or light headedness
- Often precipitated by sudden change of posture/pain/micturition

BOX 2: Rule out.

Seizure	Seizure-closest d/d favored if: • Loss of consciousness exceeds 5 minutes • Tongue bite • Stool incontinence • Confusion or focal deficit upon recovery • Witnessed focal onset or tonic-clonic movements
Pseudoseizure	• Loss of consciousness was not complete—patient says he could hear people around her/him • Recurrent episodes always in the presence of a witness • No injury—fall is always in a *safe* manner
Hypoglycemia	• It may be accompanied by focal deficit that reverses on administration of dextrose • Tremor/dizziness/palpitations/diaphoresis (drenched in one's sweat) is all clues but may be completely absent if episodes are recurrent
Cataplexy	• Triggered by extreme emotions duration similar to syncope • Loss of tone but no loss of consciousness • May also have a history of narcolepsy

BOX 3: Evaluation.

History:
- Precipitating factor
- Position before/during the event
- Activity before the event
- Eyewitness account
- Drug history—medications and substance abuse
- Comorbidities
- Prior events

BOX 4: Red flags.

- Chest pain-exertion before onset/dyspnea/palpitations—electrocardiography (ECG)/trop i -detailed cardiac evaluation
- Severe headache/focal deficit after the episode—detailed neurological evaluation/CT brain

BOX 5: Physical examination and laboratory workup.

- Systemic examination—cardiac/pulmonary and neurological
- Blood glucose
- Complete blood count (CBC)/electrolytes
- ECG (*normal ECG 99% negative predictive value)*
- *Point-of-care ultrasound (POCUS) for inferior vena cava (IVC) collapsibility or passive leg raise test*
- 8 am and 4 pm cortisol if unexplained postural drop (hyponatremia/hyperkalemia may accompany)

BOX 6: Types.

Three types:

1. Neurogenic
2. Cardiogenic
3. Orthostatic

- Cardiogenic—high risk of SCD
- Orthostatic—propensity to recur, higher mortality

BOX 7: Neurogenic/reflex.

- Excellent prognosis especially if single episode
- Situation triggered—emotional (pain/fear/anxiety/sight of blood/unpleasant sight or odour), procedures (instrumentation—airway/pleural cavity/gastrointestinal, urogenital/ocular examination/ocular pressure/carotid sinus massage/prostatic massage/rectal examination), physiological (swallow/sneeze/micturition/defecation), and exertional (weightlifting, blowing a wind instrument)

Management:

- Hydration—in ER and counsel regards increase water and electrolyte intake
- Counsel regarding identification and avoiding triggers
- TED stockings
- *Preprocedure atropinization:* 0.6 mL sc atropine 10 minutes before instrumentation in all individuals with a prior reflex syncope
- Isometric counterpressure maneuvers (hand grip/toe grip/crossing legs/tensing arms)
- Pharmacotherapy if the above are ineffective midodrine/mineralocorticoid if indicated [midodrine caution in benign prostatic hyperplasia (BPH), mineralocorticoid: Caution in CCF/left ventricular (LV) dysfunction]

BOX 8: Cardiogenic.

- *Cause:* Arrythmias/Structural heart disease/Acute coronary syndrome/Pulmonary Thromboembolism (ACS/PTE)
- High mortality, risk of sudden cardiac death (SCD)
- If ECG is inconclusive and suspicion is high—Holter (>1/week), external loop recorder (>1/month), and implantable loop recorder(<1/month)
- Bradyarrhythmias review drug list and eliminate potential culprit drugs
- ACS-revascularization
- Cardiac pacing as indicated
- Antiarrhythmics

BOX 9: Orthostatic.

- Propensity to recur and thus increased mortality
- Autonomic dysfunction may be primary [central nervous system (CNS)] or secondary to neuropathies such as associated with diabetes mellitus (DM)/ autoimmune/hereditary/paraneoplastic/amyloidosis/Human immunodeficiency virus (HIV) associated
- Generally not reversible except when drug induced
- CT/MRI brain, electroencephalography (EEG), electromyography-nerve conduction test (EMG-NCV), and tilt table

Evaluation:

- Check blood pressure (BP) and heart rate—supine, sitting (with legs dependent) at 0 minute and 2 minutes and standing at 0 minute and 2 minutes
- Postural hypotension is confirmed when systolic drop >20 and diastolic >10 mm Hg.
- If this is unaccompanied by an increase in heart rate> 20% in the absence of rate lowering drugs, autonomic dysfunction must be considered

Autonomic dysfunction:

- Review drug list and eliminate
- Supportive care as in neurally mediated syncope
- Patient education to prevent falls/injury

SUGGESTED READING

1. Loscalzo J, Fauci A, Kasper D, Hauser S, Longo D, Jameson JL. Harrison's Principles of Internal Medicine. Philadelphia: McGraw Hill LLC; 2022.

3.13 ENDOCARDITIS

Nihar Mehta, Divya A Samat

BOX 1: Definition.

- Infective endocarditis (IE) results from an infection of the endocardial surface, most often affecting the heart valves
- Although IE is a rare condition, it poses a significant diagnostic challenge and can lead to considerable morbidity and mortality if not promptly identified and treated

BOX 2: Risk factors.

Key risk factors include:
- History of previous endocarditis (the most prevalent risk factor)
- Structural heart damage
- Intravenous drug use (IVDU), with an annual risk ranging from 2 to 5%
- Compromised immune function [e.g., vasculitis, human immunodeficiency virus (HIV), diabetes, malignancy]
- Nosocomial factors (related to surgical hardware placement, surgical technique, and hematoma formation)
- Poor oral hygiene

BOX 3: Organism.

- *Staphylococcus aureus*
- *Streptococcus pneumoniae*
- *Streptococcus agalactiae (Group B strep)*
- Coagulase negative staphylococci
- *Streptococcus viridans*
- *Streptococcus intermedius*
- *Streptococcus gallolyticus* (bovis)
- Enterococci
- *Bartonella*
- *Pseudomonas*
- Fungal

BOX 4: Clinical diagnosis.

- The diagnosis of IE is established based on clinical manifestations, blood cultures (or other microbiologic data), and cardiac imaging.
- The diagnosis of IE requires:
  - Identification of the infecting pathogen by culture, serologic testing, or molecular testing
  - Cardiac imaging to identify a valvular vegetation, paravalvular abscess, or other structural complication of infection.
- The accepted criteria for diagnosis of IE are the 2023 Duke-International Society for Cardiovascular Infectious Disease (ISCVID) criteria.

Contd...

Contd...

- *Definite IE:* Definite IE is established if pathologic criteria (either microbiologic or histopathologic criteria) or clinical criteria are met
- *Possible IE:* Possible IE is defined as either of the following:
  - One major and one minor clinical criteria
  - Three minor clinical criteria

The 2023 Duke-ISCVID IE Criteria (Major)	
Major	
Microbiologic	1. Positive blood cultures i. **Microorganisms that commonly cause IE isolated from two or more separate blood culture sets** or ii. Microorganisms that occasionally or rarely cause IE **isolated from three or more separate blood culture sets** 2. Positive laboratory tests i. **Positive PCR or other nucleic acid-based technique for *Coxiella burnetii, Bartonella species, or Tropheryma whipplei* from blood** or ii. *Coxiella burnetii* antiphase I IgG antibody titer >1:800, or isolated from a single blood culture or iii. **Indirect immunofluorescence assays (IFA) for detection of IgM and IgG antibodies to *Bartonella henselae* or *Bartonella quintana* with IgG titer >1:800**
Imaging	1. Echocardiography and **Cardiac Computed Tomography** Imaging i. Echocardiography and/or **Cardiac CT** showing vegetation, valvular/leaflet perforation, valvular/leaflet aneurysm, abscess, pseudoaneurysm, or intracardiac fistula or ii. Significant new valvular regurgitation on echocardiography as compared to previous imaging. Worsening or changing of pre-existing regurgitation is not sufficient. or iii. New partial dehiscence of prosthetic valve as compared to previous imaging 2. **[18F]FDG PET/CT Imaging** **Abnormal metabolic activity involving a native or prosthetic valve, ascending aortic graft (with concomitant evidence of valve involvement), intracardiac device leads or other prosthetic material**
Surgical	**Evidence of IE documented by direct inspection during heart surgery neither Major Imaging Criteria nor subsequent histologic or microbiologic confirmation**
Note: Please note significant changes, including new microbiology diagnostics, imaging, and inclusion of surgical inspection as a new Major Clinical Criterion. *Source:* Fowler VG, Durack DT, Selton-Suty C, Athan E, Bayer AS, Chamis AL, et al. The 2023 Duke-International Society for Cardiovascular Infectious Diseases Criteria for Infective Endocarditis: Updating the Modified Duke Criteria. Clin Infect Dis. 2023;77(4):518-26.	

Contd...

Contd...

The 2023 Duke-ISCVID IE Criteria (Minor)	
Minor	
Predisposition	**Previous history of IE**—Prosthetic valve—Previous valve repair - Congenital heart disease more than mild regurgitation or stenosis of any etiology—**Endovascular CIED**—Hypertrophic obstructive cardiomyopathy—Injection drug use
Fever	Documented temperature greater than 38.0 degrees centigrade (100.4 degrees fahrenheit)
Vascular phenomena	Clinical or radiological evidence of arterial emboli, septic pulmonary infarcts, **cerebral or splenic abscess**, mycotic aneurysm, intracranial hemorrhage, conjunctival hemorrhages, Janeway lesions, purulent purpura
Immunologic phenomena	Positive rheumatoid factor, Osier's nodes, Roth's spots, or immune complex-mediated glomerulonephritis
Microbiologic evidence, Falling short of a major criterion	1. Positive blood cultures for a microorganism consistent with IE but not meeting the requirements for Major Criterion 2. **Positive culture, PCR or other nucleic acid based test (amplicon or shotgun sequencing, in situ hybridization) for an organism consistent with IE from a sterile body site other than cardiac tissue, cardiac prosthesis, or embolus; or a single finding of a skin bacterium by PCR on a valve or wire without additional clinical or microbiological supporting evidence**
Imaging	**Abnormal metabolic activity as detected by [18F]FDG PET/CT within 3 months of implantation of prosthetic valve, ascending aortic graft (with concomitant evidence of valve involvement), intracardiac device leads or other prosthetic material**
Physical examination	New valvular regurgitation identified on auscultation, if echocardiography is not available. Worsening or changing of pre-existing murmur not sufficient
Note: Please note additional predisposing conditions (transcatheter valve implants, endovascular cardiac implantable electronic devices, prior IE) were clarified. *Source:* Fowler VG, Durack DT, Selton-Suty C, Athan E, Bayer AS, Chamis AL, et al. The 2023 Duke-International Society for Cardiovascular Infectious Diseases Criteria for Infective Endocarditis: Updating the Modified Duke Criteria. Clin Infect Dis. 2023;77(4):518-26.	

BOX 5: Management.

The management of IE requires prompt diagnosis, the initiation of suitable antimicrobial therapy, and, for complicated cases, consideration of surgical intervention. Patients with IE should be treated by a multidisciplinary team, including specialists in infectious diseases, cardiology, and cardiac surgery, to ensure thorough clinical evaluation, effective antibiotic treatment, and appropriate surgical care. Key components of IE management include:

- *Antimicrobial therapy:* Prompt diagnosis and initiation of effective antimicrobial treatment to reduce complications. Antibiotic therapy should be customized based on the pathogens identified in blood cultures.
- *Evaluation of foreign material:* Assess whether removal of infected implanted devices, arteriovenous fistulas, or grafts is required.
- *Surgical consideration:* Identification of patients who may benefit from early valve surgery.
- *Monitoring:*
  - Assess the response to antibiotic therapy, ensuring the resolution of bacteremia.
  - Monitor hemodynamic and cardiac status, including periodic electrocardiograms to detect new conduction abnormalities.
- *Follow-up and prevention of recurrent IE:* Emphasize maintaining good dental hygiene, appropriate antimicrobial prophylaxis for high-risk procedures, and consider closing patent ductus arteriosus or ventricular septal defects if present.

BOX 6: Antimicrobial therapy.

- For patients exhibiting hemodynamic instability and clinical signs indicative of acute endocarditis (such as fever and a new murmur), especially when relevant cardiac risk factors or predisposing conditions are present, it is recommended to promptly start empiric antibiotic therapy
- Patients without acute symptoms may not require immediate empiric therapy. However, empiric treatment should be considered after obtaining at least two, preferably three, sets of blood cultures from separate venipunctures, ideally spaced 30–60 minutes apart
- Empiric therapy should generally provide coverage for staphylococci (both methicillin susceptible and resistant), streptococci, and enterococci. Vancomycin is an appropriate initial therapy in most cases
- The duration of therapy for native valve endocarditis (NVE) depends on the specific pathogen identified and the location of the valvular infection. Typically, treatment for NVE is recommended for up to 6 weeks

BOX 7: Drugs and their doses against the disease causing drug resistant strains.

American Heart Association (AHA)		***European Society of Cardiology (ESC)***	***British Society for Antimicrobial Chemotherapy (BSAC)***
Adult	***Pediatric***		
Methicillin susceptible strains	***Methicillin susceptible strains***	***Methicillin susceptible strains***	***Methicillin sensitive***
Nafcillin or oxacillin 12 g per 24 hours IV in four or six divided doses for 6 weeks **or** Cefazolin 6 g per 24 hours IV in three divided doses for 6 weeks	Nafcillin or oxacillin 200 mg/kg per 24 hours IV (maximum dose: 12 g per 24 hours) in four or six divided doses for 4–6 weeks **or** Cefazolin 100 mg/kg per 24 hours IV (maximum dose: 6 g per 24 hours) in three divided doses for 4–6 weeks	Oxacillin or cloxacillin or flucloxacillin 12 g per 24 hours IV in four or six divided doses for 4–6 weeks **or** Cefazolin 6 g per 24 hours IV in three divided doses for 6 weeks **or** Cefotaxime 6 g per 24 hours in three divided doses	Flucloxacillin 2 g IV every 4–6 hours for 4 weeks
Methicillin-resistant strains	***Methicillin-resistant strains***	***Methicillin-resistant strains***	***Methicillin resistant***
Vancomycin for 6 weeks **or** Daptomycin ≥ 8 mg/kg per 24 hours IV once daily for 6 weeks	Vancomycin 40 mg/kg per 24 hours IV (maximum dose: 2 g per 24 hours unless levels are inappropriately low) in two or three divided doses for 6 weeks	Vancomycin 30–60 mg/kg per 24 hours IV in two or three divided doses for 4–6 weeks **or** Daptomycin 10 mg/kg per 24 hours IV once daily for 4–6 weeks	Vancomycin 1 g IV every 12 hours for 4 weeks **plus** Rifampicin 300–600 mg orally every 12 hours for 4 weeks **or** Daptomycin 6 mg/kg IV every 24 hours for 4 weeks **plus** Rifampicin 300–600 mg orally every 24 hours for 4 weeks **or** Gentamicin 1 mg/kg IV every 12 hours for 4 weeks

BOX 8: Indications for surgery.

For left-sided native valve IE:

Indications for surgery are:

- IE-associated valve dysfunction causing symptoms or signs of heart failure (HF)
- Paravalvular extension of infection with development of annular or aortic abscess, destructive penetrating lesion (e.g., fistula), and/or heart block
- Infection due to a difficult to treat pathogen such as fungi and multidrug-resistant organisms. Persistent infection (persistent bacteremia or fever lasting >5 days after initiation of appropriate antibiotic therapy)

For patients with large vegetations, we perform an individualized risk benefit assessment

For right-sided native valve IE:

- Very large vegetations (≥20 mm in diameter)
- Recurrent septic pulmonary emboli
- Highly resistant organisms
- Persistent bacteremia

For prosthetic valve IE:

Indications are as follows:

- HF resulting from valve dehiscence, intracardiac fistula, or severe prosthetic valve dysfunction
- Complication such as heart block, annular or aortic abscess, or destructive penetrating lesion
- Prosthetic valve endocarditis (PVE) caused by fungi or other highly resistant organism despite appropriate antibiotic therapy for 5–7 days and exclusion of other sites of infection if sepsis persists.

BOX 9: Complications.

- Cardiac complications include HF, perivalvular abscess, pericarditis, and intracardiac fistula.
- Metastatic infections may present as septic embolization, metastatic abscesses, and mycotic aneurysms. Septic emboli can affect systemic or pulmonary arterial vessels, while abscesses can form in the spleen, kidneys, brain, soft tissues, or lungs. Mycotic aneurysms typically occur at vessel bifurcations in the cerebral or systemic circulation.
- Neurologic complications consist of stroke, brain abscesses, meningitis, and other neurological sequelae, which can sometimes be the initial symptoms of IE.
- Renal complications involve renal infarction or abscess following septic embolization, glomerulonephritis, and drug-induced acute interstitial nephritis.
- Musculoskeletal complications include vertebral osteomyelitis and septic arthritis.

BOX 10: Take away points.

Emergency physicians should evaluate IE in patients presenting with flu-like symptoms and relevant risk factors. Timely and appropriate assessment and treatment can greatly decrease the morbidity and mortality associated with the disease.

SUGGESTED READING

1. Baddour LM, Wilson WR, Bayer AS, Fowler VG Jr, Tleyjeh IM, Rybak MJ, et al. Infective Endocarditis in Adults: Diagnosis, Antimicrobial Therapy, and Management of Complications: A Scientific Statement for Healthcare Professionals From the American Heart Association. Circulation. 2015;132:1435-86.
2. Fowler VG Jr, Miro JM, Hoen B, Cabell CH, Abrutyn E, Rubinstein E, et al. Staphylococcus aureus endocarditis: a consequence of medical progress. JAMA. 2005;293:3012-21.
3. Fowler VG, Durack DT, SeltonSuty C, Athan E, Bayer AS, Chamis AL, et al. The 2023 DukeInternational Society for Cardiovascular Infectious Diseases Criteria for Infective Endocarditis: Updating the Modified Duke Criteria. Clin Infect Dis. 2023; 77:518-26.
4. Gould FK, Denning DW, Elliott TS, Foweraker J, Perry JD, Prendergast BD, et al. Guidelines for the diagnosis and antibiotic treatment of endocarditis in adults: a report of the Working Party of the British Society for Antimicrobial Chemotherapy. J Antimicrob Chemother. 2012;67:269-89.
5. Habib G, Lancellotti P, Antunes MJ, Bongiorni MG, Casalta JP, Del Zotti F, et al. 2015 ESC Guidelines for the management of infective endocarditis: The Task Force for the Management of Infective Endocarditis of the European Society of Cardiology (ESC). Endorsed by: European Association for CardioThoracic Surgery (EACTS), the European Association of Nuclear Medicine (EANM). Eur Heart J. 2015;36:3075-128.
6. Hoen B, Duval X. Infective endocarditis. N Engl J Med. 2013;369:785.
7. Iversen K, Ihlemann N, Gill SU, Madsen T, Elming H, Jensen KT, et al. Partial oral versus intravenous antibiotic treatment of endocarditis. N Engl J Med. 2019;380:415.
8. Long R, Koyfman A. Infectious endocarditis: An update for emergency clinicians. Am J Emerg Med. 2018;36(9):1686-92.
9. Mansur AJ, Grinberg M, da Luz PL, Bellotti G. The complications of infective endocarditis. A reappraisal in the 1980s. Arch Intern Med. 1992;152:2428-32.

Gastrointestinal Emergencies

4.1 ACUTE ABDOMEN PAIN

Judith Rebello, Vismaya KB, Sanjay Nagral

INTRODUCTION

This chapter is structured using a triage framework for an emergency service in a reasonably-equipped urban center in India. We acknowledge that the algorithm will differ based on the resources and settings and should be tailored to local conditions.

BOX 1: General triage.

- Who needs investigation? (Who can be sent home without investigations?)
- Who needs observation/admission?
- Who needs referral?
- Who can be sent home?

BOX 2: High-risk abdominal pain.

- Sudden onset with minimal signs
- Severe pain not responding to usual analgesics
- Pain with upper/lower gastrointestinal bleed
- Pain with altered mentation

Common sense alarm symptoms:
- Presenting late night or on a holiday
- Repeated visits to casualty

BOX 3: Demographics and symptoms.

- Gender—female (of childbearing age/pubertal)—last menstrual period (risk of ectopic pregnancy)
- Age >65 years
- Immunocompromised (Human immunodeficiency virus, chronic steroid, and transplant recipient)
- Alcoholism
- Smoking
- Cardiovascular disease
- Prior surgery/recent gastro-intestinal or genitourinary instrumentation (obstruction and perforation)
- Comorbidities (chronic liver disease, renal failure, and diabetes mellitus)
- Previously known abdominal illnesses (cancer, diverticula, gallstones, inflammatory bowel disease and pancreatitis)
- Medications [anticoagulants, nonsteroidal anti-inflammatory drugs]
- Recent trauma

BOX 4: Examination findings (alarm signs).

- Tachycardia
- Tachypnea
- Signs of shock
- Guarded or rigid abdomen
- Patient lying absolutely still as movement would aggravate pain
- Distension
- Auscultation for presence or absence of peristalsis is unreliable
- If in doubt best to re-examine the abdomen after a gap
- Do not examine during a rigor as one can get a false feeling of guarding

BOX 5: Who can be sent home without investigations or imaging?

- Normal vitals, no alarm symptoms and signs
- No similar past episodes
- No worrying signs on physical examination
- No high-risk abdominal pain features
- Easy access to healthcare
- Accompanied by an adult/responsible attendant

BOX 6: Blood tests.

- Complete blood count; may not be very useful though leukocytosis denotes infection
- Serum amylase if pancreatitis suspected, should be more than three times upper limit of normal, false positives and negatives are known
- Serum lipase rises after 48 hours though more specific
- Serum lactate (bowel ischemia)
- Urine routine
- Useful if urinary tract suspected as cause of acute pain

BOX 7: Imaging.

X-ray:
- Chest—Basal lung findings and air under diaphragm
- Abdomen—air under diaphragm, air fluid levels, renal stone, calcific foreign body, and pancreatic calculi

Ultrasound (USG) abdomen:
- Easily available, bedside (point-of-care), safe, but limited accuracy
- Accurate to diagnose-free fluid, gall stones, and renal stones
- Accuracy is operator dependent, limited by gaseous distension and obesity

Computed tomography (CT) abdomen plain:
- More accurate than plain X-ray or USG; we would recommend plain CT as the first radiological test if easily available
- *Better than USG for:*
  - Bowel Pancreas
  - Vessels (ischemia)
  - Small amount of free fluid, and free air
  - Retroperitoneum

Intravenous (IV) contrast with CT: Only after plain CT, if doubt of ischemia. Ideally check creatinine, if creatinine clearance abnormal weigh pros and cons of clinching diagnosis with contrast versus risk of contrast induced nephropathy

BOX 8: Over (mis) diagnosed conditions.

- Acute gastritis
- Amoebic colitis/colitis
- Appendicitis

Underdiagnosed conditions:
- *Ischemic bowel:*
  - Increasing incidence, underdiagnosed
  - Elderly patients
  - Ischemic heart disease and arrythmias
  - Symptoms out of proportion to signs
  - Quick decisions necessary to save bowel
  - CT with contrast
  - **High mortality (60%); good results only with early diagnosis and immediate intervention**
- Diverticulitis
- *Dengue related abdominal pain:*
  - Acalculous cholecystitis
  - Pancreatitis
  - Nonspecific peritonitis
  - Hemoperitoneum
  - Appendicitis
- Malaria-related abdominal pain (pancreatitis and ischemia)
  - Acute pancreatitis (rare, falciparum > vivax)
  - Splenic infarction/rupture

BOX 9: Incidence of the following is decreasing.

- Typhoid perforation
- Ulcer perforation (except elderly—NSAID)
- Amoebic/round worm complications

BOX 10: Common pitfalls.

- Blaming the pain on "malingering" if no alarm symptoms or signs
- Examination of groin (for hernia/testicular torsion) is often missed if systematic approach for examination is not adhered to resulting in a major miss
- Cultural belief of only women in reproductive age group being pregnant may miss a pregnancy in a younger female
- Acute myocardial ischemia (MI) masquerading as abdominal discomfort
- Missed diagnosis are common in the elderly especially bowel ischemia
- A normal CT abdomen does not guarantee the absence of serious pathology
  It may miss mesenteric ischemia (send for lactates), testicular torsion, early pancreatitis, and non-structural causes [acute MI and diabetic ketoacidosis (DKA)]

BOX 11: Algorithm for abdominal pain in adults.

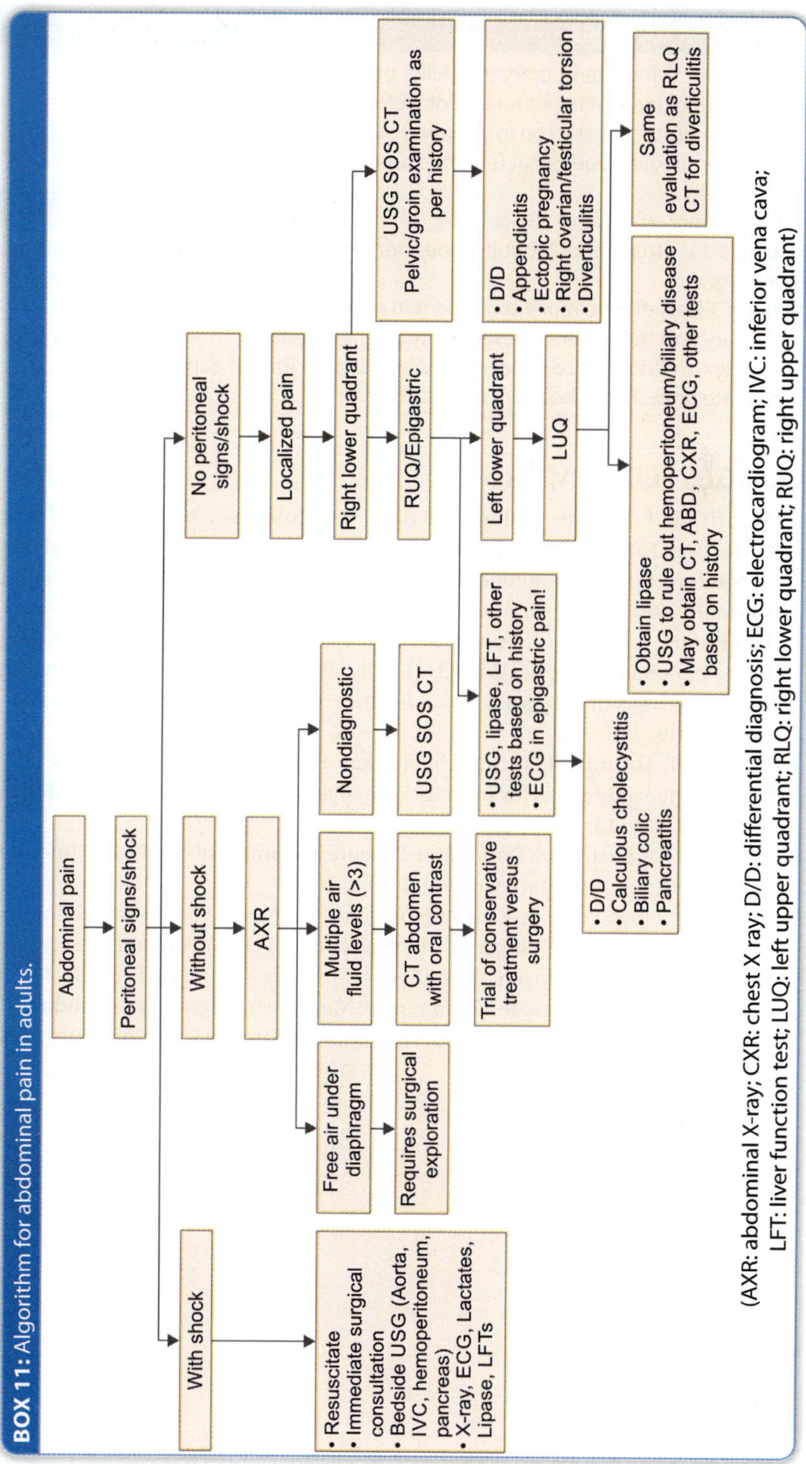

(AXR: abdominal X-ray; CXR: chest X ray; D/D: differential diagnosis; ECG: electrocardiogram; IVC: inferior vena cava; LFT: liver function test; LUQ: left upper quadrant; RLQ: right lower quadrant; RUQ: right upper quadrant)

BOX 12: Other key points.

- No harm in giving a temporary pain killer but avoid NSAIDs
- "Malingering" is a reality but rare; think before you use the label
- Develop a protocol based on local expertise and availability
- Inform sonologist about what is being suspected, emergency team performs sonography
- CT is superior to a plain X-ray or USG
- A plain CT is often enough but if it does not reveal pathology intravenous contrast maybe given
- Whilst CT is useful too much time spent in procuring it is dangerous, if CT is necessary and the patient is restless intubate and sedate
- Very few conditions need super-urgent laparotomy (bowel gangrene)
- Adequate time should be spent on resuscitation

SUGGESTED READING

1. Algorithm for acute abdominal pain in adults has been adapted from UpToDate, Townsend Jr CM. Sabiston Textbook of Surgery: The Biological Basis of Modern Surgical Practice, 21st edition. India: Elsevier—Health Sciences Division; 2021.
2. Landmann A, Bonds M, Postier R. Acute Abdomen. In: Townsend CM, Evers BM, Beauchamp RD, Mattox KL (Eds). Sabiston Textbook of Surgery: The Biological Basis of Modern Surgical Practice, 21st edition. India: Elsevier; 2021. pp. 1134-49.
3. Mayumi T, Yoshida M, Tazuma S, Furukawa A, Nishii O, Shigematsu K, et al. The practice guidelines for primary care of acute abdomen 2015. Jpn J Radiol. 2016;34(1):80-115.
4. Patterson JW, Kashyap S, Dominique E. Acute Abdomen. In: StatPearls [Internet]. Treasure Island (FL): StatPearls Publishing; 2024.
5. Pereira B, Fraga G. High-Risk Patients and Prognostic Factors for Abdominal Sepsis. In: Sartelli M, Bassetti M, Martin-Loeches I (Eds). Abdominal sepsis—A multidisciplinary approach. Philadelphia: Springer Nature; 2018. pp. 37-46.
6. Tiwari A, Haribhakti S. Acute abdomen. In: Nanavati A, Nagral S (Eds). Abdominal Trauma, Peritoneum, and Retroperitoneum. Oxford: Oxford University Press; 2023. pp. 59-68.

4.2 APPENDICITIS

Kayomars B Kapadia

BOX 1: Symptoms.

Typical triad (Murphy's) for diagnosis:
- Pain in right iliac fossa (RIF)
- Fever
- Vomiting

While all the three symptoms are present in most of the patients, they may not always be there in all the patients.

Typically, pain is periumbilical which later localizes in RIF

***Duration of pain** is important:* Within the first 24–72 hours of onset of pain, laparoscopic appendicectomy is usually straight forward. Thereafter, there may be an appendicular lump formation which makes surgery difficult and hence should be documented

Associated symptoms: Loss of appetite, constipation or loose motions, urinary symptoms, etc.

BOX 2: Clinical examination findings.

General:
- Pulse may be normal or tachycardia may be present
- Tachypnea indicates advanced stage of infection, viz., perforated appendix with Septicemia

Abdominal:
- Tenderness in RIF
- Guarding, rigidity, and rebound tenderness indicate peritonitis/perforated appendix
- Tender mass in RIF indicates an appendicular mass, abscess or very rarely associated pathologies such Ileocecal Koch, Crohn's, and malignancy
- Bowel sounds may be sluggish or absent

BOX 3: Differential diagnosis.

- Right ureteric calculi
- Pelvic inflammatory disease/salpingitis
- Torsion of tubo-ovarian mass
- Meckle's diverticulitis
- Amoebic typhlitis
- Mesenteric adenitis
- Ileocecal tuberculosis (TB), malignancy, Crohn's disease, and intussusception

BOX 4: Investigations.

Acute appendicitis was thought to be a clinical diagnosis. But now a days investigations are essential

- *Blood tests:* Complete blood count (CBC), creatinine, electrolytes, blood sugar, and C-reactive protein (CRP)
- *Radiological*—ultrasound; if needed CT scan

BOX 5: Treatment in ER.

- Patient should be kept nil-by-mouth (NBM)
- *Antibiotics:* Depending on the severity of infection, select:
  - Amoxycillin + clavulanic acid
  - Third-generation cephalosporin + metronidazole
  - Piperacillin + tazobactam
- Analgesics—paracetamol/diclofenac (if no contraindications)/opioids
- IV fluids—Ringer lactate/DNS
- Nasal Ryle's tube, urinary catheter may be needed
- Surgical reference is to be given as soon as there is a suspicion of acute appendicitis

BOX 6: Caveats.

- Clinically, a high index of suspicion should be maintained as different types of appendicitis might present in a different manner
- Like retrocecal type which is the commonest causes right loin pain
- Subcecal and pelvic type causes suprapubic pain with urinary frequency and diarrhea, with rectal or vaginal tenderness
- Preileal and postileal type signs and symptoms might be lacking, but may present with vomiting, diarrhea
- Gold standard is graded compression USG for diagnosis—typical findings in appendicitis are a thickened, noncompressible appendix >6 mm in diameter
- Some scores like Alvarado can assess the severity but clinical judgement is superficial in any decision of medical versus surgical management
- In addition, acute appendicitis at extremes of age requires prompt surgical intervention

SUGGESTED READING

1. Brunicardi FC, Andersen DK, Billiar TR, Dunn DL, Hunter JG, Kao L, et al. Schwartz's Principles of Surgery, 11th edition. USA: McGraw Hill; 2019.
2. Doherty GM. Current Diagnosis & Treatment Surgery, 15th edition. India: McGraw Hill; 2021.
3. Townsend Jr CM. Sabiston Textbook of Surgery: The Biological Basis of Modern Surgical Practice, 21st edition. India: Elsevier—Health Sciences Division; 2021.
4. Williams NS. Bailey & Love's Short Practice of Surgery, 27th edition. United Kingdom: CRC Press; 2000.

4.3 AMOEBIC COLITIS

Parnasha Chemburkar, Chintamani Godbole

BOX 1: Introduction.

- Intestinal amoebiasis is an infection caused by parasitic *Entamoeba histolytica* species
- In most cases, it is asymptomatic
- Clinical manifestations broadly are classified into amoebic dysentery and extraintestinal disease
- Extraintestinal manifestations can occur, such as, amoebic liver abscess (ALA) and rarely pulmonary, cardiac, or brain involvement may be seen

BOX 2: Clinical manifestations.

- Vary from asymptomatic disease to invasive amoebiasis
- In mild cases, it manifests as abdominal pain and diarrhea
- Amoebic dysentery is characterized by mucus in the stools and diarrhea containing visible blood
- Weight loss and fever are common symptoms
- Rarely, acute fulminant necrotizing amoebic colitis can occur, leading to life-threatening lower gastrointestinal bleeding without diarrhea, colonic perforation, or ischemia

BOX 3: Differential diagnosis.

- Intestinal ischemia, tuberculosis or malignancy, and inflammatory bowel diseases
- Appendicitis, perianal cutaneous amoebiasis, and rectovaginal fistulae

BOX 4: Complications.

- Fulminant colitis with bowel necrosis
- Can evolve into toxic megacolon, perforation, and bowel necrosis of intestine with shock (acute fulminant amoebic colitis)
- Requires surgical intervention

BOX 5: Diagnosis.

- Indirect hemagglutination (IHA) is very sensitive as a serological test
- Stool microscopy is the gold standard. The demonstration of cysts or trophozoites in the stool is diagnostic
- Antigen detection kits using enzyme-linked immunosorbent assay (ELISA), radioimmunoassay, or immunofluorescence
- Colonoscopy

BOX 6: Treatment.

- Asymptomatic infection needs treatment with intraluminal agents only. These include:
  - Paromomycin (25–30 mg/kg per day orally in three divided doses for 7 days)
  - Iodoquinol (650 mg orally three times daily for adults and 30–40 mg/kg per day in three divided doses for children for 20 days)
  - Diloxanide furoate (500 mg orally three times daily for adults and 20 mg/kg per day in three divided doses for children for 10 days)
- Symptomatic infection needs to be treated with systemic therapy first (details mentioned below) followed by intraluminal agents for complete eradication

Systemic therapy:
- Mainstay of systemic therapy is metronidazole (MTZ) or tinidazole
- Dose for MTZ is 500 mg by mouth three times daily in adults and 35–50 mg/kg per day in three divided doses in children for 7–10 days
- Dose for tinidazole is 2 g orally each day for 3 days
- Fulminant colitis/peritonitis/toxic megacolon—empirical broad-spectrum antibiotics should be added to MTZ for the risk of coexisting bacterial sepsis. Occasionally, surgical intervention, such as a colectomy, is required in the setting of toxic megacolon or colonic perforation
- Pregnant women with mild-to-moderate amoebic colitis due to *E. histolytica* without evidence of extraluminal disease, treatment with paromomycin is preferred, due to the teratogenic toxicity of MTZ
- Pregnant women with severe amebic colitis due to *E. histolytica*, MTZ needs to be given

BOX 7: Amoebic liver abscess.

- An ALA is the most common extraintestinal manifestation of invasive amebiasis and the most common form of liver abscess in tropical area
- Source of infection is water or food contaminated with cysts of *E. histolytica*
- Aspirate characterized by thick brown acellular debris that is odorless and almost always sterile. Unlike pyogenic liver abscess (PLA), which contains leukocytes and appears hot on nuclear scanning, ALA lacks leukocytes and appears as a cold lesion on technetium-99m liver scan
- The majority of ALA heal without the need for a drainage procedure

Predominant involves the right lobar as the trophozoites invade the cecum and travel to the liver *via* portal circulation. Because the right lobe of the liver receives portal blood mostly through the superior mesenteric vein, which drains the cecum, ALA more frequently affects this part of the liver

BOX 8: Caveat.

Such lobar predilection is not observed in the case of PLA, where bacterial invasion can occur through venous, arterial, or biliary systems

BOX 9: Clinical presentation.

- Uncomplicated cases have a short history of fever and abdominal pain in the right upper quadrant
- According to the severity and duration of symptoms:
  - Acute aggressive is ALA characterized by acute onset of severe symptoms, systemic toxicity, markedly deranged laboratory parameters, and high risk of rupture requiring a drainage procedure
  - Subacute mild ALA is characterized by mild-to-moderate symptoms with onset within 24 week, usually responding to the medical therapy
  - Chronic indolent ALA is characterized by late presentation (>4 week) with mild persistent symptoms including pain in abdomen

BOX 10: Complications.

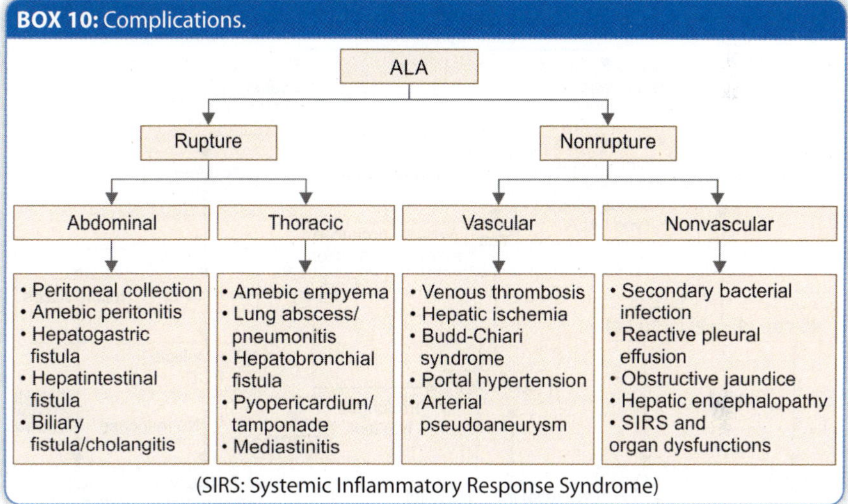

(SIRS: Systemic Inflammatory Response Syndrome)

BOX 11: Diagnosis.

- Ultrasonography for liver abscess
- Computed tomography (CT) scan is usually required for complicated ALA patients. *Characteristic:* Type I—the clinically aggressive type, absent or incomplete wall, and ragged edges with irregular enhancement; type II—complete rim enhancement and peripheral hypodense halo and was clinically less aggressive; and type III—the least common type, nonenhancing wall, and a chronic indolent course
- Endoscopic evaluation for bleeding symptoms from ileocolonic ulcerations or ruptured abscess into the gastrointestinal tract

BOX 12: Drug of choice.

- MTZ, the most widely used is the cornerstone of treatment for uncomplicated ALA. Dose as given above for 7–10 days, it resolves symptoms within 72 hours of treatment. Since the parasites can linger in the colon, MTZ treatment should be followed with a luminal agent, such as paromomycin (dose as above for 7 days) or diloxanide furoate (as given above for 20 days). The failure to take luminal medicines can result in relapse of infection in about 10% patients
- Alternative nitroimidazole compounds that have been used in the treatment of ALA include tinidazole, ornidazole, and nitazoxanide

BOX 13: Management.

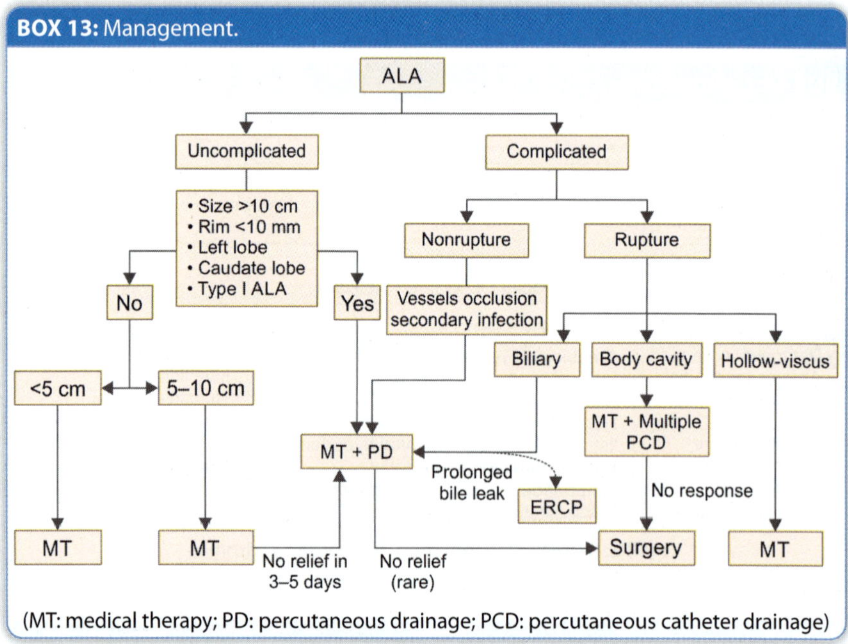

(MT: medical therapy; PD: percutaneous drainage; PCD: percutaneous catheter drainage)

SUGGESTED READING

1. Bercu TE, Petri WA, Behm JW. Amebic colitis: new insights into pathogenesis and treatment. Curr Gastroenterol Rep. 2007;9:429-33.
2. Haque R, Huston CD, Hughes M, Houpt E, Petri WA Jr. Amebiasis. N Engl J Med. 2003;348:1565-73.
3. Heredia RD, Fonseca JA, López MC. Entamoeba moshkovskii perspectives of a new agent to be considered in the diagnosis of amebiasis. Acta Trop. 2012;123:139.
4. Kumar R, Patel R, Priyadarshi RN, Narayan R, Maji T, Anand U, et al. Amebic liver abscess: an update. World J Hepatol. 2024;16(3):316-30.
5. Parija SC, Mandal J, Ponnambath DK. Laboratory methods of identification of Entamoeba histolytica and its differentiation from lookalike Entamoeba spp. Trop Parasitol. 2014;4:90-95.

6. Peterson KM, Singh U, Petri WA Jr. Enteric Amebiasis. In: Guerrant R, Walker DH, Weller PF (Eds). Tropical Infectious Diseases: Principles, Pathogens and Practice, 3rd edition. Philadelphia: Saunders Elsevier; 2011. pp. 614.
7. Shirley DT, Farr L, Watanabe K, Moonah S. A review of the global burden, new diagnostics, and current therapeutics for amebiasis. Open Forum Infect Dis. 2018;5:ofy161.

4.4 ACUTE PANCREATITIS

Nilesh Doctor, Vivek Shetty, Govind Purushothanam

BOX 1: Diagnostic criteria.

Clinical	• Upper abdominal pain, severe and persistent, can radiate to back, chest, or flank • Associated with nausea, vomiting anorexia diaphoresis • May worsen while lying flat, may improve on forward bending
Laboratory	• Serum amylase/lipase > three times upper limit of normal
Imaging	• Computed tomography/ultrasonography (CT/USG) (details in **Box 4**)

BOX 2: Etiology determination.

Personal history	• Previous acute pancreatitis • Known gallstone disease • Alcohol intake • Medication, drug intake (thiazides, sulfonamides, furosemide, estrogens, tetracycline, and azathioprine] • Hyperlipidemia, trauma • Recent endoscopic retrograde cholangiopancreatography (ERCP)
Family history	• Pancreatic diseases

BOX 3: Physical examination.

General examination: Spectrum of findings:
- Normal examination
- Fever in some patients
- Secondary to pain tachycardia, tachypnea, and diaphoresis might be noted
- In initial presentation patient might have hypertension (especially due to pain), but if in shock hypotension is noted
- *Abdominal examination:*
  - Tenderness upon palpation
  - Guarding
  - Signs of peritoneal irritation, distension, or rigidity
  - Bowel sounds—occasionally decreased
  - Jaundice—occasionally present
- *In severe cases:* Altered mental status
- Rare physical signs*:*
  - Cullen sign—bruising and swelling in the subcutaneous tissue around the umbilicus
  - Grey Turner sign—bruising of the flank

BOX 4: Investigations.

Lab	*Imaging*
• Complete blood counts (increased leukocytes and polymorphs) • Amylase, Lipase > thrice the upper normal limit • Blood sugars • Liver enzymes if biliary pancreatitis suspected • Calcium • Triglycerides • C-reactive protein (CRP) >150 at >72 hours, procalcitonin	• CT abdomen • RUQ ultrasonography (not very sensitive) • Magnetic resonance cholangiopancreatography (MRCP) (but limited in early hour as due to tachypnea in patients resulting in suboptimal scans)
	• In idiopathic pancreatitis with negative workup • Endoscopic ultrasound (microlithiasis) • Secretin stimulated MRCP (morphological abnormalities) • Genetic counseling (etiology uncertain even after second attack)

BOX 5: Prognostication of severity.

Bedside index of severity in acute pancreatitis (BISAP) score:
- Blood urea nitrogen (BUN) >25 mg/dL
- Impaired mental status
- Systemic inflammatory response syndrome (SIRS)
- Age >60
- Presence of a pleural effusion

BISAP score >5—mortality >20%

BOX 6: Imaging.

Initial CT indications	• Diagnostic uncertainty • Confirmation of severity based on clinical predictors of severe acute pancreatitis • Failure to respond to conservative treatment or clinical deterioration • Optimal timing ≥72–96 hours after onset of symptoms

BOX 7: Management in an emergency room.

- Fluid resuscitation
- Pain control
- Risk stratification
- Nutrition management

BOX 8: Fluid therapy.

Fluid of choice	Fluid of choice—isotonic crystalloid solution which contains NA and balanced/buffered crystalloid [Ringer's Lactate (RL), plasmalyte, or Hartmann's solution]
	Goal-directed, moderate fluid resuscitation (10 mL/kg bolus in hypovolemia, followed by 1.5 mL/kg/h)
Goals of resuscitation	• Urine output 0.5–1 mL/kg/h • Lactate • Mixed venous oxygen saturation • Base deficit • Pressure and flow parameters • Hematocrit (Hct) >35% within 48 hours

BOX 9: Pain management.

- Choice of analgesic largely dependent on local protocols, physician preference no one approach has been shown to be more beneficial
- Opioids may be an appropriate choice
- Compared with other analgesics, opioids may decrease the need for supplementary analgesia
- For prolonged and severe pain, opiates can be administered using a patient-controlled analgesia (PCA) pump
- Thoracic epidural analgesia—no supporting clinical trials

BOX 10: Intensive care management.

Indication	***Persistent organ failure (Atlanta criteria)***	
Organ system	***Failure***	***Treatment***
Respiratory system (RS)	Acute lung injury → hypoxemia	• Noninvasive ventilation • Mech ventilation with lung protection • Maintain SpO_2 >95%
Cardiovascular system (CVS)	Hypotension	• Volume resuscitation • Vasoactive agents
Renal	Reduced renal perfusion	• Restore circulatory volume • Hemodialysis
Gastrointestinal (GI) tract	Reduced perfusion → failure to tolerate enteral nutrition (EN) → gut barrier break → translocation → bacteremia, infected necrosis	• Early oral/enteral feeds • 20% complain pain after feed restart → EN, total parenteral nutrition (TPN) • Among EN, nasojejunal (NJ) feeds preferred nasogastric (NG) tube feeds can be used if no gastric outlet obstruction (GOO) • Contraindications—gastric stasis/Ileus/GI fistulae
Intra-abdominal hypertension	Sustained IAP >20 mm + new-onset organ failure – surrogate marker of negative outcome	• NG tube/rectal tube decompression • Percutaneous drainage of ascites • Laparotomy/subcutaneous linea alba fasciotomy

Antibiotic	• Not recommended as routine prophylaxis [International Association of Pancreatology/American Pancreatic Association (IAP/APA) 2013]
	• Subgroup of severe acute pancreatitis needing ABs—coexisting cholangitis
	• *Indication:*
	  – Severe acute pancreatitis
	  – Clinical/radiological/microbiological evidence of infected necrosis
	• *Antibiotics with adequate penetration*—imipenem, clindamycin, piperacillin, fluoroquinolones, and metronidazole	

BOX 11: Biliary tract management in biliary pancreatitis.

- ERCP—not indicated in mild biliary pancreatitis without cholangitis
- Urgent ERCP—indicated in acute pancreatitis with acute cholangitis
- MRCP and endoscopic ultrasonography (EUS) prevent unnecessary ERCPs [suspected common bile duct (CBD) stones in biliary pancreatitis without cholangitis]

BOX 12: Timing of intervention in acute pancreatitis.

Proven/suspected infected necrotizing pancreatitis, intervention (minimally invasive/percutaneous/endoscopic/surgical) delayed until at least 4 weeks after onset to allow formation of walled-off necrosis (WON)

BOX 13: Intervention strategies in acute necrotizing pancreatitis.

- Suspected/confirmed infected necrotizing pancreatitis initial image-guided percutaneous (retroperitoneal) catheter drainage or endoscopic transluminal drainage → endoscopic/surgical necrosectomy SOS
- Suspected/confirmed infected WON percutaneous catheter/endoscopic transmural drainage first step

BOX 14: Interventions for infected pancreatic necrosis.

Intervention avoided in first 2 weeks, except ischemia/bleeding/abdominal compartment syndrome

Indications:

- In secondary infection clinical/biochemical deterioration/CT evidence of infection (small gas pockets)
- Ongoing organ failure for several weeks after onset, after necrosis is walled off routine percutaneous fine-needle aspiration (FNA) of peripancreatic collections to detect bacteria: Not indicated (false-positive rates)

BOX 15: Timing of cholecystectomy in biliary pancreatitis.

- *Mild biliary pancreatitis:* Cholecystectomy during index admission—safe, recommended; interval cholecystectomy—risk of recurrence
- *Peripancreatic collections:* Interval cholecystectomy >6 weeks or after the collections subside
- *Biliary pancreatitis who have undergone sphincterotomy:* If fit for surgery, cholecystectomy advised (ERCP, sphincterotomy prevent recurrence of biliary pancreatitis, not biliary colic and cholecystitis)

SUGGESTED READING

1. Andrews RJCB, Scott JJ. Guidelines for the Management of Acute Pancreatitis. Clinical Gastroenterology and Hepatology; 2020.
2. Brandt RRG, McClain JP. Management of Acute Pancreatitis. Gastroenterology Clinics of North America. 2017.
3. Cheung KG, Anderson LT. Acute Pancreatitis: An Update on Management. The Lancet. 2022.
4. Fagan RWJ, Galli SB. Acute Pancreatitis: Clinical Features and Diagnosis. UpToDate
5. Lewis ER, Williams PJ. Surgical Interventions in Acute Pancreatitis. British Journal of Surgery. 2021.
6. Singh RM, Kumar MR. Biliary Pancreatitis: Management and Treatment. Journal of Hepatology. 2018.
7. Sutton BR, Brown TB, Howell CM. Acute Pancreatitis: Diagnosis, Classification, and Management. American Journal of Gastroenterology; 2019.
8. Yamada T, Podolsky DK, Alpers DH. Textbook of Gastroenterology, 6th edition. Philadelphia: Wiley Blackwell; 2016.

4.5 BOWEL OBSTRUCTION

Vivek Shetty

BOX 1: Introduction.

Definition	Mechanical or functional obstruction of the small or large intestines
Classification	• Small bowel obstruction (85%), large bowel obstruction (15%), and closed loop obstruction (bowel segment is occluded both proximally and distally) • Partial obstruction (gas and liquid can pass across) versus complete obstruction

BOX 2: Etiology.

	Small bowel	***Large bowel***
Intrinsic	• Crohn's disease • Bowel stricture • Malignancy • Intussusception • Intestinal malrotation	• Colonic/rectal malignancy • Inflammatory bowel disease • Diverticular stricture • Acute colonic pseudo-obstruction (Oglivie's syndrome) • Volvulus • Intussusception
Extrinsic	• Adhesions • Hernia • Compression by extra intestinal malignancy/ metastatic deposits	• Adhesions (recent/remote surgery) • Hernia • Compression
Intraluminal	• Foreign body obstruction the lumen • Gall stone ileus • Parasites • Bezoar	• Impacted fecal matter • Foreign body

BOX 3: Clinical features.

Symptoms	• Abdominal pain, colicky type, usually improves after vomiting/ passing stool • Nausea • Vomiting (bilious/feculent), usually large volume • Constipation +/obstipation • Can have paradoxical loose stools due to hyperperistalsis of the bowel distal to the block
Signs	• Dehydration (dry tongue, weak pulses, and reduced urine output) • Distended abdomen • Tenderness (should raise suspicion of peritonitis) • Increased bowel sounds (borborygmi) • Hernia orifices should always be examined • Rectal examination (usually collapsed, impacted fecal matter may be noticed)

BOX 4: Complications.

- Dehydration leading to hypovolemia and its resultant complications
- Electrolyte abnormalities, metabolic alkalosis
- Bacterial translocation from the bowel wall leading to sepsis
- Bowel edema and congestion leading to hypoperfusion
- Bowel perforation
- Aspiration due to repeated vomiting
- Respiratory embarrassment due to distended abdomen
- Bowel gangrene (in case of strangulated hernia/volvulus)

BOX 5: Differential diagnosis

Differential diagnosis	***Clues***
Medication adverse effects (diagnosis of exclusion)	Medication review (e.g., tricyclic antidepressants and narcotics)
Mesenteric ischemia	History of postprandial abdominal angina or peripheral vascular disease, hypercoagulable state, and cardiac diseases (atrial fibrillation and vegetation on valves)
Perforated viscus/intra-abdominal sepsis	Fever, leukocytosis, peritonitis, and pneumoperitoneum
Postoperative paralytic ileus	Recent abdominal surgery with no passage of flatus or bowel movement after surgery
Pseudo-obstruction (Ogilvie syndrome)	Acutely dilated large intestine, diabetes mellitus, history of intestinal dysmotility, and scleroderma

BOX 6: Investigations.

Hematology	• Complete metabolic panel, serum lactate levels, arterial blood gas (ABG) • Hypokalemic hypochloremic metabolic alkalosis (due to vomiting and fluid sequestration) • ↑ Blood urea nitrogen (BUN) hematocrit suggests dehydration • ↑ White blood cell (WBC) count sepsis/peritonitis • ↑ Lactate intestinal ischemia • Help to determine need for or urgency of surgical intervention
X-ray abdomen erect	• Air-fluid levels in a stepladder distribution, may be associated with minimal/absent gas and stool in the distal colon and rectum **(Fig. 1)** • *Sigmoid volvulus:* Hugely dilated colonic loop pointing toward the pelvis—coffee bean sign does not identify the etiology of obstruction **(Fig. 2)** • *Air under diaphragm:* Bowel perforation
Abdominal ultrasound	Limited utility due to dilated bowel loops with intestinal gas

Contd...

Contd...

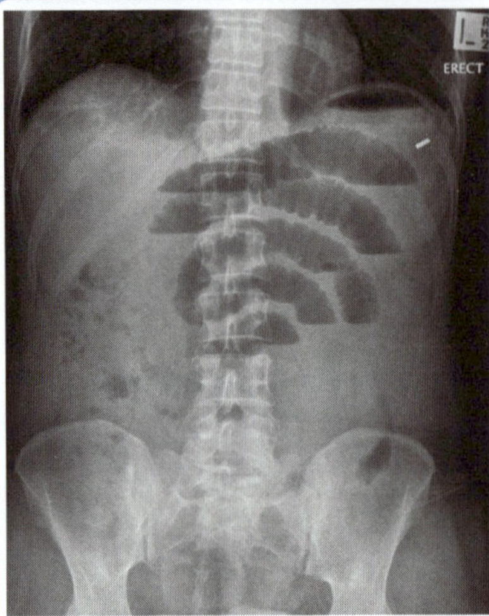

Fig. 1: Erect X-ray abdomen showing dilated small bowel loops (jejunum) with air-fluid level in a patient with intestinal obstruction.

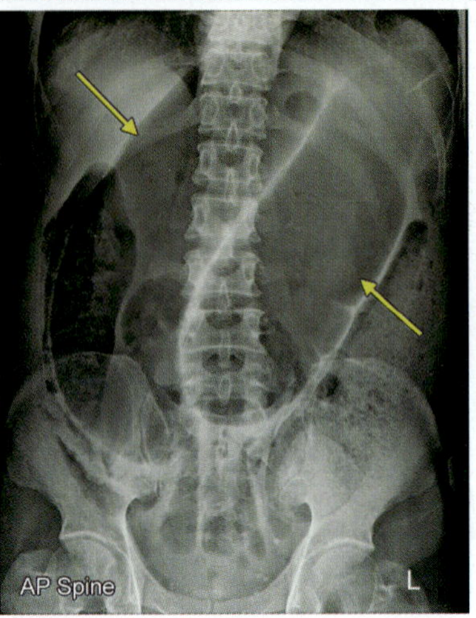

Fig. 2: X-ray abdomen supine showing hugely dilated sigmoid lops (arrows) with their apex pointing toward the pelvis suggestive of sigmoid volvulus.

Computed tomography (CT)	• Should be performed in all patients with clinical suspicion of intestinal obstruction (IO) can identify the etiology in most cases • If plain scan is suggestive IV contrast to be considered if renal function permits • Findings in patients with acute IO include intestinal dilation proximal to the site of obstruction, with collapsed bowel distally • Water soluble contrast can be administered orally/via RT can identify the zone of transition (the area where the bowel diameter changes from dilated to normal) • CT can identify most causes of IO and also assists in surgical planning wall thickening and poor flow of contrast into a segment of bowel and suggest ischemia, whereas pneumatosis intestinalis, pneumoperitoneum, and mesenteric fat stranding may suggest necrosis and perforation • CT with hypertonic enteric contrast can also help in resolving low grade IO especially in adhesive obstruction and postoperative situations
Enteroclysis	Involves intubation of the small bowel and rapidly administering a large volume of enteric contrast → used in subacute obstruction in stable patients to identify pathology

BOX 7: Management.

Medical management:

- *Stable patients:* In hemodynamically stable patients with an IO and a history of abdominal surgery, nonoperative management should be considered
- *Initial management:* For suspected acute IO, initiate intravenous isotonic fluid replacement and restrict oral intake
- *Nasogastric decompression:* Most patients will require nasogastric decompression
- *Electrolyte correction:* Aggressive correction of electrolytes is recommended after ensuring adequate renal function. Use bladder catheterization to monitor urine output and assess the adequacy of fluid resuscitation
- *Antibiotics:* Administer antibiotics to treat intestinal bacterial overgrowth and prevent bacterial translocation across the gut wall. Coverage should include gram-negative organisms and anaerobes, typically using a third-generation cephalosporin in combination with metronidazole
- *Oral contrast media:* In selected patients with adhesive or partial IO, oral hypertonic water-soluble contrast media may be therapeutic and assist in resolution, but consider the risk of vomiting and aspiration

Surgical management:

- *Exploratory laparotomy:* Recommended for patients who deteriorate clinically during hospitalization or for whom 35 days of nonoperative management is ineffective, due to the increasing risk of complications
- *Immediate surgery:* Required for patients showing signs of peritonitis, clinical instability, leukocytosis, leukopenia, or acidosis, which may indicate abdominal sepsis, ischemia, or perforation. Immediate surgery is also necessary for patients with irreducible or strangulated hernias
- *Elective hernia repair:* Schedule elective hernia repair for patients whose IO resolves after hernia reduction
- *Laparoscopy:* Suitable for initial exploration in most patients with uncomplicated or adhesive IO, offering benefits of earlier recovery and shorter hospital stay
- *Malignancy evaluation:* Stable patients with known or suspected intraabdominal malignancy should be evaluated for optimal surgical planning. Disseminated or advanced intra-abdominal malignancy causing multilevel obstruction is rarely treated operatively
- *Primary resection:* Isolated gastrointestinal or intraabdominal malignancy causing IO can be managed with primary resection and reconstruction
- *Palliative decompression:* For advanced or unresectable tumors, palliative decompression can be achieved surgically through diversion and/or insertion of venting and feeding tubes, or endoscopically with expandable stents placed by gastroenterologists

SUGGESTED READING

1. Di Saverio S, Coccolini F, Galati M, Smerieri N, Biffl WL, Ansaloni L, et al. Bologna guidelines for diagnosis and management of adhesive small bowel obstruction (ASBO): 2013 update of the evidence-based guidelines from the world society of emergency surgery ASBO working group. World J Emerg Surg. 2013;8(1):42.
2. Jackson P, Vigiola Cruz M. Intestinal obstruction: evaluation and management. Am Fam Physician. 2018;98(6):362-7.
3. Smith DA, Kashyap S, Nehring SM. Bowel Obstruction. In: StatPearls [Internet]. Treasure Island (FL): StatPearls Publishing; 2024.

4.6 ACUTE EMERGENCIES IN HERNIAS

Kayomars B Kapadia

BOX 1: Reasons for presentation to emergency room.

Complications of a hernia:
- Irreducibility
- Obstruction
- Strangulation
- Skin problems viz ulceration/skin necrosis in case of huge hernias

All obstructed hernia should be considered as strangulated unless proved otherwise.

BOX 2: Features of hernia complications.

- *Primarily hernia symptoms:* Swelling has suddenly become –
  - Painful
  - Increased in size
  - Tense
  - Skin redness
- *Secondary features due to Intestinal obstruction:*
  - Abdominal distension
  - Colicky abdominal pain
  - Vomiting
  - Constipation/obstipation

BOX 3: Clinical features.

General:
- Pulse may be normal or tachycardia may be present
- Features of dehydration due to vomiting may be present

Abdominal:
- Hernia swelling is irreducible and tender
- No impulse on coughing
- Tinkling bowel sounds in early stages and absent in late
- Scars of previous surgeries to be documented in case of incisional hernias
- Per rectum may be empty

BOX 4: Hernias that are likely to give rise to complications.

- Indirect inguinal hernias as compared to direct inguinal hernias
- Femoral, obturator hernias
- Incisional/ventral hernias with multiple loculations
- Narrow neck hernias

BOX 5: Investigations.

- Blood tests—complete blood count (CBC), creatinine, electrolytes, and blood sugar
- *Radiological:*
  - Chest X-ray to look for gas under diaphragm
  - Abdominal X-ray for features of obstruction
  - Ultrasound for vascularity (viability) of obstructed bowel loop
    - Fluid in hernia sac
    - To and fro peristalsis in bowel loop suggesting obstruction
  - Computed tomography (CT) scan with oral and intravenous (IV) contrast (if creatinine is normal) for:
    - Checking the viability of obstructed intestine
    - Those instances where there is a doubt whether the hernia is a cause of obstruction or an obstruction elsewhere in the intestine has simply made the hernia larger and painful

BOX 6: Treatment.

- Keep the patient nil-by-mouth (NBM)
- Ryles/nasogastric (NG) tube aspiration
- Urinary catheterization may be needed
- Analgesics—paracetamol/diclofenac (if no contraindications)/opioids
- IV fluids—Ringer lactate/dextrose normal saline (DNS)—dehydration to be treated aggressively
- Antibiotics for strangulated hernias
- As soon as an obstructed hernia is diagnosed
- Urgent surgical reference should be made
- Obstructed hernia if not released soon within 6–8 hours can lead to strangulation and gangrene of the intestine which may need bowel resection

SUGGESTED READING

1. Brunicardi FC, Andersen DK, Billiar TR, Dunn DL, Kao LS, Hunter JG, et al. Schwartz's Principles of Surgery, 11th edition. USA: McGraw Hill; 2019.
2. Doherty GM. Current Diagnosis & Treatment Surgery, 15th edition. India: McGraw Hill; 2020.
3. Townsend Jr CM. Sabiston Textbook of Surgery: The Biological Basis of Modern Surgical Practice, 19th edition. India: Elsevier-Health Sciences Division; 2021.
4. Williams NS. Bailey & Love's Short Practice of Surgery, 27th edition. UK: CRC Press; 2000.

4.7 DYSPEPSIA

Ajay B Jhaveri, Shweta Parekh

BOX 1: Introduction.

- Dyspepsia is a heterogenous group of symptoms located in the upper abdomen
- "Symptoms of peptic ulceration, reflux disease, and gastric dysmotility often overlap"

BOX 2: Definitions.

- *Dyspepsia:* Defined as discomfort centered in the upper abdomen characterized by abdominal fullness, early satiety, bloating, or nausea
- *Functional dyspepsia (Rome IV criteria):* Patients with one or more of the following symptoms including (1) bothersome postprandial fullness, (2) early satiation, (3) epigastric pain, and (4) epigastric burning for the previous 3 months with symptom onset at least 6 months prior are told to have functional dyspepsia, if they have no evidence of structural disease, including upper endoscopy that can explain their symptoms
- *Uninvestigated dyspepsia:* This group of patients has not yet undergone diagnostic investigations, and a specific diagnosis explaining their dyspeptic symptoms has not been established

BOX 3: Causes.

- *Gastrointestinal tract disorders:*
  - Peptic ulcer disease
  - Gastric or esophageal neoplasm
  - Gastroparesis
  - Irritable bowel syndrome
  - Malabsorption
  - Infiltrative disorders
- *Pancreatobiliary disorders:*
  - Cholelithiasis
  - Chronic pancreatitis
  - Pancreatic or gallbladder neoplasm
- *Systemic disorders:*
  - Diabetes mellitus
  - Thyroid and parathyroid disorders
  - Renal and heart failure
- *Drugs:*
  - Nonsteroidal anti-inflammatory drugs (NSAIDs)
  - Antibiotics
  - Steroids
  - Iron
  - Diuretics

BOX 4: Clinical history.

- *Onset:* Acute onset of dyspepsia indicates food intolerance, medications, and peptic ulcer disease
- *Age:* Age >45 years indicates more chances of organic cause of dyspepsia
- Recent change in character of chronic symptoms suggests organic cause of dyspepsia
- Alarming symptoms such as weight loss, bleeding, dysphagia, or protracted vomiting suggest organic etiology for dysphagia
- Associated with abdominal pain indicates pancreaticobiliary or infiltrative gastrointestinal disorders
- Medications and dietary history

BOX 5: Physical examination.

- Physical examination in patients with dyspepsia normally shows epigastric tenderness
- *Carnett's sign:* This clinical test helps distinguish between pain originating from the abdominal wall and pain due to inflammation of underlying viscera. If local tenderness increases during muscle tensing, it indicates abdominal wall pain (positive Carnett's sign). Conversely, if the pain decreases (negative Carnett's sign), it suggests that the pain originates from an intra-abdominal organ, as the tensed abdominal muscles provide protection to the viscera
- Pallor suggests organic cause for dyspepsia
- Signs of malabsorption syndrome in case of suspected chronic pancreatitis, a cause of dyspepsia
- Lymph nodes in left supraclavicular fossa suggest gastrointestinal tumor, a cause of dyspepsia
- Thorough abdominal examination to identify cause of dyspepsia

BOX 6: Diagnostic procedures.

- Usually diagnostic procedures are not required in all dyspeptic patients
- Age >45 years, alarming symptoms such as anorexia, weight loss, or anemia merits investigations to identify the cause of dyspepsia
- Routine biochemical tests, abdominal sonogram, and upper endoscopic evaluation are frequently ordered tests for patients with dyspepsia

BOX 7: Test and treat for *Helicobacter pylori*.

- The rationale for testing for *H. pylori* in patients with dyspepsia is based on the identification of *H. pylori* as a causative factor in peptic ulcer disease
- Tests for *H. pylori* infection include the urea breath test, stool antigen assay, or rapid urease test. Serologic testing is discouraged due to its low positive predictive value
- Patients who test positive for *H. pylori* infection should receive eradication therapy

BOX 8: Management.

Options for a patient who do not have risk factors for organic dyspepsia include the following:

- Do a diagnostic endoscopy
- Use noninvasive test for *H. pylori*
- Use empirical antisecretory medications

BOX 9: Management of functional dyspepsia.

Try following measures in patients with mild or intermittent symptoms:

- Reassurance and education are very essential
- Make a confident and positive diagnosis
- Eat small meals more frequently
- Avoid meals with high-fat content
- Discourage spicy food
- Reduce coffee consumption
- Avoid smoking and alcohol
- Avoid NSAID and aspirin
- Treat anxiety and depression if present

Drug therapy is recommended for patients with severe symptoms or those who do not respond to reassurance and lifestyle modifications

- *Acid suppression therapy:* A Cochrane review examined the efficacy of acid suppressants in treating functional dyspepsia. 12 randomized controlled trials comparing H2 antihistamines to placebo found these drugs to be effective. 10 trials assessing proton pump inhibitors (PPIs) also showed significant, though modest, benefit over placebo
- *H. pylori eradication:* While the benefit of eradication therapy is less pronounced in functional dyspepsia compared to peptic ulcer disease, it is still more effective than placebo
- Prokinetic agents can be tried with good safety record for patients with postprandial fullness and early satiation. Therapy with a single drug is preferable than combining PPI with prokinetic agent
- Low-dose tricyclic antidepressant can be tried in patients who fail above measures. High-dose tricyclic antidepressant can be tried, if they have features of anxiety or depression
- A referral to psychiatrist or psychologist should be arranged for patients with obvious coexisting psychiatric illness, a history of physical or sexual abuse

BOX 10: Newer drugs.

Drugs that can improve gastric fundal relaxation and that modify the visceral analgesia are newer concepts in the treatment of functional dyspepsia. Many of such drugs are still investigational drugs

BOX 11: Postprandial distress syndrome.

- *Diagnostic criteria*:* Must include one or both of the following:
  1. Bothersome postprandial fullness, occurring after ordinary-sized meals, many times per week
  2. Early satiation prevents finishing a regular meal, many times per week
- *Supportive criteria:*
  - Upper abdominal bloating or postprandial nausea or excessive belching
  - Epigastric pain syndrome may coexist

*Criteria to be fulfilled for the last 3 months with symptom onset at least 6 months prior to diagnosis.

BOX 12: Epigastric pain syndrome.

- *Diagnostic criteria*:* Must include all of the following:
  - Pain or burning localized to the epigastrium of moderate severity, at least once per week
  - Pain is intermittent
  - Pain is not generalized or localized to other abdominal or chest regions
  - Pain is not relieved by defecation or passage of flatus
  - Not fulfilling criteria for gallbladder and sphincter of Oddi disorders
- *Supportive criteria:*
  - Pain may be of a burning quality, but without a retrosternal component
  - Pain is commonly induced or relieved by ingestion of a meal, but may occur while fasting
  - Postprandial distress syndrome may coexist

*Criteria to fulfilled for the last 3 months with symptom onset at least 6 months prior to diagnosis.

SUGGESTED READING

1. Moayeddi P, Soo S, Deeks J, Delaney B, Innes M, Forman D. Pharmacological interventions for non-ulcer dyspepsia. Cochrane Database Syst Rev. 2006;4:CD001960.
2. Tack J, Bisschops R, Sarnelli G. Pathophysiology and treatment of functional dyspepsia. Gastroenterology. 2004;127:1239-55.
3. Tally NJ, American Gastroenterology Association. American Gastroenterological Association medical position statement: evaluation of dyspepsia. Gastroenterology. 2005;129:1753.

4.8 SEVERE CONSTIPATION

Manali Patel, Sachna P Shetty

BOX 1: Definition.

Constipation is diagnosed using the Rome criteria, which require the presence of two or more of the following symptoms: (1) Straining during at least 25% of bowel movements, (2) hard stools at least 25% of the time, (3) a sensation of incomplete evacuation at least 25% of the time, (4) fewer than three bowel movements per week, and (5) rarely having loose stools without the use of laxatives. These symptoms must persist for at least 3 months within the previous 6 months to be considered chronic constipation.

BOX 2: Differential diagnosis (Refer Chapter 1).

- Accurate history taking is essential for diagnosing constipation
- Determine the onset of symptoms
- Assess whether new medications, dietary supplements, reduced fiber or fluid intake, or changes in activity levels have been introduced
- Identify risk factors such as hypothyroidism, diabetes, pastabdominal surgeries, or frequent kidney stones, which might indicate hyperparathyroidism
- Investigate the patient's medical and family history to gain insights into the potential causes of constipation
- Most constipation cases are not emergencies and can be managed symptomatically on an outpatient basis
- Look for clues to more serious underlying cause, such as intestinal obstruction, especially when accompanied by alarming signs such as unexplained weight loss, rectal bleeding, unexplained iron deficiency anemia, or a family history of colon cancer, or ovarian cancer

BOX 3: Examination.

- Abdominal examination to check for distension, tenderness, and bowel sounds
- Perform an external and digital rectal examination
- Laboratories or imaging should only be considered if there is a suspicion of systemic involvement (refer to the bowel obstruction Chapter 4.5 for details)

BOX 4: Treatment.

If fecal impaction is detected during a rectal examination, it should be manually evacuated. Note that diarrhea does not exclude constipation, particularly in elderly and debilitated patients. After evacuation, continue with appropriate medications

Group	*Drugs*	*MOA onset*	*Dose*	*Caution*
Lubricant	Liquid paraffin	–	–	–
Bulk forming	Isabgol husk	12–72 hours	3.5 g three times a day	Bowel obstruction and bloating
	Methylcellulose	12–72 hours	2 g three times a day	–
Surface wetting agent	Docusate sodium	24–72 hours	100 mg/two times a day	Contact dermatitis
	Docusate calcium	24–72 hours	240 mg/day	
Osmotic laxative	Polyethylene glycol (PEG)	1–4 days	8.5–34 g	Nausea and bloating
	Lactulose	24–48 hours	10–20 g can go up to twice a day	Bloating flatulence
	Glycerin	15–60 minutes	2–3 g/PR suppository	Rectal irritation
	Magnesium sulfate	0.5–3 hours	10–20 g/up to twice a day	Watery stool, caution with renal insufficiency
Stimulant	Bisacodyl	6–10 hours	10–30 mg/po	Gastric irritation
		15–60 minutes	10 mg suppository PR	Rectal irritation
	Senna	6–12 hours	2–4 tab (up to 15 mg/day)	Melanosis coli
	Sodium picosulphate	10 mg/day	–	–
5HT 4 receptor antagonist	Prucalopride	6–12 hours	2 mg/day	Nausea, headache, and diarrhea

BOX 5: Caveats.

- Avoid phosphate enema in older adults, chronic kidney disease patients
- *Structural etiology (fissure, painful defecation):* Docusate (stool softener), mineral oil/glycerin or manual disimpaction (with adjunctive pain meds) if patient impacted with large volume of stools
- If medication or metabolic, treat the cause.

SUGGESTED READING

1. Bharucha AE, Dorn SD, Lembo A, Pressman A. American Gastroenterological Association Medical Position Statement on Constipation. Gastroenterology. 2013;144(1):211-7.
2. Drossman DA. The Functional Gastrointestinal Disorders and the Rome III Process. Gastroenterology. 2016;130(5):1377-90.
3. Lembo A, Camilleri M. (2023). Etiology and Evaluation of Chronic Constipation in Adults. [online] Available from Retrieved from https://www.uptodate.com/contents/etiology-and-evaluation-of-chronic-constipation-in-adults [Last accessed September, 2024].
4. Longstreth GF, Thompson WG, Chey WD, Houghton LA, Mearin F, Spiller RC. Functional bowel disorders. Gastroenterology. 2006;130(5):1480-91.
5. Mayo Clinic Staff. (2023). Constipation. [online] Available from https://www.mayoclinic.org/diseases-conditions/constipation/symptoms-causes/syc-20354253 [Last accessed September, 2024].
6. NIDDK. (2023). Definition and Facts for Constipation. [online] Available from https://www.niddk.nih.gov/health-information/digestive-diseases/constipation/definition-facts [Last accessed September, 2024].

4.9 SEVERE NAUSEA AND VOMITING

Ajay B Jhaveri, Shweta Parekh

BOX 1: Definitions.

- *Nausea:* Feeling of sickness with an inclination or impending desire to vomit
- *Vomiting* is a forceful expulsion of gastric contents due to contractions of gut and thoracoabdominal wall musculature
- *Retching:* Labored, abortive inspiratory movements with the glottis closed and expiratory contractions of the abdominal muscles, but no vomiting
- *Rumination:* Repeated return of small quantities of the food to the mouth, where it is chewed and swallowed again
- *Regurgitation:* Effortless expulsion of food from, or return of food to the mouth. The absence of a bitter acid taste helps to distinguish between regurgitation and vomiting

BOX 2: Causes.

- *Gastrointestinal disorders:* Peptic ulcer disease, bowel obstruction, gastroparesis, hepatitis, cholecystitis, appendicitis, pancreatitis, and gastroenteritis
- *Drugs:* NSAID, chemotherapeutic agents, digoxin, antibiotics, theophylline, and etc.
- Systemic illness
- Sepsis, myocardial infarction, renal failure, and electrolyte imbalance
- *Central nervous system:* Head trauma, raised intracranial pressure, epilepsy, stroke, meningitis, and motion sickness
- *Endocrine disorders:* Diabetes, Addison's disease, and thyrotoxicosis
- Psychogenic vomiting

BOX 3: Clinical history.

- *Onset:*
  - Acute onset vomiting indicates infections, drugs, toxins, head trauma, or visceral pain
  - Chronic vomiting indicates partial mechanical obstruction, motility disorders, endocrinopathy, metabolic disorders, brain tumor, or psychogenic cause
- *Relation to meals:*
  - Vomiting within 5 minutes after food indicates psychogenic vomiting
  - Vomiting >1 hour after food suggests gastroparesis or gastric outlet obstruction
  - Vomiting of materials eaten 12 hours before indicates gastric outlet obstruction or proximal small bowel obstruction
- *Time of day:*
  - Early morning vomiting indicates pregnancy, uremia, alcoholism or raised intracranial pressure
- *Associated abdominal pain:*
  - Relief of abdominal pain by vomiting suggests antral or small bowel obstruction
  - Vomiting has no effect on pancreatitis, appendicitis, or cholecystitis pain

Contd...

Contd...

- *Content of vomitus:*
  - Bilious vomiting excludes gastric outlet or proximal duodenal obstruction
  - Old food in the vomitus suggests gastric outlet obstruction or severe gastroparesis
  - Undigested food indicates achalasia or Zenker diverticulum
  - Presence of blood indicates peptic ulcer disease, malignancy, or portal hypertensive bleeding
  - Voluminous acidic vomiting suggests gastrinoma
  - Feculent odor indicates distal intestinal or colonic obstruction, bacterial overgrowth, or gastrocolic fistula
- *Projectile vomiting:*
  - Vomiting without hypersalivation or nausea indicates raised intracranial pressure or pyloric obstruction
- *Associated symptoms:*
  - Fever indicates systemic infection or inflammation
  - Weight loss indicates malignancy or gastric outlet obstruction. Patient with psychogenic vomiting usually maintains stable weight
  - Headache, altered mentation, convulsion, or diplopia indicates intracranial cause for vomiting
  - Vertigo, tinnitus, and deafness indicate vestibular dysfunction
  - Abdominal distension, abdominal pain, and constipation indicate small bowel obstruction
  - Prior abdominal surgery indicates mechanical obstruction or postgastrectomy status
  - History of nonsteroidal anti-inflammatory drugs

BOX 4: Physical examination.

- Assessment of Intravascular fluid loss
- Fever suggests inflammation or infection
- Loss of dental enamel in oral cavity examination suggests bulimia
- Icterus indicates hepatobiliary disease

BOX 5: Abdominal examination.

- Abdominal distension indicates ileus or intestinal obstruction
- Abdominal tenderness is noted in inflammation, infection, and luminal distension
- A succussion splash on side-to-side movement is found in gastric outlet obstruction and gastroparesis
- Look for any mass, hepatomegaly, or splenomegaly
- An absence of bowel sounds indicates ileus, whereas hyperactive, high-pitched bowel sounds with a distended abdomen suggests mechanical intestinal obstruction

BOX 6: Neurologic examination.

- Impaired mentation, focal neurological deficit, neck stiffness and papilledema suggest central nervous system disease
- Autonomic and peripheral neuropathy may be associated with gastrointestinal motility disorders

BOX 7: Diagnostic procedures.

- *Blood chemistry:*
  - Leukocytosis indicates inflammation, whereas anemia is due to either blood loss or chronic inflammation
  - Hypokalemia and elevated blood urea nitrogen with normal creatinine in patients with dehydration
  - Metabolic alkalosis may result from loss of hydrogen ions in the vomitus and contractions of the extracellular space from dehydration
  - Other endocrine and metabolic parameters in suspected cases
  - Amylase, lipase, and liver chemistry in suspected pancreatic or hepatobiliary disorders
- *Imaging studies:*
  - Plain radiograph of abdomen shows small intestinal air-fluid levels with absent colonic air suggests obstruction, while diffuse distension indicates ileus
  - Ultrasound abdomen or spiral CT abdomen for suspected hepatobiliary and pancreatic disorders
  - Contrast radiography of small intestine (barium meal follow through or enteroclysis) for partial obstruction; it may precipitate acute obstruction
- *Endoscopy study:*
  - Upper endoscopy for suspected gastric outlet obstruction. Biopsy can be obtained from suspicious lesions during endoscopic procedure. Retained food in absence of obstruction indicates gastroparesis, whereas excessive gastric contents without any food indicates Zollinger–Ellison syndrome
  - Colonoscopic examination with biopsy may be needed in suspected ileocecal tuberculosis or Crohn's disease causing luminal narrowing
- *Functional studies:*
  - Functional studies are required once luminal obstruction is excluded by either endoscopy or barium study
  - Gastroparesis is diagnosed by delayed emptying of either solid (99mTC–sulfur colloids in eggs) or liquid (111In-DTPA in water) on scintigraphy
  - Electrogastrography (EGG) measures electrical pace-maker activity of the stomach through electrodes affixed to the abdomen
  - Antroduodenal manometry for suspected intestinal pseudo-obstruction

BOX 8: Management.

- Intravenous fluid resuscitation is the most important in patients with moderate-to-severe dehydration secondary to vomiting
- Threshold for hospitalization should be lower in chronic debilitating patients and very young or old patients
- Medical management for vomiting should be directed at the underlying illness
- Many patients benefit from medications that suppress vomiting (antiemetic and prokinetic agents)

BOX 9: Drugs.

<table>
<tr><td rowspan="4">Central antiemetic agents</td><td>Dopamine D2 receptor antagonist</td><td>Metoclopramide, promethazine, and prochlorperazine</td><td>Migraine-associated nausea, postoperative nausea and vomiting and chemotherapy, and radiotherapy-induced nausea and vomiting</td></tr>
<tr><td>Antihistamines and anticholinergics</td><td>Cyclizine, meclizine, and cinnarizine</td><td>Vestibular mediated nausea, motion sickness</td></tr>
<tr><td>Antimuscarinic</td><td>Scopolamine</td><td>Vestibular mediated nausea, motion sickness</td></tr>
<tr><td>Selective serotonin antagonist</td><td>Ondansetron, granisetron, and dolasetron</td><td>Nausea and vomiting associated with radiotherapy or chemotherapy, following surgery or gastroenteritis</td></tr>
<tr><td rowspan="2">Peripheral prokinetic agents</td><td>Serotonin 5HT4 receptor agonists</td><td>Cisapride, cinitapride, and tegaserod</td><td rowspan="2">Acute nausea and vomiting associated with gastroparesis (diabetic, postsurgical, or idiopathic), to clear the stomach of retained food, secretions, and blood from the stomach before doing upper endoscopy</td></tr>
<tr><td>Motilin receptor agonist</td><td>Erythromycin</td></tr>
</table>

SUGGESTED READING

1. American Gastroenterological Association. American Gastroenterological Association medical position statement: Nausea and vomiting. Gastroenterology. 2001;120:261.
2. Hasler WL, Chey WD. Nausea and vomiting. Gastroenterology. 2003;125:1860.
3. Scorza K, Williams A, Phillips JD, Shaw J. Evaluation of nausea and vomiting. Am Fam Physician. 2007;76:76.

4.10 HEPATIC DISEASES IN EMERGENCIES AND GASTROINTESTINAL BLEED

Ravi S Shah, Aabha Nagral

BOX 1: Definition.

Acute liver failure (ALF) is a well-defined medical emergency which is defined as a severe liver injury, leading to:
- Coagulation abnormality [international normalized ratio (INR) ≥1.5] after correction with vitamin K
- Encephalopathy

In a patient without preexisting liver disease and development of encephalopathy within 12 weeks of jaundice

BOX 2: Common causes of acute liver failure.

Viral hepatitis:
- Hepatitis A, B, and E (hepatotropic viruses)
- Dengue virus
- Cytomegalovirus

Drug-induced liver injury:
- Antituberculosis drugs (isoniazid, rifampicin, and pyrazinamide)
- Paracetamol (in high doses)
- Antibacterials (dapsone, sulfonamides, and cotrimoxazole)
- Nonsteroidal anti-inflammatory drugs (NSAIDs)
- Antiepileptic drugs (aromatic)
- Antiretroviral dugs
- Complementary and alternative medications

Pregnancy:
- Hepatitis E virus
- Acute fatty liver of pregnancy
- Preeclampsia
- HELLP (hemolysis, elevated liver enzymes, and low platelet count) syndrome

Toxins:
- Yellow phosphorus (aluminum phosphide and rat poison)
- Amanita phyllodes (mushroom poisoning)

Others:
- Budd-Chiari syndrome
- Autoimmune hepatitis
- Wilson disease
- Ischemic hepatitis
- Hemophagocytic lymphohistiocytosis
- Extensive malignant infiltration of liver

BOX 3: Baseline laboratory tests to be performed in a patient with acute liver failure.

- Complete blood count (CBC)
- Liver profile
- Blood sugar
- Renal profile
- Coagulation profile [prothrombin time (PT)/partial thromboplastin time (PTT)/ INR/thromboelastography (TEG)] amongst a few
- Serum lipase
- Arterial blood sample for arterial blood gas (ABG) with lactate and ammonia level
- Urine routine and culture
- Blood culture set (BACTEC plus if patient has received prior antibiotics)
- Abdominal ultrasound with Doppler examination
- Chest X-ray
- Electrocardiogram
- Two-dimensional echocardiogram (2 D Echo)

BOX 4: The King's College criteria (used to determine consideration for liver transplantation).

King's College Hospital indicators of a poor prognosis in ALF

Acetaminophen:
- Arterial pH <7.25 >24 hours after drug ingestion or
- All of the following:
  - Prothrombin time >100 seconds or INR >6.5
  - Serum creatinine level >3.4 mg/dL (300 μmol/L) or anuria
  - Grade 3–4 encephalopathy

Nonacetaminophen:
- Prothrombin time >100 seconds or INR >6.5 or
- Any three of the following:
  - Unfavorable etiology (seronegative hepatitis or drug reaction)
  - Age <10 or >40 years
  - Duration of jaundice to encephalopathy >7 days
  - Serum bilirubin level >17.5 mg/dL (300 μmol/L)
  - Prothrombin time >50 seconds or INR >3.5

BOX 5: The dynamic ALFED score to assess and stratify patients with ALF for viral causes.

ALFED model		
Predictors of mortality	***Score on admission***	***Score on Day 3***
Hepatic encephalopathy grade ≥2	1	2
INR ≥5	1	1
Arterial ammonia ≥123 mmol/L	1	2
Serum bilirubin ≥15 mg/dL	1	1

Those with a score of 1–3 had a survival probability of about 80% or more, and those with ≥4 had a mortality risk of >80%.

(ALFED: acute liver failure early dynamic)

BOX 6: West haven criteria for semi-quantitative grading of mental state.

Grade	***Criteria***
1	• Trivial lack of awareness • Euphoria or anxiety • Shortened attention span • Impaired performance of addition
2	• Lethargy or apathy • Minimal disorientation of time or place • Subtle personality changes • Inappropriate behavior
3	• Somnolence to semistupor but responsive to verbal stimuli • Confusion • Gross disorientation
4	• Coma (unresponsive to verbal or noxious stimuli)

BOX 7: Clinical indications to determine urgent transfer to the intensive care unit.

- Hepatic encephalopathy grade 2 and higher or difficulty to manage the patient in the ward
- *Hypotension:* Mean arterial pressure (MAP) <60 mm Hg after adequate fluid resuscitation
- Oliguria despite fluid resuscitation
- Oxygen requirement >6 L/min to maintain SpO_2 >95
- Recurrent hypoglycemia

(SpO_2: peripheral oxygen saturation)

BOX 8: Management.

- *Ventilation:*
  - Intubation if grade three-fourths encephalopathy or if poor Glasgow Coma Scale (GCS)- to protect airway
  - Minimize tactile stimuli, dim ambient light, and avoid unnecessary neck rotation
- *Hemodynamics:*
  - Fluid replacement (Use plasmalyte and avoid Ringer lactate)
  - Use of inotropes when needed
  - Avoid hypervolemia
- *Renal dysfunction:*
  - Early initiation of CRRT (continuous renal replacement therapy)
- *Raised intracranial pressure:*
  - Keep head end elevated (30–40°)
  - Target sodium level: 145–155 mEq/L (Use of hypertonic saline—3% NS)
- Maintain ammonia <100 μg/mL with CRRT
- *Coagulopathy:*
  - Transfusion of blood products indicated only if clinical evidence of bleeding or any invasive procedure planned
  - Thromboelastogram (TEG)-based blood product therapy is recommended
  - Prophylactic correction of deranged coagulation can increase risk of thrombosis and volume overload
    - *Infection:* Broad-spectrum antibiotics and antifungals
- *Electrolyte balance:*
  - Hyponatremia, hypo/hyperkalemia should be aggressively corrected
  - Monitor ionized calcium if citrate-based anticoagulation used in CRRT
    - *Hypoglycemia:* Maintenance of euglycemia (140–180 mg/dL) is of utmost importance
- *Nutrition:*
  - Early enteral feeding is recommended
  - Ideal calorie intake 25–30 kcal/kg/day with protein intake 1.2–1.5 g/kg/day
- *General care:*
  - IV N-acetyl cysteine (NAC) in all cases—benefit only during early stages of encephalopathy
  - Anticonvulsants if seizure
  - Lactulose to ensure adequate bowel movements
  - Avoid enema—increased tendency of bleed
  - Deep venous thrombosis (DVT) prophylaxis
  - Pressure sores/skin peels should be looked for and taken care of
- *Extracorporeal liver assist systems:*
  - Therapeutic plasma exchange (TPE)
  - Molecular adsorbent recirculating system (MARS)
  - Extracorporeal albumin dialysis

  Note: Used mainly as a bridge to transplant in those meeting liver transplant listing criteria.
- *Liver transplantation:*
  - Patients who fulfill King's college/ALFED criteria

BOX 9: Immediate evaluation on arrival in the emergency room (ER).

- Sensorium
- Pupils
- Reflexes
- Vital parameters
- HGT
- ABG with lactate

GASTROINTESTINAL (GI) BLEED

BOX 10: Definitions.

- *Hematemesis:* Vomitus of red blood or "coffee-ground" materials
- *Melena:* Black, tarry, and foul-smelling stool. The black, tarry character of melena is caused by degradation of blood in the more proximal intestine including proximal colon
- *Hematochezia:* Passage of bright red or maroon blood per rectum
- Upper GI bleeding is bleeding from above the ligament of Treitz
- *Obscure GI bleed:* Overt GI bleeding where bidirectional endoscopy (upper endoscopy and colonoscopy) does not show an etiology of bleeding
- *Occult GI bleed:* Identification of GI bleeding in the absence of overt bleeding by special examination of the stool (e.g., guaiac testing)

BOX 11: Causes.

Upper GI Bleed:

- Peptic ulcer disease (PUD)
- Variceal bleeding related to portal hypertension
- Mallory–Weiss tear
- Portal hypertensive gastropathy
- Esophagitis or Esophageal erosion
- Arteriovenous malformation
- Duodenitis/gastritis/erosions
- Esophagogastric tumors
- Aortoduodenal fistula
- Dieulafoy's lesion

Lower GI bleed (originating in the lower GI tract):

- Hemorrhoids
- Inflammatory bowel disease
- Neoplasm
- Vascular ectasia
- Diverticular disease
- Ischemic or radiation colitis
- Colonic ulceration

Contd...

Contd...

Obscure GI bleed:
- Small bowel vascular ectasia
- Small bowel adenocarcinoma
- Small bowel stomal tumor (GIST, gastrointestinal stomal tumor)
- Meckel's diverticulum
- Ectopic varices
- Hemobilia
- Aortoenteric fistula

Occult GI bleed:
- Gastrointestinal cancer
- Crohn's disease
- Vascular ectasia
- Dieulafoy's lesion
- Worm infestation
- Gastrointestinal ulcer (at any site) colopathy
- Portal hypertensive gastropathy or colopathy

BOX 12: Initial assessment and resuscitation.

Hemodynamics	***% Blood loss***	***Bleeding type***
Normal	<10%	Minor
Postural hypotension or postural tachycardia	10–20%	Moderate
Shock (resting hypotension)	20–25%	Severe

- Intensive care admission is indicated in hemodynamically unstable patients
- Oxygen supplementation
- Close monitoring of vital signs and urine output
- Send CBC, blood grouping for crossmatching
- Secure large bore IV access and start IV fluids as soon as patient arrives to ER
- *The threshold for blood transfusion:* Hemoglobin (Hb) level of around 7.0 g/dL. Transfusion should be performed if patients with significant comorbidities (e.g., ischemic cardiovascular disease)

BOX 13: Clinical history.

Attention should turn to the clinical history only once the patient's hemodynamics is stabilized.

- *Hematemesis:*
  - Hematemesis indicates source of bleeding above the ligament of Treitz
  - Fresh blood or altered blood or "coffee-color" materials
  - Frequency and quantity are most important
  - Hematemesis of >500 mL is called severe hematemesis
- *Melena:*
  - Melena indicates that blood has been present in gastrointestinal tract for 12–14 hours
  - At least 60 mL of blood is required to produce melena
  - Black, tarry, and foul-smelling stool is due to degradation of blood in the GI tract
  - Melena indicates bleeding is from proximal source including the ascending colon
- *Hematochezia*: Hematochezia usually represents lower source of GI bleeding. Hematochezia also occurs in upper GI lesion when bleeding is very brisk and intestinal transit is fast—this will usually cause hemodynamic instability
- Recent history of NSAIDs, alcohol, or corrosive ingestion
- History of excess retching indicates Mallory–Weiss tear
- Symptoms of volume contraction such as dry mouth, dizziness, headache, decreased urine output, and postural syncope

BOX 14: Diagnosis.

- Upper GI bleeding is broadly divided into either variceal bleeding (bleeding secondary to portal hypertension) or nonvariceal bleeding (bleeding secondary to PUD, neoplasm, angiodysplasia, or erosions)
- Nasogastric lavage does not give any etiological clue for upper GI bleeding (UGIB). Thus, primary use of the nasogastric lavage to assess bleeding activity is discouraged. Lavage may help in clearing the stomach for better visualization during endoscopy. Room temperature fluid preferable for lavage

Blood chemistry:

- CBC
- Renal function test
- Liver function tests
- Coagulation parameters

Upper endoscopy: Early endoscopy (defined as endoscopy within 24 hours of patient hospital presentation) is recommended. Early endoscopy has been shown to reduce resource use, reduce hospital stay and decrease transfusion requirements

Colonoscopy:

- Colonoscopy is the best test for confirming the source of lower gastrointestinal bleeding
- Various therapeutic interventions are possible with colonoscopy; therefore, it is the most cost-effective approach to patients with lower GI bleeding

Angiography: Angiography detects bleeding with a rate of >0.5 mL/min. It also offers therapeutic possibilities such as pharmacologic vasoconstriction or selective microembolization. Usually performed for obscure GI bleed

BOX 15: Management.

Management of nonvariceal bleeding:

- *Pharmacotherapy:*
  - PPI (proton pump inhibitors) is the most important pharmacological therapy for bleeding peptic ulcer. If gastric pH is maintained above 6 by PPI, platelet aggregation is optimized and fibrinolysis relatively inhibited, leading to clot stability at an ulcer site
  - PPI bolus dose is equivalent to an infusion
- *Endoscopic injection therapy:* Major endoscopic injection therapy in patient with nonvariceal UGIB is injection of a dilute epinephrine (1:10,000)
- Endoscopic thermal therapies
- Mechanical methods (hemoclips)
- Combination of two modalities is recommended (e.g., injection therapy + thermal treatment)

Management of acute variceal bleeding:

- *Pharmacotherapy:*
  - Vasoactive agents such as terlipressin, vasopressin, somatostatin, and octreotide are used in patients with bleeding related to portal hypertension
  - If no cardiac history, a bolus dose of 1 mg IV terlipressin is advisable
- *Endotherapy:*
  - Endoscopic sclerotherapy (EST) and endoscopic variceal band ligation (EVL) are two methods to control the acute esophageal variceal bleeding and prevent rebleeding. EVL is the preferred method nowadays
  - Use of Sengstaken–Blakemore tube/Danis–Ella stent when appropriate
- *Transjugular intrahepatic portosystemic shunt (TIPS):* It is indicated in situations when bleeding varices are refractory to medical therapy. Efficacy of TIPS to control the bleeding is 95%
- *Surgery:* It is only indicated when endotherapy fails and TIPS is not available
- *BRTO (balloon-occluded retrograde transvenous obliteration):* Transvenous obliteration by instilment of sclerosants and/or liquid embolic agents into a gastro-/splenorenal collateral through the left renal vein aided by balloon occlusion
- *Balloon tamponade:* Balloon tamponade with a Sengstaken–Blakemore tube successfully achieves hemostasis in 90% of cases of bleeding varices, but it has a high recurrence rate for rebleeding once the balloon is deflated. Thus, balloon should be reserved as a rescue procedure, so that patients are stabilized for a more definitive therapy

Management of lower GI bleed:

- *Endotherapy:* Endoscopic hemostasis methods include injection therapy (epinephrine or saline), heater probe therapy, monopolar and multipolar electrocoagulation, argon plasma coagulation, hemoclip, and band ligation
- *Angiography:* Intra-arterial infusion of vasopressin or superselective embolization with various agents (gelatin sponge, microcoils, and polyvinyl alcohol particles)
- Surgery

SUGGESTED READING

1. de Franchis R, Baveno V Faculty. Expanding consensus in portal hypertension. Report of the Baveno VI Consensus Workshop: stratifying risk and individualizing care for portal hypertension. J Hepatol. 2015;63:743-52.
2. Feinman M, Haut ER. Upper gastrointestinal bleeding. Surg Clin North Am. 2014;94:43-53.
3. Garber A, Jang S. Novel therapeutic strategies in the management of non-variceal upper gastrointestinal bleeding. Clin Endosc. 2016:49:421-4.
4. Garcia-Tsao G, Abraldes JG, Berzigotti A, Bosch J. Portal hypertensive bleeding in cirrhosis: Risk stratification, diagnosis, and management: 2016 practice guidance by the American Association for the Study of Liver Diseases. Hepatology. 2017:65:310-35.
5. Garcia-Tsao G, Sanyal AJ, Grace ND, Carey W. Prevention and management of gastroesophageal varices and variceal hemorrhage in cirrhosis. Hepatology. 2007;46:922-38.
6. Groszmann RJ, Garcia-Tsao G, Bosch J, Grace ND, Burroughs AK, Planas R, et al. Beta-blockers to prevent gastroesophageal varices in patients with cirrhosis. N Engl J Med. 2005;353:2254-61.
7. Khamaysi I, Gralnek IM. Acute upper gastrointestinal bleeding (UGIB) initial evaluation and management. Best Pract Res Clin Gastroenterol. 2013:27:633-8.
8. Mehta G, Abraldes JG, Bosch J. Developments and controversies in the management of oesophageal and gastric varices. Gut. 2010;59:701-5.

4.11 ESOPHAGEAL EMERGENCIES

Ravi S Shah, Rajesh Sainani

BOX 1: Causes.

Cause of perforation	***Description***
Iatrogenic	• Intraluminal therapies • Upper gastrointestinal (GI) endoscopy • Esophageal stricture dilatation • Endoscopic variceal ligation • Intraoperative trauma
Boerhaave's syndrome	"Spontaneous", associated with transient rise in intraesophageal pressure
Trauma	• Penetrating injury • Blunt trauma (rare) • Corrosive ingestion
Foreign body	• Includes pill esophagitis
Tumor	• Intrinsic/extrinsic tumor
Aortic pathology	• Aortic aneurysm • Aberrant right subclavian artery

BOX 2: Clinical features.

- *Cervical perforation:* Neck pain, dysphagia, hoarseness, dysphonia, or subcutaneous emphysema. Systemic signs are less common
- *Intrathoracic perforation:* Sudden-onset chest pain is the main sign. The pain may radiate to the back or the left shoulder or may be accompanied by vomiting and shortness of breath
- *Intra-abdominal perforation:* Acute-onset severe epigastric pain, hematemesis, or melena
- *Associated symptoms:* Dyspnea, tachycardia, and cervical subcutaneous emphysema

BOX 3: Diagnosis.

- Obtain intravenous (IV) contrast computed tomography (CT) of the neck or chest
- Upper GI Endoscopy has a sensitivity of 95–100%, and specificity of 90–100%
- Esophagography should be performed with water-soluble contrast material initially (i.e., Gastrografin) to localize the site of perforation

BOX 4: Management.

- Nill per orally
- IV hydration with isotonic saline or Ringer's lactate solution
- To involve surgical consultant once the diagnosis is made
- To resuscitate the patient from shock
- To administer broad-spectrum IV antibiotics (ampicillin/sulbactam (3 g every 6 hours), piperacillin/tazobactam (3.375 g every 6 hours), or a carbapenem
- Endoscopy-related perforation can be treated endoscopically by primary closure with clips or suturing devices, endoscopic stenting, or endoscopic vacuum therapy
- Nonendoscopic perforations will need emergency surgery

FOREIGN BODY IMPACTION

BOX 5: Pathophysiology.

- *Children:* Children (from 1.5 years to 4 years of age) and with psychiatric disorders are the most common cases. Small objects, such as coins, crayons, and toys typically lodge in the proximal esophagus (anatomically narrowed part)
- *Adults:* Fish or chicken bone, toothpicks, or dentures are the common foreign bodies
  - Commonly seen in those with esophageal disease, dementia, prisoners, and psychiatric patients
  - Foreign body impactions usually occur above a stricture, Schatzki ring, or eosinophilic esophagitis

BOX 6: Clinical features.

- *Children:*
  - Refusal or inability to eat, vomiting, gagging and choking, stridor, neck or throat pain, and drooling
  - For unwitnessed ingestions in children (<2 years of age), high degree of suspicion is necessary
  - *Physical examination:* Airway, nasopharynx, oropharynx, neck, and chest should also be examined (which are often unremarkable). A foreign body can be directly visualized in the oropharynx occasionally
- *Adults:*
  - Retrosternal chest pain, foreign body sensation
  - Dysphagia, vomiting, choking, or odynophagia
  - Coughing or aspiration can occur if the patient tries to wash down the object with liquid or if secretions pool proximal to the obstruction
- *Complication:*
  - Airway obstruction, stricture, or perforation
  - Perforation can be secondary to the result of direct mechanical erosion (bones) or chemical corrosion (button batteries)

BOX 7: Diagnosis.

- History of type of foreign body, time of ingestion, current symptoms, and location of foreign body help decide management
- *X-ray:* Done in patients who don't have symptoms of complete esophageal obstruction such as drooling of saliva, inability to swallow liquids—anteroposterior and lateral views are used for screening radiopaque objects or coins. Food boluses are not usually visible
- *Upper GI endoscopy:* Can be directly done if obstruction is suspected in the esophagus. Patients with esophageal symptoms should undergo endoscopy even if radiological imaging is negative. If the foreign body has passed into the stomach decision is based on size of object, shape, edges, and content
- *CT scan:* It can localize the exact location of the foreign body and is usually done if perforation is suspected

BOX 8: Treatment.

- *Endoscopy:*
  - Patients who have airway compromise are resuscitated and require active airway management
  - Objects >2.5 cm in diameter and >5–6 cm in length will not pass the pylorus and will require removal by endoscopy
  - *Emergency endoscopy:*
    - Ingestion of sharp or elongated objects (toothpicks)
    - *Ingestion of button batteries:* Having a high risk of perforation
    - Ingestion of multiple foreign bodies
    - Signs of perforation
    - Object-like coin at the level of the cricopharynx in children
    - Compromised airway
    - Presence of a foreign body for >24 hours
    - Magnets
- *Laryngoscopy:*
  - In stable patients, indirect laryngoscopy using a fiberoptic scope can be used to remove the very proximal objects
  - For distal objects, imaging studies are useful for defining the location
- *Expectant treatment:*
  - If the object is distal to the pylorus and is in benign shape and patient is comfortable, who is tolerating oral intake, the treatment is expectant
  - For other foreign bodies that are in the more distal GI tract, consulting the surgeon may be necessary
- *Glucagon:* For distal esophageal foreign bodies, glucagon (1–2 mg) IV in adults relaxes the lower sphincter and allows the passage of the object into the stomach

DYSPHAGIA

BOX 9: Definition.

- It is a subjective sensation of difficulty in swallowing
- If there is a difficulty with the initiation of a swallow, it is suggestive of as oropharyngeal dysphagia and if solids or liquids are obstructed in their passage from the mouth to the stomach, it is suggestive of esophageal dysphagia

BOX 10: Types.

- *Oropharyngeal dysphagia (transfer dysphagia):*
  - Difficulty in the passage of food from the mouth to the esophagus
  - Occurs due to either mechanical or neuromuscular disorders that affect the pharynx and upper esophageal sphincter (UES).
  - Dysphagia occurs within the first few seconds of swallowing and may be associated with cough, nasal twang, nasal regurgitation, dysarthria, or hoarseness of voice.
- *Esophageal dysphagia:*
  - Difficulty in the passage of a bolus from the upper esophagus to the stomach
  - Occurs due to either mechanical or neuromuscular disorders that affect the esophageal body.
  - Patients can initiate the swallowing but complain of difficulty in transporting food down the esophagus.

BOX 11: Common causes.

Oropharyngeal dysphagia: • Retropharyngeal abscess • Zenker's diverticulum • Cricopharyngeal bar • Cervical esophagus	*Mechanical obstruction:* • Benign stricture • Neoplasm • Webs and rings • Vascular compression
Neuromuscular disorders: • Cerebrovascular stroke • Parkinson's disease • Motor neuron disease • Polymyositis • Myasthenia gravis	*Motility disorders:* • Achalasia cardia • Distal esophageal spasm • Hypercontractile esophagus • Scleroderma • Chagas disease
Miscellaneous: • Sjogren syndrome • Alzheimer disease • Eosinophilic esophagitis	*Miscellaneous:* • Diabetes • Gastroesophageal reflux • Mediastinal abnormality

BOX 12: Differences between motor and mechanical dysphagia

Character	***Motor***	***Mechanical***
Course	Intermittent	Progressive
To what	Solid/liquid at onset	Initially to solid, then both
Duration	Long	Short in malignancy
Regurgitation	Common	Uncommon
Relation to temperature	Cold precipitates, hot reduces	No relation
Relation to posture	Reduce with maneuvers	Absent
Weight loss	Absent/minimal	Marked

BOX 13: Major tests for evaluating dysphagia.

- *Oropharyngeal dysphagia:* Major role of an ER physician is to address the complaints of dysphagia which can be disturbing for the patient and help with an appropriate diagnosis.
  - *Initial assessment:*
    - History
    - Physical examination including detailed neurological examination
    - Laboratory testing to exclude Cushing's, thyrotoxicosis, myasthenia gravis, myopathy, and multiple sclerosis
    - CNS imaging
  - Video fluoroscopy (modified barium swallow)
  - Nasopharyngeal laryngoscopy
  - *Fiberoptic endoscopic evaluation of swallowing (FEES):*
    - Upper GI endoscopy
    - UES/pharyngeal high-resolution manometry (HRM)
- *Esophageal dysphagia:*
  - Barium swallow
  - Upper GI endoscopy
  - HRM esophageal manometry

BOX 14: Management of dysphagia.

- *Oropharyngeal:* Management of oropharyngeal dysphagia is directed towards the etiology.
  - Swallowing rehabilitation and reeducation by the speech pathologist
  - Nutrition and dietary modifications with the aim to maintain body weight
  - *Alternative nutritional support:* Nasogastric tube placement/percutaneous endoscopic gastrostomy (PEG) tube insertion
- *Esophageal dysphagia:* Management of esophageal dysphagia is directed towards the etiology.

SUGGESTED READING

1. Aiolfi A, Ferrari D, Riva CG, Toti F, Bonitta G, Bonavina L. Esophageal foreign bodies in adults: systematic review of the literature. Scand J Gastroenterol. 2018;53(10-11):1171-8.
2. Anderson KL, Dean AJ. Foreign bodies in the gastrointestinal tract and anorectal emergencies. Emerg Med Clin North Am. 2011;29(2):369-400.
3. Bekkerman M, Sachdev AH, Andrade J, Twersky Y, Iqbal S. Endoscopic management of foreign bodies in the gastrointestinal tract: a review of the literature. Gastroenterol Res Pract. 2016;2016:8520767.
4. Blackwell Z, Little Johns P. A review of the management of dysphagia: a South African perspective. J Neurosci Nurs. 2010;42:61-70.
5. Chen CL, Orr WC. Comparison of esophageal motility in patients with solid dysphagia and mixed dysphagia. Dysphagia. 2005;20:261-5.
6. Cook IJ, Kahrilas PJ. AGA technical review on management of oropharyngeal dysphagia. Gastroenterology. 1999;16:455-78.

7. Kupeli M, Dogan A. Successful treatment of a late diagnosed esophageal perforation with mediastinitis and pericardial abscess. J Coll Physicians Surg Pak. 2018;28(12):972-3.
8. Lind CD. Dysphagia: Evaluation and treatment. Gastroenterology Clin North Am. 2003;32:553-75.
9. Malik SA, Qureshi IA, Muhammad R. Diagnostic accuracy of plain x-ray lateral neck in the diagnosis of cervical esophageal foreign bodies keeping oesophagoscopy as gold standard. J Ayub Med Coll Abbottabad. 2018;30(3): 386-8.
10. Spechler SJ. AGA technical review on treatment of patients with dysphagia caused by benign disorders of the distal esophagus. Gastroenterology. 1999;117: 233-54.
11. Watkins JR, Farivar AS. Endoluminal therapies for esophageal perforations and leaks. Thorac Surg Clin. 2018;28(4):541-54.
12. White RK, Morris DM. Diagnosis and management of esophageal perforations. Am Surg. 1992;58(2):112-9.
13. Younes Z, Johnson DA. The spectrum of spontaneous and iatrogenic esophageal injury: perforations, Mallory-Weiss tears, and hematomas. J Clin Gastroenterol. 1999;29(4):306-17.

CHAPTER 5

Renal and Urology Emergencies

5.1 ACUTE KIDNEY INJURY

Madan M Bahadur, Ashay Shingare

BOX 1: Acute kidney injury definition.

Kidney disease: Improving Global Outcomes (KDIGO) staging of acute kidney injury		
Stage	***Serum creatinine***	***Urine output***
1	1.5–1.9 times baseline Or ≥0.3 mg/dL (>26.5 µmol/L) increase	<0.5 mL/kg/h for 6–12 hours
2	2.0–2.9 times baseline	<0.5 mL/kg/h for ≥12 hours
3	3.0 times baseline Or Increase in serum creatinine to ≥4.0 mg/dL (353.6 µmol/L) Or Initiation of renal replacement therapy Or In patients <18 years, decrease in estimated glomerular filtration rate (eGFR) to <35 mL/min per 1.73 m^2	<0.3 mL/kg/h for ≥24 hours Or Anuria for ≥12 hours

BOX 2: Causes of acute kidney injury.

Prerenal:
- *Hypovolemia:* Hemorrhage, gastrointestinal losses from vomiting, and diarrhea
- *Decreased effective circulating volume:* Congestive cardiac failure, liver failure, and nephrotic syndrome
- *Systemic vasodilatation:* Sepsis and anaphylaxis
- *Afferent arteriolar vasoconstriction:* Nonsteroidal anti-inflammatory drugs (NSAIDs), hepatorenal syndrome, radiocontrast, and hypercalcemia
- *Efferent arteriolar vasodilation:* Angiotensin-converting enzyme inhibitors (ACEi) and angiotensin receptor blockers (ARBs)

Intrinsic renal:
- *Acute tubular injury:* Ischemic and nephrotoxic (aminoglycosides, amphotericin, cisplatin, ifosfamide, radiocontrast, intravascular hemolysis, and rhabdomyolysis)
- *Acute interstitial nephritis:* Drugs, infections, and autoimmune diseases
- *Glomerular diseases:* Acute glomerulonephritis and hemolytic uremic syndrome
- *Intratubular obstruction:* Paraproteins, crystals, and tumor lysis syndrome
- *Vascular:* Renal artery thrombosis, renal vein thrombosis, and atheroembolic disease

Postrenal:
- *Intrinsic:* Bilateral urolithiasis, bladder outlet obstruction, and neurogenic bladder
- *Extrinsic:* Retroperitoneal fibrosis, metastatic cancer, and postradiation obstruction

BOX 3: Evaluation.

History and physical examination:
- Diarrhea, vomiting, fever, edema, oliguria, and hematuria
- Drug intake and contrast exposure
- Hypotension, tachycardia, dehydration, or fluid overload

Laboratory evaluation:
- Urine analysis
- Blood urea nitrogen (BUN), serum creatinine, electrolytes, bicarbonate, calcium, phosphate, and uric acid
- Complete blood count
- Arterial blood gas
- Serum creatine kinase and lactate dehydrogenase (myoglobinuria and hemolysis)
- Serum and urine osmolality
- Urine sodium

Imaging:
- Renal ultrasonography
- Renal vessel Doppler
- *CT scan:* Kidney, ureter, and bladder

Kidney biopsy (selected cases)

BOX 4: Differential diagnosis for the cause of acute kidney injury.

	Prerenal	***Intrinsic renal***
Presentation	Volume depletion, bleeding, and hypotension	Drug or toxin exposure
BUN/serum creatinine	>20	<20
Urine examination	Normal to trace proteinuria and hyaline casts	Mild to moderate proteinuria and muddy brown casts
Urine osmolality (mOsm/kg)	>500	<350
Urine sodium (mEq/L)	<20	>40
FE_{Na} (%)	<1	>1
FE_{Urea} (%)	<35	>35

(FE_{Na}: fractional excretion of sodium; FE_{Urea}: fractional excretion of urea)

$$FE_{Na} = \frac{\text{Urine sodium}}{\text{Serum sodium}} \times \frac{\text{Serum creatinine}}{\text{Urine creatinine}} \times 100$$

$$FE_{Urea} = \frac{\text{Urine urea}}{\text{Serum urea}} \times \frac{\text{Serum creatinine}}{\text{Urine creatinine}} \times 100$$

BOX 5: Complications of acute kidney injury.

- Fluid overload and pulmonary edema
- Metabolic acidosis
- Hyperkalemia and hypokalemia
- Hypernatremia and hyponatremia
- Hyperphosphatemia and hypocalcemia
- Uremic encephalopathy

BOX 6: General management.

- *Volume resuscitation:* According to fluid status, blood pressure, central venous pressure (CVP), and inferior vena cava (IVC) collapsibility
- Improvement in urine output after fluid challenge suggests prerenal acute kidney injury
- Aim for normal blood pressure. Vasopressors may be used, if required
- Replacement of electrolyte losses as per electrolyte levels
- Maintain euglycemia
- Treat infection
- Withdrawal of drugs causing acute kidney injury
- Avoid intravenous contrast and nephrotoxic agents
- Modify drug doses according to renal function
- *Intrinsic renal failure:* Glomerulonephritis and acute interstitial nephritis may require glucocorticoids and other immunosuppression
- *Postrenal acute kidney injury:* Foley catheter or suprapubic catheter for bladder outlet obstruction
- Percutaneous nephrostomy for ureteric obstruction
- Postobstructive diuresis after relief of obstruction requires appropriate fluid replacement

BOX 7: Indications for dialysis.

- *Fluid overload:* Pulmonary edema
- *Hyperkalemia:* Refractory to medical treatment
- *Metabolic acidosis:* Refractory to medical treatment
- *Uremic features:* Encephalopathy and pericarditis
- Anticipated significant fluid and/or solute derangements
- Intoxication (salicylates, ethylene glycol, methanol, lithium, metformin, and barbiturates)

MANAGEMENT OF COMPLICATIONS OF ACUTE KIDNEY INJURY

BOX 8: Fluid overload.

- Restrict fluid intake
- *Loop diuretics:* Furosemide or torsemide (40–80 mg) in intravenous bolus doses
- Continuous infusion can be started if response to bolus doses
- Diuretics are useful in cardiac failure and nephrotic syndrome
- Nitroglycerine infusion for pulmonary edema
- Supplemental oxygen and positive pressure ventilation as needed
- Hemodialysis if fluid overload is refractory to medical management

BOX 9: Hyperkalemia.

- Serum potassium >5.5 mEq/L
- *Electrocardiogram (ECG) changes:* Symmetric peaked T-wave, flattened P-wave, wide QRS, and sine wave pattern
- Rule out pseudohyperkalemia (hemolyzed blood sample and no ECG changes)
- Withdrawal of drugs causing hyperkalemia (ACEi, ARBs, spironolactone, and NSAIDs)
- Potassium-free intravenous fluid
- Potassium-free or low-potassium diet

(Further details in Chapter 8.4)

BOX 10: Hypokalemia.

- Serum potassium <3.5 mEq/L
- *Symptoms:* Weakness and leg cramps
- *ECG changes:* Flattened T-wave and prominent U-wave
- Replace volume loss with potassium-containing fluids
- Replace intravenous potassium gradually (maximum 20 mEq/h). Slower infusion rate if peripheral venous access is used
- *Oral potassium replacement:* Potassium chloride or potassium citrate solution and potassium-rich diet
- *Magnesium deficiency:* Intravenous magnesium sulfate 2–4 g

BOX 11: Sodium.

Hyponatremia:
- Rule out pseudohyponatremia (hyperglycemia, intravenous contrast, and mannitol)
- *Prerenal acute kidney injury with volume loss:* Use isotonic saline
- *Edematous state (cardiac failure, liver failure, and nephrotic syndrome):* Restrict water and salt intake
- Hemodialysis if anuria or persistent hyponatremia

Hypernatremia:
- Correct water deficit
- Intravenous dextrose or enteral free water
- Maximum sodium correction 8–10 mEq/L/day
- Hemodialysis if no response to medical management

BOX 12: Metabolic acidosis.

- Normal or high anion gap metabolic acidosis
- *High anion gap acidosis:* Lactate, ketoacids, salicylate, and glycols
- *If pH <7.2:* Intravenous sodium bicarbonate (50 mEq)
- Watch for hypocalcemia with correction
- Hemodialysis if acidosis is refractory to medical management

BOX 13: Hyperphosphatemia and hypocalcemia.

- *Oral phosphate binders:* Calcium-based (calcium acetate 667 mg or calcium carbonate 500 mg two to three times daily) or calcium-free (sevelamer carbonate 400–800 mg three times daily)
- Phosphate restricted diet
- Intravenous calcium gluconate for symptomatic hypocalcemia
- Monitor ionized calcium during correction of acidosis

BOX 14: Rhabdomyolysis.

Details in Chapter 5.2

SUGGESTED READING

1. Kellum JA, Romagnani P, Ashuntantang G, Ronco C, Zarbock A, Anders HJ. Acute kidney injury. Nat Rev Dis Primers. 2021;7(1):52.
2. Moore PK, Hsu RK, Liu KD. Management of Acute Kidney Injury: Core Curriculum 2018. Am J Kidney Dis. 2018;72(1):136-48.
3. Ronco C, Bellomo R, Kellum JA. Acute kidney injury. Lancet. 2019;394(10212): 1949-64.

5.2 RHABDOMYOLYSIS

Rushi V Deshpande, Ashwin Patil, Ashitosh R Patil

BOX 1: Introduction.

- Rhabdomyolysis is a syndrome characterized by muscle necrosis and the release of intracellular muscle constituents into the circulation
- Creatine kinase (CK) levels are typically markedly elevated, and muscle pain and myoglobinuria may be present
- The severity of illness ranges from asymptomatic elevations in serum muscle enzymes to life-threatening disease associated with extreme enzyme elevations, electrolyte imbalances, and acute kidney injury (AKI)

BOX 2: Causes.

Traumatic or compression:
- Multiple trauma
- Crush injuries
- Vascular or orthopedic surgery
- Coma
- Immobilization

Nontraumatic-nonexertional:
- Alcoholism
- Drugs and toxins
- Infections [including human immunodeficiency virus (HIV)]
- Electrolyte abnormalities
- Endocrinopathies
- Inflammatory myopathies

Nontraumatic-exertional:
- Normal muscle:
  - Extreme exertion
  - Environmental heat illness
  - Sickle cell trait
  - Seizures
  - Hyperkinetic states
- Abnormal muscle:
  - Metabolic myopathies
  - Mitochondrial myopathies
  - Malignant hyperthermia
  - Neuroleptic malignant syndrome

BOX 3: Clinical and laboratories features.

Aspect	*Details*
Clinical features	• Muscle pain, weakness, and dark urine (myoglobinuria), malaise and fever • Myalgias and tachycardia • Nausea and vomiting, abdominal pain, altered mental status
Physical findings	• Tender and swollen muscles • Weakness of muscle/groups • Limb induration, skin changes (ischemic tissue injury)
Laboratory findings	• Elevated serum muscle enzymes (including CK) • *Hallmark:* Elevation in CK and other serum muscle enzymes • Reddish-brown urine of myoglobinuria • Routine lab tests [complete blood count (CBC), erythrocyte sedimentation rate (ESR), and C-reactive protein (CRP)] marked elevation of acute phase reactants and peripheral white blood cell (WBC) count • Inflammation markers may be normal in drug-induced or electrolyte derangement cases
CK	• Levels typically exceed five times the upper limit of normal, ranging from approximately 1,500 to over 100,000 international units per liter • The majority of the enzyme present is the MM or skeletal muscle fraction, with a small proportion potentially being the MB fraction • Elevated levels of aminotransferases aspartate transaminase (AST) and alanine transaminase (ALT)] are commonly observed
Urine findings and myoglobinuria	• *Myoglobinuria:* Red to brown urine. May not be present in all cases. Myoglobin appears in plasma before CK elevation, disappears while CK is elevated or rising • Hemoglobin and myoglobin can be detected as "blood" on dipstick; microscopic evaluation may show few red blood cell (RBC) • Proteinuria may occur
Fluid and electrolyte abnormalities	• Hypovolemia the sequelae of "third-spacing", where fluid shifts into injured muscles, increasing the risk of AKI • Hyperkalemia and hyperphosphatemia arise from the release of potassium and phosphorus from damaged muscle cells • *Hypocalcemia:* Occurs initially, resolves during recovery phase • Severe hyperuricemia may develop • Metabolic acidosis common; increased anion gap possible
AKI	• Common complication of rhabdomyolysis (15–50% frequency) • *Mechanisms:* Renal ischemia, heme pigment casts, and tubular injury
Compartment syndrome	• Potential complication of severe rhabdomyolysis • May develop after fluid resuscitation, worsening limb edema
Disseminated intravascular coagulation (DIC)	• This condition arises from the release of thromboplastin and other prothrombotic substances from damaged muscle tissue

BOX 4: Diagnosis and workup.

Criteria for diagnostic testing	***Details***
Pigmenturia and myalgias	Testing in individuals experiencing both muscle pain and reddish-brown urine
Either myalgias or pigmenturia, with relevant history or exposure	Testing recommended if there is a history or recent exposure to potential causes or events related to rhabdomyolysis
Absence of myalgias or pigmenturia in high-risk settings	Suspected in situations such as prolonged immobilization, stupor, comatose patients, or those unable to provide a medical history. Criteria include muscle tenderness, skin pressure necrosis, signs of trauma, blood chemistry abnormalities, and evidence of AKI
Diagnostic evaluation	***Key diagnostic laboratory studies include***
CK	Fractionation usually not required but may be helpful in excluding other potential causes of CK elevation. Other muscle enzymes (aldolase, aminotransferases, and lactate dehydrogenase) may be elevated
Urinalysis	Routine urine dipstick and microscopic evaluation to detect evidence of myoglobinuria. Unspun or centrifuged urine tests positive for heme if myoglobinuria is present
Additional tests	CBC, blood urea nitrogen, creatinine, electrolytes (including potassium), calcium, phosphate, albumin, uric acid, and electrocardiography
When to suspect metabolic myopathy	Consider metabolic myopathy in cases of recurrent rhabdomyolysis, exercise intolerance, muscle cramps, fatigue, a family history of similar issues, and normal muscle strength between episodes
Diagnosis	Diagnosis based on acute neuromuscular illness or dark urine, plus marked acute elevation in serum CK (typically at least five times the upper limit). No absolute CK cutoff; considered in clinical context. Additional testing [electromyography (EMG), MRI, and biopsy] generally not required

BOX 5: Management of rhabdomyolysis.

Major issues	*Key actions*
Fluid and electrolyte abnormalities	• Recognize and manage fluid and electrolyte imbalances • Initiate treatment regardless of renal function to prevent severe metabolic disturbances and AKI
Identification of specific causes	• Identify underlying causes of rhabdomyolysis • Implement appropriate countermeasures targeting triggering events • Discontinue drugs or toxins contributing to rhabdomyolysis
Compartment syndrome	• Promptly recognize, evaluate, and treat compartment syndrome if present

BOX 6: Prevention and treatment of heme pigment-induced AKI.

Prevention of AKI in rhabdomyolysis

General goals:
- Correct volume depletion
- Prevent intratubular cast formation

Volume administration:
- Administer isotonic saline early and aggressively
- Adjust rate based on CK levels
- Continue until plasma CK levels <5,000 unit/L

Bicarbonate therapy:
- Consider for severe rhabdomyolysis (CK >5,000 unit/L)
- Infuse sodium bicarbonate until urine pH >6.5
- Monitor arterial pH and serum calcium

Mannitol:
- Do not routinely use
- Consider in severe rhabdomyolysis with marked CK elevation (>30,000 unit/L)
- Monitor for volume depletion, hypernatremia, and hyperosmolality

Loop diuretics:
- Do not use unless volume overload is present
- No proven impact on AKI outcomes

Dialysis:
- Reserved for established AKI with complications

Treatment of metabolic abnormalities

- Monitor and treat hyperkalemia, hypocalcemia, hyperphosphatemia, and hyperuricemia
- Use allopurinol for hyperuricemia

Contd...

Contd...

Treatment of established AKI	
Treatment aspect	***Details***
Nonoliguric AKI:	
Fluid therapy	Administer intravenous (IV) fluids judiciously to maintain euvolemia
Diuretic therapy	Diuretics generally not recommended unless volume overload occurs; use furosemide cautiously if needed
Renal replacement therapy (RRT)	Initiate RRT if renal function worsens despite conservative management; consider continuous RRT (CRRT) or hemodialysis
Urine alkalinization	Administer sodium bicarbonate cautiously to prevent myoglobin precipitation
Oliguric AKI:	
RRT	Initiate CRRT or daily hemodialysis in severe cases. Ensure extracorporeal myoglobin removal and consider cytokine adsorbers (CytoSorb)
Choice of dialysis membranes	Prefer high cutoff (HCO) membranes for better myoglobin clearance, but medium cutoff (MCO) membranes may be suitable in some cases
Combination therapy	Consider combining cytokine adsorbers with RRT methods to enhance myoglobin elimination
Prognosis: Overall favorable prognosis; most survivors recover kidney function	

SUGGESTED READING

1. Johnson RJ, Floege J, Tonelli M. Comprehensive Clinical Nephrology, 7th edition. Amsterdam: Elsevier; 2023.
2. Loscalzo J, Fauci AS, Kasper DL, Hauser SL, Longo DL, Jameson JL. Harrison's Principles of Internal Medicine, 21st edition. New York: McGraw Hill; 2022.
3. UpToDate. (2024). Rhabdomyolysis: Clinical manifestations and diagnosis. [online] Available from https://www.uptodate.com/contents/rhabdomyolysis-clinical-manifestations-and-diagnosis. [Last accessed September, 2024].
4. UpToDate. Fluid and electrolytes. [online] Available from https://www.uptodate.com/contents/table-of-contents/endocrinology-and-diabetes/fluid-and-electrolytes. [Last accessed September, 2024].

5.3 EMERGENCIES IN END STAGE RENAL DISEASE

Ashay Shingare, Madan M Bahadur

BOX 1: Chronic kidney disease (CKD) definition.

As per the Kidney Disease: Improving Global Outcomes (KDIGO), CKD is defined as abnormalities of kidney structure or function, present for >3 months, with implications for health. These may include the following:	
Markers of kidney damage	• Albuminuria [albumin excretion rate (AER) ≥30 mg/24 h; urinary albumin-to-creatinine ratio (uACR) ≥30 mg/g (≥3 mg/mmol)] • Urine sediment abnormalities • Electrolyte and other abnormalities caused by tubular disorders • Abnormalities detected through histology • Structural abnormalities detected through imaging • History of kidney transplantation
Decreased glomerular filtration rate (GFR)	GFR <60 mL/min/1.73 m^2

BOX 2: Stages of CKD [according to the Kidney Disease Outcomes Quality Initiative (KDOQI)].

Stage	*GFR (mL/min/1.73 m^2)*	*Description*
1	≥90	Kidney damage with normal or high GFR
2	60–89	Mildly decreased GFR
3	30–59	Moderately decreased GFR
4	15–29	Severely decreased GFR
5	<15 (or dialysis)	Kidney failure

BOX 3: Cardiopulmonary complications.

Acute coronary syndrome (ACS):
- Most common cause of death in CKD is cardiovascular (CV) disease
- *Traditional CV risk factors:* Aging, hypertension, diabetes, hyperlipidemia, and smoking
- *Nontraditional risk factors in CKD:* Albuminuria, chronic inflammation, fluid retention, anemia, and abnormal mineral metabolism
- *Symptoms:* Chest pain, dyspnea, nausea, vomiting, and cardiac arrhythmia
- *Evaluation:* Electrocardiogram (ECG) and echocardiography
- CKD patients may have elevated troponins; trending values are significant
- Standard ACS management, thrombolytics, or percutaneous intervention, if indicated
- No dose adjustments for antiplatelets, unfractionated heparin, or thrombolytics
- Low-molecular-weight heparins require dose adjustment

Contd...

Contd...

Hypertensive emergency and urgency:
- Due to fluid overload, salt retention, sympathetic overactivity, and erythropoietin
- Assess for target organ damage
- Blood pressure (BP) monitoring; do not measure BP in extremity with arteriovenous fistula (AVF) or graft
- Provide a quiet room and alleviate pain
- *For volume overload and pulmonary edema:* Diuretics and hemodialysis if necessary
- Intravenous medications in hypertensive emergency
- Sodium nitroprusside and metabolites (thiocyanate and cyanide) are retained in renal failure; removed by dialysis
- Oral medications for hypertensive urgency

Pulmonary edema:
- Due to noncompliance with fluid and salt restriction, missed dialysis session, ACS, and congestive cardiac failure (CCF)
- *Evaluation:* ECG, chest radiograph, electrolytes, complete blood count (CBC), and troponin
- Restrict fluid intake
- Loop diuretics and nitroglycerine infusion
- Supplemental oxygen and positive pressure ventilation as needed
- Urgent hemodialysis if fluid overload is refractory to medical management

BOX 4: Neurological complications.

Uremic encephalopathy:
- Seen in end-stage kidney disease (GFR <15 mL/min/1.73 m^2), blood urea nitrogen (BUN) often >200 mg/dL
- Due to accumulation of uremic toxins
- Impaired concentration, memory loss, tremors, asterixis, altered gait, and coma
- Neuroimaging, electroencephalography (EEG), and lumbar puncture—to rule out other causes
- *Management:* Start dialysis, increase dialysis dose if persistent symptoms

Dialysis disequilibrium syndrome:
- During or after initial hemodialysis session
- With urea removal, serum osmolality decreases, hence water shifts into brain cells causing edema
- *Symptoms:* Headache, restlessness, confusion, seizures, and coma
- Neuroimaging—to rule out other causes
- *Mild symptoms:* Self-resolve after few hours, supportive care
- *Severe symptoms:* Stop dialysis if ongoing, airway protection and ventilation if necessary, intravenous hypertonic saline or mannitol, and antiepileptics
- *Prevention:* Slow urea removal in first hemodialysis

BOX 5: Hematological and immune system complications.

Anemia:

- Due to insufficient erythropoietin, iron deficiency, chronic inflammation, hyperparathyroidism, decreased red blood cell (RBC) survival, and blood loss
- *Symptoms:* Fatigue, decreased cognitive function, and exacerbation of angina
- *Treatment:* Erythropoiesis-stimulating agents (erythropoietin and darbepoetin), intravenous iron, and hypoxia-inducible factor prolyl hydroxylase (HIF-PH) inhibitors

Abnormal hemostasis:

- Due to decreased platelet function, decreased activity of von Willebrand factor (vWF), increased endothelial nitric oxide, and prostacyclin
- *Symptoms:* Increased bleeding after trauma, easy bruisability, epistaxis, gastrointestinal hemorrhage, and hemorrhagic pericarditis
- *Treatment:* Adequate dialysis, desmopressin (DDAVP), and cryoprecipitate if life-threatening hemorrhage

Infections:

- *Increased infection risk:* Due to impaired leukocyte function, chronic inflammation, and catheters
- Infection is the most common cause of hospitalization in end-stage renal disease (ESRD)
- *Presentation:* Catheter-associated infection, lower respiratory tract infection, and urinary tract infection
- *Management:* Blood culture testing, fluid resuscitation if shock, and broad-spectrum antimicrobials

BOX 6: Gastrointestinal complications.

- *Anorexia, nausea, and vomiting:* Due to uremia
- *Gastritis management:* Proton pump inhibitors or histamine H_2-receptor antagonists

Gastrointestinal hemorrhage:

- *Etiology:* Peptic ulcer, gastritis, angiodysplasia, uremic abnormal hemostasis, and anticoagulation during hemodialysis
- *Evaluation:* GI endoscopy, angiography, and capsule endoscopy
- *Management:* Fluid replacement, transfusions, optimum dialysis, desmopressin, cryoprecipitate, heparin-free hemodialysis, and specific treatment for underlying cause of hemorrhage

Acute abdomen:

- *Etiology:* Renal calculi, cyst rupture or infection in polycystic kidney disease, retroperitoneal hemorrhage, peritonitis (in patients on peritoneal dialysis), ischemic bowel, and pancreatitis
- *Evaluation:* Radiological imaging of the abdomen
- Serum amylase and lipase may be elevated up to threefold in renal failure
- Peritoneal fluid cell count and culture in suspected peritonitis
- Specific treatment for underlying cause

BOX 7: Electrolyte disorders.

Hyperkalemia:
- *Presentation:* Nonspecific symptoms, muscle weakness, paresthesia, and cardiac arrhythmia
- Check serum potassium and monitor ECG
- Dietary potassium restriction
- *Emergency anti-potassium measures:* Calcium gluconate, glucose with insulin infusion, intravenous sodium bicarbonate, and β-adrenergic agonist nebulization
- *Hemodialysis:* For emergency potassium removal

BOX 8: Hemodialysis.

Vascular access thrombosis:
- Most common complication in AVF and arteriovenous graft (AVG)
- Due to endothelial injury, stasis, and hypercoagulability
- *Presentation:* Absence of thrill or bruit and thrombophlebitis in AVF (redness, pain, and tenderness)
- *Ultrasonography Doppler evaluation:* Site and extent of thrombosis
- Correct hypotension if present
- *Treatment:* Percutaneous mechanical thrombolysis or surgical thrombectomy

Vascular access hemorrhage:
- Due to rupture of AVF or AVG, accidental removal of central venous catheter (CVC), and uncapped ports
- *Aneurysms:* Focal dilations of vessel wall
- *Pseudoaneurysms:* Composed of hematoma and fibrous tissue
- *Signs of imminent rupture in aneurysm:* Ulceration, thin or shiny skin, and infection
- *Management:* Direct continuous pressure on the site for 15–20 minutes
- Avoid applying tourniquet or BP cuff on the extremity
- Surgical correction or ligation of ruptured AVF/AVG

Catheter-related bloodstream infection (CRBSI):
- Due to intraluminal contamination during dialysis, migration of skin flora, and colonization during bacteremia from remote site
- Fever, chills during dialysis, septic shock, and metastatic infection (endocarditis and septic arthritis)
- *Investigations:* Blood and catheter tip culture
- Urgent catheter removal, if septic shock
- *Empirical therapy:* Intravenous antibiotics after each dialysis session
- *Gram-positive organisms:* Vancomycin 20 mg/kg loading dose followed by 500 mg after each subsequent dialysis
- *Gram-negative organisms:* Gentamicin 1 mg/kg or ceftazidime 1 g after each dialysis
- Subsequent therapy as per sensitivity report
- Antibiotic lock solutions if catheter salvage is attempted

BOX 9: Peritoneal dialysis.

Peritonitis:
- Major complication of peritoneal dialysis
- Due to breaches in sterile technique, migration along the catheter or bacterial translocation from intestine
- Cloudy effluent, abdominal pain, fever, and abdominal tenderness
- Peritoneal fluid cell count (white cell count >100/mm^3 and >50% neutrophils), Gram staining, and culture
- *Empirical therapy:* Intraperitoneal antibiotics added to dialysate in one exchange
- *Gram-positive organisms:* Vancomycin 15–30 mg/kg every 5–7 days or cefazolin 15–20 mg/kg daily
- *Gram-negative organisms:* Amikacin 2 mg/kg daily or ceftazidime 1–1.5 g daily
- Subsequent therapy as per sensitivity report

Hernia and leak:
- Incisional, umbilical, and inguinal hernias are common
- *Abdominal wall leak:* Asymmetric abdominal swelling, weight gain, and absence of generalized edema
- *Genital edema:* Due to patent processus vaginalis (hydrocele) or abdominal wall leak
- *Hydrothorax:* Due to defects in the hemidiaphragm, common on right side
- *Evaluation:* Ultrasonography and CT peritoneography (contrast agent is added to dialysate and instilled into peritoneal cavity)
- *Management:* Surgical repair along with temporary hemodialysis or automated peritoneal dialysis with low volumes in supine position

BOX 10: Kidney transplantation.

Acute rejection:
- *Presentation:* Rapid rise in serum creatinine, oliguria, edema, fever, and graft tenderness
- *Differential diagnosis:* Bacterial pyelonephritis, urine leak (early posttransplant phase), urinary tract obstruction, vascular thrombosis, renal artery stenosis, and calcineurin inhibitor toxicity
- *Evaluation:* Renal function tests, urine analysis, blood and urine cultures, ultrasonography and Doppler evaluation of kidney allograft, and transplant kidney biopsy

SUGGESTED READING

1. Greenberg KI, Choi MJ. Hemodialysis Emergencies: Core Curriculum 2021. Am J Kidney Dis. 2021;77(5):796-809.
2. Long B, Koyfman A, Lee CM. Emergency medicine evaluation and management of the end stage renal disease patient. Am J Emerg Med. 2017;35(12):1946-55.
3. Venkat A, Kaufmann KR, Venkat K. Care of the end-stage renal disease patient on dialysis in the ED. Am J Emerg Med. 2006;24(7):847-58.

5.4 ACUTE URINARY TRACT INFECTION

Santosh Gawali

BOX 1: Acute urinary tract infection (UTI).

One of the common infection, if not treated urgently might lead to urosepsis, especially in diabetic or immunocompromised individuals

BOX 2: Symptoms.

- Frequency
- Urgency with occasional urge incontinence
- Dysuria
- Fever with or without chills
- Sometimes, especially in elderly males and females, can additionally have symptoms of bladder outlet obstruction such as poor flow, straining, intermittency, and sense of incomplete void

BOX 3: Associated history to be asked for differential diagnosis.

- Child below 10 years—congenital malformation
- Child till puberty—rule out sexual abuse and stone disease
- 15–30 years—rule out recent sexual activity, especially in females (honeymoon cystitis)
- 30–50 years males—rule out stricture disease
- Age >50 years:
  - Rule out prostatomegaly in males
  - Rule out urethral stenosis, caruncle, and prolapse in postmenopausal females

BOX 4: Important history to be asked in all age groups.

- Constipation
- Water intake
- Stone disease
- Diabetes
- Any previous history of urinary instrumentation

BOX 5: Investigations.

- Complete blood count (CBC)
- Random blood sugar level (RBSL)
- Serum creatinine
- Urine routine microscopy (midstream sample)
- Urine culture (midstream sample)
- Serum electrolytes ultrasonography (USG) kidneys, ureters, and urinary bladder (KUB) with postvoid residual (PVR)
- USG KUB with PVR
- Uroflow (if suspecting bladder outlet obstruction)

BOX 6: Treatment.

- Plenty of oral fluids and intravenous (IV) fluids if sick
  - Broad spectrum antibiotic (to be started only after taking urine sample): IV if indicated
    - IV cefoperazone + sulbactam 1.5 g 1-0-1 × 5 days
    - IV aminoglycosides (amikacin) 500–750 mg OD × 3 days (if creatinine normal)
- Followed by oral antibiotics:
  - Cefuroxime/cefixime × 10 days
  - Nitrofurantoin/Septran/doxycycline 1-0-1 × 10 days then 0-0-1 × 20 days
- Repeat urine culture and urine routine post 48 hours after completion
  - Alpha blockers like tamsulosin/silodosin
  - Anticholinergics like solifenacin/oxybutynin only if indicated
  - Urinary alkalizer like syrup Cital/Potrate MB6 × 1 month
  - Treatment of underlying causes
  - Catheterization whenever indicated

SUGGESTED READING

1. McAninch JW, Lue TF. Smith and Tangho's General Urology, 19th edition. New York: McGraw Hill; 2020. p. 201.
2. Partin AW, Peters CA, Kavoussi LR, Dmochowski RR, Wein AJ. Campbell-Walsh-Wein Urology, 12th edition. Amsterdam: Elsevier; 2020. p. 1129.

5.5 HEMATURIA

Percy J Chibber

BOX 1: Hematuria.

- Hematuria, or blood in the urine, can be gross or microscopic
- Common causes include urinary tract infections (UTIs), renal stones, trauma, and malignancy
- Evaluation includes history, physical examination, urine analysis, and imaging (CT scan or ultrasound)
- The American College of Physicians guidelines for hematuria recommend workup for all adults (18 years or older), including repeat assessment of urinalysis and consideration for CT imaging
- Management depends on underlying etiology and may involve conservative measures or urological intervention
- Depending on the patient's hemodynamics, initiate initial stabilization
- Treat UTI if present
- Avoid catheterization if the patient is voiding normally
- Assess bladder emptying status
- If the bladder is not emptying, consider catheterization with a 22Fr, 3-way Foley catheter
- If a catheter is already in place and the patient presents with hematuria, it is likely blocked; perform bladder irrigation
- If ultrasound reveals clots, urgent intervention in the operating theater is necessary for clot evacuation
- Important consideration for hematuria: All patients with gross hematuria should undergo a comprehensive evaluation to determine the cause, even if bleeding stops spontaneously

SUGGESTED READING

1. Davis R, Jones JS, Barocas DA, Castle EP, Lang EK, Leveillee RJ, et al. Diagnosis, evaluation and follow-up of asymptomatic microhematuria (AMH) in adults: AUA guideline. J Urol. 2012;188(6 Suppl):2473-81.
2. Grossfeld GD, Litwin MS, Wolf JS Jr, Hricak H, Shuler CL, Agerter DC, et al. Evaluation of asymptomatic microscopic hematuria in adults: the American Urological Association best practice policy recommendations. Part I: definition, detection, prevalence, and etiology. Urology. 2001;57(4):599-603.

5.6 ACUTE URINARY RETENTION

Percy J Chibber

BOX 1: Urinary retention.

- Acute urinary retention is characterized by the inability to void despite a full bladder
- Causes include anatomical obstruction (e.g., benign prostatic hyperplasia and urethral stricture) or functional (e.g., medications and neurological disorders)
- Management involves catheterization for immediate relief, followed by investigation and treatment of the underlying cause
  - *History:*
    - Previous voiding patterns (prior to this episode)
    - History of catheterization or previous endourological procedures and recent surgeries
    - Bowel history
    - Current medications
    - Use of antithrombotic or antiplatelet medications
    - Presence of neurological diseases (e.g., stroke, Parkinson's disease, and spinal pathology)
  - *Examination:*
    - Confirm presence of retention
    - Perform bedside ultrasound if uncertainty exists
    - Inspect the prepuce, external urethral meatus, or female introitus
    - Conduct digital rectal examination to assess prostate size, hardness, and presence of impacted feces
    - If prostate cancer is suspected, obtain serum prostate-specific antigen (PSA) levels before catheterization
  - *Management catheterization:*
    - Explain the procedure to the patient and consider sedation if necessary
    - Ensure all necessary equipment is readily available
    - After sterile preparation, apply 5–10 mL of lidocaine jelly and allow 3–5 minutes for anesthesia
    - Select catheter size and type based on expected pathology
    - Slowly insert the catheter until resistance is met
    - Confirm free urine flow
    - Inflate the balloon with water and secure the catheter in place
  - *Failure to catheterize:*
    - Determine the level of obstruction
    - Assess ease of jelly introduction
    - Consider using a different catheter:
      - Smaller or larger size
      - Catheter with a stiffer coude tip
      - Filiform bougie set or metal dilator set with catheter introducer
    - Consider cystoscopy (rigid or flexible) if needed
    - Suprapubic catheterization may be an alternative

Contd...

Contd...

Disposition

Postcatheterization:

- Administer a single dose of IV antibiotics
- Decide on the need for admission
- If discharged, provide a detailed management plan for the underlying condition
- Educate patients on Foley catheter care, bag drainage, and symptoms requiring immediate medical attention (e.g., fever, persistent vomiting, abdominal pain, decreased urine output, or penile pain)
- Prolonged Foley catheter drainage may be necessary for patients with retention volumes exceeding 1.3 liters to optimize voiding outcomes

BOX 2: Oliguria/anuria.

- Oliguria (reduced urine output) or anuria (complete absence of urine output) requires urgent evaluation
- Causes range from prerenal (e.g., hypovolemia) to renal (e.g., acute kidney injury) and postrenal (e.g., urinary tract obstruction)
- Management includes fluid resuscitation, diagnostic imaging (renal ultrasound, CT scan), and nephrology consultation for severe cases

SUGGESTED READING

1. Bellomo R, Ronco C, Kellum JA, Mehta RL, Palevsky P. Acute renal failure—definition, outcome measures, animal models, fluid therapy and information technology needs: the Second International Consensus Conference of the Acute Dialysis Quality Initiative (ADQI) Group. Crit Care. 2004;8(4):R204-12.
2. Lepor H. Pathophysiology of lower urinary tract symptoms in the aging male population. Rev Urol. 2005;7(Suppl 7):S3-11.
3. Rossert J, Wauters JP. Recommendations for the screening and management of patients with chronic kidney disease. Nephrol Dial Transplant. 2002;17(Suppl 11):19-28.
4. Selius BA, Subedi R. Urinary retention in adults: diagnosis and initial management. Am Fam Physician. 2008;77(5):643-50.

5.7 ACUTE STONE DISORDERS

Shailesh Raina, Sachna P Shetty

BOX 1: Emergency goals.

Emergency management of stone disorders focuses on pain relief, evaluation of kidney function, and determining the likelihood of spontaneous stone passage

BOX 2: Risk factors.

- Metabolic diseases or disturbances
- Laxative misuse
- Family history of kidney stones
- Hot and arid climates
- Male gender
- Previous kidney stones
- Dehydration

BOX 3: Clinical features.

- Kidney stone commonly presents with the sudden onset of crampy and intermittent flank pain that radiates toward the groin
- In men, the pain may extend to the testicles, while in women, it may extend to the labia majora
- A constant, dull ache in the flank often persists between episodes of colic
- Patients typically exhibit significant discomfort and are unable to find a comfortable position
- Other clinical signs include:
  - Rebound abdominal tenderness (29%)
  - Guarding (61%)
  - Rigidity (8%)
  - Nausea and vomiting (50%)
  - Rebound response to pain might lead to tachycardia, hypertension, and diaphoresis
  - Hematuria in 85% of patients, with 30% showing gross hematuria

The location of pain often correlates with the stone's position:
- Upper ureter stones cause flank pain
- Midureter stones cause lower anterior quadrant abdominal pain
- Distal ureter stones cause groin pain and are the most common, accounting for 75% of diagnoses
- Stones at the ureterovesical junction can mimic urinary tract infections, causing frequency, urgency, and dysuria in 3–24% of patients

BOX 4: Differential diagnosis.

(Details are given in Chapter 1)
Caveat: Few important ones are
- Aortic dissection or ruptured aortic aneurysm (most critical)
- A calcified aortic aneurysm might appear like a calculi

BOX 5: Laboratory evaluation.

Laboratory tests focus on detecting infection, assessing kidney function. Essential tests include:

- Pregnancy test for women of childbearing age to guide imaging choices and exclude ectopic pregnancy
- Urinalysis to rule out infection, followed by urine culture and sensitivity tests if infection is detected
- Renal function tests to check for reduced creatinine clearance

BOX 6: Imaging.

Noncontrast helical CT scans are the preferred imaging modality to confirm the presence, size, and location of kidney stones and to guide management decisions

- CT scan (noncontrast)
  - *Advantages:* Speed
  - *Disadvantages:* Radiation and no evaluation of renal function
- Ultrasonography (USG)
  - *Advantages:* No radiation, can be safely done in pregnancy, no contrast, and cost-effective
  - *Disadvantages:* Insensitive in middle third of the ureter and may miss smaller stones (<5 mm)

BOX 7: Treatment.

Management of symptomatic kidney stones in the emergency room includes:

- *Pain and nausea control:*
  - Paracetamol through the intravenous (IV) route is the safest choice of drug for pain relief
  - Nonsteroidal anti-inflammatory drugs (NSAIDs) like diclofenac/ketorolac (IV) although provide effective pain relief and when administered intravenously but should be avoided in patients with coagulopathies, or renal impairment and should be given only if patient has a normal serum creatinine
  - Opioids, such as tramadol (IV), are commonly used for pain control, often requiring concurrent antiemetics to manage opioid induced vomiting
  - Further drugs are mentioned in Chapter 22
  - Forced IV hydration shows no significant difference in pain control or stone passage rates compared to minimal IV hydration; fluids should correct any fluid deficit due to vomiting or limited oral intake
- *Antibiotic therapy:*
  - Patients with ureteral stones and signs of systemic infection (fever and renal insufficiency) should receive IV antibiotics and be admitted for further management. Initial options include piperacillin tazobactam, cefepime, ticarcillin clavulanic acid, or ciprofloxacin. Gentamicin or tobramycin, combined with ampicillin, may be considered based on local antibiotic sensitivities
  - Outpatients with less severe infections should receive antibiotics targeting gram-negative rods, tailored to local resistance patterns, with follow-up in 48–72 hours
- *Medical expulsion therapy:* Tamsulosin, an α-blocker, is commonly used, especially for stones >5 mm. It may shorten stone expulsion times and increase the likelihood of successful passage. The typical dose is 0.4 mg PO once daily. Patients should be informed of the limited benefits and potential side effects, such as orthostatic hypotension, dizziness, and headache

BOX 8: Disposition.

Indications for admission

Absolute indications:

- Intractable pain or vomiting
- Fever
- Urosepsis
- Solitary or transplanted kidney with obstruction
- Acute kidney injury
- Urinary extravasation
- Hypercalcemic crisis
- Significant medical comorbidities

Relative indications:

- Severe pain unlikely to be managed as an outpatient
- Large stone above the pelvic brim

BOX 9: Special considerations in pregnancy.

CT scans should be used only if necessary. Narcotics are typically the preferred pain management option

BOX 10: Optimal therapy.

After initial pain management and diagnosis, urologist should be involved, who further decides on the choice of therapy depending on the stone's size, location, and composition

Common techniques include:

- *Ureteroscopy:* Achieves a higher stone free rate and reduces the need for retreatment compared to extracorporeal shockwave lithotripsy (ESWL), though it has a higher complication rate and longer hospital stay
- *ESWL*: Less invasive but may require retreatment
- Caveat
- ESWL not used much often, mostly useful if Housefield unit (HU) <800
- **Percutaneous Nephrolithotomy:** Used for stones too large (higher HU) or hard for ESWL or ureteroscopy, involving the direct removal of stones from the renal pelvis
- In case of small stones in the calyces the new technique of retrograde intrarenal surgery (RIS) with laser fragmentation is effective
- In difficult high acute small stones a mini percutaneous nephrolithotomy can be done

SUGGESTED READING

1. American Urological Association. (2016). Guideline for the Management of Ureteral Calculi. [online] Available from https://www.auanet.org/guidelines/kidney-stones. [Last accessed September, 2024].
2. Goldman L, Schafer AI. Goldman-Cecil Medicine. 26th edition. Philadelphia: Elsevier; 2020.

3. Miller NL, Lingeman JE. Management of Kidney Stones. BMJ. 2007;334(7591): 468-72.
4. Smith-Bindman R, Aubin C, Bailitz J, Bengiamin RN, Camargo CA Jr, Corbo J, et al. Ultrasonography versus computed tomography for suspected nephrolithiasis. N Engl J Med. 2014;371:1100-10.
5. Tintinalli JE, Ma OJ, Yealy DM, Meckler GD, Stapczynski JS, Cline DM, et al. Tintinalli's Emergency Medicine: A Comprehensive Study Guide, 9th edition. New York: McGraw Hill; 2020.
6. Weiner ID, Rosenberg E. Kidney Stones: Medical and Surgical Management. New York: Humana Press; 2014.

5.8 ACUTE MALE GENITAL DISORDERS

Percy J Chibber

BOX 1: Fournier's gangrene.

Fournier's gangrene is a severe infective necrotizing fasciitis affecting the genital, perineal, or perianal regions. It is characterized by polymicrobial infection involving both aerobic and anaerobic bacteria

Risk factors:
- Diabetes mellitus
- Alcohol use disorder
- Immunosuppression
- Obesity
- Peripheral vascular disease

Clinical features:
- Early symptoms include severe pain, swelling, erythema, and fever
- Some patients may initially present with nonspecific symptoms such as malaise and discomfort in the affected area
- Advanced disease may manifest with crepitus and skin discoloration due to tissue necrosis and additionally might present in shock

Diagnosis:
- Clinical suspicion based on symptoms and physical examination
- Bedside ultrasound can reveal thickened scrotal wall with gas (dirty shadowing) suggesting tissue necrosis
- CT scan helps in assessing the extent of the infection and involvement of surrounding structures

Management:
- Immediate stabilization with attention to airway, breathing, and circulation
- Broad-spectrum antibiotic therapy covering gram-positive, gram-negative, and anaerobic bacteria should be initiated promptly
  - Recommended agents include piperacillin tazobactam, 3.375–4.5 g intravenous (IV) every 6 hours, or imipenem, 1 g IV every 24 hours, or meropenem, 500 mg to 1 g IV every 8 hours, plus vancomycin
  - Along with clindamycin, 600–900 mg IV every 8 hours, or metronidazole, 1 g IV, then 500 mg IV every 8 hours may be beneficial
- Surgical intervention with extensive debridement is crucial to remove necrotic tissue and control the infection
- Supportive measures include aggressive fluid resuscitation and pain management
- Close monitoring in an intensive care setting may be necessary for hemodynamically unstable patients

BOX 2: Phimosis.

- Phimosis is the inability to retract the foreskin over the glans penis
- It can lead to urinary retention and balanitis (inflammation of the glans penis)
- Management includes topical corticosteroids for mild cases and circumcision for severe or recurrent cases

BOX 3: Paraphimosis.

- Paraphimosis occurs when a retracted foreskin cannot be returned to its original position
- It is a medical emergency due to potential vascular compromise of the glans penis
- Immediate reduction with manual compression or aspiration followed by gentle repositioning is essential
- Severe cases may require surgical intervention to relieve pressure and prevent further complications

BOX 4: Entrapment issues.

- Reduce edema
- Use topical anesthesia and lubrication
- Sos circumcision

(*See* details in Chapter 37.3.2)

BOX 5: Testicular diseases.

Testicular torsion versus epididymitis

Clinical presentation:

- Testicular torsion is a urological emergency characterized by sudden onset severe testicular pain (not relieved on scrotum elevation) and swelling
- Examination asymmetrical testicles and high riding testis is noted
- Epididymitis presents with gradual onset of scrotal pain and swelling, often accompanied by urinary symptoms
- Diagnosis is confirmed by physical examination and ultrasound (decreased flow in torsion)
- Prompt surgical exploration is necessary for testicular torsion to prevent testicular loss

Management:

- Management of torsion testis: Immediate surgical exploration is essential within 6 hours of symptom onset to salvage testicular viability
- Management of epididymitis:
  - Empiric antibiotic therapy targeting likely pathogens such as Enterobacteriaceae and sexually transmitted organisms
  - Empiric outpatient treatment of epididymitis and epididymo-orchitis
  - For acute epididymitis most likely caused by sexually transmitted chlamydia or gonorrhea
  - Ceftriaxone, 250 mg intramuscular (IM) single dose, plus doxycycline, 100 mg PO twice a day for 10 days
  - For acute epididymitis most likely caused by sexually transmitted chlamydia, gonorrhea, or enteric organisms (men who practice insertive anal sex)
  - Ceftriaxone, 250 mg IM single dose, plus doxycycline, 100 mg PO twice a day for 10 days

Contd...

Contd...

- Also treat for gram-negative bacilli with:
  - Levofloxacin, 500 mg PO every day for 10 days
    Or
  - Ofloxacin, 300 mg PO twice a day for 10 days
  - For acute epididymitis most likely caused by enteric organisms
  - Levofloxacin,500 mg PO every day for 10 days
    Or
  - Ofloxacin, 300 mg PO twice a day for 10 days
- European Association of Urology Guidelines recommend 500 mg of ceftriaxone IM and 200 mg of doxycycline as first dose
- Analgesics and scrotal support help relieve symptoms
- Follow-up evaluation to assess response to therapy and exclude complications like abscess formation

Disposition:

Scrotal pain emergencies

- Timely diagnosis of testicular torsion is crucial to prevent testicular loss
- Admission criteria for epididymitis include severe pain, systemic symptoms, or suspicion of complications like abscess
- Outpatient management with scrotal support and close urological follow-up is appropriate for mild cases

BOX 6: Priapism.

- Priapism is a persistent, often painful erection unrelated to sexual stimulation
- Low-flow priapism is associated with sickle cell disease and other hematologic disorders, while high-flow priapism typically follows trauma
- Management involves immediate aspiration and irrigation of corpora cavernosa, followed by blood gases of the same to determine the etiology, classification, and management of priapism
  - It is low flow:
    - If pH is <7.25, partial pressure of carbon dioxide (pCO_2) is >60, and partial pressure of oxygen (pO_2) is <30, proceed with corporal aspirations and irrigation, along with injection of an alpha adrenergic agonist
  - Failure/recurrence:
    - In case of failure or recurrence, consider shunting
  - It is high flow if arterial blood:
    - For high-flow situations involving arterial blood, perform pelvis angiogram embolization
- Refractory cases may require surgical shunting to decompress the corpora cavernosa and restore normal blood flow

SUGGESTED READING

1. Baker LA, Sigman D, Mathews RI, Benson J, Docimo SG. An analysis of clinical outcomes using color Doppler testicular ultrasound for testicular torsion. Pediatrics. 2000;105(3 Pt 1):604-7.
2. Broderick GA. Priapism and intracavernous injection. Urol Clin North Am. 1995;22(4):809-20.
3. Eke N. Fournier's gangrene: a review of 1726 cases. Br J Surg. 2000;87(6):718-28.
4. Griffiths DM, Atwell JD, Freeman NV. A prospective study of the incidence of phimosis in boys. Br J Urol. 1985;57(2):148-52.
5. Montague DK, Jarow J, Broderick GA, Dmochowski RR, Heaton JP, Lue TF, et al. American Urological Association guideline on the management of priapism. J Urol. 2003;170(4 Pt 1):1318-24.
6. Shankar KR, Rickwood AM. The incidence of phimosis in boys. BJU Int. 1999;84(1):101-2.
7. Sorensen MD, Krieger JN, Rivara FP, Klein MB, Wessells H. Fournier's gangrene: management and mortality predictors in a population based study. J Urol. 2009;182(6):2742-7.
8. Trojian TH, Lishnak TS, Heiman D. Epididymitis and orchitis: an overview. Am Fam Physician. 2009;79(7):583-7.

CHAPTER 6

Neurological Emergencies

6.1 ACUTE HEADACHE

Joy D Desai

BOX 1: Clinical assessment of headaches in the emergency room (ER).

The analysis of headaches presenting in the emergency medical services is to be broken down into its clinical characteristics, the company it keeps, and inputs from appropriately directed investigations.

The key tenets of headache that are mandatory in the clinical assessment are *location, character, duration, severity, and to some extent the response to an analgesic*. The accompanying features that require assessment are *fever, photophobia, phonophobia, vomiting, dizziness, loss of consciousness, seizures, and the presence of any focal neurological symptom*. There is some value in the ascertainment of the presence of specific signs on clinical examination of the nervous system. The presence of an elevated systemic blood pressure (BP), papilledema on fundoscopy, neck stiffness or signs of meningeal irritation, and focal pyramidal or cerebellar signs all herald an ominous pathological alteration within the nervous system in general.

The analysis of headaches in the ER can be subcategorized into clinical subsets as follows:

- *The first and worst headache of a lifetime* (irrespective of location over the head) narrated by a patient warrants consideration of a sentinel leak from a cerebral aneurysm versus the possibility of reversible cerebral vasoconstriction syndrome (RCVS)
- The presence of splinter hemorrhages/papilledema on fundoscopy and/or neck stiffness would point to the former possibility
- A perception of "la belle indifference" in a neurologically normal individual may rarely be a clue to a functional headache in this situation too

BOX 2: Clinical assessment.

Triad of Headache, Vomiting, and Seizures

- Warrant the consideration of differing diagnostic possibilities based on the clinical accompaniments:
  - The presence of fever and photophobia are typical of meningitis or meningoencephalitis, especially on a background of otorrhea or traumatic brain injury
  - An elevated systemic BP and focal limb weakness suggests the possibility of an intracranial hypertensive parenchymal hemorrhage or a hemorrhage within a space occupying lesion
  - The presence of dehydration or a history of oral contraceptive usage suggests cerebral venous sinus thrombosis
  - In the absence of focal signs but apparent gait dysfunction or urinary urgency, one must consider the possibility of an acute hydrocephalus

Headache with Visual Symptoms

- A patient generally above 50 years age group, predominantly female sex presents with a headache [often is of 2–3 months' duration]
- Pain can be continuous or intermittent; it can worsen at night or on exposure to cold mostly as sharp, throbbing, boring, or aching and usually is localized to the temporal region but may occur anywhere in the head
- Main associated feature is visual symptom, such as Amaurosis fugax preceding permanent visual loss or diplopia
- The most significant clinical feature is visual loss accompanied by tenderness of the temporal artery, primarily located just anterior and slightly superior to the tragus of the ear, along with jaw claudication
- Systemic features along with signs and symptoms of other vascular disorder might be present as associated symptoms
- Biomarkers such as ESR/CRP are very sensitive
- Temporal artery biopsy is the final diagnostic test
- Thrombocytosis and anemia is also noted. Ophthalmology examination should be conducted
- Patients who present with visual symptoms must be treated emergently with glucocorticoids that is IV pulse therapy (e.g., 1000 mg of methylprednisolone per day for 3 consecutive days)
- For patients without visual symptoms, lower doses of steroids, in the range of 40 to 60 mg/day of prednisone should be used

BOX 3: Occurrence in various settings.

- The occurrence of headache or nuchal pain in the setting of an apparent acute *hemiparesis* without elevated BP or in the absence of known vascular risk factors in a young person should raise the possibility of an arterial dissection
- *In a person known to have trigger linked headaches,* increasing severity or frequency of stereotyped headaches should raise the suspicion of analgesic abuse, or lifestyle aberrations such as cocaine usage or binging on alcohol (with or without sleep deprivation)
- *Drug-induced headaches* need to be considered when new onset headaches occur on a background of recently prescribed nitrate therapy for coronary artery disease or vasodilators for peripheral arterial ischemia

BOX 4: Investigations in the ER.

In a person known to have previous headaches responsive to medications:
- *If papilledema or focal neurological signs are present:* MRI brain with contrast and a venogram
- *If new onset fever and/or meningeal signs present:* CT scan of the brain with contrast followed by a lumbar puncture (LP)
- *If systemic BP is elevated:* CT scan of the brain with blood sample for hemogram and renal parameters

In a person with the first and worst headaches of a lifetime:
- Look for papilledema and signs of meningeal irritation followed by a CT angiogram of the brain and a LP for evidence of subarachnoid hemorrhage (SAH)
- If a CT scan and LP fail to demonstrate evidence of SAH consider possibilities of RCVS or functional headaches

In a person with new onset headaches and focal or systemic constitutional symptoms:
- Collect a blood sample for a complete renal profile, organize a brain MRI with contrast and ensure that a MR angiogram and venogram is performed

The management of headaches in the ER is entirely dependent on the above algorithm of assessment and results of the guided investigative approach. In the interim, symptomatic therapy with a kidney-safe analgesic is justified.

SUGGESTED READING

1. Baraness L, Baker AM. Acute Headache. Treasure Island (FL): StatPearls Publishing; 2024.

6.2 ACUTE GIDDINESS

Azad M Irani

BOX 1: Introduction.

- The term giddiness in the medical terminology is possibly the symptom with the most varied diagnostic possibilities along the neuroaxis and often outside the neuroaxis
- The Indian patient often calls it chakkar. Everyone has their own description and more importantly many various medical problems (some benign and some serious) are communicated to the doctor as "giddiness"
- Giddiness is a sense a sensation of whirling and a tendency to fall or stagger
- Dizziness on the other hand is a term used to describe a multitude of subjective feelings by the patients such as feeling faint, lightheaded, foggy, just overall a weak feeling, or unsteadiness
- Dizziness that gives a feeling of a sense that you or your surroundings are spinning or moving is called vertigo
- Dizziness is one of the most common symptom, a patient presents to an emergency or outpatient room
- It is important to enquire what is the patient's exact description of the chakkar

BOX 2: Common conditions termed as chakkar/giddiness.

- True vertigo and it is various causes
- Presyncopal events
- Postural blood pressure (BP) drop
- Peripheral neuropathy
- Dorsal column—spinal cord pathology
- High BP
- Cerebral ataxia (early)
- *Hypoglycemia*: It can do anything
- Drugs, e.g., antiepileptics

BOX 3: To get a basic idea of the rough localization ask what is the description of the chakkar/giddiness.

		Possible etiology
1.	Is it a sense of rotation of self or surroundings	Vertigo
2.	Is it a blackout	Syncopal events, high blood pressure (BP), and postural low BP
3.	Is it imbalance mainly on walking only	Peripheral neuropathy, spinal cord problem, and cerebellar ataxia

BOX 4: Approach to patient management.

- When a patient presents to the emergency room (ER)—the first question the doctor wants to answer is—Is the vertigo central or peripheral
- Central vertigo must be scanned [magnetic resonance imaging (MRI) preferably, as computed tomography (CT) scan is often blind to posterior fossa which here would be the main area of interest]
- If in doubt it is always better to err on the side of caution and do an MRI brain scan with a contrast or noncontrast angiography to rule out a posterior fossa stroke or basilar occlusion
- Some basic pointers/red flags that suggest a central vertigo necessitating urgent imaging to rule out posterior circulation stroke are presented in **Box 5**

BOX 5: Red flags for central vertigo/when should we consider doing an urgent MRI scan.

- Vertigo plus brainstem symptoms/signs—double vision difficulty in speech, and difficulty in swallowing, however, transient and blackouts
- Vascular risk factors—Diabetes, HTN, and smoking
- History of vascular disease elsewhere—coronary artery disease (CAD), peripheral vascular disease (PVD), and previous cerebrovascular accident (CVA)
- Obesity or any symptom suggesting obstructive sleep apnea (OSA)
- *Central nystagmus*: Bidirectional nystagmus, vertical nystagmus, and torsional nystagmus

Caveat: If there is a posterior circulation ischemic stroke do not lower the BP too precipitously as it can further reduce the blood follow to the already ischemic penumbra resulting in further infarction and possibly quadriparesis. Further management—thrombolysis or digital subtraction angiography (DSA) intervention, etc., will depend on the entire clinical and imaging profile, most importantly the time window.

BOX 6: Clinical examination.

- Amongst the various clinical examination points, nystagmus remains the most common finding but also the most difficult to fathom
- The basic difference between central and peripheral nystagmus is shown in **Box 7**
- However, a more useful and better yield quick test is the head impulse test, HINTS, and HINTS plus **(Boxes 8 and 9)**

BOX 7: Difference between central and peripheral nystagmus.

Findings	***Peripheral nystagmus***	***Central nystagmus***
Latency	Often 3–10 seconds	No latent period
Fatigability (habituation)	Often lasts 10–30 seconds and then stops	It is continuous
Consistency (reproducibility)	Less consistent—becomes lesser when tested repeatedly/ provokes less of response each time	Consistent—persists even if repeated several times
Nystagmus direction	• Direction fixed • Typically has mixed directional components; quick phase of intorsion movement toward the dependent ear, upbeat toward forehead	• Direction can change • Often purely vertical (either upbeating or downbeating) or purely horizontal
Suppression of nystagmus by visual fixation	Suppressible	Not suppressible
Severity	More severe, marked vertigo, intense nystagmus, nausea, and vomiting	Less severe symptomatically milder vertigo, minimal nausea

BOX 8: Head impulse test.

- The head impulse test is a test used to diagnose peripheral vestibular disorder
- The test involves the patient sitting upright in front of the examiner and fixing his/ her gaze on the nose of the examiner
- The patient must be told to continue to gaze at the nose even during the test
- Then examiner holds the patient's head and then gives a rapid jerk to the head by 10–20° to one side while the patients continue to fix gaze on the examiners nose (as has been instructed already)
- The head is now gently moved back to the center and the test is repeated by turning/jerking the head to the opposite side
- A patient with a normal healthy vestibular system will have his/her gaze fixed on the examiner's nose during the jerking of the head
- However, a patient with a pathology of the peripheral/vestibular apparatus will have a short saccade (short rapid catch up movement of the eye before refixing to examiners nose) during the jerky head movement made by the examiner
- The head impulse test hence helps to diagnose a peripheral cause of vertigo. Meaning to say, it will be normal in a patient with a central cause of vertigo
- Prior to the test ensure patient has no major neck pain or pathology. Hence, an abnormal head impulse test/a saccade during the test is indeed reassuring in the ER as it points toward a peripheral and not a central cause

The HINTS is a combination of Head Impulse Test plus Nystagmus plus Test of Skew

BOX 9: HINTS test.

Head impulse test	As above
Nystagmus	A unidirectional nystagmus continues to have the fast component in the same direction (for example leftward fast component) despite the eye gazing in either direction (left or right) is reassuring for a peripheral nystagmus (left-sided pathology in this example). A bidirectional nystagmus that is beating leftward on left gaze and rightward when patient is asked to look rightward is suspicious of a central nystagmus. A vertical or a torsional nystagmus is also worrisome for a central nervous system (CNS) cause
Test of Skew	The test of skew is done rather simply with a cover-uncover test where the examiner asks the patient to fixate the gaze onto the examiner's nose and then alternately covers one eye field with his own hand, while asking the patient to continue trying to fixate on his nose. Here, a patient who gets an eye movement or skew during the alternating cover uncover is suspicious of a central cause

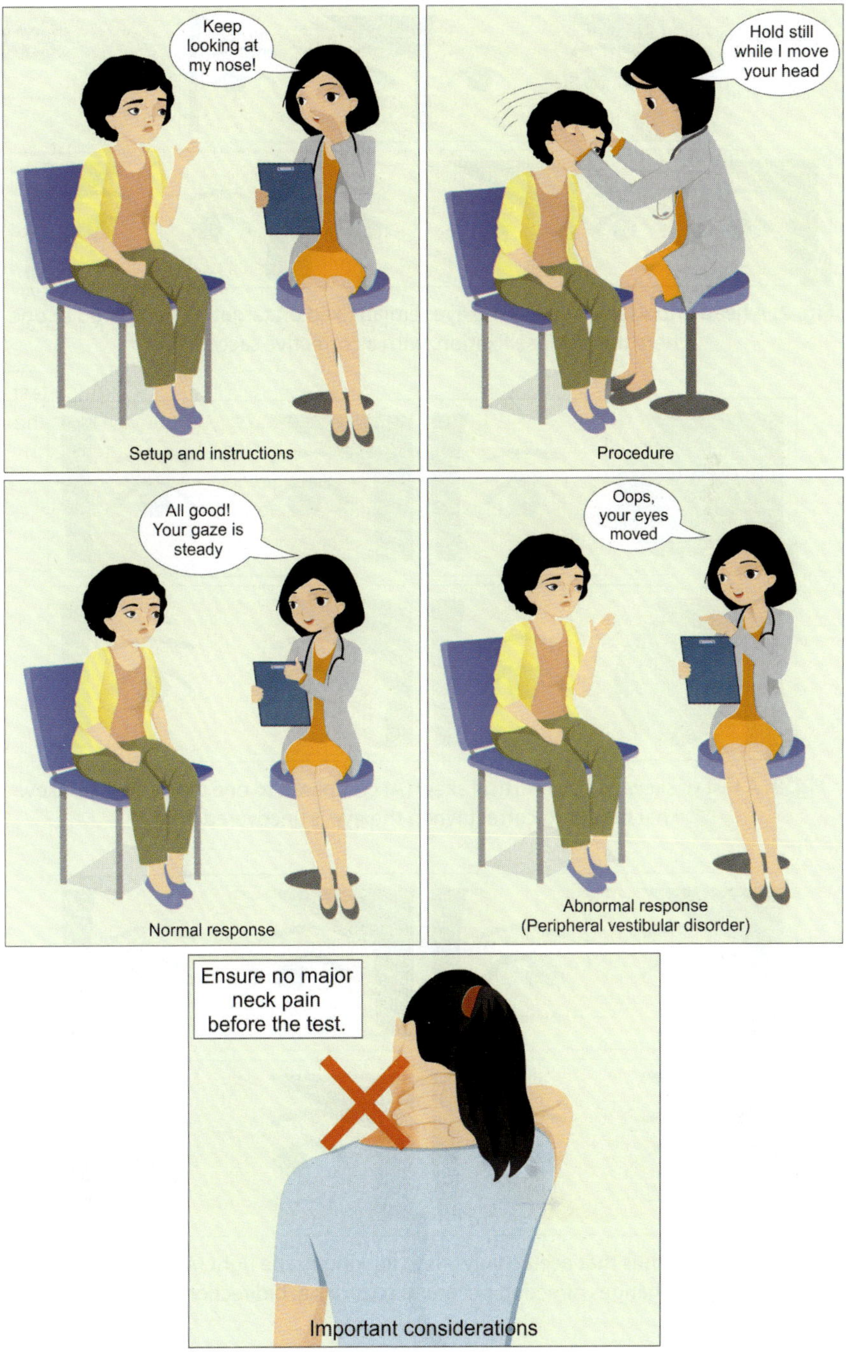

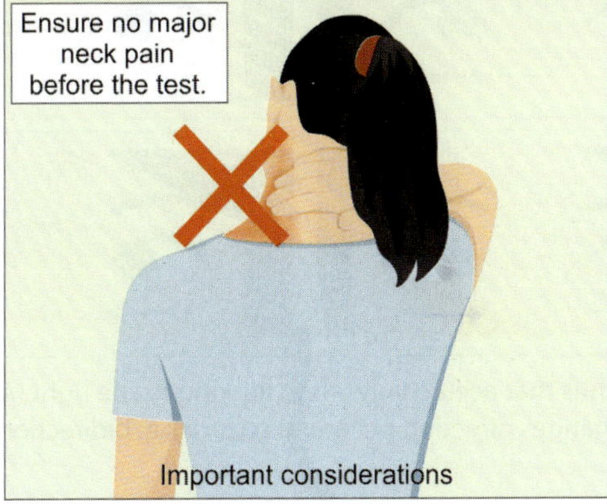

Fig. 1: Head impulse test.

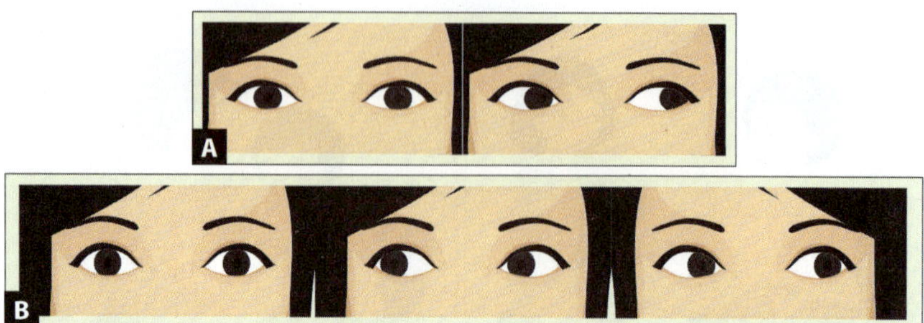

Fig. 2: A head impulse test where the eye remian fixed on target (A) compared to one where the eye lose fixation, with a corrective saccade (B).

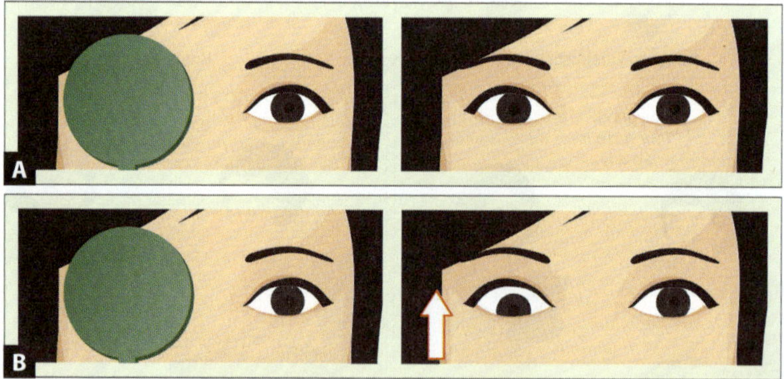

Fig. 3: A test of skew with no vertical skew (A) compared to one with a vertical skew that begins to correct when the eye is uncovered (B).

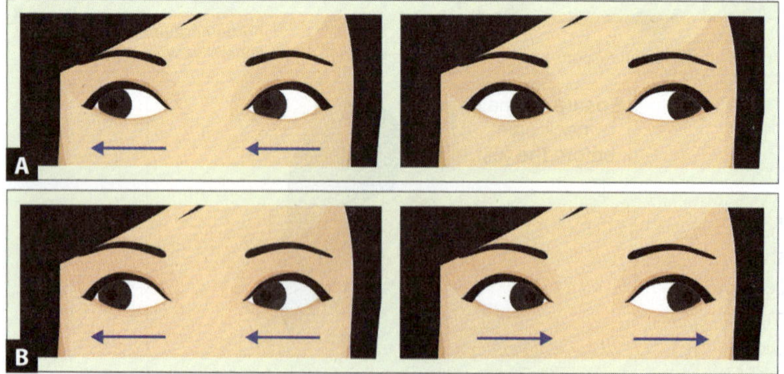

Fig. 4: Nystagmus that occurs only when looking to the right (A) compared to nystagmus that changes direction on lateral gaze, a.k.a. bidirectional nystagmus (B).

BOX 10: HINTS test analysis—peripheral versus central.

	Peripheral vertigo	***Central vertigo***
Head Impulse Test	Abnormal; corrective saccade to midline with rotation of head	Normal; no corrective saccade
Nystagmus	Unidirectional; horizontal	Horizontal and direction—changing; vertical; and torsional
Test of Skew	No skew deviation	Skew deviation present

BOX 11: Interpretation.

Hence, to have a reassuring result suggesting a peripheral cause of the vertigo (and not central), we must have a combination of all three results, i.e., (1) unidirectional nystagmus, (2) an abnormal head impulse test, and (3) no vertical skew deviation during cover-uncover testing.

Once a central cause of vertigo is ruled out by adequate clinical examination or imaging we can turn our attention to the various but common peripheral cause of vertigo that may present to the ER.

BOX 12: Common causes of peripheral vestibular disorders.

Vestibular neuritis, benign paroxysmal positional vertigo, and Meniere's disease

BOX 13: Nonpharmaceutical treatment of benign paroxysmal positional vertigo (BPPV).

Here, it is important to discuss two important procedures: The Dix–Hallpike test to diagnose BPPV and the Epley's maneuver for treating the BPPV by repositioning the otolith that has gone astray.

- *Dix–Hallpike maneuver:*
  - The Dix–Hallpike maneuver is done when patients have recurrent episodes of vertigo and BPPV is considered as the probable diagnosis. These patients experience vertigo in brief short lasting episodes most often triggered by turning/jerking the head from side to side or at times up down
  - The Dix–Hallpike maneuver involves hyperextending the neck and hence should not be done in patients with certain head and neck problems such as cervical instability, acute neck trauma, cervical disc prolapse, Arnold–Chiari malformation and those with a past history of arterial dissection
  - During the Dix–Hallpike maneuver, the patient sits upright on a bed/table with legs extended. The clinician will now rotate the head 45° toward the ear that will be tested. The patient is then swiftly laid with back down with the head hanging off the edge of the examination table. The patient's neck being extended approximately 20° below the horizontal plane while the head is still in the initial 45° rotation. The position should be held for at least next 30 seconds. During this time, the clinician observes the patient's eyes for any nystagmus

Contd...

Contd...

- In posterior canal BPPV, the nystagmus seen during this maneuver is torsional and upbeating. The vertical quick phase of the nystagmus being directed upward toward the forehead. In contrast, the torsional quick phase of the nystagmus is in a downward direction
- There is often a latency period of 2–5 seconds between the positioning of the head and the onset of nystagmus. The Dix–Hallpike maneuver is the gold standard for diagnosing posterior canal BPPV

- *Epley maneuver:* In very simple terms, BPPV occurs due to the otolith crystals migrating into the semicircular canals. Aim is to reposition this otolith back into the utricle-saccule
  - Patient is to be seated comfortably on a bed
  - Turn the head by 45° to the right
  - Quickly make the patient lie on the back, keeping the head turned at 45°
  - Next turn the head by 90° to the left
  - Next turn the head and body by 90° to the left, means now patient on his left lateral position
  - And next make the patient sit up on the left side
- *Caveat:* The Epley maneuver needs training to be done in the right way. Otherwise, it can be counterproductive. Also first turn is toward the affected ear. Between each step do not wait too less nor too long!!!!

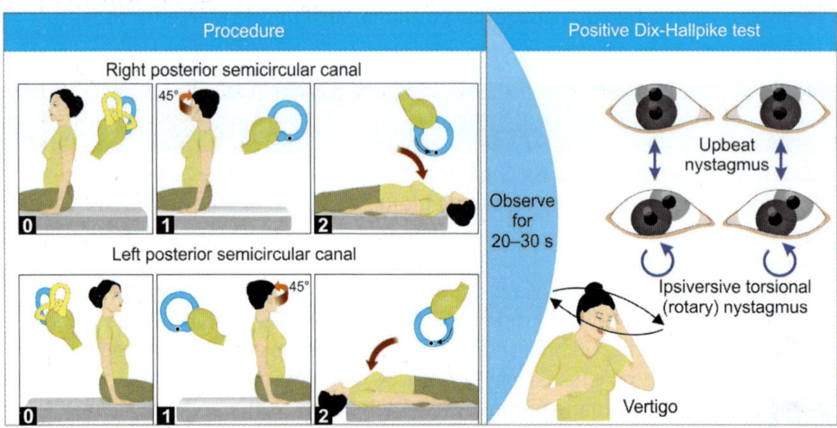

Fig. 5: Dix-Hallpike maneuver.

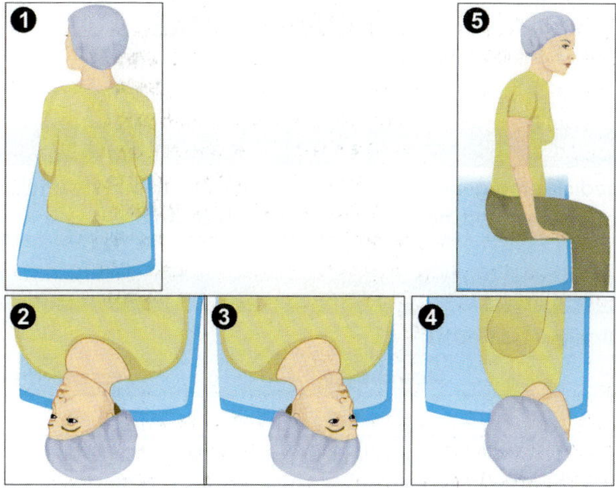

Fig. 6: Epley maneuver.

BOX 14: Pharmacological management of peripheral vertigo.

Vestibular suppressants remain the mainstay of treatment. It must be noted also that many patient who may be having relentless vomiting due to the vertigo, may be dehydrated, and will require fluid and electrolyte correction. Antiemetics and thiamine supplementation (in case of long term emesis) may also be needed.

Vestibular suppressants used in vertigo:

1.	Betahistine	Oral	8–16 mg TID	Rarely nausea/ indigestion
2.	Cinnarizine	Oral	25 mg BD or TDS	Sedation
3.	Prochlorperazine	Oral or IV	5–20 mg BD OR QDS	Extrapyramidal effects
4.	Dimenhydrinate	Oral	50 mg BD	Urinary retention, dry mouth

Note: If prochlorperazine causes the rare side effect of oculogyric crisis, use injectable promethazine 25 mg intramuscular.

BOX 15: Summary.

- Giddiness may have varied causes—neurological or non-neurological.
- We must learn basic bedside examination tests to differentiate between central or peripheral causes of vertigo.
- If any red flags exist to suggest an acute central pathology an urgent MRI brain may be needed.

Solving the difficult case of a giddy patient may make the doctor giddy too!!!! (Another unknown cause of giddiness).

SUGGESTED READING

1. Campbell WW. DeJong's The Neurologic Examination, 7th Edition. Philadelphia: Wolters Kluwer; 2012.

6.3 ACUTE STROKE

Fali Poncha

BOX 1: Introduction.

Stroke is a medical emergency. 1.9 million neurons die per minute until arterial blood flow can be restored, hence the term "**time is brain**".

BOX 2: Classification and clinical presentation.

Stroke is broadly classified as:

Stroke type	***Mechanism***	***Presentation***
Ischemic		
Thrombosis	In situ clot formation on a stenosed vessel or plaque	Transient ischemic attack (TIA) may occur before stroke
Embolic	Obstruction of a vessel secondary from a clot dislodged from a remote source (heart/aortic arch)]	Sudden
Hypoperfusion	Vascular border zone infarct [anterior cerebral artery (ACA)/middle cerebral artery (MCA)/posterior cerebral artery (PCA)]	Diffuse watershed areas, with waxing and waning
Hemorrhagic/ nonischemic (discussed in Chapters 6.7 and 6.8)	Hypertensive and other causes	Intracranial pressure (ICP) might be increased, more severe in nature

BOX 3: Clinical presentation by area of infarct.

Ischemic strokes are also divided based on the area of infarct:

Circulation	***Major arteries***	***Major region of brain supplied***	***Most common presentation***
Anterior [internal carotid artery (ICA)]	Ophthalmic	Optic nerve and retina	• TIA (amaurosis fugax) • Visual loss
	Anterior cerebral	• Frontal pole • Anteromedial cerebral cortex • Anterior corpus callosum	• Leg weakness • Urinary retention
	Middle cerebral	Frontoparietal Anterotemporal	Speech defect with facial weakness/ dropping

Contd...

Contd...

Ischemic strokes are also divided based on the area of infarct:

Circulation	***Major arteries***	***Major region of brain supplied***	***Presentation***
Posterior (vertebral system)	Vertebral	Brainstem	• Giddiness • Ataxia sensory dysfunction • Diplopia • Dysphagia
	Posteroinferior cerebral	Cerebellum	
	Basilar	Thalamus	
	Posterior cerebral	Auditory/vestibular	
	Middle temporal lobe	Visual occipital cortex	

Caveat:

BE-FAST acronym:
- *Balance:* Check for sudden loss of balance or coordination.
- *Eyes:* Look for sudden changes in vision, such as double vision or loss of vision in one or both eyes
- *Face:* Ask the person to smile. Check if one side of the face droops
- *Arms:* Ask the person to raise both arms. See if one arm drifts downward
- *Speech:* Ask the person to repeat a simple phrase. Listen for slurred or strange speech
- *Time:* If you observe any of these signs, it is time to call emergency services immediately

BOX 4: Examination.

When assessing a patient with suspected ischemic stroke, a quick neurological examination should be done briefly [National Institutes of Health Stroke Scale (NIHSS)] and the following signs and symptoms should be assessed:
- Level of consciousness (LOC) [Glasgow Coma Scale (GCS)]
- Speech
- Eye deviation
- Hemiparesis
- Ataxia
- Sensory loss
- Visual field

BOX 5: Management.

Steps to follow:
- Stabilize airway, breathing, and circulations (ABCs)
- Quick clinical assessment (NIHSS)
- Blood sugar, complete blood count (CBC) (platelets), creatinine, prothrombin time/International Normalized Ratio (PT/INR) (if the patient is not on anticoagulants and has no history of liver disease, do not wait for results), electrocardiogram (ECG) [for any arrhythmia/acute myocardial infarction (MI)], and cardiac markers
- Keep nil by mouth (NBM) until initial evaluation and stabilization
- *Immediate imaging:* Acute stroke flow chart
- Decide on endovascular thrombectomy (EVT) versus chemical thrombectomy

BOX 6: Key considerations.

In 1995, the National Institute of Neurological Disorders and Stroke (NINDS) trial was the first to show that recombinant tissue plasminogen activator (rtPA) given within 3 hours of stroke onset significantly improved outcomes. Double the number of patients were independent at 3 months compared to placebo group or arm of study.

Five subsequent trials have shown that large artery occlusion (MCA stem/M1) benefits significantly more from endovascular thrombectomy (EVT) compared to intravenous thrombolysis.

The American Heart Association (AHA) and European Stroke Organization recommend EVT in addition to best medical management for:
- Adults with anterior circulation stroke presenting within 6 hours of symptom onset
- Causative occlusion of internal carotid artery (ICA)/middle cerebral artery (MCA)
- Age >18 years
- The Alberta Stroke Program Early CT Score (ASPECTS) and NIHSS >6 (preferable but can be considered even if ASPECTS 3–5)
- If >6 hours presentation meets DAWN/DIFFUSE 3 trials, EVT is recommended

Caveat:

As further evidence from trials come in time limits, the decison regarding thrombolysis will change periodically. All these guidelines are to be used by the ER physician in conjunction with neurologists/stroke specialists.

BOX 7: Requirements for successful endovascular thrombectomy (EVT).

- Target vessel occlusion
- Salvageable tissue
- Fast and effective reperfusion

BOX 8: Algorithm in acute stroke management.

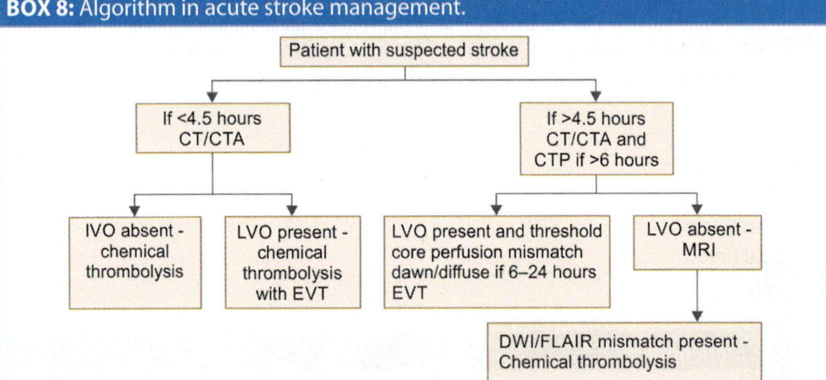

(CTA: computed tomography angiography; CTP: computed tomography perfusion; DWI: diffusion-weighted imaging; EVT: endovascular thrombectomy; FLAIR: fluid-attenuated inversion recovery; LVO: large vessel occlusion)

As per hours of presentation, decide on the choice of imaging:
- CT with angiography (unless known chronic renal failure, no need to wait for creatinine)
- MRI with magnetic resonance angiography (MRA)
- Exclude bleed
- Grade severity of ischemic stroke (ASPECTS score)
- **Unless ASPECTS score <6, patient can be given IV rtPA or tenecteplase within 4.5 hours of stroke onset**

Fibrinolysis Indication and Contraindications (Chapter 3.1)

BOX 9: Blood pressure targets.

- Hypertension and blood sugar targets should be achieved before chemical thrombolysis
- Blood pressure <180/110 mm Hg before thrombolysis should be achieved
- Blood sugars should be maintained between 140 and 180 mg/dL

For more details blood pressure target in ischemic stroke especially when patients are not thrombolysed refer to the Chapter 3.6 on hypertension

Blood pressure monitoring frequencies	
Time after start of rtPA infusion	*Frequency of blood pressure monitoring*
0–2 hours	Every 15 minutes
3–8 hours	Every 30 minutes
9–24 hours	Every 60 minutes
Drug treatment of hypertension during and after administration of thrombolytics or other acute reperfusion therapy	
If systolic blood pressure is >180–230 mm Hg Or diastolic blood pressure is >105–120 mm Hg	Labetalol, 10 mg IV followed by infusion at 2–8 mg/min Or Nicardipine infusion, 5 mg/hour, titrate up by 2.5 mg/hour at 5- to 15-minute intervals; maximum dose 15 mg/hour Or Clevidipine infusion, 1–2 mg/hour, titrate up by doubling dose every 2–5 minutes; maximum dose 21 mg/hour
If blood pressure is not controlled by above measures or if diastolic blood pressure >140 mm Hg	Consider sodium nitroprusside infusion (0.5–10 µg/kg/min). Continuous arterial monitoring advised; use with caution in patients with hepatic or renal insufficiency. Increases ICP. Pregnancy category C.

Source: Tintinalli JE, John Ma O, Yealy DM, Meckler GD, Stapczynski JS, Cline DM, et al. Tintinalli's Emergency Medicine: A Comprehensive Study Guide, 9th edition. McGraw Hill Professional; 2019.

BOX 10: Dosage.

- *Tenecteplase:* 0.25 mg/kg bolus, maximum 25 mg
- *Alteplase:* 0.9 mg/kg IV, with a maximum dose of 90 mg; administer 10% of the dose as a bolus over 1 minute, with the remaining amount infused over 60 minutes
- *Antiplatelets:* Loading dose with dual antiplatelets of aspirin and clopidogrel should be administered 24 hours post-thrombolysis if not being lysed.
- If not being lysed, administer antiplateltes immediately along with statins

Consider anticoagulation (time to start depends on size of stroke) if embolic:
- 0/immediately-in TIA
- 3 day-in minor stroke
- On 6th day in moderate stroke
- On 9th day in major stroke

BOX 11: Terminology.

- TIA is defined as a transient episode of neurological dysfunction caused by focal brain/spinal cord/retinal ischemia without acute infarction
- Symptoms typically lasts 1–2 hours
- Risk of stroke 8-12% within 7 days and 11–15% within 1 month hence TIA is an emergency
- MRI to be done to rule in/out a stroke

BOX 12: Disposition.

- All acute stroke patients should be managed initially in the intensive care unit (ICU)
- Close monitoring post-thrombolysis
- Repeat imaging should be done in 24 hours or earlier if deterioration occurs
- Monitor and document GCS and NIHSS closely

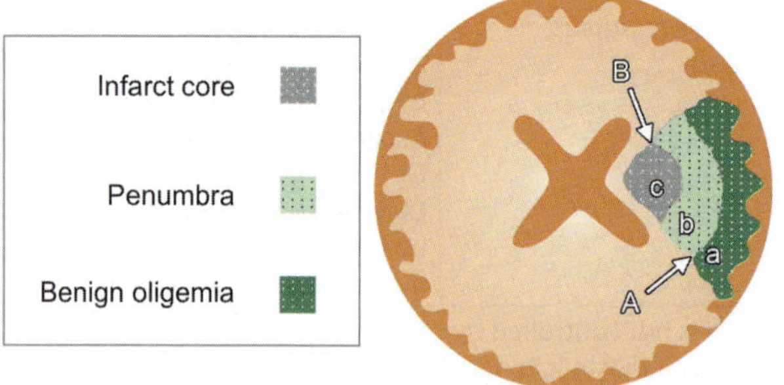

Fig. 1: Hyperacute stroke in the left middle cerebral artery region.

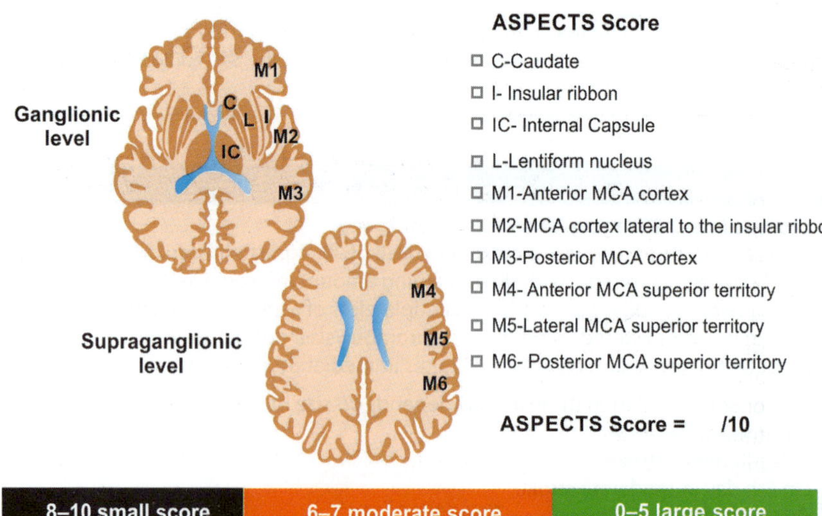

Fig. 2: ASPECTS score in the acute stroke.

BOX 13: NIHSS scoring scale.

Instructions	*Scale definition*
1a. *LOC* The investigator must choose a response if a full evaluation is prevented by such obstacles as an endotracheal tube, language barrier, or orotracheal trauma/ bandages. A 3 is scored only if the patient makes no movement (other than reflexive posturing) in response to noxious stimulation	0 = Alert, keenly responsive 1 = Not alert, but arousable by minor stimulation to obey, answer, or respond 2 = Not alert; requires repeated stimulation to attend or is obtunded and requires strong or painful stimulation to make movements (not stereotyped) 3 = Responds only with reflex motor or autonomic effects or is totally unresponsive, flaccid, and areflexic
1b. *LOC questions* The patient is asked the month and his or her age. The answer must be correct-there is no partial credit for being close. Aphasic and stuporous patients who do not comprehend the questions are given a score of 2. Patients unable to speak because of endotracheal intubation, orotracheal trauma, severe dysarthria from any cause, language barrier, or any other problem not secondary to aphasia are given a score of 1. It is important that only the initial answer be graded and that the examiner not "help" the patient with verbal or nonverbal cues	0 = Answers both questions correctly 1 = Answers one question correctly 2 = Answers neither question correctly
1c. *LOC commands* The patient is asked to open and close the eyes and then to grip and release the nonparetic hand. Substitute another one-step command if the hands cannot be used. Credit is given if an unequivocal attempt is made but not completed due to weakness. If the patient does not respond to command, the task should be demonstrated to him or her (pantomime) and the result scored (i.e., follows no, one, or two commands). Patients with trauma, amputation, or other physical impediments should be given suitable one-step commands. Only the first attempt is scored	0 = Performs both tasks correctly 1 = Performs one task correctly 2 = Performs neither task correctly

Contd...

Contd...

Instructions	*Scale definition*
2. *Best gaze* Only horizontal eye movements are tested. Voluntary or reflexive (oculocephalic) eye movements are scored, but caloric testing is not done. If the patient has a conjugate deviation of the eyes that can be overcome by voluntary or reflexive activity, the score is 1. If a patient has an isolated peripheral nerve paresis (cranial nerve III, IV, or VI), the score is 1. Gaze is testable in all aphasic patients. Patients with ocular trauma, bandages, preexisting blindness, or other disorder of visual acuity or fields should be tested with reflexive movements, and a choice made by the investigator. Establishing eye contact and then moving about the patient from side to side will occasionally clarify the presence of a partial gaze palsy	0 = Normal 1 = Partial gaze palsy, gaze is abnormal in one or both eyes, but forced deviation or total gaze paresis is not present 2 = Forced deviation, or total gaze paresis not overcome by the oculocephalic maneuver
3. *Visual* Visual fields (upper and lower quadrants) are tested by confrontation, using finger counting or visual threat, as appropriate. Patients may be encouraged, but if they look at the side of the moving fingers appropriately, this can be scored as normal. If there is unilateral blindness or enucleation, visual fields in the remaining eye are scored. Score 1 only if a clear-cut asymmetry, including quadrantanopia, is found. If the patient is blind from any cause, score 3. Double simultaneous stimulation is performed at this point. If there is extinction, patient receives a score of 1, and the results are used to respond to item 11	0 = No vision loss 1 = Partial hemianopia 2 = Complete hemianopia 3 = Bilateral hemianopia (blind including cortical blindness)
4. *Facial palsy* Ask or use pantomime to encourage the patient to show teeth or raise eyebrows and close eyes. Score symmetry of grimace in response to noxious stimuli in the poorly responsive or noncomprehending patient. If facial trauma/bandages, orotracheal tube, tape, or other physical barriers obscure the face, these should be removed to the extent possible	0 = Normal symmetric movements 1 = Minor paralysis (flattened nasolabial fold and asymmetry on smiling) 2 = Partial paralysis (total or near-total paralysis of lower face) 3 = Complete paralysis of one or both sides (absence of facial movement in the upper and lower face

Contd...

Contd...

Instructions	***Scale definition***
5. *Motor arm* The limb is placed in the appropriate position: Extend the arms (palms down) 90° (if sitting) or 45° (if supine). Drift is scored if the arm falls before 10 seconds. (Count out loud and use fingers to show the patient the count.) The aphasic patient is encouraged using urgency in the voice and pantomime, but not noxious stimulation. Each limb is tested in turn, beginning with the nonparetic arm. Only in the case of amputation or joint fusion at the shoulder, the examiner should record the score as untestable (UN) and clearly write the explanation for this choice. 5a. Left arm 5b. Right arm	0 = No drift, limb holds 90° (or 45°) for full 10 seconds 1 = Drift, limb holds 90° (or 45°), but drifts down before full 10 seconds; does not hit bed or other support 2 = Some effort against gravity, limb cannot get to or maintain (if cued) 90° (or 45°), drifts down to bed, but has some effort against gravity 3 = No effort against gravity; limb falls 4 = No movement
6. *Motor leg* The limb is placed in the appropriate position: Hold the leg at 30° (the patient is always tested supine). Drift is scored if the leg falls before 5 seconds. (Count out loud and use fingers to show the patient the count.) The aphasic patient is encouraged using urgency in the voice and pantomime, but not noxious stimulation. Each limb is tested in tum, beginning with the nonparetic leg. Only in the case of amputation or joint fusion at the hip, the examiner should record the score as UN and dearly write the explanation for this choice. 6a. Left leg 6b. Right leg	0 = No drift: Leg holds 30° position for full 5 seconds 1 = Drift; leg falls by the end of the 5 seconds period but does not hit bed 2 = Some effort against gravity, leg falls to bed by 5 seconds, but has some effort against gravity. 3 = No effort against gravity; leg falls to bed immediately 4 = No movement
7. *Limb ataxia* This item is aimed at finding evidence of a unilateral cerebellar lesion. Test with the patient's eyes open. In case of visual defect, ensure that testing is done in the intact visual field. The finger-nose-finger and heel-shin tests are performed on both sides, and ataxia is scored only if present out of proportion to weakness. Ataxia is absent in the patient who cannot understand or is paralyzed. Only in the case of amputation or joint fusion, the examiner should record the score as UN and clearly write the explanation for this choice. In case of blindness, test by having the patient touch the nose from an extended arm position.	0 = Absent 1 = Present in one limb 2 = Present in two limbs

Contd...

Contd...

Instructions	***Scale definition***
8. *Sensory* Sensation or grimace to pinprick when tested, or withdrawal from a noxious stimulus in the obtunded or aphasic patient. Only sensory loss attributed to stroke is scored as abnormal, and the examiner should test as many body areas [arms (not hands), legs, trunk, and face] as needed to check accurately for hemisensory loss. A score of 2, "severe or total sensory loss", should be given only when a severe or total loss of sensation can be clearly demonstrated. Stuporous and aphasic patients will therefore probably score 1 or 0. The patient with brainstem stroke who has bilateral loss of sensation is scored 2. If the patient does not respond and is quadriplegic, score 2. Patients in a coma (item la score 3) are automatically given a 2 on this item	0 = Normal; no sensory loss 1 = Mild-to-moderate sensory loss; patient feels pinprick is less sharp or is dull on affected side, or there is loss of superficial pain with pinprick, but patient is aware of being touched 2 = Severe to total sensory loss; patient is not aware of being touched on face, arm, and leg
9. *Best language* A great deal of information about comprehension is obtained during the preceding sections of the examination. For this scale item, the patient is asked to describe what is happening in the test picture, to name the items on the test naming sheet, and to read from the test list of sentences. Comprehension is judged from responses here as well as responses to all of the commands in the preceding general neurologic examination. If vision loss interferes with the tests, ask the patient to identify objects placed in the hand, repeat, and produce speech. The intubated patient should be asked to write. The patient in a coma (item la score = 3) automatically scores 3 on this item. The examiner must choose a score for the patient with stupor or limited cooperation, but a score of 3 should be used only if the patient is mute and follows no one-step commands	0 = No aphasia; normal 1 = Mild-to-moderate aphasia; some obvious loss of fluency or facility of comprehension, without significant limitation on ideas expressed or form of expression. However, reduction of speech and/or comprehension makes conversation about provided materials difficult or impossible. For example, in conversation about provided materials, examiner can identify picture or naming card content from patient's response 2 = Severe aphasia; all communication is through fragmentary expression; great need for inference, questioning, and guessing by listener. Range of information that can be exchanged is limited; listener carries burden of communication. Examiner cannot identify materials provided from patient's response 3 = Mute, global aphasia; no usable speech or auditory comprehension

Contd...

Contd...

Instructions	Scale definition
10. *Dysarthria* If the patient is thought to be normal, an adequate sample of speech must be obtained by asking the patient to read or repeat words from the test list. If the patient has severe aphasia, the clarity of articulation of spontaneous speech can be rated. Only if the patient is intubated or has other physical barriers to producing speech, the examiner should record the score as UN and clearly write an explanation for this choice. Do not tell the patient why he or she is being tested	0 = Normal 1 = Mild-to-moderate dysarthria; patient slurs at least some words and, at worst, can be understood with some difficulty 2 = Severe dysarthria; patient's speech is so slurred as to be unintelligible in the absence of or out of proportion to any dysphasia, or is mute/anarthric
11. *Extinction and inattention* Sufficient information to identify neglect may be obtained during the prior testing. If the patient has a severe vision loss preventing visual double simultaneous stimulation and the responses to cutaneous stimuli are normal, the score is 0. If the patient has aphasia but does appear to attend to both sides, the score is 0. The presence of visual spatial neglect or anosognosia may also be taken as evidence of abnormality. Because the abnormality is scored only if present, the item is never scored as UN	0 = No abnormality 1 = Visual, tactile, auditory, spatial, or personal inattention or extinction to bilateral simultaneous stimulation in one of the sensory modalities 2 = Profound hemi-inattention or extinction in more than one modality, patient does not recognize own hand or orients to only one side of space

SUGGESTED READING

1. American Heart Association/American Stroke Association. Guidelines for the Early Management of Patients with Acute Ischemic Stroke. Stroke. 2019;50(12):e344-418.
2. European Stroke Organisation (ESO) Executive Committee; ESO Writing Committee. Guidelines for management of ischaemic stroke and transient ischaemic attack 2008. Cerebrovasc Dis. 2008;25(5):457-507.
3. Goyal M, Menon BK, van Zwam WH, Dippel DW, Mitchell PJ, Demchuk AM, et al. Endovascular thrombectomy after large-vessel ischaemic stroke: a meta-analysis of individual patient data from five randomised trials. Lancet. 2016;387(10029):1723-31.
4. Hacke W, Kaste M, Bluhmki E, Brozman M, Dávalos A, Guidetti D, et al. Thrombolysis with alteplase 3 to 4.5 hours after acute ischemic stroke. N Engl J Med. 2008;359(13):1317-29.
5. Jovin TG, Nogueira RG, Lansberg MG, Gupta R. DAWN and DEFUSE 3 Trials: Implications for Stroke Care. Stroke. 2018;49(3):900-4.

6. National Institute of Neurological Disorders and Stroke rt-PA Stroke Study Group. Tissue Plasminogen Activator for Acute Ischemic Stroke. N Engl J Med. 1995;333(24):1581-7.
7. Powers WJ, Rabinstei AA, Ackerson T, Adeoye OM, Bambakidis NC, Becker K, et al. 2018 Guidelines for the Early Management of Patients with Acute Ischemic Stroke: A Guideline for Healthcare Professionals from the American Heart Association/American Stroke Association. Stroke. 2018;49(3):e46-99.

6.4 ACUTE SEIZURE

Natasha Tipnis

BOX 1: Definition.

- *Status epilepticus:* A seizure lasting longer than 5 minutes or having more than one seizure within a 5 minute period without returning back to a normal state of consciousness between the two seizures
- *Current timelines for defining SE:*
  - Developing SE—seizures leading up to SE
  - Established SE—seizures ≥5 minutes in duration [5–15 minutes is the recommended time to administer two doses of benzodiazepines—intravenous (IV)/buccal/nasal] (after 15 minutes, if not responsive to benzodiazepines—second-line antiseizure medication needs to be given intravenously)
- *Refractory SE:* Failure of two appropriately chosen and dosed antiseizure medication (benzodiazepine + second line)—this is at around 30 minutes post the beginning of the seizure. Usually at this point we proceed with intubation and IV anesthetic agents. Also, an electroencephalogram (EEG) should have been ideally performed by this time)
- *Super refractory SE:* SE persisting despite 24 hours of IV anesthesia

BOX 2: History.

The first step is to ascertain how long the seizure has been ongoing and at what stage of SE is the patient

Questions to ask the patient/relative:

- How long has the patient been seizing?
- Have any medications—oral/IV/nasal/buccal been given either at home or in the ambulance?
- Is the patient a known case of seizure disorder? If yes ask the following:
  - What is the seizure disorder?
  - What medicines is the patient taking?
  - Has the patient missed any medications?
  - Have any new medications been recently added or reduced?
  - Has the patient ever had SE in the past?
- Does the patient have fever/nausea/vomiting/visual disturbances/diplopia/loss of awareness?

BOX 3: Classification of status epilepticus (SE).

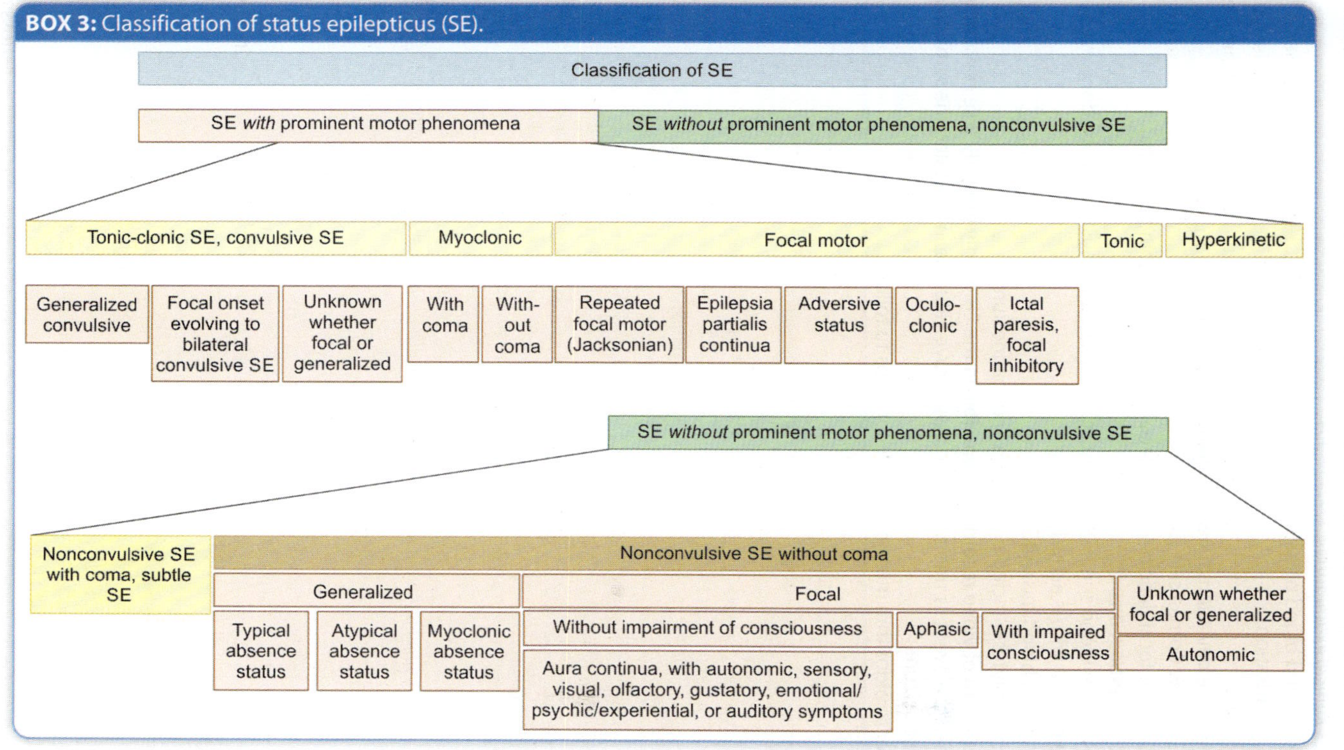

Source: https://onlinelibrary.wiley.com/doi/10.1111/epi.13121

BOX 4: Clinical examination and investigation.

- *Quick clinical examination:*
  - Pulse and blood pressure (BP)
  - O_2 saturation
  - Pupils
  - Any eye deviation or head deviation to one side
  - Glasgow Coma Scale (GCS)
  - Look for focal deficits—limbs/facial deviation/up going plantars
- *Blood investigations:*
  - Random blood sugar (RBS)—most important and must always be done even in a patient who is actively seizing
  - Arterial blood gas (ABG)
  - Electrolytes—including calcium and magnesium
- If any form of video recording is possible in the ER, kindly urgently take consent to record the event as this information will prove valuable in assessing the semiology of the seizure.
- Refer to algorithm mentioned here for steps to follow.

Treatment algorithm for tonic-clonic status epilepticus in adults

Timeline

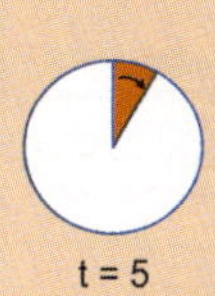

t = 0

t = 5

t = 15

Initial patient management 0–5 minutes

- Protect the patient. Do not restrain
- Consider *airway* adjunct
- Administer *oxygen*
- Place patient in a semi-prone position, head down
- Gain IV access
- Obtain BM. If hypoglycemic →

Give 150–200 mL 10% glucose IV stat

If seizures continue repeat this step AND commence 10% glucose infusion at 100 mL/hour

If suspicion of alcohol excess or malnutrition commence 1 pair Pabrinex IV BEFORE glucose replacement

1st line treatment 5–15 minutes

If IV access	If no IV access
DOSE 1 – IV lorazepam 4 mg bolus	DOSE 1 – Buccal midazolam 10 mg (Alternative IM midazolam 10 mg)
Wait 5 minutes	Wait 5 minutes
DOSE 2 – IV lorazepam 4 mg bolus	DOSE 2 – Buccal midazolam 10 mg (Alternative IM midazolam 10 mg)
Wait 5 minutes	Wait 5 minutes

2nd line treatment 15 minutes onwards

IV or IO access
Escalate to Critical Care as per local policy

DOSE 3

IV Levetiracetam 60 mg/kg, maximum 4,500 mg (In 100 mL sodium chloride 0.9% over 10 minutes)
OR IV Phenytoin 20 mg/kg, maximum 2 g (rate 50 mg/min, 25 mg/min for elderly or patients with cardiac history, give undiluted)
OR IV Valproate 40 mg/kg, maximum 3000 mg (In 100 mL sodium chloride 0.9% over 5 minutes)

Caution: Phenytoin administration requires cardiac monitoring and wide bore IV access due to risk of extravasation and phlebitis

	Preferred if	*Avoid it*
Levetiracetam (Keppra)	Polypharmacy (fewest drug interactions)	• Mood or behavioral disorder (may worsen symptoms)
Phenytoin		• Cardiac montoring not available • Known or suspected generalized epilepsy (genetic eplepsy) • Hypotension/bradycardia heart block • Porphyria • Known or suspected overdose of recreational drugs/alcohol withdrawal
Valproate	• Known or suspected Idiopathic generalized epilepsy (genetic epilepsy) • Co-morbid mood disorder/migraines	• Women of childbearing (potential consider pregnancy test) • Liver disease • Pancreatitis nown or suspected metabolic disorder/imitochondrial disease (risk of hepatotoxicity)

If ongoing seizures following the completion of the infusion consider 2nd IV antiepileptic drug infusion of a different drug from the same list (levetiracetam, phenytoin, valproate as above) OR phenobarbital

Phenobarbital can be given 15 mg/kg as a single dose, maximum rate 100 mg/min
If at any point >30 minutes since seizure onset move to 3rd line treatment

Ongoing management

Regular observations

12 lead ECG

Obtain FBC, U&Es, LFTs, Ca^{2+}, Mg^{2+} clotting studies and if applicable antiepileptic drug levels and blood gas

Treat acidosis if severe (discuss with critical care)

Determine if diagnosed epilepsy, medication history and acute seizure care plan

Consider neuroimaging and EEG

Consider possibility of non-epileptic seizures

Consider and treat potential causes:

- Medication related (poor compliance, poor absorption, recent antiepileptic drug changes, medication interactions or subtherapeutic levels)
- Infection
- Electrolyte disturbance
- Toxicity or drug withdrawal (including alcohol withdrawal)
- CNS pathology (tumor, stroke, encephalitis, PRES, neurodegenerative diseases etc.)

Seizure terminated

↓

ABCDE assessment of patient at regular intervals

Consider escalation to Critical Care setting if indicated

Start supportive medical care and look for underlying cause of status epilepticus

Caution when using multiple agents with similar mechanism of action in view of potential adverse effects.

Treatment algorithm for tonic-clonic status epilepticus in adults (cont.)

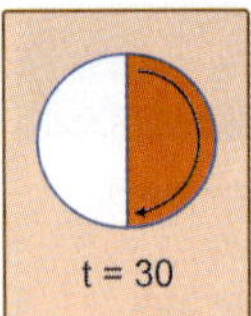

t = 30

The following stages must occur with anesthetic input, airway support and early arrangements for transfer to ITU

3rd line treatment 30 minutes onwards (refractory status)

General anesthesia – induction and maintenance

The properties of each drug should be considered when selecting induction and maintenance agents (these may be different)

	Induction	*Maintenance*
Propofol	1–2 mg/kg bolus	Up to 4 mg/kg/hour titrated to effect, continuous infusion for minimum 24 hours
Thiopental sodium	3–5 mg/kg bolus	3–5 mg/kg/hour titrated to effect, continuous infusion for minimum 24 hours
Ketamine	3 mg/kg bolus	1 mg/kg/hour titrated to effect maximum 10 mg/kg/hour, continuous infusion for minimum 24 hours
Midazolam	0.2 mg/kg bolus	0.05–0.5 mg/kg/hour titrated to effect, continuous infusion for minimum 24 hours

- General anesthesia maintenance is typically with propofol and/or midazolam in the first instance
- If first maintenance agent is unsuccessful at terminating seizures a second anesthetic agent should be used
- As a minimum, intermittent *EEG* to be performed aiming for suppression of electrographic epileptic activity
- Maintenance doses of *antiepileptic drugs* (commence 10–14 hours after loading dose to allow regular ongoing dosing)

24 hours+

4th line treatment 24+ hours (Super-Refractory Status)

Seizures that continue or recur 24 hours after third line treatment are considered Super Refractory Status Epilepticus. Treatment at this stage should be guided by specialists using an MDT approach. There is no high quality randomized controlled trial evidence to guide treatment decisions

- Look for an *underlying cause and treat* (e.g., infectious/autoimmune encephalitis, systemic infection, electrolyte disturbance, toxicity)
- *Neurosurgical intervention* (e.g., lesional resection)
- If no underlying cause identified in a first presentation of seizures, *immunotherapy* can be considered: high dose steroids, IVIG and/or therapeutic plasmapheresis
- *Alternative treatments* at this stage include therapeutic hypothermia, ketogenic diet and magnesium infusion

Treatments considered to be ineffective should be discontinued to minimize risk of adverse effects.

Ongoing management in critical care unit

At point of admission to ITU all patients should have an up-to-date ECG

Ensure regular antiepileptic drugs are prescribed alongside any additional treatment as part of this pathway

It is important to document why treatment decisions have been made and ensure detailed communication with next of kin regarding treatment plan and prognosis

Caution

Midazolam exhibits multiple drug interactions which should be considered: See **Appendix 2**

Patients on propofol should be monitored for PRIS–propofol infusion syndrome (metabolic acidosis, rhabdomyolysis, renal failure, hypertriglycerid–aemia, refractory bradycardia and cardiac failure)

Interpretation of processed EEG monitoring such as bispectral index (BIS) may become unreliable when using ketamine infusion

Caution when using multiple agents with similar mechanism of action in view of potential adverse effects.

Source: Walton Centre NHS. Guidelines for the management of status epilepticus. July 2020. Available from: https://www.thewaltoncentre.nhs.uk/downloads/information%20for%20healthcare%20professionals/status%20epilepticus%20guidelines%20july%202020.pdf

BOX 5: Rule of 1, 2, 3, 4, and 5.

- **1** essential blood test—blood sugar
- Maximum **2** doses of benzodiazepines before commencing with second-line treatment
- **3** drugs for second-line treatment (>15 minutes ongoing seizures)—levetiracetam, sodium valproate, and fosphenytoin
- **4** drugs for refractory status (>30 minutes ongoing seizures)—propofol, thiopental sodium, ketamine, and midazolam
- **5** treatment options for super-refractory seizures (>24 hours after beginning of seizures after treatment for underlying cause has been initiated)—high dose steroids, intravenous immunoglobulin (IVIg), therapeutic hypothermia, ketogenic diet, and surgical intervention

BOX 6: Doses of drugs used in management of status epilepticus (SE).

- Lorazepam—4 mg IV bolus followed by 4 mg IV bolus after 5 minutes if seizures do not stop
- Midazolam—nasal spray available in India—5 mg/mL—one spray in a single nostril followed by another in the other nostril after 5 minutes if seizures do not stop. Buccal or intramuscular (IM) midazolam is dosed at 10 mg per dose
- Levetiracetam—60 mg/kg (maximum 4,500 mg) in 100 mL 0.9% NS over 10 minutes
- Sodium valproate—40 mg/kg (maximum 3,000 mg) in 100 mL 0.9% NS over 5 minutes
- Fosphenytoin—20 mg PE/kg (maximum 2 g PE) at 50 mg PE/min
- Midazolam—0.2 mg/kg bolus followed by—start at 0.05 mg/kg/hour and up titrate to maximum 0.5 mg/kg/hour
- Propofol—1–2 mg/kg bolus followed by 4 mg/kg/hour
- Thiopental sodium—3–5 mg/kg bolus followed by 3–5 mg/kg/hour
- Ketamine—3 mg/kg bolus followed by—start at 1 mg/kg/hour and slowly up titrate to maximum 10 mg/kg/hour

BOX 7: Investigation specific to seizures.

Role of imaging:

- MRI brain is the investigation of choice for a patient with seizure; however, this should be considered only after the initial airway, breathing, and circulation (ABC) management has been done and the patient has been moved to the intensive care unit (ICU)

Role of EEG:

- EEG monitoring is mandatory for all patients with SE. Even after the patient has stopped visible seizures, EEG can be used to rule out nonconvulsive SE.

BOX 8: Disposition.

Patients who come to the ER with seizures lasting >10 minutes need ICU admission regardless of whether they meet other criteria or not.

BOX 9: Seizures which do not fit criteria for status epilepticus (SE).

Either the patient has had a seizure at home or the seizure has been controlled with a benzodiazepine

- Check ABC
- Check RBS and perform an ABG if breathing or consciousness is impaired
- Routine blood investigations—complete blood count (CBC), renal function test (RFT), liver function test (LFT), ionized Ca, serum Mg, and serum ammonia
- EEG whenever possible at the earliest
- MRI brain urgently if there is a focal neurological deficit, else within 24 hours.
- Todd's paralysis is transient motor weakness in the affected limb/s after a seizure. This may last from minutes to hours to even up to 2 days. In case a patient presents with a motor deficit, an MRI done immediately does not reveal any acute event, the weakness may be attributed to Todd's paralysis and the patient needs to be observed for the same
- If known case of epilepsy—ask for missed doses and start with a loading dose of the medication the patient was on
- If not a known case, or no history of epilepsy, the first seizure does not warrant any treatment except for a benzodiazepine
- The patient may be admitted for 24 hours to investigate further

History of alcohol intake is important and must always be obtained. Patients who have had binge drinking episodes or alcohol withdrawal seizures must always be administered injectable thiamine in large doses along with glucose.

SUGGESTED READING

1. Trinka E, Cock H, Hesdorffer D, Rossetti AO, Scheffer IE, Shinnar S, et al. A definition and classification of status epilepticus - Report of the ILAE Task Force on Classification of Status Epilepticus. Epilepsia. 2015;56(11):1515-23. doi:10.1111/epi.13121.
2. Walton Centre NHS. Guidelines for the management of status epilepticus. July 2020. Available from: https://www.thewaltoncentre.nhs.uk/downloads/information%20for%20healthcare%20professionals/status%20epilepticus%20guidelines%20july%202020.pdf

6.5 MOVEMENT DISORDER EMERGENCIES

Heli S Shah, Pettarusp M Wadia

BOX 1: Introduction to movement disorders (MD) emergencies.

- Movement disorder emergencies can rapidly evolve from hours to days wherein delay in diagnosis and treatment may lead to significant morbidity or mortality
- Based on phenomenology, it can be subdivided into **hypokinetic** or **hyperkinetic** movement disorders
- **Hypokinetic disorders** are characterized by akinesia or bradykinesia—the absence or paucity of movement. The hyperkinetic disorders are characterized by excess of movements and can be divided into dystonia, chorea, tics, myoclonus, and tremor
- **Hypokinetic MD** emergencies include drug-induced movement disorder emergencies neuroleptic malignant syndrome (NMS), malignant hyperthermia, parkinsonism-hyperpyrexia syndrome (PHS), serotonin syndrome (SS) as well as emergent complications of Parkinson disease (PD) including PD psychosis
- Common hyperkinetic movement disorder emergencies include acute dystonic reaction, status dystonicus, and acute onset chorea/ballismus
- Identification of phenomenology and clinical pattern recognition and removal of offending agents and triggers are key factors for appropriate recognition and management in the emergent situation

BOX 2: Neuroleptic malignant syndrome (NMS).

- NMS results from exposure to antipsychotics or antiemetic neuroleptics or its rapid withdrawal
- The syndrome typically presents within 4–6 weeks of exposure to antipsychotics, with a clinical tetrad of altered mental status, hyperthermia, rigidity, and dysautonomia
- The exact pathogenesis of NMS is not entirely clear but "**central**" dopaminergic hypofunction and "**peripheral**" sympathoadrenergic hyperactivity are suggested
- **Major criteria:** Fever, rigidity, and ↑ CK level (four times the upper limit of normal)
- **Minor criteria:** Encephalopathy, hypertension, tachycardia, diaphoresis, and leukocytosis
- *High likelihood of NMS*: All three major criteria or two major + four minors
- **Risk factors:**
  - Higher doses of neuroleptic drugs
  - Hyponatremia and hypokalemia
  - Thyroid disease
  - Catatonia
  - Parkinsonism
- Withdrawal of the causative agent is the key to management
- **Management of NMS**

Clinical features	***Management***
Mild rigidity; catatonia or confusion; hyperthermia (100.4°F); and tachycardia (≤100/min)	Lorazepam 1–2 mg IM or IV every 4–6 hours
Moderate rigidity, mutism, and catatonia; confusion, stupor, hyperthermia (100–104°F), and tachycardia (100–120/min)	• Lorazepam 1–2 mg IM or IV Every 4–6 hours • Bromocriptine 2.5–5 mg PO or by nasogastric tube (NG) tube, every 8 hours

Contd...

Contd...

Clinical features	***Management***
Severe rigidity, catatonia, or coma; hyperthermia (≥104°F) and tachycardia (≥120 bpm)	• Dantrolene 1–2.5 mg/kg body weight, IV every 6 hours for 48 hours, tapered • Bromocriptine 2.5–5 mg PO or by NG tube, every 8 hours • Amantadine 100 mg PO or by NG tube every 8 hours

BOX 3: Serotonin syndrome (SS).

- **Serotonin syndrome** (serotonin toxicity) is a potentially life-threatening condition associated with increased serotonergic activity in the central nervous system **(Fig. 1)**.
- SS may develop in patients taking two or more drugs with serotonergic actions (tricyclic antidepressants or selective serotonin reuptake inhibitors (SSRIs) plus nonselective monoamine oxidase inhibitor (MAOI), cocaine, opiates, amphetamines, lithium, etc.) **(*See* Box 4)**.
- **Hunter toxicity criteria for diagnosis of SS include:**
  - A serotonergic agent has been administered in the past 5 weeks plus.
  - One or more of the following combination of symptoms is seen:
    - Spontaneous clonus
    - Inducible clonus + agitation or sweating
    - Opsoclonus + agitation or sweating
    - Tremor + hyperreflexia
    - Hypertonia + temperature >38°C (100.4°F) + opsoclonus or inducible clonus

Management involves withdrawal of offending agents:
- Supportive therapy including normalization of vital signs, oxygenation, IV fluids, cardiac monitoring
- Management of hyperthermia including immediate sedation, standard rapid sequence intubation
- Management of autonomic instability—hypotension/hypertension and tachycardia
- Sedation with benzodiazepines (Lorazepam 2–4 mg IV or diazepam 5–10 mg IV) can be repeated based on patient response
- Cyproheptadine, serotonin antagonist via nasogastric tube—12 mg bolus followed by 2 mg every 2 hourly for persistent symptoms up to 32 mg in 24 hours

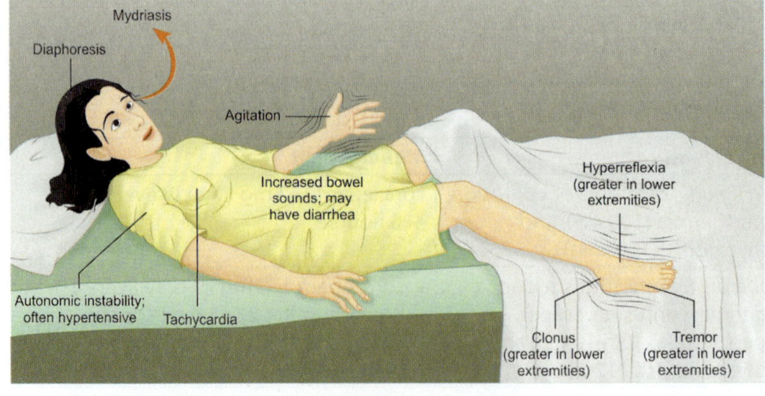

Fig. 1: Clinical features in a patient with severe serotonin syndrome.

BOX 4: Common drugs and interactions associated with serotonin syndrome.

Drug class	***Example of drugs***
Selective serotonin reuptake inhibitors (SSRIs) and selective serotonin and norepinephrine reuptake inhibitors (SNRIs)	Sertraline, paroxetine, fluoxetine, citalopram, escitalopram, venlafaxine, desvenlafaxine, and duloxetine
Monoamine oxidase inhibitors (MAO)	Amitriptyline, nortriptyline, clomipramine, and imipramine
Other psychiatric medications	Lithium, trazodone (serotonin modulator), and bupropion (dopamine/ norepinephrine reuptake inhibitor)
Antiepileptic	Valproic acid
Antiemetic and properistaltic	Ondansetron and metoclopramide
Antibiotics and antiviral	Linezolid and ritonavir
Analgesics, relaxants	Fentanyl, Tramadol, Meperidine
Cough and cold	Dextromethorphan
Dietary supplements	St John's Wort and tryptophan
Recreational and "street" drugs	Cocaine "Ecstasy" [methylenedioxymethamphetamine (MDMA)]. Lysergic acid diethylamide (LSD)
Drug–drug interactions	SSRI with antipsychotics, SSRI with MAO inhibitors, SSRI and amphetamine (serotonin releaser), paroxetine and buspirone, tramadol, venlafaxine, and mirtazapine, linezolid, and citalopram

BOX 5: Key differentiating features of serotonin syndrome, neuroleptic malignant syndrome, malignant hyperthermia, Parkinson hyperpyrexia syndrome, and anticholinergic toxicity.

Drug-induced movement disorders	***Key clinical features***	***Causative drugs/triggers***	***Management***
Serotonin syndrome (SS)	Delirium, agitation, akathisia, *neuro-muscular hyperactivity* (tremor, rigidity, myoclonus, hyperreflexia, and clonus), hyperthermia (>41.1°C), tachycardia, *hyperactive bowel,* and *mydriasis*	Serotonergic drugs, SSRI, SNRI, TCA, MAO inhibitors, bupropion, cocaine, amphetamine, tramadol, lithium, tryptophan, and linezolid	Removal of offending agent, supportive care and hydration, BZD, cyproheptadine, 5-HT2A antagonist-olanzapine, and chlorpromazine (resistant cases)
Neuroleptic malignant syndrome (NMS)	Hyperthermia, tachycardia, delirium, *neuromuscular hypoactivity* (rigidity and bradykinesia), and hypoactive bowel	DRBA, promethazine, prochlorperazine, metoclopramide, and antipsychotic agents	Discontinue causative agent, cooling blankets, supportive care, BZD, dantrolene, bromocriptine, and amantadine
Malignant hyperthermia (MH)	Severe hyperthermia, hypertension, agitation, rigor mortis like rigidity, hyporeflexia, hypoactive bowel, mottled skin with flushing, cyanosis, and ↑ end-tidal CO_2	Inhalational anesthetics and depolarizing muscle relaxants (succinyl choline)	Remove triggering agent, optimize oxygenation and ventilation, cooling agents, dantrolene, and ECMO (refractory case)
Parkinson hyperpyrexia syndrome	Worsening of parkinsonism, hyperpyrexia, autonomic instability, and ↑ CK	Abrupt withdrawal or dose reduction of DA, levodopa, amantadine, and cessation of deep brain stimulation	Replacing antiparkinsonian medications to previous dose orally or via nasogastric tube, transdermal rotigotine, apomorphine by injection/ continuous infusion
Anticholinergic toxicity	Hyperthermia, tachycardia, agitation, dry flushed skin, delirium, hallucination, normal muscle tone and reflexes, myoclonus, urinary retention, and *mydriasis*	Trihexyphenidyl, benztropine, atropine, ipratropium, promethazine, chlorpromazine, and darifenacin	Hemodynamic stabilization, BZD physostigmine, activated charcoal, and oral/transdermal rivastigmine (delirium)

(BZD: benzodiazepine; DA: dopamine agonist; DRBA: dopamine receptor blocking agent; ECMO: extracorporeal membrane oxygenation; MAO: monoamine oxidase inhibitor; SSRI: selective serotonin reuptake inhibitor; SNRI: serotonin norepinephrine reuptake inhibitor; TCA: tricyclic antidepressant)

BOX 6: Management of psychosis in Parkinson disease (PD).

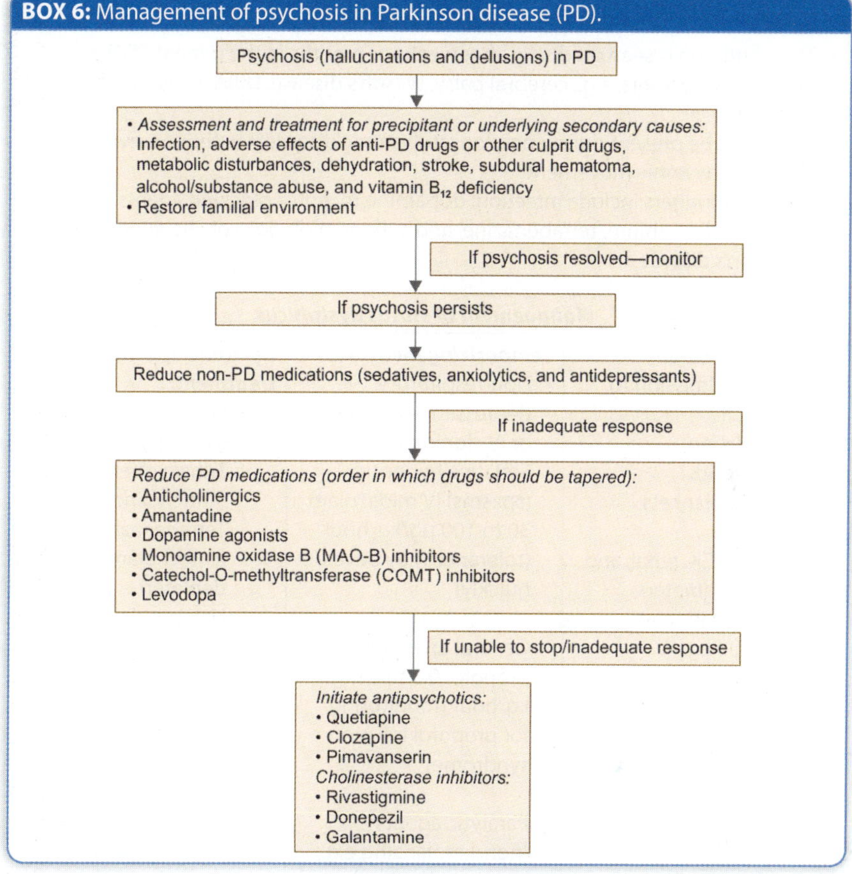

BOX 7: Acute dystonic reaction.

- **Acute dystonic reaction** is commonly seen after exposure to dopamine receptor blockers, depleters mainly neuroleptics, and antiemetics
- Dystonia typically begins within 24 hours of exposure, 90% of reactions may occur within 5–7 days
- **Risk factors:** Younger age, male gender, recent cocaine use, history of mood disorders, metabolic abnormalities issues such as electrolyte disturbances, and dehydration
- High-potency dopamine D2 receptor antagonists such as fluphenazine and haloperidol are the most likely causative drugs but notably for the emergency room, metoclopramide is a common culprit for acute dystonic reactions especially when the dose exceeds 30 mg
- Drug-related dystonic reactions can occur after a single dose of the drug or after repeated use
- **Clinical manifestations** are variable usually affecting head and neck involving oromandibular dystonia, oculogyric crisis, laryngeal dystonia, blepharospasm, cervical dystonia, and focal limb dystonia have all been reported
- **Treatment** with an intravenous anticholinergic agent such as *benztropine* (1–2 mg), promethazine (25–50 mg), or *diphenhydramine* (25–50 mg) is very effective
- Owing to the possibility of a reoccurrence, a short oral course of an anticholinergic (4–7 days) may be necessary

BOX 8: Status dystonicus.

- This condition is seen gradually after weeks or months in the patient with an underlying dystonia, e.g., cerebral palsy, Wilson's disease, NBIA, and mitochondrial disorders
- It can also be present during new-onset dystonic disorders without previous or only mild dystonic movements
- Common triggers include infection, dopamine receptor blocking agents, sudden withdrawal of lithium, tetrabenazine, and sudden high dose of chelation therapy in Wilson's disease

Management of status dystonicus		
Supportive care: • Urgent admission to ICU • IV hydration • Antipyretics • Cooling blankets • Analgesia • Monitor (CK, renal, and other parameters) • Identify and treat triggers (e.g., IV antibiotics)	***Temporizing measures:*** • Non-respiratory depressant e.g., enteral or IV clonidine • Sedative hypnotic (spasms) IV midazolam 30 to 100 µg/kg/hour (tolerance may develop quickly) ± • General anesthesia e.g., propofol 0.3 to 3 mg/kg/hour (monitoring for propofol infusion syndrome) ± Paralytic agents (nondepolarizing e.g., pancuronium)	***Dystonia-specific treatment:*** • *Noninvasive:* Initial oral polytherapy – Trihexyphenidyl (anticholinergic) – Tetrabenazine (catecholamine depleter) – Haloperidol (dopamine receptor blocker) • *Consider trial:* – Baclofen – Benzodiazepine – Gabapentin (Wilson) – L-dopa • *Invasive (consider early refractory cases):* – ITB (test before pump) – Bilateral GPi DBS – Pallidotomy

(DBS: deep brain stimulation; Gpi: globus pallidus internus; ITB: intrathecal baclofen; NBIA: neurodegeneration with brain iron accumulation)

BOX 9: Hemichorea-hemiballismus (HH).

- HH is a violent and distressing movement disorder characterized by high amplitude, flinging movements of limbs on one side of the body in which ballismus, and chorea represent a continuum of hyperkinetic movements with different velocity and amplitude
- In children, Sydenham chorea in the setting of rheumatic fever is the most common cause which is due to group A streptococcal infection. Chorea may be unilateral or bilateral, and brain imaging typically lacks specific finding. In addition to antibiotics, a course of steroids has been shown to be beneficial
- In adults, basal ganglia stroke is the most common cause of acute chorea-ballism. Ischemic/hemorrhagic stroke may cause hemichorea-ballism, with causative lesions usually affecting the contralateral basal ganglia (most commonly the thalamus) and adjacent white matter. The movements typically subside over a period of months after the stroke
- The second most common cause of hemiballismus is nonketotic hyperglycemia. Chorea or ballism may be unilateral or bilateral with this condition. It may be the initial presentation of diabetes mellitus in some cases. Magnetic resonance T1-weighted images demonstrate hyperintensity in the putamen, caudate nucleus, and globus pallidus. Abnormal movements often reverse when the glucose level is normalized. Resolution of magnetic resonance imaging signal change often correlates with clinical improvement in chorea
- VMAT-2 inhibitors (tetrabenazine, deutetrabenazine, and valbenazine), dopamine receptor blocking agents (haloperidol and pimozide), and antiepileptics (valproate) are effective in symptomatic treatment of chorea. VMAT-2 inhibitors have a more favorable side effect profile and are best chosen as first line therapy initially
- If movements are violent, self-injurious, exhausting, or distressing despite adequate medical treatment pallidotomy or GPi DBS may be considered in select cases
- For majority of such cases, as the movements usually resolve over time, medication should be tapered after 3 months and the patient should be reevaluated

(DBS: deep brain stimulation; Gpi: globus pallidus internus; VMAT-2: vesicular monoamine transporter type 2)

BOX 10: Differential diagnosis of acute chorea and ballismus.

Category	***Examples***
Vascular	Ischemic/hemorrhagic stroke, malformations, cerebral anoxia, post pump chorea, polycythemia vera
Metabolic	Nonketotic hyperglycemia, hypoglycemia, uremic encephalopathy hyperthyroidism, and hypoparathyroidism
Infectious	Cryptococcal granuloma, toxoplasmosis, tuberculoma, and HIV encephalitis
Structural	Basal ganglia lesion or mass, thalamotomy/subthalamotomy
Autoimmune	Postinfectious/Sydenham chorea/chorea gravidarum, systemic lupus erythematosus, antiphospholipid antibody syndrome, scleroderma, Behcet disease, polyarteritis nodosa, sarcoidosis, and multiple sclerosis paraneoplastic (CV2/CRMP-5 antibodies)
Drug induced	Anticonvulsants, oral contraceptives, levodopa, cocaine, amphetamines morphine, methadone, and alcohol

SUGGESTED READING

1. Allen NM, Lin JP, Lynch T, King MD. Status dystonicus: a practice guide. Dev Med Child Neurol. 2014;56(2):105-12.
2. Boyer EW, Shannon M. The serotonin syndrome. N Engl J Med. 2005;352(11):1112-20.
3. Chen JJ. Treatment of psychotic symptoms in patients with Parkinson disease. Ment Health Clin. 2018;7(6):262-70.
4. Ganti L, Rosario J. Movement Disorder Emergencies. In: Ganti L, Goldstein J (eds). Neurologic Emergencies. Edinburgh: Springer, Cham; 2018.
5. Munhoz RP, Scorr LM, Factor SA. Movement disorders emergencies. Curr Opin Neurol. 2015;28(4):406-12.
6. Rajan S, Kaas B, Moukheiber E. Movement disorders emergencies. Semin Neurol. 2019;39(1):125-36.
7. Robottom BJ, Factor SA, Weiner WJ. Movement disorders emergencies Part 2: hyperkinetic disorders. Arch Neurol. 2011;68(6):719-24.

6.6 COMA IN ER—A CLINICAL APPROACH

SM Katrak, Jamshed D Sunavala

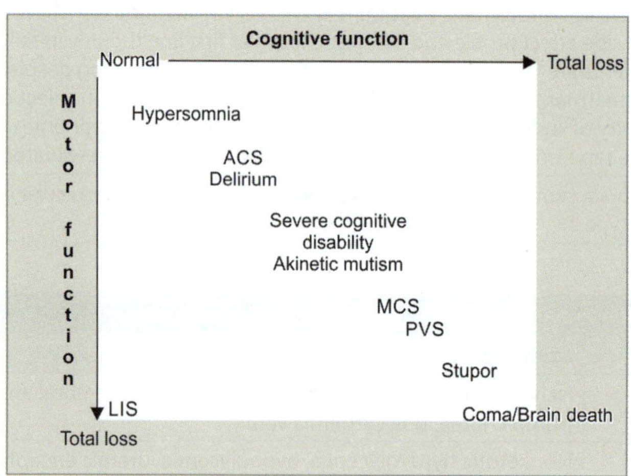

Fig. 1: Graph for differential diagnosis of coma. (ACS: acute confusional state; LIS: locked-in state; MCS: minimal conscious state; PVS: persistent vegetative state)

BOX 1: Coma—neurological examination.

- Position, posture, and spontaneous movements
- Respiratory pattern—see **Box 2**
- Rule out fracture of skull and/or spine
- Then check for neck stiffness
- *Fundal examination:*
  - Signs of hypertension
  - Signs of diabetic retinopathy
  - Signs of SAH
- Level of consciousness—see **Box 3**
- Level of lateralization—see **Box 4**
- Brain activity—see **Box 5**

BOX 2: Respiratory patterns in coma.

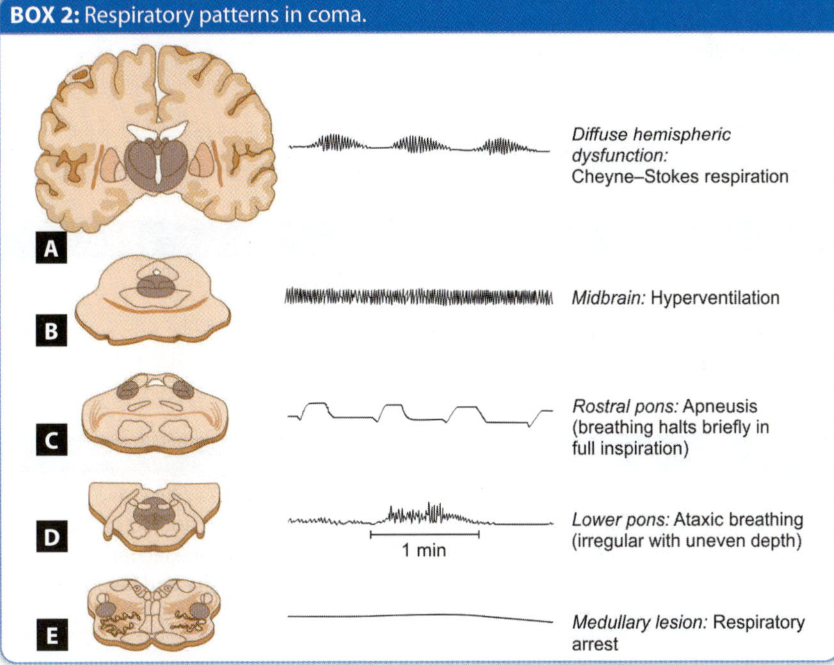

BOX 3: Coma—level of consciousness.

Glasgow Coma Scale		
Eye opening: 1. Nil 2. To pain 3. To speech 4. Spontaneous	*Motor response:* 1. Nil 2. Extensor 3. Flexor 4. Withdrawal 5. Localizing 6. Voluntary	*Verbal response:* 1. Nil 2. Groans 3. Inappropriate 4. Confused 5. Orientated

BOX 4: Coma—lateralizing and motor signs.

- Weakness, grasp reflex, or focal seizures
- *Plucking or clutching:* Intact corticospinal tracts
- *Grimacing:* Intact corticobulbar tracts up to pons
- *Roving eye movements:* Pons and midbrain intact
- *Multifocal myoclonus:* Hypoxic/ischemic or metabolic encephalopathy
- *Orofacial dyskinesia:* Metabolic encephalopathy

BOX 5: Coma—brainstem function.

Brainstem function judged by brainstem reflexes:

- Pupillary reaction*
- Corneal reflex
- Spontaneous eye movements
- *Reflex eye movements:* Oculocephalic maneuver (OCM) and oculovestibular reflex (OVR)
- Gag reflex
- Respiration

**Note:* Position of upper eyelids and edema

BOX 6: Coma—clinical groups.

Neurological assessment divides patients into three groups:

1. Coma with focal signs
2. Coma without focal signs but with meningeal signs
3. Coma without focal or meningeal signs

BOX 7: Coma—with focal signs.

- Focal trauma (history available)
- Cerebral or cerebellar hemorrhage or infarct (acute history and risk factors)
- Space-occupying lesion (SOL) or tumors (subacute or chronic headache)
- Abscess or herpes simplex virus (HSV) encephalitis (acute history and fever)
- Rarely hypoglycemic hemiplegia

BOX 8: Coma—no focal but meningeal signs.

- *With fever:* Meningitis/encephalitis
- *Without fever:*
  - Subarachnoid hemorrhage (SAH)
  - Diffuse trauma with SAH
- *Red flags:*
  - Midline posterior fossa tumors
  - Acute rise of intracranial pressure (ICP) with hydrocephalus may mimic the above conditions
  - Rule out trauma to the cervical spine

BOX 9: Coma—no focal or meningeal signs.

- Anoxic ischemic encephalopathy
- Metabolic encephalopathy
- Toxic encephalopathy
- Nonconvulsive status epilepticus
- Drug intoxication or poisoning
- Hypo- or hyperthermic brain damage

BOX 10: Coma—prognosis.

- *Etiology:* Traumatic versus nontraumatic (traumatic has better prognosis)
- Duration (shorter duration of coma has better prognosis)
- Pupillary light reflex (PLR), corneal reflex (CR), OCM, and OVR—early return has better prognosis
- *Motor response:* Absence of motor response to pain predicts poor prognosis
- Combination of above four
- Prognosis at day 1:
  - *Good outcome:* BS reflex present, purposeful movement, and nystagmus
  - *Poor outcome:* BS reflex absent and flaccidity/reflex
- Electroencephalogram (EEG), evoked potentials, neuron-specific enolase (NSE) levels

TABLE 1: Drug-induced seizures and coma.

Antibiotics	*Encephalopathy*	*Seizures*	*Nonconvulsive status epilepticus*	*Delirium/ psychosis*	*Coma*
Cephalosporins (cefepime)	+	++	+	+	– +
Piperacillin Tazobactam	+	+	+	+	–
Carbapenems	–	++	–	–	–
Quinolones	+	++	+	++	–
Linezolid	+	–	–	–	–
Metronidazole*	+	+	–	–	–

Risk factors: Elderly, renal failure, prior central nervous system (CNS) disease, *hepatic failure
Cefepime: 1–10 days administration, 2–7 days resolution

Source: Adapted from Grill MF, Maganti RK. Neurotoxic effects associated with antibiotic use: management considerations. Br J Clin Pharmacol. 2011;72:381-93.

BOX 11: Coma—emergent therapy.

Principles:
- Ensure and maintain airway, breathing, and circulation (ABC)
- Adequate nutrition and vitamins
- Lower ICP
- Control seizures and infection
- Maintain fluid, electrolyte, and acid-base balance
- Poisoning—specific antidotes
- Control agitation and pain
- Protect eyes

SUGGESTED READING

1. Bates D, Caronna JJ, Cartlidge NE, Knill-Jones RP, Levy DE, Shaw DA, et al. A prospective study of non-traumatic coma: methods and results in 310 patients. Ann Neurol. 1977;2:211-20.
2. Edlow IA, Newman-Toker DE, Savitz SL. Diagnosis and initial management of cerebellar Infarction. Lancet Neurol. 2008;7:951-64.
3. Grill MF, Maganti RK. Neurotoxic effects associated with antibiotic use: management considerations. Br J Clin Pharmacol. 2011;72:381-93.
4. Hosting MWB, Franken MD, Meulenbelt I, van Klei WA, de Lange DW. The etiology and outcome of non-traumatic coma in critical care: a systemic review. BMC Anesthesiol. 2015;15:65.
5. Multi-Society Task Force on PVS. Medical aspects of the persistent vegetative state (1). N Engl J Med. 1994;330:1499-508.
6. Plum E, Poser JB. The diagnosis of stupor and coma. Brain Nerve. 2015;67(3):344-5.
7. Rates D. Coma in Clinical Neurology. New York: Churchill Livingstone; 1991. pp. 188-204.
8. Wijdicks EF, Hijdra A, Young GB, Bassetti CL, Wiebe S. Practice parameters: prediction of outcome in comatose survivors after cardiopulmonary resuscitation (an evidence based review): report of the Quality Standards Subcommittee of the American Academy of Neurology). Neurology. 2006:67:203-10.
9. Wijdicks EFM, Bamlet WR, Maramattom BV, Manno EM, McClelland RL. Validation of a new coma scale: the FOUR score. Ann Neurol. 2006;58:585-93.

6.7 INTRACRANIAL HEMORRHAGE

Nikhil S Chamankar, Sudheer Ambekar

BOX 1: Introduction.

- Intracerebral hemorrhage (ICH) involves sudden onset spontaneous bleeding within the brain parenchyma
- Second most common type of stroke (15–30%)
- ICH may be caused because of hypertensive bleed, amyloid angiopathy, aneurysmal rupture, arteriovenous malformation, or may be idiopathic
- *Risk factors:*
  - Common in elderly
  - Asian population is more susceptible
  - More common in men
  - Patients on anticoagulation
  - Patients with history of previous bleed or untreated vascular malformation
  - Hypertensive patients not on regular medications
  - Liver dysfunction leading to bleeding diathesis
  - Alcohol, smoking, or any other drug addiction

BOX 2: Classification.

Based on etiology:

- Primary—idiopathic
- Secondary—due to underlying causes such as hypertension, amyloid angiopathy, drug abuse, venous or dural sinus thrombosis or vascular malformations

Based on location:

- Lobar—depending on location of hemorrhage can be frontal, parietal, temporal, occipital, or cerebellar
- Intraventricular—hemorrhage within the ventricular system

Location of ICH	***Percentage***
Striate body (basal ganglia); putamen most common; also includes lenticular nucleus, internal capsule, and globus pallidus	50
Thalamus	15
Pons	10–15
Cerebellum	10
Cerebral white matter	10–20
Brainstem	1–6

BOX 3: Signs and symptoms.

Patients present with the following symptoms:
- Slow-onset weakness of one side of body
- Altered sensorium or unconsciousness
- Seizures
- Aphasia if bleeding on left side of cerebral hemisphere

Signs:
- Hemiplegia or hemiparesis
- Low Glasgow Coma Scale (GCS) score
- Unequal pupils
- Papilledema in case of posterior fossa bleed
- Raised blood pressure with irregular respiration and bradycardia in cases with raised intracranial pressure (ICP)

BOX 4: Investigation.

Blood investigations:
- Complete hemogram
- Liver function test
- Renal function test
- Coagulation profile
- Blood grouping and cross match

Radiological investigations:
- CT scan—most easily available and quick investigation in patients with suspected ICH. Hyperdensity in the intraparenchymal or intraventricular region is noted
- MRI—gives information similar to CT scan but is time and cost consuming. Blood in different stages shows different intensities in T1 and T2 sequences

Stage	***Time since onset***	***Hemoglobin (Hb) state***	***T1***	***T2***
Hyperacute	0–6 hours	Oxy Hb (intracellular)	Iso	Bright
Acute	6–72 hours	Deoxy Hb (intracellular)	Iso	Dark
Early subacute	3–7 days	Met Hb (intracellular)	Bright	Dark
Late subacute	7–14 days	Met Hb (extracellular)	Bright	Bright
Chronic	>2 weeks	Hemosiderin (intracellular)	Dark	Dark

BOX 5: ICH score.

Graded feature	***Criteria***	***Points***	***Score***
Glasgow Coma Scale	3–4 5–12 13–15	2 1 0	0–2
Age	>80 <80	1 0	0–1
Location	Infratentorial Supratentorial	1 0	0–1
ICH volume	>30 <30	1 0	0–1
Intraventricular blood	Yes No	1 0	0–1
ICH score total			0–6

Mortality based on ICH score

ICH score	***Mortality***
0	0%
1	13%
2	26%
3	72%
4	97%
5	100%
6	?100%

BOX 6: In the emergency room (ER).

In the ER once a patient is received with the signs and symptoms suggestive of ICH the following steps are initiated:

- Wide bore intravenous cannula and fluid resuscitation
- Intubation if GCS is <8
- Antihypertensive to control blood pressure
- Antiepileptics drugs in patients presenting with seizures
- Anti-edema measures such as propped up position, hyperventilation to intubated patient, mannitol or 3% saline
- Stop any anticoagulation or antiplatelet drugs and give appropriate antidote to the drug or blood products

BOX 7: Treatment.

Medical management:
- In patients whose GCS score is good can be managed conservatively
- Once the clot has stabilized and there is no mass effect noted requiring surgical intervention patient is started on feeds, physiotherapy and rehabilitation. Speech therapy is given to those with aphasia

Surgical management:
- In patients with poor GCS score and mass effect on imaging are offered surgical intervention
- Patients with obstructive hydrocephalus due to intraventricular hemorrhage need external ventricular drainage and drainage of cerebrospinal fluid (CSF)
- Patient with infratentorial hemorrhage need urgent decompression as the posterior fossa has a smaller volume
- In patients with supratentorial hemorrhage, large volume of bleed with mass effect decompressive craniectomy with evacuation of clot may help in reducing ICP

SUGGESTED READING

1. De Oliveira Manoel AL, Goffi A, Zampieri FG, Turkel-Parrella D, Duggal A, Marotta TR, et al. The critical care management of spontaneous intracranial hemorrhage: a contemporary review. Crit Care. 2016;20:272.
2. Giray S, Sen O, Sarica FB, Tufan K, Karatas M, Goksel BK, et al. Spontaneous primary intraventricular hemorrhage in adults: clinical data, etiology and outcome. Turk Neurosurg. 2009;19(4):338-44.
3. Hemphill JC, Greenberg SM, Anderson CS, Becker K, Bendok BR, Cushman M, et al. Guidelines for the management of spontaneous intracerebral hemorrhage: a guideline for healthcare professionals from the American Heart Association/American Stroke Association. Stroke. 2015;46(7):2032-60.
4. Jolink WMT, Wiegertjes K, Rinkel GJE, Algra A, de Leeuw FE, Klijn CJM, et al. Location-specific risk factors for intracerebral hemorrhage: systematic review and meta-analysis. Neurology. 2020;95(13):e1807-18.
5. Qureshi AI, Palesch YY, Barsan WG, Hanley DF, Hsu CY, Martin RL, et al. Intensive blood pressure lowering in patients with acute cerebral hemorrhage. N Engl J Med. 2016;375(11):1033-43.

6.8 SUBARACHNOID HEMORRHAGE

Nikhil S Chamankar, Sudheer Ambekar

BOX 1: Definition.

Aneurysm describes a pathologic condition of vessels wherein there is a permanent localized dilatation of the blood vessel. Subarachnoid hemorrhage (SAH) denotes the presence of blood in the subarachnoid space. It often presents as headache which is frequently described by patients as the worst headache of their life also known as *thunderclap headache*. Trauma and aneurysm rupture are the most common causes of SAH.

BOX 2: Clinical presentation.

Warning symptoms also called as "sentinel symptoms" consisting of headache, retrobulbar pain, and nuchal pain occur in 60–70% patients prior to frank bleed.

Thunderclap headache: Sudden onset severe headache classically described as worst headache of life. Patients may also describe a change in the characteristics of headache in terms of location, duration severity, and type of headache as compared to any previous episodes of headache in life.

The presentation of aneurysm can be divided into two parts:
1. Ruptured aneurysm
2. Unruptured aneurysm

Ruptured aneurysm may present with the following clinical features:
- Sudden-onset loss of consciousness or altered sensorium
- Hemiplegia or hemiparesis
- Severe sudden-onset headache (thunderclap headache)
- Focal neurological deficit or cranial nerve deficit
- Seizures either generalized tonic-clonic or focal seizures
- Vomiting
- Terson syndrome which is intraocular extension of subarachnoid blood

Systemic manifestations:
- Acute hypertension as part of Cushing's triad
- Acute hypotension due to stunned neurogenic myocardium
- Cardiac Arrhythmia
- Hypoxia due to aspiration following altered sensorium, vomiting, seizures, or respiratory depression

Unruptured aneurysm may present with the following clinical features:
- Focal neurological deficit or cranial nerve deficit
- Headache
- Seizures
- Incidental pick up on scans done for any other symptoms

BOX 3: Depending on the site of aneurysmal rupture the patient presentation might vary.

Anterior cerebral artery (ACA)	Weakness of both lower extremities
Middle cerebral artery (MCA)	Hemiparesis, paresthesia, hemianopsia, and dysphasia. Seizures occur more commonly in MCA aneurysms
Internal carotid artery (ICA)	Third nerve palsy or unilateral retro-orbital pain
Posterior communicating artery (PComm)	Third nerve palsy or unilateral retro-orbital pain
Superior cerebellar artery (SCA)	Third nerve palsy
Carotid-ophthalmic aneurysms and superior hypophyseal artery	Unilateral visual loss or bilateral field defects

BOX 4: Assessment.

The *Ottawa SAH* rule tells to investigate if one or more variables are present of the following:

- Age >40 years
- Neck pain or stiffness
- History of loss of consciousness
- Onset during exertion
- Thunderclap headache reaching maximum intensity within 1 minute
- Limited neck flexion on examination

The rule is applicable for patients aged 15 years or more with new severe nontraumatic headache reaching maximum intensity within 1 hour.

The *Hunt and Hess Scale* (1968) or the World Federation of Neurological Surgeons Scale (1988) (WFNSS) is most commonly used to measure the severity of SAH. They predict the surgical risk and mortality in SAH. Clinical severity scores is one of the strongest predictors of functional outcome in various epidemiological studies.

Grade	*Hunt and Hess Scale*	*WFNSS*
1	Asymptomatic or mild headache, minimal or no nuchal rigidity	Glasgow Coma Scale (GCS) score of 15, motor deficit absent
2	Moderate to severe headache, nuchal rigidity and no neurologic deficit other than cranial nerve palsy	GCS score of 13–14, motor deficit absent
3	Mild alteration in mental status (confusion and lethargy), with or without mild focal neurologic deficit	GCS score of 13–14, motor deficit present
4	Stupor and/or hemiparesis	GCS score of 7–12, motor deficit absent or present
5	Comatose and/or decerebrate rigidity and/or no motor response	GCS score of 3–6, motor deficit absent or present

BOX 5: Investigation.

CT brain: Most commonly and easily available diagnostic modality to diagnose SAH. Hyperdensity in the cisternal spaces indicates SAH due to rupture of aneurysm.

CT scan classification of SAH—Fischer scale	
Grade 1	No blood detected
Grade 2	Diffuse deposition or thin layer of blood with all vertical layers of blood (interhemispheric fissure, insular cistern, and ambient cistern) <1 mm thick
Grade 3	Localized clots or vertical layers of blood 1 mm or greater in thickness
Grade 4	Diffuse or no SAH but with intraparenchymal or intraventricular clots

Other radiological grading scale in SAH		
	Modified Fischer scale	***Hijdra scale***
Grade 1	No SAH or intraventricular hemorrhage (IVH)	No blood in the cistern or ventricle
Grade 2	Localized or diffuse thin SAH, with no IVH	Small amount of blood in cistern, sedimentation of blood in the posterior part of ventricle
Grade 3	Localized or diffuse thin SAH, with IVH	Moderate amount of blood in cistern, ventricle partly filled with blood
Grade 4	Localized or diffuse thick SAH, with no IVH	Cistern completely filled with blood, ventricle completely filled with blood
Grade 5	Localized or diffuse thick SAH, with IVH	NA

MRI: Less frequently done in view of cost, availability and time taken to perform complete sequence

Lumbar puncture (LP): In cases with high suspicion of SAH with negative CT/MRI LP may be performed. The presence of xanthochromia is the diagnostic criteria on laboratory spectrophotometry analysis. While performing a lumbar we may also evaluate the opening pressure which helps us in estimating the intracranial pressure.

Transcranial Doppler (TCD): TCD assesses the cerebral artery flow velocity. It is both a low-risk and noninvasive tool to monitor for the presence of cerebral vasospasm. The proximal segments of the MCA and ICA as part of circle of Willis are much reliably seen on TCD as compared to the ACA branches and posterior circulation arteries. The Lindegaard ratio is defined as the ratio of mean MCA flow velocity divided by mean ICA flow velocity. It helps in the diagnosis of vasospasm in the MCA when the ratio is above 3. TCD is however operator dependent.

CT angiography: High sensitivity of 90% in detecting aneurysmal rupture.

MR angiography (MRA): It has high sensitivity to the flow phenomena and, therefore, cerebral vessels can be displayed without contrast medium administration. The average sensitivity and specificity of MRA for the detection of intracranial aneurysms (IAs) is, respectively, 87% and 95%.

Intra-arterial digital subtraction angiography (IADSA): Gold standard for diagnosing SAH due to aneurysmal rupture and for planning further course of definitive treatment both for coiling and clipping.

BOX 6: Treatment.

In the emergency room:

- *Elective intubation* of all patients with poor GCS score
- Securing broad gauge intravenous (IV) line and starting fluid resuscitation if patient is hypotensive
- To prevent vasospasm calcium channel blocker like *nimodipine* is started 60 mg every 4th hourly
- *Antiedema measure like 20% mannitol or 3% hypertonic saline is started.*
- *Antiseizure medication like levetiracetam 1 g loading followed by 500 mg twice a day is started in patients presenting with seizures. Other antiepileptics that may be considered are lacosamide, sodium valproate, brivaracetam, and phenytoin*
- *The old hypervolemia, hemodilution, and hypertension (HHH) therapy consisting of hypertension hypervolemia and hemodilution has now given way to normovolemic mild hypertension. Hypervolemia has been found to not decrease the incidence of vasospasm on the contrary increases the chances of complications*

Clipping versus coiling: Definitive treatment for aneurysm should be done within 48 hours of diagnosing aneurysm. As per the International Subarachnoid Aneurysm Trial (ISAT) both the treatment modalities are equally efficacious.

External ventricular drain insertion: In patients presenting with SAH with hydrocephalus may need insertion of external ventricular drain to reduce intracranial pressure.

BOX 7: Complications.

Delayed cerebral ischemia (DCI): It is defined as the development of delayed neurological deficit, decline in GCS of at least 2 points, and/or cerebral infarction unrelated to aneurysm or other causes. Typically occurs between 4th to 7th day post ictus and may need intra-arterial nimodipine. Delayed ischemic neurologic deficit (DIND) or clinical vasospasm or symptomatic vasospasm is development of delayed ischemic neurologic deficit following SAH and is clinically characterized by confusion, decreased level of consciousness with motor or sensory deficit. Vasospasm is considered in the following setting:

- Delayed onset or persistent neurologic deficit
- Onset 4–20 days post SAH
- Deficit appropriate to involved arteries
- Other causes of deterioration such as rebleeding, hydrocephalus, cerebral edema, seizure, hyponatremia, hypoxia, and sepsis have been ruled out
- Radiological evaluation with TCD or CT angiography showing vasospasm

Hydrocephalus: Persistent hydrocephalus in patients with IVH may need to be addressed with ventriculoperitoneal (VP) shunt.

Hyponatremia: Hyponatremia may develop in patients with SAH due to syndrome of inappropriate antidiuretic hormone secretion (SIADH) and needs sodium correction with hypertonic saline and fluid restriction. Few patients may need tolvaptan.
In patients with diabetes insipidus (DI), desmopressin intranasal spray may be considered.

SUGGESTED READING

1. Connolly ES, Rabinstein AA, Carhuapoma JR, Derdeyn CP, Dion J, Higashida RT, et al. Guidelines for the management of aneurysmal subarachnoid hemorrhage: a guideline for healthcare professionals from the American Heart Association/ American Stroke Association. Stroke. 2012;43(6):1711-37.
2. Findlay JM, Nisar J, Darsaut T. Cerebral vasospasm: a review. Can J Neurol Sci. 2016;43(1):15-32.
3. Kao L, Al-Lawati Z, Vavao J, Steinberg GK, Katznelson L. Prevalence and clinical demographics of cerebral salt wasting in patients with aneurysmal subarachnoid hemorrhage. Pituitary. 2009;12:347-51.
4. Liu-DeRyke X, Rhoney DH. Cerebral vasospasm after aneurysmal subarachnoid hemorrhage: an overview of pharmacologic management. Pharmacother J Hum Pharmacol Drug Ther. 2006;26(2):182-203.
5. Mayberg MR, Batjer HH, Dacey R, Diringer M, Haley EC, Heros RC, et al. Guidelines for the management of aneurysmal subarachnoid hemorrhage. A statement for healthcare professionals from a special writing group of the Stroke Council, American Heart Association. Circulation. 1994;90(5):2592-605.

CHAPTER 7

Infections

7.1 SEPSIS

Jamshed D Sunavala

DEFINITIONS

BOX 1: Sepsis-1 (1992) definition.

Sepsis	Systemic infection manifested by two or more of the SIRS criteria, secondary to a suspected or known source of infection
SIRS	*Systemic inflammatory response syndrome (SIRS):* • White blood cell (WBC) >12,000 mm^3 or <4,000/mm^3 or >10% immature bands • Respiratory rate >20 or partial pressure of arterial carbon dioxide ($PaCO_2$) <32 mm Hg • Body temperature >38°C or <36°C • Heart rate >90 beats/minute
Severe sepsis	Sepsis with any organ dysfunction (including hypotension, lactic acidosis, oliguria, or altered mental status)
Septic shock	Sepsis + systolic blood pressure (BP) <90 mm Hg despite adequate volume challenge and requiring vasopressor support

BOX 2: Sepsis-3 (2016) definition.

Sepsis	Life-threatening organ dysfunction caused by a dysregulated host response to an infection
Criteria of organ dysfunction	Acute change in the Sequential Organ Failure Assessment (SOFA) score by 2 or more points from the baseline
Septic shock	It is subset of sepsis with persistent hypotension requiring vasopressors to maintain mean arterial pressure (MAP) ≥65 mm Hg and serum lactate ≥2 mmol/L despite adequate volume resuscitation

BOX 3: Sequential organ failure assessment (SOFA) score.

	0	*1*	*2*	*3*	*4*
Respiratory partial pressure of arterial oxygen (PaO_2)/fraction of inspired oxygen (FiO_2) mm Hg peripheral arterial oxygen saturation (SaO_2)/FiO_2	>400	<400 221–301	<300 142–220	<200 67–141	<100 <67
Coagulation Platelets $10^3/mm^3$	>150	<150	<100	<50	<20
Liver Bilirubin (mg/dL)	<1.2	1.2–1.9	2.0–5.9	6.0–11.9	>12.0
Cardiovascular Hypotension	No hypotension	MAP <70	Dopamine ≤5 or dobutamine any dose	Dopamine >5 or Norepinephrine/epinephrine ≤0.1	Dopamine >15 or Norepinephrine/epinephrine >0.1
Central nervous system (CNS) Glasgow coma score	15	13–14	10–12	6–9	<6
Renal Creatinine (mg/dL)	<1.2	1.2–1.9	2.0–3.4	3.5–4.9 or urine output (UO) <500 mL/day	>5.0 or UO <200 mL/day

PaO_2/FiO_2 ratio used preferentially. If not available SaO_2/FiO_2 ratio used.
Vasoactive medication administered for at least 1 hour (dopamine and norepinephrine doses in μg/kg/min)

BOX 4: Quick sequential organ failure assessment (qSOFA).

qSOFa is used to identify high-risk patients for in-hospital mortality with suspected infection at the bedside

Criteria:
- Respiratory rate ≥22 breaths/min
- Acute change in mental state [Glasgow Coma Scale (GCS) <15]
- Systolic BP ≤100 mm Hg

A positive qSOFA ≥2 suggests high risk of poor outcome in patients with suspected infection.

DIAGNOSIS

BOX 5: Diagnosis.

- **Boxes 1 and 2** vividly describe the clinical and biochemical manifestations of sepsis and severe sepsis
- Using the 1992 definition **(Box 1)** is to risk refuting a significant false positives because signs of inflammation are often seen in patients of bloodstream infection with no evidence of sepsis. However, it helps in early detection of sepsis in many cases
- Though sepsis-3 (1966) definition is more specific and minimizes false positive, it at times cannot differentiate between sepsis induced organ failure and that resulting from associated comorbidities
- Hypotension not responding to fluid challenge or signs of tissue perfusion such as lactic acidosis and/or encephalopathy are hallmark of severe sepsis

BOX 6: Biomarkers.

1. C-reactive protein (CRP)
2. Procalcitonin (PCT)

- CRP is nonspecific, in that it is increased in all inflammatory states and appears late (12–24 hours)
- *"PCT, as a biomarker, is more useful to rule out than to rule in"*—hence a normal PCT level would by and large exclude infection, but a raised PCT does not necessarily confirm infection because of its poor specificity; hence it is a poor indicator regarding decision to commence antibiotics
- *"Greater the concentration of PCT, greater the severity"*—hence it is useful for patient triage in identifying a high-risk group
- *"Trend over time"*—It is useful to evaluate response to therapy reflected by a falling trend in the PCT levels
- *"PCT kinetics is the key word"* for diagnosis of bacterial infection. Delta change in values (before and after the onset of fever) of over 0.76 ng/dL has a sensitivity of 80% and specificity of 86%
- *PCT can remain normal in the early course of bacterial infections* and also in localized infections [empyema, osteomyelitis or localized collection, subacute bacterial endocarditis (SBE)]
- The following *noninfective causes of raised PCT* could be misleading:
  - Major surgery, trauma, and burns
  - Drugs that stimulate cytokine release
  - Medullary thyroid and small cell lung carcinomas
  - Chronic kidney disease (CKD)
- *With recurrent infections* encountered during prolonged intensive care unit (ICU) stays, the value of PCT is unreliable and makes detection of new infection very difficult
- Biomarkers cannot be used as standalone in decision-making; they only complement clinical suspicion and other laboratory parameters

MANAGEMENT

BOX 7: Early resuscitation.

- Includes hemodynamic and respiratory support. This includes fluid challenge, inotropic, and ventilator support
- Early intervention is of prime importance and improves survival
- Early resuscitation is targeting predefined parameters such as MAP, central venous pressure (CVP), and mixed venous oxygen saturation (SvO_2) within a predefined period of 6 hours
- Septic shock is defined as hypotension not responding to fluid challenge; hence, initial approach should be toward volume challenge
- Vasopressors are considered when fluid challenge has failed to correct hypotension. Hypotension if persistent may contribute to impaired oxygenation and poor peripheral tissue perfusion. Hence, imperative to target a MAP of 65–70 mm Hg. Persistent lower MAP is associated with acute kidney injury (AKI); however, higher MAP above 75 mm Hg has not shown any survival benefit

BOX 8: Fluid resuscitation.

- Rapid infusion of 30 mL/kg or crystalloid fluid (normal saline or Ringer lactate) to be given within first 3 hours
- Once hemodynamic stability is achieved further aggressive fluid resuscitation is not necessary, in fact it could be harmful. However maintenance fluid need to be continued
- As of date the recommendation is to prefer giving Ringer lactate or Ringer acetate. Normal saline (0.9% NaCl) if given rapidly in large volume is associated with metabolic acidosis due to chloride load and there is also a concern of potential chloride-induced nephropathy
- Albumin (4%) may be used for resuscitation if there is a poor response to crystalloids
- Clinical endpoint of resuscitation should be stabilization of BP, heart rate (HR), improving cognition, urine output, and serum lactate. Decreasing trend in CVP and inferior vena cava (IVC) collapsibility index on Echo should be monitored simultaneously if there is a high risk of volume overload as in elderly patients or patients with history of cardiac compromise
- The maxim here is to give larger volume in the early phase of sepsis and avoid positive fluid balance beyond 24 hours when alveolar capillary leak becomes more prominent

BOX 9: Mechanical ventilation (MV).

- All patients in septic shock with respiratory distress should be intubated and supported on MV as part of early resuscitation
- Patients with sepsis but hemodynamically stable with no respiratory affliction can be maintained on nasal oxygen or noninvasive ventilation (NIV)
- Delaying intubation and in patients who are worsening on NIV with persistent hypoxia will adversely influence the outcome
- Recruitment strategies (like proning or advanced modes of ventilation) may be used for severe lung injury
- Lung protection strategies to safeguard against ventilator-induced lung injury (VILI) are imperative to prevent ventilator-associated pneumonia (VAP)

BOX 10: Contraindication for noninvasive ventilation (NIV).

- Unconscious or semiconscious patients
- Poor respiratory effort
- Uncontrolled seizures
- Life-threatening circulatory or respiratory failure
- Copious tracheal secretions
- Vomiting/hemoptysis
- Serious injuries of the face and neck
- Laryngeal edema or obstruction

BOX 11: Hemodynamic profile in shock.

Type of shock	***CVP***	***PCWP***	***SVR***	***CO***
Distributive (septic or anaphylactic)	↓N	↓N	↓↓	↑↑ (low in terminal stage)
Cardiogenic	↑↑	↑↑	↑	↓↓
Hypovolemic (hemorrhagic)	↓↓	↓↓	↑	↓↓
Pericardial tamponade	↑↑	↑↑	↑	↓ or ↓↓
Obstructive massive air embolism	↑↑	N↓	↑	↓↓

(CO: cardiac output; PCWP: Pulmonary capillary wedge pressure; SVR: systemic vascular resistance)

BOX 12: Doses and effects of vasopressors.

Norepinephrine
Effect: Mainly vasopressor effect
Dose: 0.1 µg/kg/min as starter and increase as needed up to 3 µg/kg/min
Remarks: It is the first drug of choice. Add dopamine if desired MAP is not achieved with 3–3.5 µg/kg/min

Dopamine
Effect: Dopaminergic effect
- Probable splanchnic and renal perfusion in dose up to 5 µg/kg/min
- Vasoconstriction is predominant effect in dose above 10 µg/kg/min

Dose: 5 µg/kg/min up to 15 µg/kg/min
Remarks: Tachycardia and arrhythmias

Vasopressin
Effect: Vasopressor effect
Dose: 0.01–0.03 units/min
Remarks: Pure vasoconstrictor and can promote splanchnic and digital ischemia if given in higher doses or for prolonged period.
It is always given in addition to norepinephrine and not alone.

Epinephrine
Effect: Strong alpha and beta adrenergic effects
Dose: The initial dose recommended is 0.01–0.02 µg/kg/min and the usual effective dose to correct hypotension or augment CO is 0.1–0.2 µg/kg/min
Remarks: Main side effect—tachycardia, increased insulin requirement, and lactic acid acidosis when given in higher doses

BOX 13: Choice of antimicrobials for empiric therapy in sepsis using the mnemonic "SEPSIS".

Site	Location of infection is specific to contain pathogens which are susceptible to selective antibiotics which should be used in symptomatic patients. These sites are also home to colonizers; hence disregard cultures in asymptomatic patients, e.g., urinary tract infection (UTI) with Foley's catheter, wounds with nonpurulent discharge, respiratory secretions in intubated patients with no imaging evidence of lower respiratory tract infection (LRTI).
Environment	Community, healthcare facility or ICU-acquired infections including VAP. To be familiar with hospital flora and antibiogram—community and regional flora.
Previously used antibiotics	Best to avoid antibiotics used in last 3 months.
Severity	In patients with septic shock and severe sepsis a multidrug approach—covering gram-negative bacteria (GNB) + *Pseudomonas* [if strongly suspected also to cover methicillin-resistant *Staphylococcus aureus* (MRSA) and antifungal] Using blanket, broad-spectrum combination therapy for all patients admitted to ICU with severe sepsis may be counter-productive. Empiric treatment must be based on the host factor/community-hospital acquired and site of infection regardless of severity.
Immunologically compromised	• Age, comorbidities, depressed immunity. • Broad-spectrum coverage with GNB + *Pseudomonas* cover, (if indicated antifungal and MRSA cover)
Side effects	Avoid nephrotoxic drugs (aminoglycosides, colistin in patients with kidney dysfunction, or high serum creatinine).

BOX 14: Antibiotic usage.

- Guidelines for appropriate antibiotics—see **Box 13**
- *Timing:* There is overwhelming evidence in clinical studies to administer antibiotics with the first hour of sepsis detection or on arrival to emergency medical services (EMS). This should always be preceded by collection of blood and other relevant specimens for aerobic, anaerobic, and fungal cultures
- Choice of empirical antibiotics—see **Box 13**
- Dosing should be based on the pharmacokinetic/pharmacodynamic (PK/PD) properties of the drug, renal clearance, rate of infection, and the severity of underlying infection

SOURCE CONTROL

BOX 15: Source control.

- Site of infection should be identified at the earliest
- Necessary source control should be implemented as soon as possible
- Withdrawal of central lines and catheter is mandatory if suspected to be the source of infection
- Abscesses or collection should be drained or aspirated
- Surgical reference should be immediately sought for any internal source of infection requiring surgical intervention

OTHER STRATEGIES

BOX 16: Other strategies.

- Control of blood sugar level. Preferably maintain at 150 mg%
- *Corticosteroids:* Only indication is in septic shock not responding to vasopressor or requiring high dose of vasopressin for over 24 hours

SUGGESTED READING

1. Dellinger P, Roy A, Paririllo J. Severe sepsis and septic shock. In: Parrillo J, Dellinger P (Eds). Critical Care Medicine: Principles of Diagnosis and Management in Adults, 5th edition. New York: Elsevier; 2019.
2. Dellinger RP, Schorr CA, Levy MM. A users' guide to the 2016 Surviving Sepsis Guidelines. Intensive Care Med. 2017;43(3):299-303.
3. Levy MM, Evans LE, Rhodes A. The surviving sepsis campaign bundle: 2018 update. Intensive Care Med. 2018;44(6):925-8.

7.2 ACUTE GASTROENTERITIS

Indraneel P Raut

BOX 1: Definition of diarrhea.

Passage of loose, watery stools typically at least three times in a 24-hour period:
- *Acute:* <14 days or fewer in duration
- *Persistent diarrhea:* >14 days, <30 days
- *Chronic:* >30 days

BOX 2: Etiology.

Most are due to infections and self-limited.

Causes:
- *Viruses:*
  - Norovirus
  - Adenovirus
  - Astrovirus
- *Bacteria:*
  - *Salmonella*
  - *Campylobacter*
  - *Shigella*
  - *E. coli*
  - *Clostridium difficile*
- *Protozoa:*
  - Cryptosporidium
  - Giardia
  - Cyclospora
  - Entamoeba

Acute diarrhea:
Virus: Most common cause (stool culture positive in only 1.5–5.6% of cases)

Severe diarrhea: Usually bacteria

Noninfectious causes:
- Drug induced
- Occlusive or nonocclusive ischemic colitis
- Graft-versus-host disease (GVHD)

BOX 3: Evaluation.

History:
- Duration of symptoms
- Frequency and characteristics of stool
- Associated symptoms
- Evidence of extracellular volume depletion (concentrated urine, oliguria, decreased skin turgor, orthostatic hypotension)

Food history:

Occupational exposure
- Travel history
- Pets
- Hobbies

Character of symptoms
- *Diarrhea of small bowel:*
  - Large volume
  - Abdominal cramp
  - Bloating
  - Gas
- *Diarrhea of large bowel:*
  - Frequent
  - Regular
  - Small volume
  - Painful bowel movements
  - Fever
  - Bleeding/mucoid stool
  - Red blood cell (RBC) and inflammatory cells on microscopy

BOX 4: Causes of large bowel diarrhea with fever, bloody, or mucoid stools.

Bacterial:
- *Salmonella*
- *Shigella*
- *Campylobacter*

Enteric virus:
- Cytomegalovirus (CMV)
- Adenovirus
- *Entamoeba histolytica*
- *C. difficile*

Visibly blood diarrhea:
- *E. coli* [shiga toxin-producing *E. coli* (STEC)]
- *Shigella*
- *Campylobacter*
- *Salmonella*

BOX 5: Evaluation.

Food history–impact
- *Within 6 hours:*
  - Preformed toxin
  - *Staphylococcus aureus*
  - *Bacillus cereus*
- *8–16 hours:*
  - Clostridium perfringens
- *More than 16 hours:*
  - Viral or other bacterial infection [enterotoxigenic *E. coli* (ETEC) or STEC]

Exposure history:
- *Salmonella*—exposure to animals
- Bacterial—travel to resource limited settings
- History of occupation in day care centers:
  - Shigella, Cryptosporidium, Giardia

BOX 6: Medical history.

- *Recent antibiotic use: C. difficile*
- Pregnancy and consumption of contaminated meat: *Listeria*
- Proton pump inhibitor
- *Immunodeficiency [primary IgA, secondary–acquired immunodeficiency syndrome (AIDS) immunosuppressive drug]*
- Common pathogens cause severe diarrhea and opportunistic infections: (*Cryptosporidium*, adenovirus, *Isospora belli*, CMV, microsporidia)

BOX 7: Diagnosis.

Physical examination:
To look for volume status and identify complications

- Sign of volume depletion
- Dry mucous membranes
- Diminished skin turgor
- Hypotension
- Tachycardia
- Altered sensorium
- Look for tenderness and rigidity in abdomen

Laboratory tests:
- General laboratory tests warranted when signs of volume depletion
- Stool tests for pathogens are indicated with acute diarrhea with following:
  - Severe illness (hypovolemia, >6 unformed stools in 24 hours pain)
  - Inflammatory diarrhea: (bloody diarrhea, small volume stool with blood and mucus)
  - High risk host features (>70 years, comorbidities like ischemic heart disease (IHD), Immunocompromised status, inflammatory bowel disease (IBD), and pregnancy)
  - Symptoms >1 week
  - Public, health concerns, e.g., food handlers, healthcare workers

Contd...

Contd...

Stool culture:
Should be inoculated as soon as possible
May help in Identifying:
- *Salmonella*
- *Campylobacter*
- *Shigella*
- *E. coli* (O157:O7)

Multipathogen molecular panels
Clinical correlation necessary as tests detect genetic material which may not always reflect infection with a viable organism
- If possible–stool culture

If bloody diarrhea
Test for:
- STEC (Shiga toxin)
- Entamoeba histolytica (if fecal leukocytes or lactoferrin test is negative)

Persistent diarrhea and nonresponding diarrhea
- Tests for parasite organism [*Giardia*, *Cryptosporidium*, and *Entamoeba histolytica*]
- Microscopy of stool for ova and parasites on three specimens on consecutive days

If history of antibiotic or healthcare exposure test for C. difficile toxin
If CMV diarrhea suspected: Endoscopy with biopsy
Imaging: Warranted in patients with clinical signs of peritonitis

BOX 8: Management.

Fluid repletion	• Rehydration most important • Oral route preferable • Oral rehydration solution (ORS) is standard fluid • Severe hypovolemia—intravenous (IV) hydration
Empiric antibiotic therapy	Indications: 1. Severe illness 2. Inflammatory diarrhea 3. High risk host features
To be avoided	1. Most patients with acute nonbloody diarrhea 2. Stable patients with concern for Shiga toxin producing *E. coli* pending stool testing

BOX 9: Fluid replacement with acute diarrhea causing severe volume depletion or hypovolemic shock.

At least 1 to 2 liters of isotonic IV fluids given as rapidly as possible.

Fluid replacement continued at rapid rate till the clinical signs of hypovolemia decreases (hypotension, decreased urine/altered mental status)

Cholera with severe dehydration:
- 100 mL/kg IV over 3 hours
- 30 mL/kg IV over 30 minutes
- 70 mL/kg IV over 2.5 hours

BOX 10: Choice of agent.

Azithromycin:

In patients with fever or dysentery and in patients with suspicion of fluoroquinolone-resistant diarrhea

- 1 g single dose patients without dysentery
- 500 mg once a day for 3 days for patients with or without dysentery

Fluoroquinolones:

- *Ciprofloxacin*
  - 50 mg single dose
  - 500 mg twice daily for 3–5 days
- *Levofloxacin*
  - 500 mg as a single dose for 3–5 days

BOX 11: Specific circumstances.

- *Empiric therapy for C. difficile* in setting of diarrhea with prior antibiotic therapy
- *Empiric treatment for Listeria monocytogenes in pregnant* women with diarrhea, fever, or systemic illness and exposure to Listeria
- *Empiric cover for Vibrio cholerae* in patients with profuse watery diarrhea and patient exposure to cholera
- In severe illness and suspected Shigellosis with risk of drug resistant infection [e.g., people with human immunodeficiency virus (HIV)]: Carbapenems
  - Vibrio cholerae
    - Doxycycline 300 mg single dose
    - Ciprofloxacin 1,000 mg single dose
    - Azithromycin 20 mg/kg single dose

BOX 12: Symptomatic treatment.

Agents (loperamide) cautious use in patients without fever and bloody diarrhea

Dose:

4 mg, but it is preferred to administer 2 mg initially to avoid side effects after each unformed stool for <2 days

Alternative options in patients with dysentery

1. Bismuth subsalicylate
2. Racecadotril

BOX 13: Dietary guidance.

- Adequate nutrition important for enterocyte renewal
- Dietary modifications
- Avoidance of dairy products
- Boiled starches and cereals with salt are indicated

BOX 14: Major foodborne microbes by principal gastrointestinal symptom.

Vomiting

- *Staphylococcus aureus:*
  - Incubation period: 1–6 hours
  - Likely food sources: Prepared foods, such as salads, dairy products, and meats
- *Bacillus cereus:*
  - Incubation period: 1–6 hours
  - Likely food sources: Rice and meat
- *Norovirus (Norwalk-like viruses):*
  - Incubation period: 24–48 hours
  - Likely food sources: Shellfish, prepared foods, salads, sandwiches, and fruit

Watery diarrhea

- *Clostridium perfringens:*
  - Incubation period: 8–16 hours
  - Likely food sources: Meat, poultry, and gravy
- Enterotoxigenic Escherichia coli (ETEC):
  - Incubation period: 1–3 days
  - Likely food sources: Food or water contaminated with feces
- Enteric viruses:
  - Incubation period: 10–72 hours
  - Likely food sources: Food or water contaminated with feces
- *Cryptosporidium parvum:*
  - Incubation period: 2–28 days
  - Likely food sources: Vegetables, fruit, unpasteurized milk, and water
- *Cyclospora cayetanensis:*
  - Incubation period: 1–11 days
  - Likely food sources: Imported berries and basil

Inflammatory diarrhea

- *Campylobacter species:*
  - Incubation period: 2–5 days
  - Likely food sources: Poultry, unpasteurized milk, and water
- *Nontyphoidal Salmonella:*
  - Incubation period: 1–3 days
  - Likely food sources: Eggs, poultry, meat, unpasteurized milk or juice, and fresh produce
- STEC:
  - Incubation period: 1–8 days
  - Likely food sources: Ground beef, unpasteurized milk and juice, raw vegetables, and water
- *Shigella species:*
  - Incubation period: 1–3 days
  - Likely food sources: Food and water contaminated with feces
- *Vibrio parahaemolyticus:*
  - Incubation period: 2–48 hours
  - Likely food sources: Raw shellfish

BOX 15: Approach to acute nonbloody diarrhea in adults in resource rich settings.

1. Clinical evaluation:
   - Assess the duration and frequency of diarrhea
   - Examine stool characteristics (e.g., watery or abdominal pain)
   - Measure stool volume status and signs of dehydration
   - Evaluate for associated symptoms to determine the need for further intervention
   - Focus on fluid replacement and maintenance
   - Symptomatic therapy may be considered if needed
2. Indications for stool testing (microscopy, molecular testing, and additional tests):
   - Persistent diarrhea lasting more than seven days
   - Advanced HIV infection (CD4 count <200 cells/μL)
   - Men who have sex with men
   - A history of a community-wide waterborne outbreak
3. Severe symptoms requiring immediate testing:
   - Fever ≥38.5°C (101.3°F)
   - Signs of hypovolemia or dehydration
   - More than six stools in a 24-hour period
   - Severe abdominal pain
   - High-risk groups, including individuals aged 70 years or older
   - Coexisting comorbidities such as cardiac disease or immunocompromising conditions (e.g., advanced HIV infection)

   If any of these severe symptoms are present, the following should be done:
   - Test stool for bacterial culture
   - Conduct molecular testing based on clinical suspicion (e.g., *Clostridioides difficile* if associated with antibiotic use)
   - Perform testing for parasites if clinically relevant
   - Consider starting empiric antibiotic therapy based on test results
4. Exclusions to consider testing or antibiotics are;
   If the patient has inflammatory bowel disease (IBD), is pregnant, or has symptoms persisting for more than one week despite conservative measures, public health concerns (e.g., being a food handler) should guide testing and management.

In the absence of symptoms warranting testing, stool testing and antibiotic therapy are not indicated.

SUGGESTED READING

1. Jameson JL, Kasper DL, Fauci AS, Hauser SL, Longo DL, Loscalzo J, et al. Harrison's Principles of Internal Medicine, 20th edition. New York: McGraw Hill Education; 2018.
2. UpToDate. Acute viral gastroenteritis in adults [Internet]. Available from: https://www.uptodate.com/contents/acute-viral-gastroenteritis-in-adults.

7.3 TROPICAL INFECTIONS IN THE EMERGENCY ROOM

Mala Kaneria

BOX 1: Definition of tropical fevers.

- Febrile infections that are prevalent in or unique to tropical and subtropical regions are collectively referred to as tropical fevers
- They are caused by a multitude of viruses, bacteria, and protozoa and often get transmitted by a vector, commonly mosquitoes
- Some occur perennially, while some are greatly influenced by the seasons (especially rainy season) and geography
- Mumbai witnesses torrential rains during the monsoon and hospitals are inundated with infectious fevers which are also termed as *monsoon-related illnesses*
- Acute febrile illness (AFI) or undifferentiated fever is another term which is often used synonymously

These fevers comprise of:

- The big three viz. malaria, dengue, and leptospirosis
- Acute viral hepatitis
- Enteric fever
- Rickettsiosis including scrub typhus
- Cholera and other acute diarrheal illnesses
- Chikungunya
- Japanese encephalitis

BOX 2: Reasons why tropical fevers are challenging.

- Overlapping clinical presentations pose a diagnostic dilemma
- Serological tests which are frequently used for diagnosis may be negative in the first week or may be false-positive due to a remote infection
- In spite of extensive and appropriate workup, these infections may remain undiagnosed and enter the nebulous basket of undifferentiated fevers
- The presence of underlying comorbidities like alcoholic liver disease with its associated liver and kidney dysfunction (acute kidney injury, hepatorenal syndrome, and sepsis), sickle cell disease with hemolytic anemia, etc., may further create a diagnostic conundrum
- Infections may coexist leading to one of them remaining occult and to synergistic organ damage
- Noninfectious causes of fever such as hemophagocytic lymphohistiocytosis (HLH) and DRESS syndrome (drug rash, eosinophilia and systemic symptoms) can cause declining counts and ongoing fever and compound the confusion
- Empirical treatment with versatile drugs, covering more than one organism may often be required
- A large number of these patients require intensive care unit (ICU) care for mechanical ventilation, renal replacement therapy, vasopressor support, blood, and blood component therapy

Contd...

Contd...

- Pregnant patients pose further challenges in both diagnosis (the altered physiology may interfere with the interpretation of reports) and management
- Even if the underlying infectious agent does not have a specific therapy, identifying it is important for limiting unnecessary testing
- A syndromic approach is favored by most guidelines, in the absence of a definitive diagnosis. Most of the tropical infections can be clubbed into:

Fever with thrombocytopenia	• Malaria • Leptospirosis • Dengue • Scrub typhus • Viral infections
Fever with acute respiratory distress syndrome (ARDS)	• Malaria • Leptospirosis • Dengue • Hemorrhagic fevers • Scrub typhus
Fever with hepatorenal involvement	• Malaria • Leptospirosis • Acute fulminant hepatitis • Hemorrhagic fevers (Hanta virus, Ebola virus, Marburg virus, etc.) • Scrub typhus
Fever with neurological involvement	• Any of the previous fevers • Japanese encephalitis • Herpes simplex virus (HSV) encephalitis/meningitis
Fever with diarrhea	• Enteric fever • Cholera • Acute gastroenteritis • Amebiasis • Drug fever
Fever with rash	• Viral fevers • Dengue • Drug fever • Chikungunya • Scrub typhus
Fever with joint pains	• Chikungunya • Dengue • Scrub typhus • Drug fever

BOX 3: Clinical presentation.

- Brief period of high fever (may be intermittent in malaria, continuous in enteric fever, saddle back in dengue and biphasic in leptospirosis)
- Body ache (severe in dengue, hence called break bone fever)
- Myalgia (severe in leptospirosis, often mimicking acute abdomen or even paraparesis due to severe calf pain)
- Dry cough (observed in all tropical fevers, especially enteric fever)
- Jaundice (the intensity may vary and may be a clue to the diagnosis)
- Bleeding manifestations [epistaxis, gastrointestinal (GI) bleed, and petechiae]; related to thrombocytopenia or hypoprothrombinemia
- Rash (maculopapular); eschar in scrub typhus
- Oliguria (renal involvement in malaria, leptospirosis, and scrub typhus)
- Right hypochondrial pain and tenderness in amoebic liver abscess (ALA)
- Acute watery diarrhea is a presenting feature of cholera, *Giardia*, rotavirus, *Cryptosporidium*, *Isospora*, etc.

BOX 4: Clues/pointers to the diagnosis (clinically and laboratory parameters wise).

- Altered sensorium may be a manifestation of cerebral malaria, hypoglycemia caused by malaria or antimalarial drugs, aseptic meningitis in leptospirosis, Japanese encephalitis, typhoid fever encephalopathy, dengue, scrub typhus or chikungunya encephalopathy, etc.
- Bradycardia is commonly observed in enteric fever, typhus, and in dengue during resolution of symptoms
- Dengue has a primary and a secondary rash. Drugs taken for fever can lead to a drug rash, which is violaceous and intensely pruritic
- Subconjunctival hemorrhage is commonly seen in leptospirosis
- Hyperbilirubinemia disproportionately high as compared to liver enzymes, suggests leptospirosis
- Transaminitis is present in all tropical fevers with aspartate transaminase (AST) and alanine transaminase (ALT) in the range of hundreds
- Very high AST and ALT (in thousands) is a feature of acute viral hepatitis. However, certain clades of dengue serotypes can occasionally cause a similar picture. In addition, hemophagocytic lymphohistiocytosis (HLH) can complicate dengue and cause a steep rise in transaminitis
- AST >ALT is a feature of dengue and helps distinguish it from viral hepatitis, in situations where liver enzymes are significantly elevated with certain dengue genotypes. In dengue, the source of AST is the muscles
- Cytopenias and persistent high fevers in dengue may be due to HLH
- Acute calculus cholecystitis and gallbladder wall thickening (GBWT) (on ultrasound) is often seen in dengue
- Serositis (mild pleural effusion or ascites) is commonly observed in dengue due to capillary leak syndrome
- Lymphocytosis is commonly seen in dengue by day 4–5 of fever

Contd...

Contd...

- Significantly low platelets are a feature of all tropical fevers; in enteric fever and chikungunya, platelets are usually not lower than 100,000/cmm
- Hemoglobin is usually low in malaria due to hemolysis of parasitized red blood cells (RBCs), whereas it is high in dengue due to hemoconcentration
- Creatine phosphokinase (CPK) is elevated in leptospirosis and may help in case of a diagnostic dilemma
- Acute renal involvement is common in many tropical fevers. However, hypokalemia, and nonoliguric renal failure are hallmarks of leptospirosis
- Lung involvement in the form of ARDS may occur in all tropical fevers. Additionally, leptospirosis can cause intra-alveolar pulmonary hemorrhages, which can mimic viral pneumonia, miliary tuberculosis, bacterial pneumonia, and even pneumocystis jirovecii pneumonia. These hemorrhages clear completely with timely and judicious administration of steroids
- Physiologic changes in pregnancy, confound the usual manifestations and laboratory findings in tropical fevers, e.g., gestational thrombocytopenia

BOX 5: Complications.

- *Hemophagocytic lymphohistiocytosis:* Secondary HLH should be considered when a patient with dengue has persistent high fevers beyond day 5–7 or a relapse of fever
- *Idiopathic thrombocytopenic purpura (ITP):* This should be considered if platelets do not start increasing in 7–10 days after fever onset in dengue
- *Secondary bacterial infection/sepsis:* This usually occurs in the second week and is thought to be due the translocation of bacteria from the gut
- Drug fever should always be considered, especially in the presence of rash and eosinophilia
- Recurrent fever after treatment of malaria can be due to *R*ecrudescence, *R*elapse (*Plasmodium vivax* and *P. ovale* only) and *R*einfection

BOX 6: Diagnosis.	
Definitive tests	• Peripheral smear for malarial parasite (thick smear for the parasite load and thin for species identification) • Rapid malaria antigen test (RMAT) • NS1Ag for dengue (in the first 5–7 days of fever) • Dengue polymerase chain reaction (PCR) (in the first 5–7 days of fever) • Dengue immunoglobulin M (IgM) and dengue IgG (after day 7 of fever) • *Leptospira* PCR (in the first 5–7 days of fever) • Leptospira IgM (after day 7 of fever) • IgM scrub typhus—rapid immunochromatographic test • Blood culture (for enteric fever; in the first 7 days after fever onset) • Widal test (after day 7 of fever onset) • Chikungunya PCR (in the first 5–7 days of fever) • Chikungunya IgM (after day 7 of fever) • IgM anti-hepatitis A virus (HAV) • IgM anti hepatitis E virus (HEV)
Ancillary tests	• Complete blood count with differential count • Liver function test • Renal function test [blood urea nitrogen (BUN), serum creatinine, uric acid, etc.) • Serum electrolytes • Blood sugar • CPK • Serum lactate dehydrogenase (LDH) (raised in hemolysis of malaria) • Chest radiograph (look for blunting of the costophrenic angle in dengue, ARDS, and pulmonary hemorrhages in leptospirosis) • Sonography of the abdomen • Stool examination for cysts and trophozoites of *Entamoeba histolytica*
Others	• Serum ferritin and serum triglyceride • Immature platelet fraction in ITP secondary to dengue • Glucose-6-phosphate dehydrogenase (G6PD) • Indirect hemagglutination test for ALA

BOX 7: Management.

- Often, in the absence of a definitive diagnosis, a combination of antimalarials and antibiotics has to be empirically administered, in order to include common tropical infections. Initiate empirical therapy based on the initial presentation
- The World Health Organization (WHO) guidelines recommend combination therapy for falciparum malaria and complicated vivax malaria (artemisinin combination therapy or ACT)
- In severe malaria, parenteral artesunate [2.4 mg/kg intravenous (IV) bolus at admission, 12 hours and 24 hours; followed by once a day for 7 days] should be started and once the patient can take orally, a shift should be made to a WHO approved combination therapy, such as artemether plus lumefantrine one tablet (80/480 mg) bd for 3 days
- Vivax malaria can be treated with chloroquine (total 25 mg/kg over 3 days)
- Primaquine (an 8-aminoquinoline) 7.5 mg bd for 14 days should be given for radical treatment of vivax malaria; single dose of 45 mg is sufficient in falciparum malaria. A G6PD test should be done prior to this
- Adequate hydration is paramount in dengue with warning signs, and can make the difference between life and death
- Watch out for the red flags in dengue, such as abdominal pain, tender hepatomegaly, persistent vomiting, bleeding manifestations, etc., which warrant admission to the ICU
- Bleeding in dengue is multifactorial and thrombocytopenia is just one of the causes. Theoretically, bleeding due to thrombocytopenia occurs only if platelets drop below 10,000/cm. Platelet transfusions should be given judiciously as they can cause complications like transfusion-related acute lung injury (TRALI)
- If the undifferentiated fever does not resolve by day 5, doxycycline is recommended to cover scrub typhus, which is underdiagnosed. Azithromycin is an alternative drug
- For enteric fever, depending on the severity of the infection, oral cefixime (20 mg/kg) or oral azithromycin or a combination can be given. If the patient requires admission, then ceftriaxone 50–75 mg/kg/day for 10–14 days with or without azithromycin should be given
- Oral or IV metronidazole 750 mg tds for 7–10 days for ALA. Oral tinidazole 2 g once a day for 5 days is a suitable alternative. After a response to initial therapy, diloxanide furoate 500 mg tds orally for 10 days should be given, to clear the luminal cysts

SUGGESTED READING

1. Banukumar S, Kannan I, Premavathi RK, Shantha S. Study on incidence of leptospirosis by serodiagnosis in rural population in the district of Kanchipuram, Tamilnadu, India. Int J Pharm Clin Res. 2016;8(3):189-92.
2. Chaudhry D, Tyagi D, Jakka S. Severe tropical infections. In: Chawla R, Todi S (Eds). ICU Protocols. Singapore: Springer; 2020.
3. Karnad DR, Amin P. An Approach to a patient with tropical infection in the intensive care unit. Indian J Crit Care Med. 2021;25(Suppl 2):S118-21.
4. Singhi S, Chaudhary D, Varghese GM, Bhalla A, Karthi N. Tropical fevers: management guidelines. Indian J Crit Care Med. 2014;18(2):62-9.
5. World Health Organization. (2012). Handbook for Clinical Management of Dengue. [online] Available from http://apps.who.int/iris/bitstream/10665/76887/1/9789241504713_eng. pdf?ua=1 [Last accessed September, 2024].

7.4 VIRAL INFECTION IN THE EMERGENCY ROOM

Mala Kaneria

BOX 1: Introduction.

Viral infections form a substantial part of the emergency workload, even before the recent coronavirus disease-2019 (COVID-19) pandemic.

The growing availability of molecular diagnostics for viral infections has led to increased recognition of these pathogens.

Viral infections have protean clinical presentations including upper respiratory symptoms, pneumonia, acute respiratory distress syndrome (ARDS), respiratory failure, gastrointestinal disturbances, skin vesicles and pustules, central or peripheral nervous system manifestations, and viral-induced shock.

Many viruses can efficiently spread within hospital environment leading to inhospital outbreaks, sometimes with high rates of mortality and morbidity, thus infection control measures are of paramount importance.

BOX 2: History.

- Knowledge of the underlying comorbidities and the immune status of the patient are crucial as some viruses such as cytomegalovirus (CMV) and Epstein–Barr virus (EBV) enter a latent period and reactivate during periods of immunosuppression.
- Animal bites (dog, cat, etc.) can transmit rabies
- Viral illness in other family members and close contacts
- Immunization status of the host
- Travel history, including travel history of recent close contacts
- Many bacterial/parasitic and viral pathogens are transmitted by ticks, and a history of insect bites preceding an acute febrile illness and/or encephalitis may suggest an arboviral infection

Caveat: Since antiviral therapies are known for just a few viral infections, the pillar of treatment for most serious viral infections is symptomatic and supportive, and therefore critical care is of utmost importance for the management of severe viral infections.

BOX 3: Transmission.

Like bacterial infections, these too spread in four ways:

- They could be transmitted by vectors (vector borne), e.g., dengue, chikungunya, and Zika virus and are transmitted by mosquitoes
- Close contact with an infected individual, through coughing, sneezing, touching, kissing, or sexual contact
- Ingestion of contaminated food or water
- Contact with fomites such as a bed railings, water faucet, or a doorknob
- Congenital infections due to mother to child transmission

BOX 4: Respiratory viruses.

Types:
- Viruses are frequently identified in patients with severe community-acquired pneumonia, where they may be the culprit pathogens along with bacteria or just colonizers in patients without clinical pneumonia
- The most frequently isolated viruses are influenza A viruses (including H1N1 and H3N2), influenza B viruses (B/Yamagata and B/Victoria), human coronaviruses [HCoV and severe acute respiratory syndrome coronavirus 2 (SARS-CoV-2)] and noninfluenza viruses such as respiratory syncytial virus, human rhinoviruses, human metapneumovirus, human parainfluenza viruses, and adenoviruses

Respiratory viral infections may have myriad presentations:
- Usually, an acute exacerbation of an underlying comorbidity such as chronic obstructive lung disease and acute severe bronchial asthma
- Viral pneumonia precipitating ARDS
- Nonpulmonary complications arising from viral triggered systemic inflammation causing organ failure, direct viral pathology leading to myocarditis, heart failure, myocardial infarction due to viral coronary vasculitis, rhabdomyolysis, and encephalitis
- Viral infections can occasionally be followed by autoimmune conditions such as Guillain–Barré syndrome and chronic autoimmune diseases such as type 1 diabetes
- The terminologies influenza-like illness (ILI) and severe acute respiratory infection (SARI) are used to define the typical presentation of viral pneumonias

Testing:
- As a consequence of the recent pandemics of H1N1 and COVID-19, and due to vigorous molecular testing, both influenza (H1N1 and H3N2) and SARS-CoV-2 are easily identified in the intensive care unit (ICU). However, it is essential to identify other lesser known respiratory viruses, especially in children and immunosuppressed patients

Various single target and multiplex assays are available point of care and are recommended by both the American Thoracic Society (ATS) and the Infectious Diseases Society of America (IDSA) to diagnose influenza and noninfluenza respiratory viruses. Both upper and lower respiratory panel may be utilized, as indicated. Upper respiratory tract molecular panels may not be sensitive enough to exclude lower respiratory tract infections, especially in critically ill and immunocompromised patients

BOX 5: Blood-borne viruses.

Types and presentation:

- Blood-borne viruses such as human immunodeficiency virus (HIV), hepatitis B virus (HBV), and hepatitis C virus (HCV) are transmitted via body fluids, commonly blood, vaginal secretions, semen, amniotic fluid, and less commonly other body fluids
- The HIV positive patients may present acutely to the emergency room (ER) in acute seroconversion or with some opportunistic infections (depending on the CD4 counts) or with drug–drug interactions
- Hepatitis B and C, though usually responsible for chronic liver damage, may present with acute fulminant hepatitis

Diagnosis:

- Diagnosis is usually done by serology initially
- Quantitative polymerase chain reaction (PCR) assays for viral nucleic acids are used to diagnose active viral replication or sometimes as the initial test in immunocompromised patients who may not seroconvert

BOX 6: Viral hemorrhagic fever (VHF).

- Viral hemorrhagic fevers, caused by an array of different viruses, present with fever, body ache, and capillary leak syndrome with hypotension
- Thrombocytopenia, leukopenia, bleeding diathesis, and respiratory distress are all features of VHFs, especially when the disease is severe
- The important VHFs in India spread by arthropod vectors are dengue fever/ dengue hemorrhagic fever and Kyasanur forest disease
- Another VHF is caused by Hanta virus infection and for this there is no known vector
- With increasing global interconnectedness, VHFs may present to nonendemic areas

BOX 7: Enteric viruses.

- Multiple viruses from different families produce gastrointestinal symptoms viz., norovirus, rotavirus, human astrovirus, hepatitis A, hepatitis E, and enteroviruses including poliovirus
- Respiratory viruses too can produce enteral infection with gastrointestinal symptoms (e.g., SARS-CoV-2)
- Extraintestinal manifestations of some viruses may lead to specific syndromes, e.g., flaccid paralysis due to polio and enterovirus D86
- Multiplex PCR of stool samples, the most reliable method to determine the causative pathogen, is however, more useful and cost effective in the immunocompromised host

BOX 8: Herpesviridae infections and reactivations.

- The eight herpesviruses which can cause infections in humans are herpes simplex virus (HSV) 1 and 2; varicella zoster virus (VZV); CMV; EBV; and human herpes virus 6, 7, and 8
- The primary infections usually occur in childhood and early adulthood, after which these viruses lie dormant and get reactivated under conditions of immunosuppression, stress, and critical illness
- Reactivation may be asymptomatic or fulminant causing encephalitis or malignant transformation
- HSV 1 commonly presents as gingivostomatitis or pharyngitis, with painful vesicular lesions or with HSV encephalitis
- The detection of HSV 1 in the respiratory secretions of ventilated patients is not uncommon, and is attributed to a decline in host immune control, leading to reactivation
- Treatment is usually not required in this situation
- Severely immunocompromised patients, such as those with advanced HIV infection, hematopoietic stem cell and organ transplant recipients and profoundly neutropenic patients are at increased risk of HSV 1 infection and may need acyclovir prophylaxis
- HSV 2, which is predominantly transmitted sexually, has a similar clinical presentation but occurs only in the high-risk immunocompromised group
- Similarly, CMV infection too is latent until reactivated by immunosuppression, when it can cause CMV viremia, colitis, retinitis, hepatitis, and pneumonitis
- Solid organ and hemopoietic stem cell transplant patients need prophylaxis and treatment
- High titers of CMV copies are commonly found in the bronchoalveolar lavage fluid of mechanically ventilated, critically ill patients, and treatment in these situations has not been shown to be beneficial
- **EBV** infection may present to the ER with fever, lethargy, cervical lymphadenopathy, pharyngitis, macular rash, and hepatosplenomegaly, with a concurrent peripheral blood lymphocytosis and transaminitis, suggestive of infectious mononucleosis (IM)
- CMV may present similarly with IM-like illness. Acute seroconversion in HIV may have a similar CMV may present similarly with IM-like illness
- HHV 6 is commonly associated with drug reactions and DRESS (drug rash, eosinophilia and systemic symptoms) and is thought to be due to a complex interplay between the offending drug and HHV 6 reactivation
- Asymptomatic patients with antibodies to these viruses suggest past infection and do not require treatment

BOX 9: Fever with rash.

- Many viral fevers present with fever and rash which may be maculopapular, generalized diffuse erythema, vesicular, pustular, nodular, petechial, and purpuric, depending on the characteristic morphology, distribution, and accompanying symptoms.
  - *Measles:* Rash progresses from face to body; the fever disappears when the rash stops evolving; a brownish desquamation remains after the rash disappears. Koplik spots (enanthem) in the oral cavity appear either 12 hours before or within 24 hours of rash appearance
  - *Rubella:* It has a similar rash which is lighter, though with a faster evolution, and no residual desquamation. Lymph nodes behind the ears or below the occiput may be observed.
  - *Exanthema subitum (6th disease):* Caused by HHV 6 and causes a 3-day fever, with rash appearing after fever resolution.
  - *Erythema infectiosum (5th disease):* Caused by human parvovirus B19, causes a slapped cheek appearance and is seen in school children.
  - *Hand, foot, and mouth disease (HFMD):* Caused by coxsackievirus A type 16 and other strains of coxsackieviruses and enteroviruses, is seen in children (more often) and adults. Fever, sore throat and blisters on the hands, mouth, feet, and sometimes thighs and bottoms are characteristic.
  - *Varicella zoster:* Causes chickenpox as a primary infection and reactivation due to immunosuppression or immunosenescence results in shingles or herpes zoster. Chickenpox in adults may be severe and complicated by pneumonia, hepatitis, encephalitis, etc.
    - **Prompt treatment with acyclovir 10 mg/kg 8 hourly (oral or IV) may reduce the severity of infection**
- *Neurological involvement*
  - This is a feared complication of viral infection with the common offenders being HSV 1, VZV, arboviruses (Dengue and Zika), chikungunya, Japanese encephalitis virus, rabies, and nonpolio enteroviruses
  - Patients should be subjected to a detailed history taking emphasizing on travel to endemic areas, exposure to ticks and mosquitoes and a sexual history, along with a dedicated clinical examination to look for tick bites in hidden areas
  - An attempt should be made to identify aseptic meningitis, encephalitis, and acute disseminated encephalomyelitis (ADEM), a postinfectious sequela of viral encephalitis
  - MRI brain, electroencephalograph (EEG) and cerebrospinal fluid (CSF) multiplex PCR may provide clues

BOX 10: Unusual and emerging viruses.

- Imported and emerging viruses will be the fallout of globalization
- SARS-CoV-2 and monkeypox (renamed mpox by the WHO in late 2022) are two such examples
- When the initial investigations are unrevealing, a careful history taking to identify exposures and a continued search for causative agents should be maintained, in order to diagnose outbreaks of emerging viruses such as Nipah and Hendra viruses

BOX 11: Postviral syndromes.

- Viral infections can trigger an uncontrolled immunological response leading to secondary hemophagocytic lymphohistiocytosis (HLH), with EBV being implicated most commonly
- HLH is characterized by fever, cytopenias, organomegaly, raised ferritin, triglyceride, and bone marrow aspirate usually confirms hemophagocytosis
- Viral infections may also trigger autoimmune diseases, commonly Guillain–Barré syndrome and ADEM
- **Treatment and prevention:**
  - Infection control measures go a long way in the prevention of viral infection transmission, within hospital settings. Droplet and contact precaution measures, specialized airborne infection isolation room, source control (face mask) and use of various levels of personal protective equipment (PPE) are important interventions
  - Vaccination of exposed health workers as indicated
  - Vaccination with varicella zoster vaccine within 72–96 hours of exposure, can act as a postexposure prophylaxis in susceptible individuals
  - Antirabies vaccine (ARV) with or without human rabies immunoglobulin (HRIG) in case of animal bites, according to the category of bite
  - Neuraminidase inhibitors such as oseltamivir, zanamivir, peramivir and baloxavir, a novel inhibitor of the cap-dependent endonuclease activity, should be initiated within 48 hours, depending on the severity of the pneumonia, for 5–10 days
  - The role of corticosteroids in ARDS due to viral infections has been proved only in SARS-CoV-2 (RECOVERY trial), whereas it remains controversial in other viral infections
  - Management of COVID-19 (with Paxlovid, remdesivir, and molnupiravir) keeps evolving as the virus keeps mutating and data on the use of newer drugs emerges
  - Superadded bacterial (mainly *Staphylococcus aureus*) and fungal infections (*Aspergillus*, *Candida*, and mucormycosis) should be watched for, especially when the fever is unrelenting
  - Cytokine storm and ARDS, which usually occur in the second week, after the viremia declines, should be anticipated and managed in the ICU
  - Intravenous acyclovir may be started empirically when viral encephalitis is suspected
  - Early ICU admission, fever control, and treatment of seizures/status epilepticus) or adjunctive immunomodulatory therapies (i.e., steroids and intravenous immunoglobulins) may improve neurologic outcomes

SUGGESTED READING

1. Chi-Chung Cheng V, Fuk-Woo Chan J, FN Hung I, Yuen KY. Viral Infections, an Overview with a Focus on Prevention of Transmission. Reference Module in Biomedical Sciences. 2016:B978-0-12-801238-3.90174-0.
2. Fragkou PC, Moschopoulos CD, Karofylakis E, Kelesidis T, Tsiodras S. Update in Viral Infections in the Intensive Care Unit. Front Med (Lausanne). 2021;8:575-80.
3. Grech AK, Foo CT, Paul E, Aung AK, Yu C. Epidemiological trends of respiratory tract pathogens detected via mPCR in Australian adult patients before COVID-19. BMC Infect Dis. 2024;24(1):38.
4. Morris AC, Smielewska A. Viral infections in critical care: a narrative review. Anaesthesia. 2023;78:626-35.

7.5 SOFT TISSUE INFECTION IN THE EMERGENCY ROOM

Hemant P Thacker, Kunal Srivastava

BOX 1: Introduction.

- Skin and soft tissue infections (SSTIs) encompass a variety of conditions affecting the epidermis, dermis, subcutaneous tissue, or superficial fascia
- Uncomplicated infections are typically caused by gram-positive bacteria, such as *Streptococcus* and *Staphylococcus*, which infiltrate the skin after minor injuries like scratches or insect bites
- Complicated infections are more likely to be polymicrobial. SSTIs usually present with painful, warm, erythematous skin lesions and may also result in purulent fluid collections or necrosis of the affected tissue
- Systemic symptoms, such as fever, often indicate more severe infections. Risk factors for developing SSTIs or more severe forms of SSTIs include diabetes mellitus, immunodeficiency, and chronic edema
- Diagnosis is primarily clinical, though some patients may need imaging or laboratory studies. Purulent infections, like abscesses, are mainly treated with incision and drainage, whereas nonpurulent infections, such as erysipelas and cellulitis, require antibiotic therapy
- Necrotizing soft tissue infections (NSTIs) have a high mortality rate and are considered a surgical emergency, necessitating immediate wound debridement

BOX 2: Overview of SSTIs.

Condition	***Most common pathogens***	***Tissue involvement***	***Clinical features***
Impetigo	*Staphylococcus aureus* (bullous and nonbullous)	Superficial epidermis	Highly contagious superficial infection with honey yellow crusts
	Streptococcus pyogenes (nonbullous)		Bullae formation (common in staphylococcal infection)
Staphylococcal scalded skin syndrome (generalized form of impetigo)	Exotoxin of *S. aureus*	Superficial epidermis	• Erythematous rash • Fever • Heals completely

Contd...

Contd...

Condition		***Most common pathogens***	***Tissue involvement***	***Clinical features***
Nonpurulent SSTIs	Erysipelas	Group A *Streptococcus*	• Superficial dermis • Lymphatic vessels	Sharply demarcated, erythematous skin lesion
	Cellulitis	• Group A *Streptococcus* (nonpurulent) • *S. aureus* (purulent)	• Deep dermis • Subcutaneous tissue	• Rapidly spreading infection • Erythematous skin lesion with indistinct margins • With or without purulent exudate
Purulent SSTIs	Skin abscess	*S. aureus* [often methicillin-resistant *S. aureus* (MRSA)]	Deeper layers of the skin	• Walled-off infection with a collection of pus
	Folliculitis, furuncles, carbuncles	• *S. aureus* • *Pseudomonas aeruginosa*	Hair follicle	• Localized papules and pustules on the base of hair follicles • Usually containing a central hair
NSTIs		• *Mixed infection:* Group A streptococci + Anaerobic bacteria • *Clostridial myonecrosis: Clostridium* spp. (gas gangrene)	• *Necrotizing cellulitis:* Deep dermis and subcutaneous tissue • *Necrotizing fasciitis:* Superficial fascia • *Necrotizing myositis:* Muscular tissue	• Severe, rapidly progressive infection with necrosis • Possible crepitus, bullae, and purple skin discoloration • High risk of systemic complications, high mortality

BOX 3: Diagnostic evaluation of SSTIs.

Suspected SSTI

- Evaluate whether the infection involves the hand or face
- **If the hand is involved:**
  - Tests: Perform blood cultures and imaging (X-ray)
  - If warranted, consider procedures such as surgical exploration or lumbar puncture, depending on clinical findings
- **If the face is involved:**
  - Tests: Similar to hand involvement, include blood cultures and imaging (X-ray)
  - Additionally, consider CT imaging if complications like orbital involvement are suspected
- **If the SSTI is non-hand/non-face:**
  - Tests:
    - Conduct blood cultures and imaging (as needed)
    - Evaluate for severe conditions or other systemic signs (e.g., fever, elevated white blood cell count, hypotension)
    - Perform additional imaging (e.g., ultrasound or CT) for deeper or poorly defined infections
- **General guidance:**
  - At all stages, prioritize clinical evaluation and decide whether immediate surgical consultation is necessary for potential drainage or debridement
  - Advanced imaging (e.g., MRI or CT) may be necessary to assess the extent of infection or complications

BOX 4: Evaluation algorithm for severity of SSTI.

Step 1: Initial assessment

- Suspect SSTI based on clinical signs, including:
  - Redness
  - Warmth
  - Swelling
  - Pain
  - Dysfunction (e.g., impaired movement or organ involvement)

Step 2: Check for comorbidities

- Assess for high-risk conditions such as:
  - Chronic liver or renal disease
  - Vascular insufficiency
  - Asplenia
  - Immunocompromised states
  - Necrotizing peripheral infections

If any of these are present, the infection may require closer monitoring or specialized care.

Step 3: Evaluate for severe symptoms

- Check for systemic signs of severe infection, including:
  - Fever (≥38°C or ≥40°C)
  - Hypotension
  - Heart rate >100 beats/min
  - Altered mental status

Presence of any of these suggests a need for more intensive management.

Step 4: Assess specific sites and extent of infection

- Is the infection in the hand and/or face?
- Does the lesion cover >9% of the body surface area?

If yes, it may indicate a moderate-to-severe infection.

Step 5: Check for critical symptoms or rapid progression

- Look for signs such as:
  - Bullae formation
  - Hemorrhage
  - Rapid progression
  - Crepitus (gas under the skin)
  - Anesthesia (loss of sensation)

These symptoms could signal necrotizing or severe infection.

Outcome determination:

- Mild cases: Managed with outpatient therapy.
- Moderate-to-Severe Cases: Consider hospital admission or close observation for 2–3 days, especially if risk factors or severe symptoms are present.

BOX 5: Severity of SSTI.

There is no universally accepted classification system for the severity of SSTI **(Table 1)**. The Infectious Diseases Society of America (IDSA) 2014 guidelines on SSTIs use a system based on the presence or absence of systemic symptoms

TABLE 1: SSTI severity grading.

Grade	***Characteristics***
Mild SSTI	Locally confined
Moderate SSTI	Systemic symptoms
Severe SSTI	• Unsuccessful initial treatment • Systemic inflammatory response syndrome (SIRS) criteria (the difference between moderate and severe infections is poorly defined in the IDSA criteria. SIRS criteria are specifically mentioned by the IDSA) • Any NSTI • Immunocompromised patients • Signs of deep tissue infection • Organ failure

"Necrotizing infections are always considered severe!"

BOX 6: Empiric antibiotic therapy for SSTIs.

Based on the 2014 IDSA guidelines and LAGICON (Levonadifloxacin in Management of Resistant Gram-positive Infections: An Indian Consensus)

Recommendations in this section are based on the 2014 IDSA guidelines and LAGICON. However, depending on the patient's individual risk profile, even patients with locally confined infections may require admission for intravenous antibiotic therapy.

- Choice of empiric antibiotic therapy should include the following factors:
  - Severity (see "SSTI severity grading")
  - Presence of purulence
  - Local resistance patterns
  - Risk for complications
  - Risk factors for SSTIs (many risk factors predispose individuals not only to the development of SSTIs but also to more complicated courses of disease)
- Variants that may require a more specialized treatment include:
  - Bite wounds
  - Recurrent or complex skin abscesses
  - Orbital and periorbital cellulitis
  - Device-associated infections (e.g., dialysis catheters and prosthetic joints)
  - Patients at risk for endocarditis (e.g., patients with a prosthetic heart valve)

BOX 7: Empiric antibiotic therapy.

S1: Levonadifloxacin is a preferred therapy for acute bacterial skin and skin structure infections (ABSSSI) in patients with existing kidney disease or history of kidney disease or high risk for kidney diseases
S2: Levonadifloxacin is a preferred therapy for ABSSSI in patients with existing liver disease or history of liver diseases
S3: Alalevonadifloxacin stands out as a preferred oral stepdown therapy for patients with ABSSSI who have received initial hospital treatment
S4: Levonadifloxacin is the preferred therapy for ABSSSI patients concurrently experiencing bacteremia
S8: Levonadifloxacin stands as the preferred treatment for managing NSTIs in patients with compromised immune systems

Empiric antibiotic therapy for SSTIs (based on the 2014 IDSA guidelines)			
	Mild infection	***Moderate infection***	***Severe infection***
Purulent SSTI (e.g., furuncle, carbuncle, and skin abscess)	• Incision and drainage usually sufficient • Consider topical antibiotics (e.g., mupirocin). (Mupirocin 2% topical ointment every 8 hours)	• Incision and drainage with cultures • One of the following: – Trimethoprim/ sulfamethoxazole (trimethoprim/ sulfamethoxazole DS 160 mg/800 mg PO 1–2 tablets every 12 hours) – Doxycycline (doxycycline 100 mg PO every 12 hours)	• Incision and drainage with cultures • One of the following: – Vancomycin (vancomycin 15 mg/kg IV every 12 hours) – Daptomycin (daptomycin 4 mg/kg IV every 24 hours) – Linezolid (linezolid 600 mg IV every 12 hours) – Telavancin (telavancin 10 mg/kg IV once daily) – Ceftaroline (Ceftaroline 600 mg IV every 12 hours)

Contd...

Contd...

Empiric antibiotic therapy for SSTIs (based on the 2014 IDSA guidelines)			
	Mild infection	***Moderate infection***	***Severe infection***
Nonpurulent SSTI (e.g., erysipelas and cellulitis)	• Oral therapy with one of the following: – Penicillin V (Penicillin VK 250–500 mg PO every 6 hours) – Cephalexin (Cephalexin 500 mg PO every 6 hours) – Dicloxacillin (Dicloxacillin 500 mg PO every 6 hours) – Clindamycin (clindamycin 300–450 every 6 hours)	• Intravenous therapy with one of the following: – Penicillin G (penicillin 2–4 million units IV every 4–6 hours) – Ceftriaxone (ceftriaxone 1–2 g IV once daily) – Cefazolin (cefazolin 1 g IV every 8 hours) – Clindamycin (Clindamycin 600 mg IV every 8 hours)	• Rule out necrotizing infections (consider surgical exploration and samples for cultures) • Intravenous combination therapy – Vancomycin (vancomycin 15 mg/kg IV every 12 hours) – Plus one of the following: - Piperacillin/tazobactam (piperacillin/tazobactam 3.375 g IV every 6–8 hours) - Meropenem (meropenem 1 g IV every 8 hours)
Necrotizing SSTI (e.g., necrotizing fasciitis, necrotizing cellulitis, necrotizing myositis, and clostridial myonecrosis**)**	• Necrotizing infections are always considered severe		• Emergency surgical debridement with cultures • Broad-spectrum intravenous combination therapy with one of the following (MRSA coverage): – Daptomycin (daptomycin 4–6 mg/kg IV once daily) – Linezolid (linezolid 600 mg IV every 12 hours) – Vancomycin (vancomycin 15 mg/kg IV every 12 hours)

Contd...

Contd...

Empiric antibiotic therapy for SSTIs (based on the 2014 IDSA guidelines)			
	Mild infection	***Moderate infection***	***Severe infection***
			• Plus one of the following: – A carbapenem (e.g., meropenem) (meropenem 1 g IV every 8 hours) – Piperacillin/tazobactam (piperacillin/tazobactam 3.375 g IV every 6–8 hour) – A fluoroquinolone (e.g., ciprofloxacin) (ciprofloxacin 500 mg IV every 12 hours) • PLUS metronidazole (metronidazole 500 mg IV every 6 hours) – Ceftriaxone (ceftriaxone 1–2 g IV once daily) – Plus metronidazole (metronidazole 500 mg IV every 6 hours) • If linezolid is not part of the regimen consider the addition of clindamycin (clindamycin 600 mg IV every 8 hours) to reduce the risk of toxic shock syndrome (TSS) (antitoxin activity)

BOX 8: Nonpurulent SSTIs.

Definitions:
- *Erysipelas:* A superficial skin infection involving the upper dermis
- *Cellulitis:* A local infection affecting the deep dermis and subcutaneous tissue

Clinical features:
- *Local signs:* Include erythema, edema, warmth, and tenderness
  - *Specific to erysipelas:* Lesions are raised and sharply demarcated
  - *Specific to cellulitis:* Lesions are poorly defined with induration
- *Cutaneous lymphatic edema:* Historically referred to as "peau d'orange"
- *Common locations:* Primarily affect the lower limbs and face
- Additional features may include:
  - *Lymphangitis:* Red streaks extending from the skin lesion following lymphatic vessels
  - *Lymphadenitis:* Swollen and tender regional lymph nodes
  - *Bullae:* Blistering of the skin
  - *Purulent exudate:* Presence of pus
- *Systemic symptoms in moderate to severe infections:* Fever, chills, confusion, nausea, headache, muscle, and joint pain
- Bilateral cellulitis is rare. Evaluation of patients with bilateral leg erythema should consider alternative diagnoses such as stasis dermatitis and lymphedema

Etiology:
- Includes pathogens mentioned earlier
- *Pasteurella multocida:* A gram-negative encapsulated coccobacillus often associated with infections secondary to dog and cat bites

Diagnostics:
- Diagnosis is primarily clinical
- In cases with systemic symptoms, laboratory studies like complete blood count (CBC), inflammatory markers, cultures (not routinely recommended only in specific cases), and imaging ultrasonography, is the first choice
- CT/MRI with or without IV contrast consider if there is concern for complications such as pyomyositis or osteomyelitis
- MRI is particularly sensitive for detecting soft tissue inflammation and necrosis. May be necessary to evaluate severity and guide treatment

Treatment of nonpurulent SSTIs:
- General principles:
  - Empiric antibiotic therapy effective against streptococci and *Staphylococcus aureus* is the primary treatment for nonpurulent SSTIs
  - Management should address any predisposing factors such as edema or fungal infections
  - Most patients with cellulitis or erysipelas who are clinically stable can be treated as outpatients
  - Patients with systemic symptoms often require hospitalization and intravenous antibiotic therapy
  - Follow sepsis management guidelines for severe infections

Contd...

Contd...

- Antibiotic therapy:
  - Systemic antibiotics are typically necessary for treatment
  - Empiric regimens should usually cover *Streptococcus* spp. and *S. aureus* (*See* **Box 7** "Antibiotic therapy for skin and soft tissue infections" for detailed recommendations)
  - Criteria for inpatient management or coverage for MRSA antibiotics (given in above boxes)

Supportive care:

- Elevation of the affected limbs
- Rest and acute pain management as needed

SUBTYPES AND VARIANTS

BOX 9: Perianal streptococcal dermatitis.

- **Definition:** An infection of the perianal skin with group A *Streptococcus* characterized by pain, pruritus, and rash
- **Epidemiology:** Most common in children between 6 months and 10 years of age
- **Etiology:** Group A *Streptococcus* infection
- **Clinical features:**
  - Signs of systemic infection are rare
  - Pruritus, rectal pain, and blood streaked stools
  - Sharply demarcated, erythematous perianal rash with pseudo exudate, crusting, and/or superficial anal fissures/cracks
- **Diagnosis:** Clinical
- **Differential diagnosis:**
  - *Candida* diaper dermatitis
  - Irritant contact diaper dermatitis
- **Treatment:** Penicillin; in pediatric patients—amoxicillin (oral emulsion is tolerated better)
- **Other:**
  - Orbital cellulitis; periorbital (preseptal) cellulitis
  - Ludwig angina
- **Complications:**
  - Complications are generally rare; the majority of affected individuals respond well to treatment
  - *In orbital cellulitis:* Blindness, cavernous sinus thrombosis, and intracranial abscess

PURULENT SKIN AND SOFT TISSUE INFECTIONS

BOX 10: Folliculitis, furuncles, and carbuncles.

Definitions:
- *Folliculitis:* Localized inflammation of the hair follicle or sebaceous glands, restricted to the epidermis. Despite the hair follicle extending beyond the epidermis, folliculitis denotes a purulent infection primarily affecting the superficial layers
- *Hot tub folliculitis:* Pseudomonal folliculitis appearing 848 hours postexposure to contaminated water. It typically resolves on its own without requiring antibiotic treatment
- *Furuncle:* Deep folliculitis extending into the dermis, often forming an abscess in the subcutaneous tissue
- *Carbuncle:* A confluent form of folliculitis resulting in an inflammatory mass. It may involve abscess formation and skin necrosis

Clinical features:
- Tender papules and/or pustules, often causing itching
- Located at the hair follicle sites, with lesions containing one or more hairs
- Possible drainage of pus from follicular openings
- Potential for multiple lesions
- Variable locations, with carbuncles most commonly found on the back of the neck

Differential diagnoses:
- Ecthyma
- Acne vulgaris
- Eosinophilic folliculitis

Facial furuncles can lead to severe complications such as periorbital cellulitis or cavernous sinus thrombosis

Skin abscess:
Definition: An accumulation of white yellow pus containing proteins, leukocytes (particularly neutrophils), bacteria, and cellular debris, typically located in the dermis and subcutaneous tissue

Clinical features:
- Manifests cardinal signs of inflammation
- Presents as painful, tender, and fluctuant red nodules
- Pain usually diminishes following rupture or drainage of the abscess
- May be surrounded by erythema and induration. (The frequently used term "purulent cellulitis" is not applicable to a drainable abscess. Treatment should focus on incision and drainage of the abscess, if possible, and not antibiotic therapy of cellulitis)

Differential diagnosis: Inflamed epidermoid cyst and carbuncle

Etiology: Mentioned earlier

Diagnostics: Diagnosis is usually clinical. In patients with systemic symptoms, laboratory studies, cultures, and imaging may be indicated to assess severity and tailor treatment (similar to other soft tissue infections)

BOX 11: Microbiology.

- Gram stain and cultures are not routinely recommended, even if community-acquired MRSA (CA-MRSA) is suspected. **(The 2014 guidelines on SSTIs from the IDSA recommend abscess cultures in general but emphasize that their use is mainly for the management of patients with systemic symptoms. The American College of Emergency Physicians specifically discourages collecting cultures in uncomplicated SSTIs that can be treated with incision and drainage)**
- Indications for abscess and blood cultures include:
  - **Systemic symptoms, severe infections** (see "severity of SSTI")
  - Immunocompromised patients
  - Recurrent skin abscess
  - Carbuncles

Caveat

Additional evaluation: Consider additional evaluation for underlying conditions in patients with recurrent abscess and/or complex skin abscess:

- Colonization with resistant pathogens (e.g., MRSA)
- Local causes (e.g., foreign body, pilonidal cyst, and hidradenitis suppurativa)
- Systemic predisposing conditions (e.g., neutrophil disorders)

BOX 12: Treatment of purulent SSTIs.

General principles:

- Incision and drainage are the mainstay of treatment for purulent SSTIs and are usually sufficient for mild infections
- Patients with systemic signs of infections require empiric antibiotic therapy. (If performed, microbiological studies can be used to tailor antibiotic regimens)
- Outpatient management is appropriate for clinically stable patients
- Consider inpatient management for patients with systemic symptoms. (Especially for patients who have severe infection, are immunocompromised, or for whom treatment has been unsuccessful)
- Follow management of "sepsis" for more details on the management of severe infections

Interventional therapy

Incision and drainage:

- Bedside procedure
- *Indications:* Small skin abscesses (the decision of bedside incision and drainage versus surgical drainage in the operation room depends on the experience and preference)
- Carbuncles, large furuncles (spontaneous rupture and drainage will sometimes occur without incision and can be facilitated with moist heat)
- Inflamed epidermoid cysts
- *See* Chapter 37.1 for detailed procedural guidance.

Antibiotic therapy:

- *Topical antibiotics*: Consider in MRSA folliculitis (e.g., mupirocin) (mupirocin 2% topical ointment every 8 hours)
- *Systemic antibiotic therapy for purulent SSTIs*: Usually *not indicated* after successful drainage in otherwise healthy individuals
- *Caveat:* Following the publication of the IDSA guidelines on SSTIs in 2014, multiple studies have suggested that administering systemic antibiotic treatment even after the drainage of small abscesses may be beneficial
- Consequently, the decision to administer antibiotics following drainage requires weighing the risks and benefits of a more aggressive antibiotic therapy.
- The 2020 Surgical Infection Society (SIS) guidelines suggest that the administration of adjuvant antibiotics after drainage of complex abscesses is increasingly supported by evidence)
- *Indications:* Moderate/severe infections, recurrent or complex abscesses, according to risk factors and comorbidities (e.g., diabetes mellitus)
- Regimens often include coverage for MRSA (*See* **Box 7** "Antibiotic therapy for skin and soft tissue infections" for detailed recommendations)

Supportive measures:

- Warm compresses (in folliculitis, furuncles, and carbuncles)
- Rest and acute pain management as needed
- Keep the affected area clean and dry (Some physicians recommend the use of antibacterial soaps or chlorhexidine)
- Consider MRSA decolonization for recurrent abscesses

BOX 13: Necrotizing soft tissue infections.

Definitions:
- *Necrotizing soft tissue infection:* An aggressive, life-threatening infection involving necrosis of the tissue. Superficial and/or deep tissue may be affected (i.e., necrotizing cellulitis, necrotizing fasciitis, and necrotizing myositis)
- *Fournier gangrene:* Necrotizing fasciitis of the external genitalia that can spread rapidly to the anterior abdominal wall and gluteal muscles
- *Clostridial myonecrosis:* A rapidly spreading necrotizing infection caused by *Clostridium perfringens* or *Clostridium septicum*

Etiology: Mentioned earlier

Clinical features:
- *Systemic symptoms*: Fever, chills, and altered mental status
- *Cutaneous findings*:
  - Diffuse erythema, often initially mistaken for cellulitis that does not respond to initial antibiotic therapy
  - Extreme tenderness and pain disproportionate to the visible erythema
  - Significant induration of the subcutaneous tissue, with the affected area of the subcutaneous tissue being larger than the area of skin involvement
  - *Crepitus:* Caused by bacterial production of methane and CO_2
  - Purple skin discoloration indicating skin necrosis or ecchymosis
  - Bullae formation
  - Loss of sensation in the affected area (paresthesia)
- *Caveat:* Necrotizing fasciitis initially spreads along the fascial planes before involving superficial cutaneous tissues. Therefore, local findings may not be initially remarkable, with patients experiencing disproportionate pain

- *Red flags for necrotizing deep tissue infection:*
  - Presence of crepitus
  - Formation of bullous lesions
  - Skin necrosis or discoloration
  - Pain that is out of proportion to physical examination findings
  - Signs of systemic toxicity, especially altered mental status

Diagnostics:
- A definitive diagnosis is usually made during the visualization of the tissue during surgery
- Do not delay surgical consultation and definitive surgical intervention for imaging and laboratory studies

Laboratory studies:
- CBC, metabolic panel, and inflammatory markers
- Assess organ failure and severity

Microbiology:
- Blood cultures (two sets)
- Gram stain and cultures from **deep tissue** (obtain samples during surgical exploration)
- *Caveat:* Superficial wound cultures may not accurately represent the pathogens found in deep tissue and should not be used to guide management

Contd...

Contd...

Imaging:
- Not routinely indicated and should **not delay treatment**
- CT/MRI with/without IV contrast (contrast enhancement is useful for the identification of necrotic areas. CT has a higher sensitivity than MRI for detecting gas in soft tissue but MRI has a higher sensitivity for detecting inflammation and necrosis)
- *Ultrasound:* Bedside ultrasound can sometimes provide a quick and easy first impression of the extent and depth of the inflammation, supplementing clinical findings, and helping to confirm the diagnosis

Management:
- Admit all patients with suspected or confirmed NSTI to hospital for treatment
- If clinical features suggest NSTI, start **immediate surgical and medical treatment**. (Distinguishing regular cellulitis from NSTI can be challenging. When in doubt, an urgent surgery consult can help determine adequate treatment as soon as possible)
- Surgical exploration with debridement (confirms the diagnosis and the mainstay of treatment)
- Broad-spectrum antibiotic therapy
- ICU for admission and aggressive supportive care for sepsis, if present
- Provide immediate hemodynamic support, e.g., fluid resuscitation, vasopressors (following surgical debridement, fluid loss through the wound is significant and needs to be replaced)
- Begin sepsis management
- Consider respiratory support as needed, e.g., oxygen therapy and mechanical ventilation
- Consider adjuvant therapy on an individual basis (e.g., hyperbaric oxygen, negative pressure wound therapy, intravenous immunoglobulin therapy). Adjuvant therapies are not routinely recommended and there is limited evidence to support their use. Consider on a case-by-case basis (e.g., intravenous immunoglobulin for patients with necrotizing infections caused by GAS)

Necrotizing soft tissue infections are a surgical emergency. Expedite and prioritize **surgical exploration** for diagnostic confirmation and debridement as much as possible!

BOX 14: Surgical exploration and debridement.

Antibiotic therapy:
- See "Antibiotic therapy for skin and soft tissue infections" for detailed recommendations
- Consider polymicrobial infections (provide coverage against aerobes, anaerobes, and MRSA)
- If there is evidence of TSS, include antitoxin active antibiotics (e.g., levonadifloxacin, clindamycin, and linezolid)

Complications:
- Severe necrosis requiring amputation of the affected limb
- Sepsis
- Disseminated intravascular coagulation
- Organ dysfunction (e.g., acute kidney injury)
- *Death:* High mortality rate even with adequate treatment (>30%) (reported mortality rates vary but are generally high)

Differential diagnoses:
- *Gas gangrene:* Caused by *C. perfringens*
- Severe SSTI without necrosis

BOX 15: Differential diagnoses of skin and soft tissue lesions.

Disease entity	*Description*
Superficial thrombophlebitis	• Inflammation of superficial vein associated with thrombus • Usually caused by intravenous needle or catheter; may become secondarily infected • Red, indurated area; tender, palpable vein
Deep venous thrombosis	Blood clot formation in deep veins leading to venous obstruction and inflammation
Contact dermatitis	• Irritant or allergic skin reaction to environmental agents • Sharply demarcated area of erythema and pruritus; may become secondarily infected
Pyoderma gangrenosum	• Ulcerative skin condition associated with systemic disease with unknown etiology • Commonly occurs with inflammatory bowel disease (IBD), leukemia, monoclonal gammopathies and rheumatoides • Papule or pustule progress to ulceration with violaceous or vesiculopustular borders
Drug reactions	• Erupt secondary to hypersensitivity reaction to consumption of specific medication • Usually associated with sulfur-based antibiotics and anti-inflammatory agents • Pruritic or burning, well-demarcated plaque that recurs at the same site and spreads slowly
Eosinophilic cellulitis (Wells' syndrome)	• Idiopathic acute dermatitis with dermal eosinophilic infiltration and eosinophilia • Associated with myeloproliferative, immunological and infectious disorders • Recurrent; 2–8 weeks' duration; multiple, pruritic, erythematous plaques
Acute febrile neutrophilic dermatosis (Sweet's syndrome)	• Idiopathic neutrophilic skin plaque eruption • Associated with hematological malignancy (acute myelogenous leukemia) • Red, tender plaques on face, neck and arms; fever; ocular, oral and joint pathology
Gouty arthritis	• Joint inflammation causing cutaneous erythema • Caused by joint space urate crystal precipitate induced inflammatory response • Erythema, warmth and tenderness; mild fever, chills and leukocytosis; urate crystals
Erythromelalgia	• Idiopathic paroxysmal foot or hand cutaneous disorder • Associated with myeloproliferative disorders; triggered by heat, fever and exercise • Foot and hand burning, erythema and elevated skin temperature

Contd...

Contd...

Disease entity	***Description***
Relapsing polychondritis	• Idiopathic inflammatory disease affecting cartilaginous structures • Commonly affects the ears, with ear lobe sparing • Inflammatory lesions, nonerosive polyarthritis, ocular disease and aortic insufficiency
Carcinoma erysipeloides (inflammatory carcinoma)	• Metastatic disease invading into skin lymphatic vessels • Associated most with breast carcinoma • Erythematous plaque on or under breast without fever or leukocytosis
Familial Mediterranean fever	• Autosomal recessive disease with self-limited fever, synovitis and serositis • Self-limited, recurrent, erysipelas-like skin lesions commonly below the knee • Responds well to colchicines
Familial Hibernian fever	• Idiopathic, genetic disease with fever and similar symptoms as above • Erysipelas-like lesion on limb, which migrates distally from origin • Does not respond to colchicines
Foreign body reactions	• Rare hypersensitivity reactions to metallic implants • Associated with hypersensitivity to nickel, chromium and cobalt • Reaction causes overlying cutaneous, cellulitis like erythema
Polyarteritis nodosa	• Multisystemic, necrotizing vasculitis • Subcutaneous, inflammatory nodules along affected artery that coalesce into plaques • Often bilateral and involve lower extremities
Erythema nodosum	Septal panniculitis, usually secondary to systemic disease Associated with IBD, sarcoidosis and Behçet's syndrome Coalescent raised, painful lesions, usually in arms and legs bilaterally; 4–6 weeks' duration

IMAGE GALLERY

- *Nonbullous impetigo:* Multiple red papules of varying sizes are visible around the mouth and on the left cheek. The characteristic honey colored crusts have, for the most part, been scratched off; remnants visible in the left corner of the mouth **(Fig. 1)**.

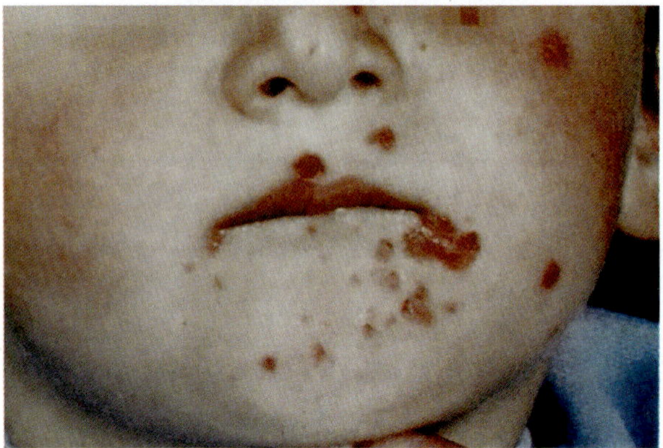

Fig. 1: Nonbullous impetigo.

- *Staphylococcal scalded skin syndrome*: Perioral, cervical and axillary reddening of the skin is visible, resulting in a scalded appearance on this child's face. In some areas, the superficial epidermal layer is detached (e.g., on the chin). On the right side of the neck, several flaccid blisters can be seen. The lips appear dry, with several rhagades in the corners of the mouth **(Fig. 2)**.

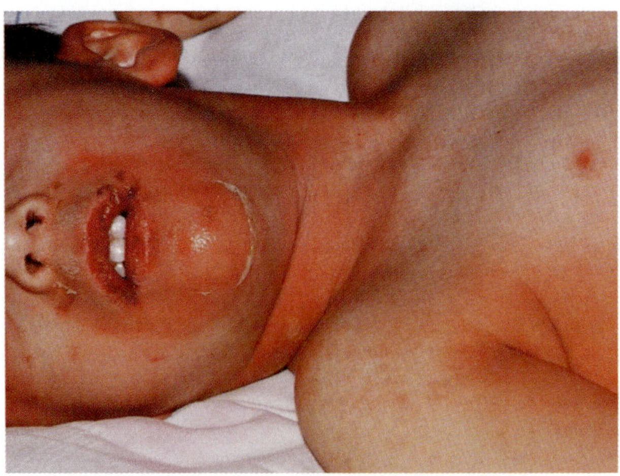

Fig. 2: Staphylococcal scalded skin syndrome.

- *Erysipelas:* A sharply demarcated erythematous rash with discrete narrowing extensions is visible on the lower leg of this patient. Location and appearance of the lesion are typical of a bacterial infection with group A *Streptococcus* affecting the upper dermis and lymphatic vessels **(Fig. 3)**.

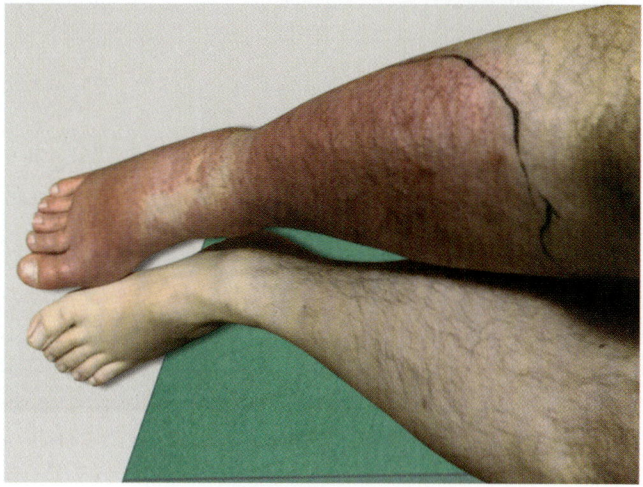

Fig. 3: Erysipelas.

- *Cellulitis in superinfected scabies:* Diffuse, poorly demarcated erythema and edema associated with small, crusted red patches are visible over the left leg. These findings are consistent with cellulitis due to scabies infection **(Fig. 4)**.

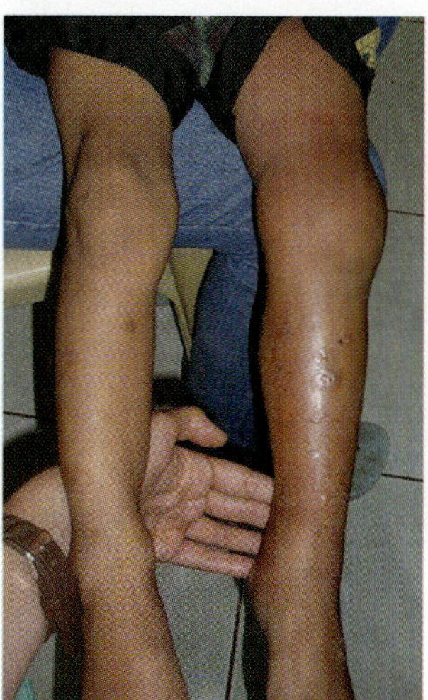

Fig. 4: Cellulitis in superinfected scabies.

- *Skin abscess:* There is marked erythema and swelling with pus and a large comedone **(Fig. 5)**.

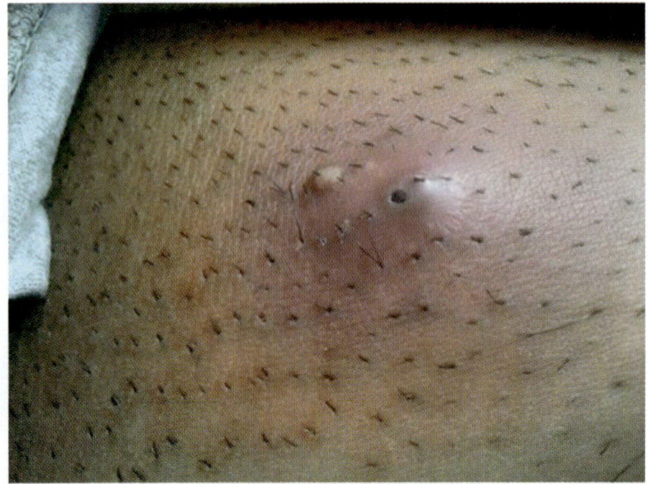

Fig. 5: Skin abscess.

- *Folliculitis:* A solitary pustule with surrounding erythema is visible in the center of the image. In many cases of folliculitis, a single hair can be seen in the middle of the lesion **(Fig. 6)**.

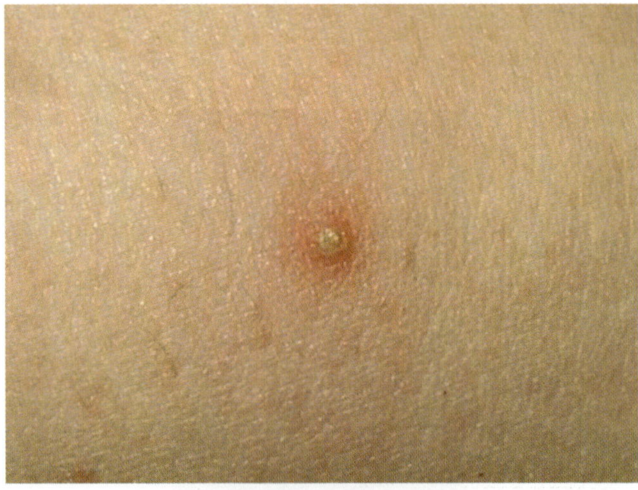

Fig. 6: Folliculitis.

- *Necrotizing fasciitis:* Posterolateral aspect of the left thigh, gluteal region, and popliteal fossa. There is significant diffuse edema and erythema across the entire visible region, with well-defined areas of necrosis, desquamation, and hemorrhagic bullae **(Fig. 7)**.

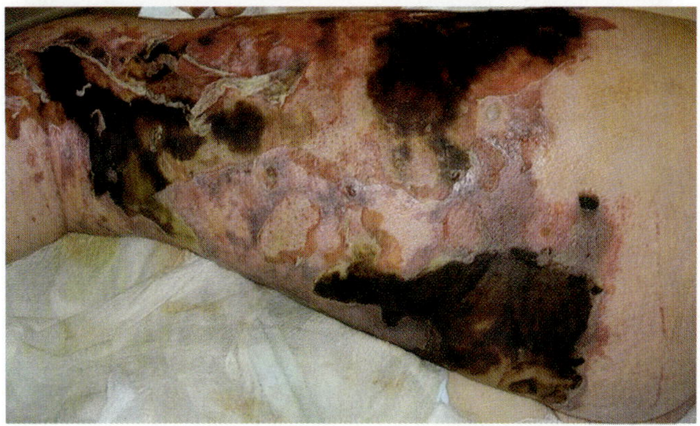

Fig. 7: Necrotizing fasciitis.

- *Orbital cellulitis:* The left upper and lower eyelids are red and severely swollen, resulting in the patient not being able to open the eye. Orbital cellulitis is an emergency requiring immediate treatment **(Fig. 8)**.

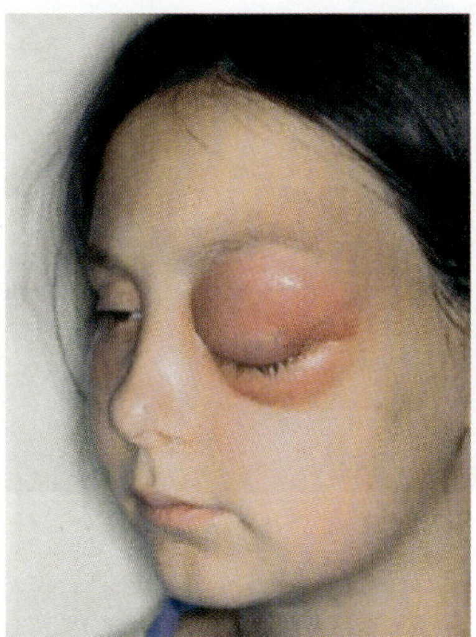

Fig. 8: Orbital cellulitis.

- *Furuncle:* Thigh of a male patient. A solitary purulent lesion surrounded by erythematous and edematous skin is visible **(Fig. 9)**.

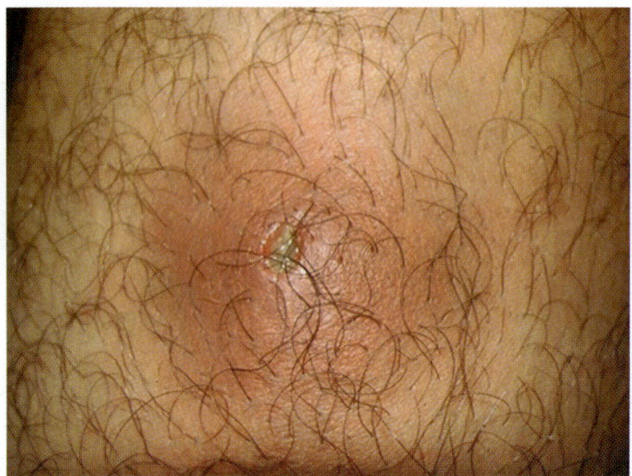

Fig. 9: Furuncle.

- *Carbuncle:* A large, inflammatory, subcutaneous mass can be seen over the right gluteal region **(Fig. 10)**.

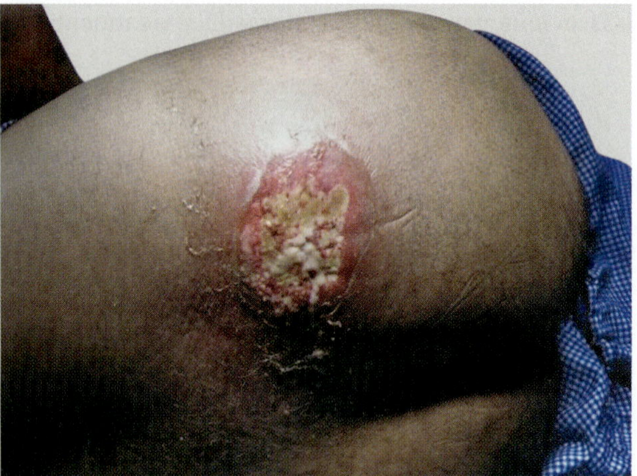

Fig. 10: Carbuncle.

SUGGESTED READING

1. Brook I, Frazier EH. Clinical and microbiological features of necrotizing fasciitis. J Clin Microbiol. 1995;33(9):2382-7.
2. Chitalia VC, Kothari J, Wells EJ, Livesey JH, Robson RA, Searle M, et al. Cost-benefit analysis and prediction of 24-hour proteinuria from the spot urine protein-creatinine ratio. Clin Nephrol. 2001;55(6):436-47.

3. Daum RS, Miller LG, Immergluck L, Fritz S, Creech CB, Young D, et al. A Placebo-Controlled Trial of Antibiotics for Smaller Skin Abscesses. N Engl J Med. 2017;376(26):2545-55.
4. Duane TM, Huston JM, Collom M, Beyer A, Parli S, Buckman S, et al. Surgical Infection Society 2020 Updated Guidelines on the Management of Complicated Skin and Soft Tissue Infections. Surg Infect (Larchmt). 2021;22(4):383-99.
5. Expert Panel on Musculoskeletal Imaging; Beaman FD, von Herrmann PF, Kransdorf MJ, Adler RS, Amini B, Appel M, et al. ACR Appropriateness Criteria® Suspected Osteomyelitis, Septic Arthritis, or Soft Tissue Infection (Excluding Spine and Diabetic Foot). J Am Coll Radiol. 2017;14(5S):S326-37.
6. Fitch MT, Manthey DE, McGinnis HD, Nicks BA, Pariyadath M. Abscess Incision and Drainage. N Engl J Med. 2007;357(19):e20.
7. Gottlieb M, DeMott JM, Hallock M, Peksa GD. Systemic Antibiotics for the Treatment of Skin and Soft Tissue Abscesses: A Systematic Review and Meta-Analysis. Ann Emerg Med. 2019;73(1):8-16.
8. Jameson JL, Fauci AS, Kasper DL, Hauser SL, Longo DL, Loscalzo J. Harrison's Principles of Internal Medicine, 20th edition. New York: McGraw Hill Education; 2018.
9. Ki V, Rotstein C. Bacterial skin and soft tissue infections in adults: A review of their epidemiology, pathogenesis, diagnosis, treatment and site of care. Can J Infect Dis Med Microbiol. 2008;19(2):173-84.
10. Klevens RM, Morrison MA, Nadle J, Petit S, Gershman K, Ray S, et al. Invasive methicillin-resistant *Staphylococcus aureus* infections in the United States. JAMA. 2007;298(15):1763-71.
11. Liu C, Bayer A, Cosgrove SE, Daum RS, Fridkin SK, Gorwitz RJ, et al. Clinical Practice Guidelines by the Infectious Diseases Society of America for the Treatment of Methicillin-Resistant *Staphylococcus aureus* Infections in Adults and Children. Clin Infect Dis. 2011;52(3):e18-55.
12. Mermel LA, Allon M, Bouza E, Craven DE, Flynn P, O'Grady NP, et al. Clinical practice guidelines for the diagnosis and management of intravascular catheter-related infection: 2009 Update by the Infectious Diseases Society of America. Clin Infect Dis. 2009;49(1):1-45.
13. Miller LG, Quan C, Shay A, Mostafaie K, Bharadwa K, Tan N, et al. A Prospective Investigation of Outcomes after Hospital Discharge for Endemic, Community-Acquired Methicillin-Resistant and Susceptible *Staphylococcus aureus* Skin Infection. Clin Infect Dis. 2007;44(4):483-92.
14. Raff AB, Kroshinsky D. Cellulitis. JAMA. 2016;316(3):3-25.
15. Ramakrishnan K, Salinas RC, Agudelo Higuita NI. Skin and Soft Tissue Infections. Am Fam Physician. 2015;92(6):474-83.
16. Sartelli M, Guirao X, Hardcastle TC, Kluger Y, Boermeester MA, Raşa K, et al. 2018 WSES/SISE consensus conference: recommendations for the management of skin and soft tissue infections. World J Emerg Surg. 2018;13:58.
17. Saseedharan S, Dubey D, Singh RK, Zirpe K, Choudhuri AH, Mukherjee DN, et al. Treatment challenges in the management of difficult-to-treat gram-positive infections: A consensus view apropos therapeutic role of novel anti-MRSA antibiotics, levonadifloxacin (IV) and alalevonadifloxacin (oral). Indian J Med Microbiol. 2024;47:100528.

18. Stevens DL, Bisno AL, Chambers HF, Dellinger EP, Goldstein EJ, Gorbach SL, et al. Practice guidelines for the diagnosis and management of skin and soft tissue infections: 2014 update by the Infectious Diseases Society of America. Clin Infect Dis. 2014;59(2):e10-52.
19. Summanen PH, Talan DA, Strong C, McTeague M, Bennion R, Thompson JE Jr, et al. Bacteriology of skin and soft-tissue infections: comparison of infections in intravenous drug users and individuals with no history of intravenous drug use. Clin Infect Dis. 1995;20 (Suppl 2):S279-82.
20. Talan DA, Moran GJ, Krishnadasan A, Abrahamian FM, Lovecchio F, Karras DJ, et al. Subgroup Analysis of Antibiotic Treatment for Skin Abscesses. Ann Emerg Med. 2018;71(1):21-30.
21. Walls R, Hockberger R, GauscheHill M. Rosen's Emergency Medicine. Amsterdam, Netherlands: Elsevier Health Sciences; 2018.

7.6 SEXUALLY TRANSMITTED DISEASES IN THE EMERGENCY ROOM

JK Maniar, Resham Vasani

KEY POINTS

- Sexually transmitted infections (STIs) are common, most patients with STIs are evaluated and treated in primary care settings; however, many also present to the emergency rooms (ERs) for initial care.
- Management of STIs in the ER includes appropriate testing and treatment as per standard guidelines for Disease Control and Prevention Sexually Transmitted Diseases Treatment.
- ERs are often the only point of healthcare access for many individuals at risk for STIs, ER visit for STI exposure or STI-related complaints are very common.
- Failure to test for syphilis and human immunodeficiency virus (HIV) in the ER is a missed opportunity that can contribute to delay in diagnosis, treatment and/or image to medical care and has public health implications.

BOX 1: Approach to a patient with Sexually transmitted disease (STD).

- Complete in-depth history—should be conducted in privacy and with assistance of a chaperone
- Sexual history taking skills present at www.cdc.gov/std/treatment/sexualhistory.pdf
- Focus on 5 "Ps" of sexual health—partners, practices, protection from STDs, past history of STDs, and prevention of pregnancy
- Examination—review of vital signs—tachycardia, hypotension, and fever should suggest possible pelvic inflammatory disease (PID)/sepsis

Categorize:

- Genital ulcerative disease (GUD)
- Genital discharge
- Genital area lumps and bumps

BOX 2: Clinical diagnosis of genital ulceration.

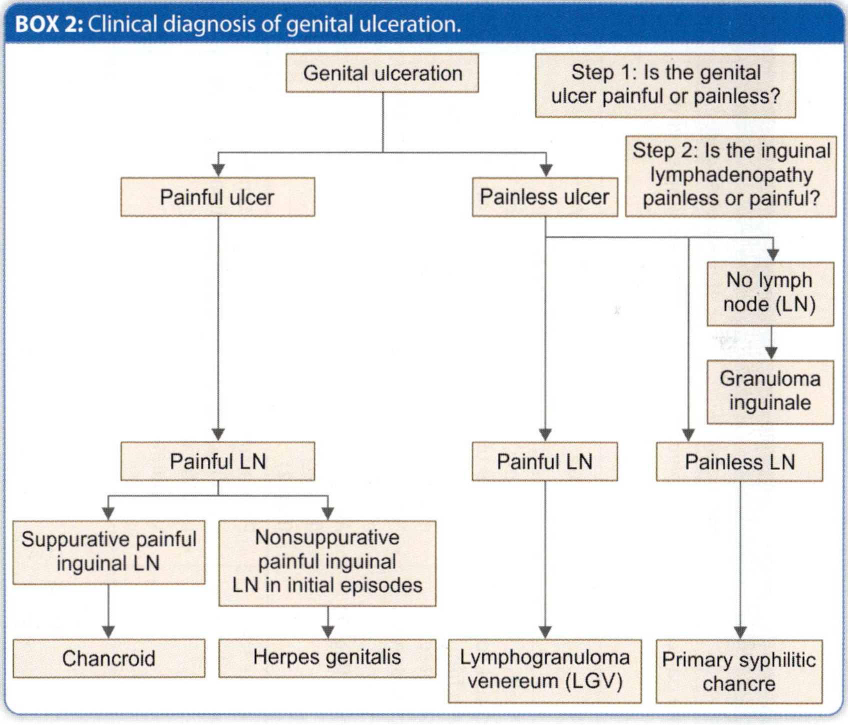

BOX 3: Clinical characteristics of genital ulceration with investigations and treatment.

Features	***Chancre***	***Chancroid***	***Herpes genitalis***	***LGV***	***Donovanosis***
Causative organism	Treponema pallidum	*Haemophilus ducreyi*	Herpes simplex virus (HSV) 2 >1	*Chlamydia trachomatis* serovars L1, L2, and L3	*Klebsiella granulomatis/ Calymmatobacterium granulomatis*
Incubation period	9–90 days	3–10 days	2–20 days	10–30 days	8–80 days
Ulcer features	• Single, well demarcated, round ulcer with firm indurated base • Cartilaginous feel, button like • Nontender **(Fig. 1)**	• Multiple, soft, painful tender ulcers with ragged undermined edges • Nonindurated base, bleed easily • Autoinoculation (kissing ulcers) **(Fig. 2)**	• Grouped vesicles which on rupturing produce grouped erosions • Recurrent **(Fig. 3)**	Transient ulcers not noticed by the patient	• Beefy red hypertrophic granulation tissue on ulcer floor • Bleeds easily • Painless **(Fig. 4)**
Inguinal area	Bilateral, nontender, shotty nonsuppurative LN	• Painful and tender lymph nodes (bubo) • Unilateral, often suppurates **(Fig. 5)**	Bilateral tender in initial primary episode	• Painful and tender lymph nodes (bubo+) • Sign of groove+ **(Fig. 6)**	Granulomatous nodules in the inguinal area forming pseudobuboes not true lymphadenopathy

Contd...

Contd...

Features	***Chancre***	***Chancroid***	***Herpes genitalis***	***LGV***	***Donovanosis***
Diagnosis	• DGI on smear from ulcer/lymph node aspirate • Direct fluorescent antibody test • If DGI cannot be done then serology • Sensitivity • EIA > TPPA = FTA-Abs	• Gram stain on smear from ulcer—school of fish or rail road track appearance • PCR if facilities available	Tzanck smear–multinucleate giant cells	• Nucleic acid amplification test (NAAT)—test of choice • Complement fixation test–MC done • Micro-immunofluorescence testing	Crush smear of fresh biopsy material stained with Wright or Giemsa stain shows parasitized histiocytes containing Donovan bodies (showing closed safety pin appearance: prominent staining at poles) **(Fig. 7)**
Treatment	• Injection benzathine penicillin 2.4 million units intramuscularly • Single dose after test dose (ATD)	Tablet azithromycin 1 g single dose or injection cefuroxime 250 mg IM stat or tablet ciprofloxacin 500 mg twice daily for 3 days or tablet erythromycin 500 mg TDS for 7 days	Tablet acyclovir 400 mg TDS for 7 days for a primary episode and 5 days for secondary episodes	• Doxycycline 100 mg BD for 21 days • For inguinal buboes–needle aspiration or incision and drainage	Azithromycin 1 g orally once per week or 500 mg daily for at least 3 weeks and until all lesions have completely healed

(DGI: dark ground illumination; EIA: enzyme immunoassay; FTA-Abs: fluorescent treponemal antibody-absorption; IM: intramuscular; MC: most common; PCR: polymerase chain reaction; TPPA: treponema pallidum particle agglutination)

BOX 4: Causes of genital discharge.

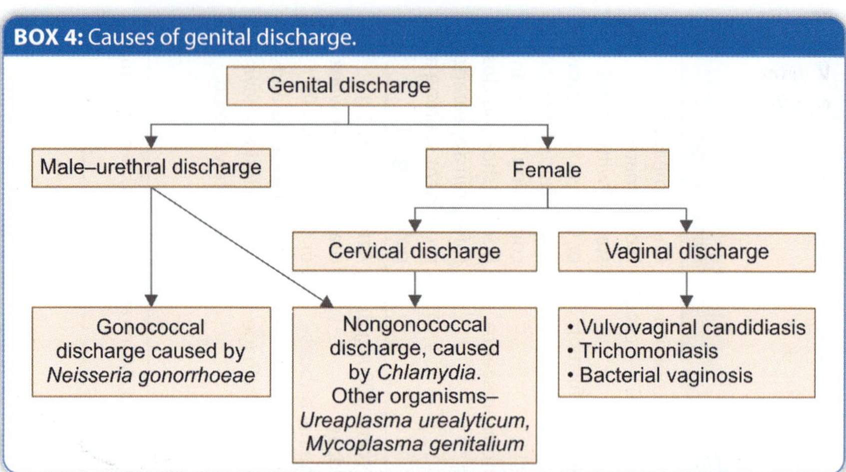

BOX 5: Clinical characteristics of urethral or cervical discharge with diagnosis and treatment.

Gonococcal discharge	***Nongonococcal discharge***
Incubation period: 2–8 days	Incubation period: 1–3 weeks
Clinical features: • In males—thick, profuse, purulent urethral discharge. Others have prostatitis, epididymo-orchitis • In females—primary infection is in the endocervix, often asymptomatic but can cause cervical discharge, salpingitis, PID	*Clinical features:* • Watery or thin mucopurulent discharge • Can also cause epididymitis, PID
Diagnosis: • Gram stain microscopy for gram negative diplococci • Culture–gold standard • NAAT on urine, urethral discharge, cervix, vagina	*Diagnosis:* NAAT on urethral swab or first void urine
Treatment: • Ceftriaxone 250 mg IM a single dose or cefixime 400 mg • Single dose plus azithromycin 1 g as a single dose	*Treatment:* • Tablet azithromycin 1 g stat dose or • Capsule doxycycline 100 mg BD for 7 days

BOX 6: Clinical features, diagnosis and treatment of vaginal discharge.

Vulvovaginal candidiasis	***Trichomoniasis***	***Bacterial vaginosis***
Caused by *Candida albicans*	Caused by *Trichomonas vaginalis*	Caused by overgrowth of commensals like *Gardnerella vaginalis, mycoplasma hominis,* anaerobic bacteria, and *Ureaplasma*
Thick, curdy white, minimal vaginal discharge	Yellow green copious discharge	Homogenous thin vaginal discharge
Vulval itching, swelling, and redness	Itching, dysuria, strawberry cervix	Fishy odor, no inflammation, no itching
Wet mount/Gram stain–shows budding yeasts, hyphae, pseudohyphae	Wet mount, culture, NAAT, pH elevated >4.5	• Clinical criteria–Amsel criteria • Homogenous thin white discharge • Clue cells • Whiff test positive • Vaginal pH >4.5
Treatment: Topical azole creams or suppository Oral–tablet fluconazole 150 mg stat	Tablet metronidazole 2 g or tablet tinidazole 2 g stat or tablet secnidazole 2 g stat	Drug of choice–tablet metronidazole 500 mg BD for 7 days Or Tablet tinidazole 2 g OD for 1–2 days Or Tablet secnidazole 2 g stat Or Capsule clindamycin 300 mg BD for 7 days Or Metronidazole gel 0.75% intravaginally once a day for 5 days Or Clindamycin cream 2% intravaginally at bedtime for 7 days

BOX 7: Approach to STD-induced genital lumps and bumps.

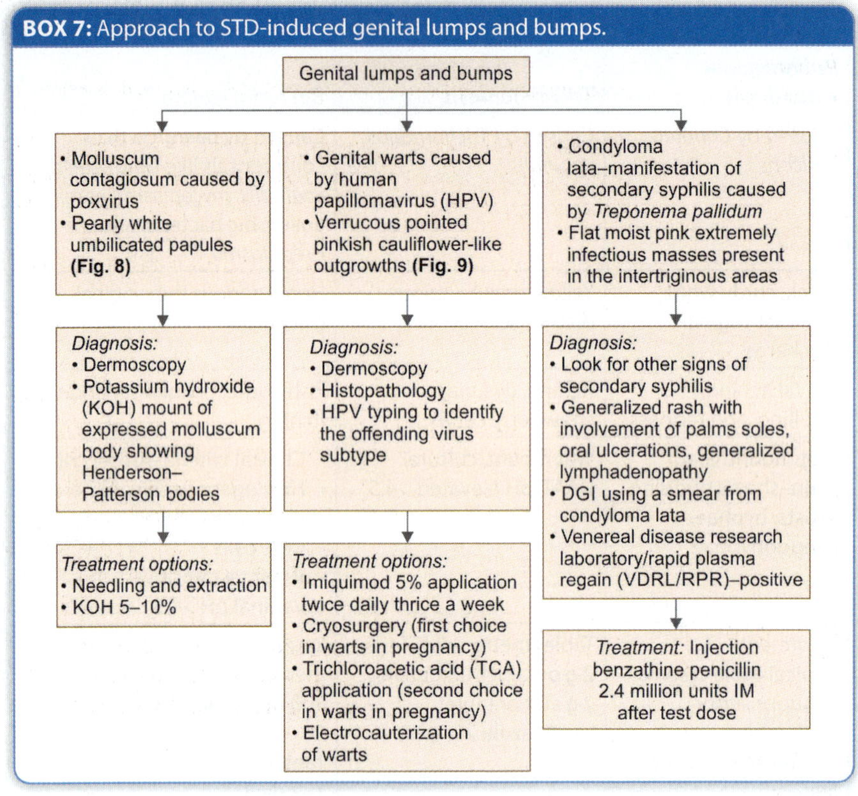

BOX 8: Complications of sexually transmitted conditions that can present to the emergency room (ER).

- Primary episode of herpes genitalis in female—can present as acute urinary retention on account of severe burning and pain
- As a complication of chancroid, especially in patients co infected with HIV, there can be superinfection by anaerobes such as *Fusobacterium* or *Bacteroides*—called as Phagedenic chancroid—causes extensive destruction of genitalia **(Fig. 10)**
- Lues maligna–severe form of secondary syphilis with ulceronodular appearance unlike the classic mucocutaneous eruption of secondary syphilis
- Prepuce when retracted in genital warts or STD ulcers on the coronal sulcus/glans in uncircumcised males can cause paraphimosis leading to strangulation of glans as well painful vascular compromise. Manual reduction of paraphimosis may be attempted in such cases
- In chancroid/LGV, the bubo (inguinal lymph node swelling) can present as an intensely painful abscess that may need drainage via a wide bore needle
- Jarisch Herxheimer reaction—it is a transient clinical phenomenon that occurs in patients with syphilis (especially when the load of spirochetes is higher like in secondary syphilis) who undergo treatment with penicillin. It manifests with fever, chills, rigors, nausea, vomiting, headache, tachycardia, hyperventilation, flushing, myalgia, and exacerbation of skin lesions. Mild reactions may recover spontaneously within 24 hours and symptomatic treatment is necessary. In pregnant patients, those with neurosyphilis and those having severe symptoms a short course of steroids can be considered

BOX 9: Management of special populations.

Pediatrics:

- The presence of STI in a pediatric patient should always raise concern of sexual abuse
- Transmission from mother to child of gonorrhea, chlamydia trachomatis, trichomonas, HPV, and HSV are all possible in the neonate and can present as nongenital infections such as conjunctivitis, pneumonia and in case of HSV–encephalitis
- Sexually active adolescents are at high risk of STIs due to biological, cognitive and behavioral factors

Pregnant women:

- Complications of STIs in pregnancy include, preterm labor, premature rupture of membranes, low birth weight, still birth and congenital infections in newborn
- Approach to diagnosis and treatment is essentially unchanged from non-pregnant patients except to avoid tetracyclines in pregnancy
- New lesions suspicious of HSV should be addressed and started on acyclovir or valacyclovir with close follow up especially if late into the third trimester.
- Pregnant patients with syphilis need treatment and close follow up. Those with penicillin allergy should undergo desensitization therapy

Men having sex with men and transgender:

- Sexual history should be direct, inclusive and respectful
- Testing at all sites of sexual contact is very important and hence in addition to the urine/urethral testing, extragenital testing pharyngeal and rectal sites are important

Sexual assault victims:

The Centers for Disease Control and Prevention (CDC) STD treatment guidelines recommend following for treatment and prophylaxis:

- Since there is a low rate of follow-up–single dose empiric treatment is recommended
- Emergency contraception
- Postexposure hepatitis B vaccination if assailant is not known or victim is unvaccinated
- Female victims 9–26 years and male victims 9–21 years [men who have sex with men (MSM) up to 26 years] should receive HPV vaccination

Consider postexposure prophylaxis:

- If patient presents within 72 hours of assault
- If the assailant/s has high risk behavior for HIV (MSM/IV drug abuse)
- Local epidemiology for HIV/acquired immunodeficiency syndrome (AIDS)
- Exposure characteristics for assault:
  - Vaginal or anal penetration
  - Ejaculation on mucus membranes
  - Multiple assailants
  - Presence of mucosal lesions
  - Any other characteristics that increase risk of HIV transmission

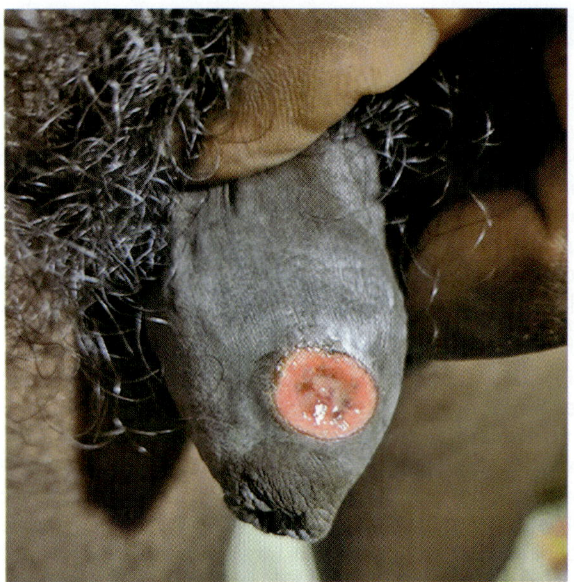

Fig. 1: Solitary well-defined, clean looking ulceration on penis—primary chancre of syphilis.

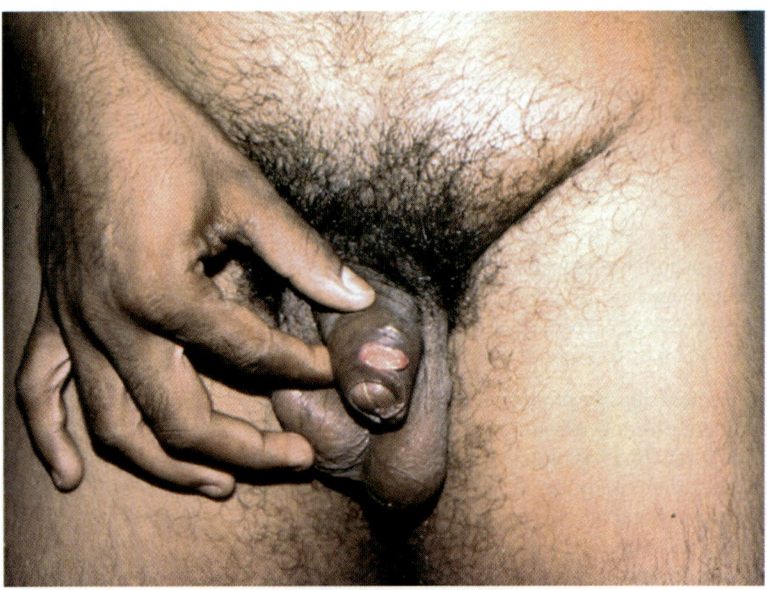

Fig. 2: Dirty looking ulceration with slough—chancroid.

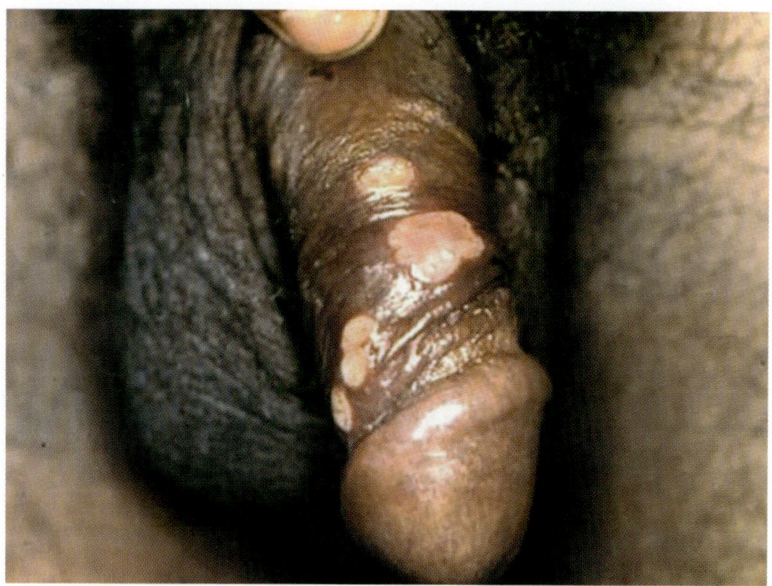

Fig. 3: Polycyclic-shaped erosions on the inner aspect of the prepuce—herpes genitalis.

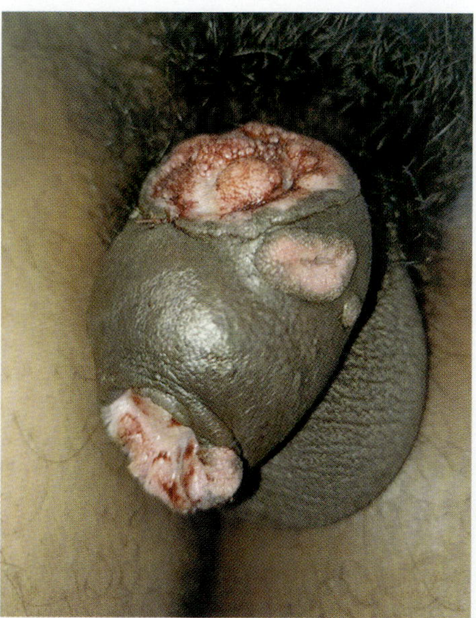

Fig. 4: Ulceration on the penile shaft and outer preputial skin with red beefy granulation tissue that bleeds on touch.

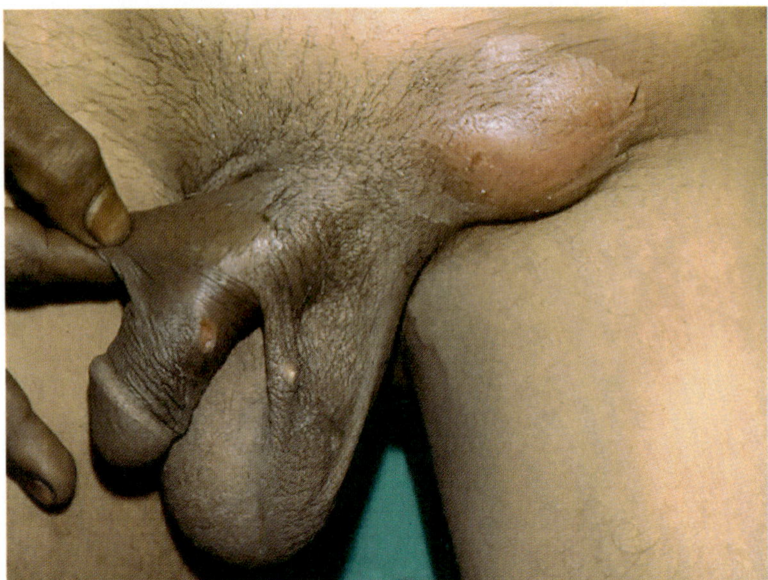

Fig. 5: Autoinoculation of chancroid ulcer on the scrotum with associated tender unilateral lymphadenopathy.

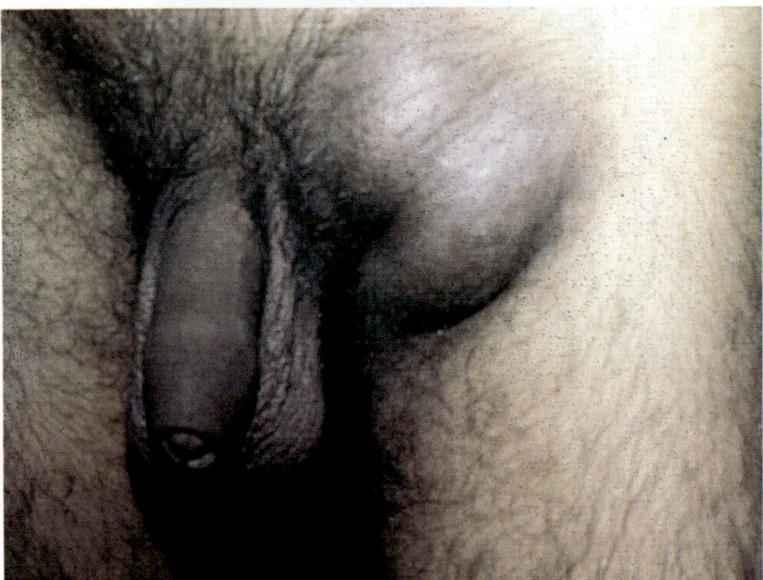

Fig. 6: Inguinal swelling separated from each other by the inguinal ligament forming a groove—groove sign of Greenblatt–seen in the inguinal stage of lymphogranuloma venereum.

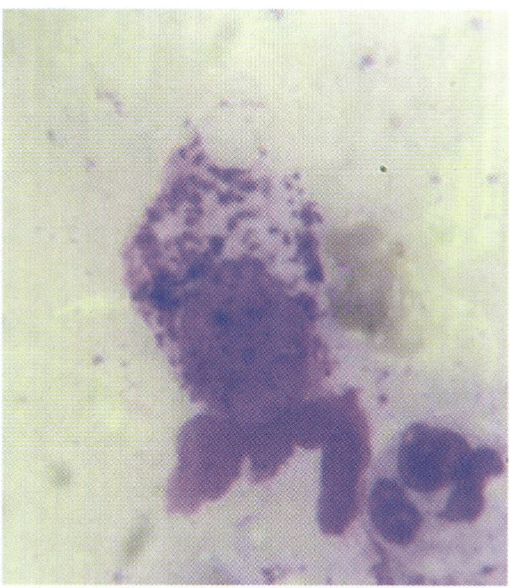

Fig. 7: Crush smear of donovanosis showing Donovan bodies which demonstrate bipolar staining called as closed safety pin appearance.

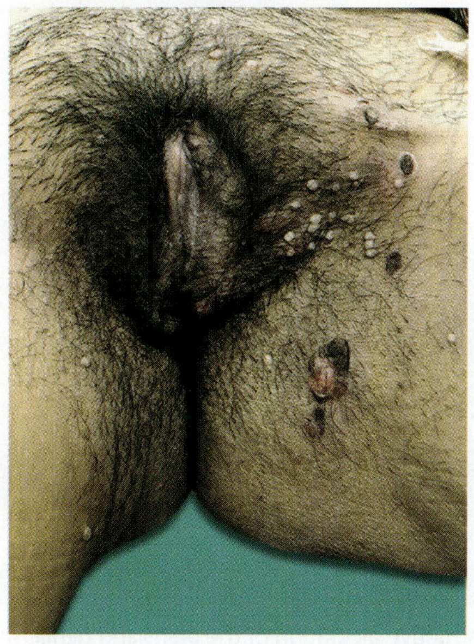

Fig. 8: Pearly white umbilicated papules on the right labia majora and perineal area—molluscum contagiosum.

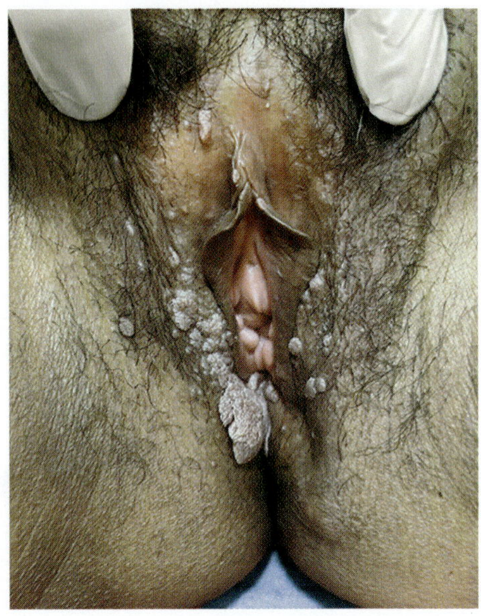

Fig. 9: Verrucous pointed pink outgrowths on the inner aspects of the labia majora and clitoris—condyloma accuminata.

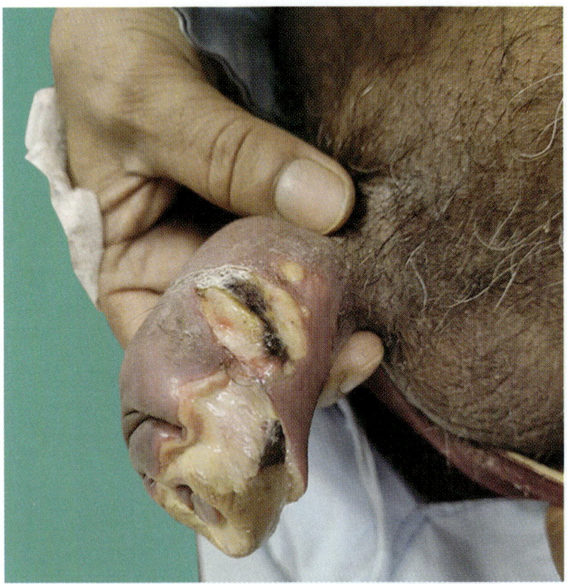

Fig. 10: Large destructive ulceration of the glans and penile shaft suggestive of phagedenic chancroid.

SUGGESTED READING

1. Hilbert SM, Reno HEL. Management of Patients with Sexually Transmitted Infections in the Emergency Department. Emerg Med Clin North Am. 2018;36(4):767-76.
2. Pfennig CL. Sexually Transmitted Diseases in the Emergency Department. Emerg Med Clin North Am. 2019;37(2):165-92.

7.7 CENTRAL NERVOUS SYSTEM AND SPINAL INFECTION IN THE EMERGENCY ROOM

Ayesha J Sunavala

BOX 1: Introduction.

- Central nervous system (CNS) infections including meningitis, encephalitis, and brain abscess, are relatively uncommon but time-sensitive emergency room diagnoses
- A minority of patients will present with the classic triad of fever, neck stiffness, and altered mental status. Most patients present with a host of non-specific signs and symptoms based on various factors such as age, duration of illness, immune status, exposure and prior receipt of antibiotics in the community
- The diagnosis and treatment of CNS infections requires vigilance and a high index of suspicion based on the history and physical examination corroborated with appropriate imaging and laboratory evaluation
- An initial dose of appropriate empirical antimicrobials based on clinical suspicion in the emergency room is justified as a delay in treatment negatively impacts outcomes especially in acute bacterial meningitis and herpes simplex viral encephalitis

BOX 2: CNS infections commonly encountered in the emergency medical service (EMS).

Type of infection	*Etiology*	*Characteristic features*
Acute bacterial meningitis/ meningoencephalitis	*Community acquired:* *Streptococcus pneumoniae*, *Neisseria meningitidis*, *Listeria monocytogenes* *Haemophilus influenzae*, *Streptococcus agalactiae* *Healthcare acquired:* *Staphylococcus aureus*, Coagulase-negative, *Staphylococcus*, Gram-negative bacilli, *Candida spp.*	• Classical triad—fever, neck rigidity, change in mental status • Meningismus • *Streptococcus pneumoniae*—cerebral infarcts • *L. monocytogenes*—early seizures, focal neurological deficit (FND), ataxia, nystagmus • *N. meningitidis*—petechial-purpural rash

Contd...

Type of infection	***Etiology***	***Characteristic features***
Acute viral meningitis	• Enteroviruses (coxsackie, echovirus), varicella zoster virus (VZV), herpes simplex virus (HSV) 2, Epstein–Barr virus (EBV), arthropod-borne viruses*, human immunodeficiency virus (HIV) • Less common-HSV 1, human herpesvirus (HHV) 6, CMV, mumps	• Headache, fever, mild nuchal rigidity • Viral prodrome-malaise, myalgia, nausea, abdominal pain, diarrhea
Acute viral encephalitis	• HSV 1 (most common) • Cytomegalovirus (CMV), HSV 2, HHV 6, VZV, EBV, arthropod borne viruses*, rabies, enteroviruses, tick borne encephalitis, rickettsiosis	Profound alteration in consciousness-stupor, coma, marked confusion, seizures, FND
Subacute-chronic meningitis	• Tubercular meningitis, cryptococcal meningitis, histoplasmosis, neurobrucellosis, Lyme's disease, syphilis • Partially treated bacterial meningitis	Days-weeks: unrelenting headache, stiff neck, low-grade fever, lethargy
Brain abscess	*Immunocompetent host: Streptococcal spp.* aerobic, anaerobic and viridans group, enterobacteriaceae, anaerobes (*Bacteroides spp, Fusobacterium spp.), S. aureus,* tuberculoma, neurocysticercosis *Immunocompromised host: Nocardia spp., Toxoplasma gondii, Candida spp.,* cryptococcomas, mold infections (*Aspergillus spp, Mucor spp.)*	Progressive headache, focal/generalized seizure, focal neurological deficit ± fever

*Arthropod-borne viruses include chikungunya, dengue, Japanese encephalitis, West Nile virus, Zika virus

Flowchart 1: Algorithmic approach to evaluation of a suspected CNS infection in the EMS.

Headache ± fever ± neck stiffness

↓

Altered mental status/new-onset seizures/focal neurological deficit

- Yes → Meningoencephalitis/encephalitis/encephalopathy/ADEM/mass lesion/abscess
  - → Obtain blood cultures and start empirical antimicrobials
  - → CNS imaging-CT or MRI (preferred)
    - → Mass lesion (tumor/abscess) → Appropriate surgical/medical
    - → No mass lesion → Obtain blood cultures and immediate lumbar puncture*
- → Meningitis
  - → Papilledema present, immunocompromised, recent head trauma, known malignancy/CNS neoplasm/sinusitis, platelet count <20,000/mm^3
    - Yes → CNS imaging-CT or MRI (preferred)
    - No → Obtain blood cultures and immediate lumbar puncture*
      - → CSF: Pleocytosis with polymorphonuclear leukocytes (PMNs), elevated protein, decreased glucose → Bacterial process
      - → Cerebrospinal fluid (CSF): Pleocytosis with mononuclear cells (MNCs), normal/elevated protein, normal/decreased glucose → Mycobacterial/viral/fungal/partially treated bacterial process

Note: If lumbar puncture is not immediately feasible/delayed, collect blood cultures and start first dose of appropriate empirical antimicrobials in EMS.

BOX 3: CSF analysis and interpretation.

	Normal	***Bacterial***	***Viral***	***Fungal***	***Tubercular***
Appearance	Clear	Cloudy and turbid	Clear	Fibrin web	Cloudy and viscous
White blood cells (WBCs) (/μL)	<5	100–50,000	5–100	0–1,000	<500
Predominant WBC	Mainly lymphocytes, 5% neutrophils	Neutrophils	Lymphocytes	Lymphocytes	Lymphocytes
Red blood cells (RBCs) (/μL)	Normal <10				
Proteins (mg/dL)	<40	>100	40–100	20–500	100–500 or higher
Glucose (CSF: blood ratio)	>0.5	Low (<0.5)	Normal*	Low (<0.5)	Low (<0.5)
Opening CSF pressure (cmH_2O)	<20	High	Normal-slightly elevated	High-very high	High

*CSF glucose may be low in viral infections such as mumps and lymphocytic choriomeningitis virus (LCMV)

In addition to the above routine CSF analysis, the fluid should be collected for Gram stain and culture. HSV deoxyribonucleic acid (DNA) polymerase chain reaction (PCR), multiplex PCR panels, Adenosine deaminase (ADA), GeneXpert MTB/RIF Ultra and TB MGIT C/S, CSF cryptococcal antigen etc. may be carried out depending on host factors and the level of concern for atypical or opportunistic etiologies of meningitis/meningoencephalitis.

BOX 4: Empirical antimicrobial treatment for suspected acute bacterial CNS infection.

Host factor (risk)	***Suspected pathogen(s)***	***Recommended antibiotic(s)***
Age <1 month	*S. agalactiae, E. coli, Listeria monocytogenes*	Ampicillin + cefotaxime/aminoglycoside
1 month to 2 years	*S. pneumoniae, S agalactiae, N. meningitidis, H. influenzae, E. coli*	Vancomycin + ceftriaxone/cefotaxime
2–55 years	*S. pneumoniae, N. meningitidis*	Vancomycin + ceftriaxone/cefotaxime
>55 years	*S. pneumoniae, N. meningitidis, L. monocytogenes*, aerobic gram-negative bacilli	Vancomycin + ceftriaxone/cefotaxime + ampicillin
Adult of any age (head trauma/post neurosurgery/debilitating illness/immunocompromised/alcohol abuse)	*Staphylococcus aureus*, coagulase-negative staph, aerobic gram-negative bacilli (including *Pseudomonas aeruginosa*), *H. influenzae*, group A beta-hemolytic streptococci, *L. monocytogenes*	Vancomycin + ceftazidime/cefepime/meropenem ± ampicillin

Note: Adjunctive dexamethasone 0.15 mg/kg q6h should be given shortly before or at the same time as the first dose of antibiotics, in adults with suspected community-acquired meningitis. Dexamethasone should be continued for 2–4 days if the CSF Gram stain and/or the CSF or blood cultures reveal *S. pneumoniae.*

BOX 5: Viral infections of the CNS.

- Some viral agents typically cause aseptic meningitis, whereas others are more likely to cause encephalitis
- Encephalitis involves the parenchyma of the brain and is characterized by abnormalities in brain function such as an altered mental status, behavior or personality changes, motor or sensory deficits, and speech or movement disorders
- Patients with meningitis may be lethargic, irritable or distracted by headache, but their cerebral function remains normal. Seizures may be seen with meningitis alone.
- Differentiating between the two entities may often be challenging as some patients have overlapping features of a parenchymal and meningeal process termed as meningoencephalitis

BOX 6: Initial treatment of agents causing encephalitis.

	Etiology	*Agent of choice*
1.	**Viral**	
	HSV 1*, VZV	Acyclovir
	CMV, HHV 6	Ganciclovir ± foscarnet
	Influenza	Oseltamivir
	Acute HIV	ART
	Measles, Nipah virus, Crimean–Congo hemorrhagic fever (CCHF)	Ribavirin
	Japanese B encephalitis, EBV, dengue	Supportive treatment
2.	**Bacterial**	
	Listeria	Ampicillin + gentamicin; trimethoprim/sulfamethoxazole (TMP/SMX)
	Mycoplasma	Macrolide or tetracycline or FQN
3.	**Tubercular**	AKT + steroids**
4.	**Fungal**	
	Cryptococcus	Liposomal amphotericin B plus 5 FC
	Histoplasmosis	Liposomal amphotericin B
5.	**Rickettsial**	
	Spotted fever/scrub typhus	Doxycycline
6.	**Protozoa**	
	Plasmodium falciparum	Initial IV artesunate followed by artemisinin-based combination therapy (ACT) to complete treatment course
	Toxoplasma gondii	Pyrimethamine + sulfadiazine/clindamycin

*In a patient with community-acquired acute encephalitis syndrome, empiric treatment for HSV 1 infection should always be initiated as soon as possible as early therapy is vital in decreasing mortality and morbidity. It may be discontinued if an alternative cause is identified and CSF HSV PCR is negative.

**For tuberculosis (TB) meningitis, adjunctive dexamethasone is recommended at 0.4 mg/kg/d IV for 2 weeks followed by gradual taper @ 0.1 mg/kg/week.

BOX 7: Appropriate doses of antimicrobials for adults with CNS infections.	
Amikacin*	5 mg/kg q8h (dose based on ideal body weight, ideally dosage and intervals to be individualized based on peak and trough concentrations)
Ampicillin*	2 g q4h (12 g/day)
Ceftazidime*	2 g q6–8h
Ceftriaxone	2 g q12h
Meropenem*	2 g q8h
Vancomycin*	Loading dose (20–35 mg/kg) not exceeding 3 g, followed by 15–20 mg/kg every 8–12 hours. Dose and interval adjustments are based on area under the curve (AUC)-guided or trough-guided serum concentration monitoring.
Acyclovir*	10 mg/kg/q8h
*Renal dose adjustment required.	

SUGGESTED READING

1. Archibald LK, Quisling RG. Central nervous system infections. In: Layon AJ, Gabrielli A, Friedman WA (Eds). Textbook of Neurointensive Care. Berlin, Germany: Springer Nature; 2013. pp. 427-517.
2. Dorsett M, Liang SY. Diagnosis and treatment of central nervous system infections in the emergency department. Emerg Med Clin North Am. 2016;34(4):917-42.
3. Roos KL, Tyler KL. Meningitis, encephalitis, brain abscess and empyema. In: Jameson JL, Fauci A, Kasper D, Hauser S, Longo D, Loscalzo J (Eds). Harrison's Principles and Practice of Internal Medicine, 19th edition. New York: McGraw Hill Education; 2017.

7.8 ANTIBIOTICS IN THE EMERGENCY ROOM

Jamshed D Sunavala

BOX 1: Cephalosporins.

Drug	***Dosage [intravenous (IV)]***	***Remarks***
First-generation cefazolin	• 1 g q6h IV • 2 g q8h for deep seated/bone infections*	• Drug of choice for methicillin-susceptible *Staphylococcus aureus* (MSSA) infections and preoperative surgical prophylaxis • Affected by inoculum effect in deep seated Staphylococcal infections in which case cloxacillin/flucloxacillin are preferred • Most effective for aerobic gram-positive cocci (GPC) and also effective against *Haemophilus influenzae*. No activity against methicillin-resistant *Staphylococcus aureus* (MRSA) and methicillin-resistant coagulase-negative staphylococci (MRCoNS)
Second-generation cefuroxime axetil	1.5 g q6–8h IV*	• Drug of choice for preoperative surgical prophylaxis • Effective against both GPC and to some susceptible gram-negative bacteria (GNBs) • No activity against *P. aeruginosa*
Third-generation ceftazidime	2 g q6–8h IV for central nervous system (CNS)/severe infections* 2 g q12h IV [no renal dose adjustment except in patients on hemodialysis (HD)]	• Most effective against GNB but only ceftazidime has activity against *P. aeruginosa*; however all in this group are inactivated by extended spectrum beta-lactamase (ESBL) producing organisms. Third-generation cephalosporins are effective against ESBL producers when combined with beta-lactamase inhibitors like sulbactam or avibactam • Ceftazidime has limited activity against *Staphylococcus aureus*. Ceftriaxone is a drug of choice for *Salmonella*. Good activity against *H. influenzae* • Useful in meningitis, intracranial abscesses as they penetrate inflamed meninges and achieve adequate concentrations in the CNS

Contd...

Contd...

Drug	***Dosage [intravenous (IV)]***	***Remarks***
Third-generation ceftriaxone		• Ceftazidime and ceftriaxone both may elevate international normalized ratio (INR) • Neonates <28 days do not give any Ca containing IV drugs within 48 hours of ceftriaxone • >28 days—Ca can be given after flushing the line but not simultaneously (chemically incompatible)
Fourth-generation cefepime	1–2 g q8h IV*	• Has excellent activity against *P. aeruginosa* and other susceptible GNB but practically no staphylococcal activity • Use with caution in patients with a history of seizure disorder • May elevate INR
Fifth-generation ceftaroline	600 mg q12h*	It has excellent activity against gram-positive (GP) organisms including MRSA; its activity against GNB is as good as 3rd generation cephalosporins. Its main advantage may be targeting both GNB + MRSA in empirical therapy especially for community acquired pneumonia and skin and soft tissue infections (SSTIs)
Cefoperazone + sulbactam **(Table 1)**	1.5–3 g TDS 1 g cefoperazone + 0.5 sulbactam	• Good activity against all GNB including *P. aeruginosa* • Good safety profile. Not inactivated by ESBL producing organisms
Ceftazidime + Avibactam **(Table 1)**	2.5 g TDS 1.25 g TDS or BID [renal failure (RF)] 0.94 g OD [creatinine clearance (CrCl) <15 mL]	• It is effective against GNBs and *P. aeruginosa* and is stable against most ESBLs (unlike ceftazidime used alone) and AmpC beta-lactamases but unstable in the presence of metallo-beta-lactamases • Administer over 2 hours

*Renal dose adjustment required

TABLE 1: Beta-lactam beta-lactamase inhibitors (BLBLIs).

Piperacillin tazobactam	4.5 g q6–8h IV*	• Broad-spectrum activity against ESBL producing GN organisms including *P. aeruginosa,* anaerobes, and GP organisms except MRSA and penicillin resistant enterococci • *Stenotrophomonas maltophilia* is highly resistant • There is divergent clinical evidence as to whether piperacillin-tazobactam should be used to treat bacteremia or other high inoculum infections due to ESBL producing GNOs • Carbapenems may be considered in the above setting especially if piperacillin tazobactam minimal inhibitory concentration (MICs) are >16 mg/L • Cerebrospinal fluid (CSF) penetration is poor
Cefoperazone + sulbactam	1.5–3 g q12h IV 1 g Cefoperazone + 0.5 sulbactam*	• Good activity against all GNB including susceptible strains of *P. aeruginosa* and *Acinetobacter baumannii* • Intrinsically resistant to all enterococci • Good safety profile • Not inactivated by ESBL producing organisms
Ceftazidime/ avibactam (CAZ/AVI)	2.5 g TDS*	• This combination is active against carbapenemase-producing (KPC, AmpC and OXA-48-like) GN enterobacteriaceae and *Pseudomonas*. It has no activity against NDM producers. However, combination of CAZ/AVI + aztreonam may be used for NDM producing isolates. [This drug should be used only as a *reserve* drug for patients with proven carbapenems resistance (CR) infections] • Poor activity against *Acinetobacter spp.* and anaerobes. Additional anaerobic cover advised in patients with intra-abdominal/other anaerobic infections

*Renal dose adjustment required

BOX 2: Carbapenems.

Drugs	*Dosage (IV)*
Meropenem	1–2 g q8h*
Imipenem	0.5 g q6h*
Doripenem	0.5 g q8h*
Ertapenem	1 g q24h*

Usage

- **All carbapenems require renal dose adjustment*
- Excellent broad-spectrum activity against GNBs and provides adequate cover against MSSA, MSCoNS and anaerobes including *Bacteroides fragilis*.
- They are not hydrolyzed by ESBLs.
- Not active against MRSA, MRCoNS, and penicillin-resistant enterococci.
- Except for ertapenem they have good activity against *P. aeruginosa*.
- Meropenem and imipenem are drugs of first choice for empiric use in septic shock for their broad-spectrum activity and also useful for pelvic infections because of their effective mixed aerobic–anaerobic activity.
- Imipenem is rapidly destroyed in the kidney by an enzyme hydropeptidase hence it is combined with cilastatin.
- Carbapenems rely on time-dependent killing hence pharmacokinetic-pharmacodynamic (PKPD) may be optimized by extended infusions over 3 hours [data exists supporting stability of extended and continuous infusion when admixed with normal saline (NS) at a concentration of 14.3 mg/mL at room temperature] or using a long-acting agent like ertapenem.
- Carbapenems can develop resistance to GNB following hydrolysis by carbapenemases. Combination of carbapenems with polymyxins, tigecycline, Fosfomycin, aminoglycosides may be used for CR infections if the carbapenem MIC <16 mg/L.
- They have good CNS penetration. Meropenem is the drug of choice for GN meningitis.
- Carbapenems, especially imipenem, have seizurogenic potential especially in elderly patients. They may decrease the serum concentration of divalproex sodium/valproic acid increasing the risk of breakthrough seizures. Doripenem: Not approved for ventilator-associated pneumonia (VAP), increased mortality when compared with imipenem and the clinical response rates is lower.

Note: Faropenem (penem-class oral beta-lactamase agent), has a different structure from carbapenems and should not be considered an oral carbapenem. Although active against most GP and ESBL-producing GN Enterobacteriaceae, it has a lower potential for development of resistance. It has no activity against *Pseudomonas*, *Acinetobacter*, MRSA and *Enterococcus faecium*.

BOX 3: Aminoglycosides.

Drug: Amikacin

Dose: 15 mg/kg q24h (dosing interval extended for reduced renal clearance)
- Ideal body weight and adjusted body weight formulas should be used for determining dosage in obese and morbidly obese patients, respectively
- Once daily, extended interval dosing as compared to traditional thrice daily dosing offers the potential advantages of reduced nephrotoxicity, ease of administration and serum concentration monitoring. This administration rationale is based on the pharmacodynamics properties of aminoglycosides—concentration dependent killing and postantibiotic effect
- Aminoglycoside infusion should be given over 60 minutes
- Avoid coadministration of beta-lactams in the same solution as they may inactivate the aminoglycoside (based on in vitro data)
- Therapeutic drug monitoring is not routinely recommended. Consider through monitoring in patients at higher risk of nephrotoxicity, e.g., intensive care unit (ICU), elderly, and concomitant use of nephrotoxic agents

Usage in ICU
- Most active of the aminoglycosides
- Good activity against GNB including *P. aeruginosa* and *Acinetobacter baumannii,* may show susceptibility to some carbapenem-resistant strains
- Aminoglycosides have no anaerobic activity
- Traditionally used for neutropenic patients and those in septic shocks combined with a beta-lactam drug. However, superiority of combination therapy has not been established and should be weighed against potential for drug toxicity and selection of drug resistance
- Higher loading dose up to 25–30 mg/kg are advised to achieve adequate concentrations in critically ill patients due to increased volume of distribution and unpredictable clearance
- Nephrotoxic, hence dose adjustment required as per creatinine clearance
- *Adverse reactions:* Neurotoxicity, ototoxicity
- Avoid concomitant use with other nephrotoxic agents (colistin, vancomycin, amphotericin B, and mannitol). Avoid loop diuretics as concomitant use may enhance cochlear toxicity
- Use with caution in patients with neuromuscular disorders (myasthenia gravis/ parkinsonism). Neuromuscular blockade and respiratory paralysis have been reported following use soon after anesthesia or muscle relaxants
- Avoid use of mannitol with amikacin as it enhances its nephrotoxic effect

Gentamicin: The place of gentamicin in the ICU is now restricted to select indications like part of a combination regimen for prosthetic valve endocarditis due to enterococci or *S. aureus* and for neonatal sepsis and meningitis.

BOX 4: Antibiotics against MRSA.

Drugs	***Dosage (IV)***
Vancomycin	*Loading dose:* 20–35 mg/kg in critically ill/meningitis (not to exceed 3 g) *Maintenance dose:* 15 mg/kg q8–12h (as per therapeutic drug monitoring) Target trough concentrations (before fourth dose): *Mild-mod infections:* 10–15 μg/mL *Severe/CNS/deep-seated infections:* 15–20 μg/mL
• Most effective if used in the highest possible dose recommended as per the creatinine clearance • Other than nephrotoxicity, flushing due to vasodilation (red man's syndrome) and thrombocytopenia may occur occasionally. Vancomycin infusion over 2 hours to avoid red man's syndrome. IV vancomycin is an irritant, extravasation and thrombophlebitis may occur (slow infusion rates, dilute solution 5 mg/mL and rotate injection site) • Broad aerobic and anaerobic gram-positive coverage. Should be reserved for MRSA/CoNS and resistant enterococcal species • Inferior option for methicillin sensitive staphylococcal isolates (cloxacillin, first-generation cephalosporins are preferred options)	
Teicoplanin	• Loading dose 12 mg/kg (400 mg q12h) × three doses • Maintenance dose—6 mg/kg (400 mg q24h) • Higher maintenance doses of 12 mg/kg/d (400 mg q12h) have been recommended for serious/deep-seated infections
Spectrum of activity similar to vancomycin. Inferior option for methicillin sensitive staphylococcal isolates.	
Linezolid	600 mg BID (no renal/hepatic dose adjustment recommended)
Daptomycin	• 4–6 mg/kg OD for soft tissue infections • 8–10 mg/kg/d for deep-seated/complicated infections
Usage: • Linezolid and daptomycin are alternatives to vancomycin and may be useful in strains with reduced vancomycin susceptibility. • Linezolid has good lung penetration unlike daptomycin which is inactivated by surfactants in the lungs. However, daptomycin may be used in infections with lung involvement due to a hematogenous source of infection, e.g., IE with pulmonary emboli. • Drug reaction with eosinophilia and systemic symptoms (DRESS) has been reported with daptomycin use. Myopathy/rhabdomyolysis has also been reported. • Statins may enhance the adverse effects of daptomycin. It is advisable to temporarily stop statins prior to initiating daptomycin. If continued, monitor CPK levels. • Linezolid–lactic acidosis, cytopenias, peripheral neuropathy, and optic neuritis are among the important adverse effects reported. • Avoid coadministration of linezolid with serotonergic psychiatric drugs [selective serotonin reuptake inhibitor (SSRI), serotonin and norepinephrine reuptake inhibitor (SNRI), tricyclic antidepressant (TCA), monoamine oxidase inhibitor (MAOI)] unless indicated due to increased risk of serotonin syndrome. May increase serotonin CNS levels by MAO-A inhibition.	

BOX 5: Antibiotics for multidrug-resistant GNBS (polymyxin B and E).

Drugs	***Dosage***	***Usage***
• Colistin (Polymyxin-E) • Colistin is available as the prodrug colistimethate sodium (CMS)	• CMS 9 MIU stat followed by 4.5 MIU twice a day after 12–24 hours of the stat dose as maintenance dose • Renal dose adjustment is necessary and recommended dosing in patients on renal replacement therapy must be adhered to see International Consensus Guidelines for the Optimal Use of the Polymyxins. (*Tsuji et al. Pharmacotherapy. 2019;39(1):10-39.)*	• The polymyxins (colistin/polymyxin E and polymyxin B) have the identical spectrum of activity and should be used as reserve antibiotics for carbapenem resistant gram-negative organisms particularly CR *Pseudomonas* and *Acinetobacter* spp. • Polymyxins are intrinsically resistant to gram-positive organisms, anaerobes, and many gram-negative agents such as *Burkholderia* spp., *Proteus* spp., *Morganella* spp. *Serratia* spp., *Brucella* spp., etc. • MIC using the broth microdilution technique is the only recommended method for drug susceptibility testing • Polymyxins have a narrow therapeutic index with major dose limiting nephrotoxicity and neurotoxicity. They should be avoided in cases with myasthenia, and in patients on neuromuscular blocking agents • Combination therapy with other susceptible agents (carbapenems/ tigecycline/fosfomycin, etc.) is encouraged in critically ill patients especially in infections where polymyxins achieve suboptimal drug concentrations, for example, lung, CNS, and bones • Unlike polymyxin B, colistin achieves levels in the urine and is preferred in treatment of urinary tract infections (UTIs)
Polymyxin B	*Loading:* 20,000–25,000 units/kg *Maintenance:* 12,500–15,000 units/kg every 12 h (no renal dose adjustment is recommended)	• Polymyxin B is not a prodrug, hence achieves rapid steady-state concentration in the blood unlike colistin which can take up to 36 hours. It is, hence, a preferred option in critically ill ICU patients • It does not achieve levels in urine and hence to be avoided in urosepsis

Contd...

Contd...

Drugs	***Dosage***	***Usage***
Fosfomycin	12–24 g/day IV (higher doses in critically ill patients) oral 3 g sachets for uncomplicated carbapenem-resistant GN UTI	• Reserve antibiotic for carbapenem-resistant GN infections. Must be used in combination with another effective drug for complicated/ deep-seated infections due to early development of resistance when used as monotherapy • Monotherapy may be considered in uncomplicated UTI due to resistant organisms • Achieves good concentrations in the lung and CSF and has excellent biofilm activity making it an attractive option for implant associated infections • Broad-spectrum GN and GP activity including MRSA and vancomycin-resistant Enterococci (VRE) • Higher MICs for *Klebsiella oxytoca, Enterobacter spp., Pseudomonas aeruginosa, Morganella morganii*, and *Providencia rettgeri* • No activity against *Acinetobacter* spp., *Stenotrophomonas* spp., *Bacteroides* spp., *Burkholderia cepacia, Bordetella, Brucella, Borrelia, Legionella, and Moraxella* spp.

BOX 6: Tetracyclines for ICU use.

Drugs	***Dosage (IV)***
Doxycycline	100 mg BID
Minocycline	200 mg stat then 100 mg BID

Usage:

- No dose adjustment for renal or hepatic failure (doxycycline may be preferred in patients with renal insufficiency)
- Contraindicated in pregnancy and children
- Usual indication—community-acquired infections such as atypical pneumonia *(Chlamydia and Mycoplasma)*, scrub typhus, rickettsial infections, Lyme disease, brucellosis, leptospirosis, cholera, nocardia, sexually transmitted infections (STIs) and pelvic inflammatory diseases
- Useful agents in GN sepsis due to *Acinetobacter, E. coli, Enterobacter* spp. when susceptible
- For SSTIs due to *S. aureus* if susceptible on culture
- Minocycline should be infused over 60 minutes to avoid reaction
- *Retinoids:* Administration of isotretinoin should be avoided shortly before, during and shortly after minocycline therapy. Each drug alone has been associated with pseudotumor cerebri (benign intracranial hypertension)
- Absorption impaired with concomitant administration with Fe, Ca, Mg bismuth, AL, and Zn

BOX 7: Glycylcycline.

Drugs	***Dosage (IV)***
Tigecycline	Loading dose (LD) 100 mg stat; maintenance dose—50 mg BID

Usage

- Has a reduced potential for resistance, as it is not affected by the ribosomal protection proteins and many efflux pumps. Thus, tigecycline may have activity against tetracycline-resistant organisms
- *Broader spectrum of activity compared to other tetracyclines including DR GN and GP organisms including MRSA and VRE.* Not active against *P. aeruginosa* but activity against *Acinetobacter* species has been reported in studies
- No dose adjustment for patients in renal failure
- In patients with hepatic failure (Child-Pugh C), loading dose 100 mg stat, maintenance 25 mg BID
- Best used for SSTIs, complicated intra-abdominal infection
- The Food and Drug Administration (FDA) black box warning stating that tigecycline should be reserved for use in situations when alternative agents are not suitable, based on a 2013 meta-analysis showing greater mortality with tigecycline use in community-acquired pneumonia (CAP), complicated intra-abdominal, SSTIs. However, higher doses of tigecycline (200 mg LD, followed by 100 mg 12 hourly), to achieve optimum concentrations, have been safely and successfully used for the above indications in multiple clinical studies

SUGGESTED READING

1. Sunavala J. Essentials of Critical Care Medicine for the Physician, 1st edition. New Delhi: Jaypee Brothers Medical Publishers (P) Ltd.; 2022.

Endocrine and Metabolic Disorder Emergency

8.1 DIABETES MELLITUS-RELATED EMERGENCIES

8.1.1 Diabetic Ketoacidosis and Hyperosmolar Hyperglycemic State

Hemraj B Chandalia

BOX 1: Introduction.

Diabetic ketoacidosis (DKA) and hyperosmolar hyperglycemic state (HHS) are grave acute emergencies in diabetes

BOX 2: Etiology, clinical antecedents.

Etiology	***Insulinopenia***
Clinical antecedents	• Omission of insulin dose • Undiagnosed type 1 diabetes mellitus (DM) • Stress situations with increase in contrainsulin hormones in both type 1 and type 2 DM • *Drugs (rare):* Psychotropic (clozapine), recreational drugs (ecstasy—methylenedioxymethamphetamine), and antiretroviral drugs: indinavir, lamivudine, pentamidine, L-asparaginase

BOX 3: Clinical presentation.

- Diabetic ketoacidosis is characterized by hyperglycemia, dehydration, ketosis, and metabolic acidosis with increased anion gap
- Hyperglycemia can cause polydipsia polyuria initially
- As acidosis sets in ventilation is stimulated causing CO_2 depletion
- Prostaglandins are the main reasons for unexplained nausea, vomiting, pain in abdomen
- Impaired mental status may be related to metabolic acidosis, hyperosmolarity, low extracellular fluid volume, and poor hemodynamics, mostly seen with elevated serum osmolality (>320 mOsm/L or >320 mmol/kg) than with severity of metabolic acidosis
- Tachycardia, orthostasis or hypotension, poor skin turgor, and dry mucous membranes result from volume depletion
- Kussmaul respirations, increased rate and depth of breathing, may be observed

Caveat:

- Type 1 diabetes may be diagnosed with an initial episode of DKA
- Patients of type 2 diabetes may go into DKA with sepsis or severe stress with resultant increased insulin demand produced by the surge of contrainsulin hormones
- A variety of drugs can precipitate DKA **(Box 6)**

BOX 4: Typical clinical presentation and laboratory parameters in DKA and HHS.

	DKA			***HHS***
Severity	***Mild***	***Moderate***	***Severe***	
Plasma glucose (mg/dL)	>250	>250	>250	>600
Arterial pH	7.25–7.30	7–7.24	<7	>7.30
Serum bicarbonate (mEq/L)	<15	10–15	<10	>15
Urine and serum ketones	Positive (+++)	Positive (+++)	Positive (+++)	Trace/small (±)
Serum osmolarity (mOsm/L)	Variable	Variable	Variable	>320
Anion gap	>10	>12–16	>16	<12
Mental status	Alert	Alert/drowsy	Stupor/coma	Stupor/coma
Sodium (mmol/L)	125–135	125–135	125–135	135–145
Potassium (mmol/L)	Normal to high	Normal to high	Normal to high	Normal
Creatinine (mg/dL)	Minimal increase	Minimal increase	Minimal increase	Moderate increase

Biochemical abnormalities.

- **Box 4** shows a typical profile of biochemical abnormalities in DKA contrasted with HHS
- In HHS, hyperglycemia and dehydration are more severe, but significant ketosis and acidosis is absent
- Patients can present with a variable admixture of the features of DKA and HHS and will need individualization of treatment

BOX 5: Caveats.

The average deficits of water and electrolytes per kg of body weight in DKA: Water 100 mL, Na 7–10 mEq, Cl 3–5 mEq, K 3–5 mEq, Mg 1–2 mEq, and PO_4 1–2 mEq. About half of the deficit should be corrected in the first 24–48 hours, remaining over the next 1–2 weeks

BOX 6: Protocol for the management of DKA (moderately severe).

On admission—Initial treatment:

- Obtain complete blood count (CBC), blood glucose (BG), electrolytes, creatinine, and urine
- Glucose and ketone, plasma ketone (β-hydroxybutyrate), and blood gases
- *Secure two intravenous (IV) lines:* Line 1 for insulin infusion and Line 2 for IV fluids and electrolytes

Line 1

- Give 10–20 units human regular insulin IV bolus
- *100 mL normal saline + 100 units regular human insulin:* Infuse at the rate of 5–10 units/h
- *Caution:* Flush out first 10 mL fluid rapidly in order to saturate insulin adsorption sites in the plastic syringe and tubing

Line 2: Normal saline 1 L over 1 hour; simultaneously infuse (through piggyback or bivalve) sodium bicarbonate 50–100 mEq in 250–500 mL of normal saline over 1 hour (if pH <7.2)

***0–4 hours:* Monitor BG and K hourly**

Line 1: Continue insulin infusion

Line 2

- May infuse 500–1,000 mL of half normal saline or change to 5% dextrose when BG drops to about 200 mg/dL
- **Start potassium chloride (KCl) 40 mEq for each liter of IV fluids if serum K >4.0 mEq/L or if urine output is good and BG is dropping**

4–24 hours:

- Monitor BG and K^+ 2 hourly
- *Line 1:* Reduce insulin infusion rate to 2–5 units/h IV when BG drops to 200 mg/dL
- *Line 2:* 5% dextrose solution IV to correct half of calculated fluid requirement
- KCl 40 mEq/L of IV fluids

24–48 hours: Repeat CBC, electrolytes, and creatinine once a day

Line 1: If able to eat or drink per os (PO), plan to discontinue IV insulin infusion; give 10–20 U subcutaneous (SC) human regular insulin 2 hours before discontinuation of insulin infusion. Put patient on basal + bolus (4–8 U regular insulin) SC regime

Line 2: If patient is unable to eat or drink PO, continue a 5% dextrose infusion and IV insulin infusion. Reduce IV fluids infused when able to retain fluids PO and start SC insulin (basal-bolus)

After 48 hours:

- Shift to oral feeds
- Start basal-bolus insulin regime SC
- Start KCl PO
- *During treatment, following complications are possible:* Hypoglycemia, hypokalemia, cerebral edema (especially in children), and hyperchloremic acidosis (due to excessive saline infusion). To avoid afore-mentioned complications, the following strategy is employed
  - *Water and salt replacement:* Proportionately, there is higher deficit of water than salt; hence the fluids used are: Initially saline, later half normal saline followed by water with dextrose
  - ***Use of alkali:* Soda bicarbonate should also be considered if pH <7.2 and be definitely used if pH <7.0. The dose used is half of the calculated deficit**
  - ***Soda bicarbonate (mEq) required:* Half of bicarbonate deficiency X (1/3 body water)**
- Alkali used is minimized for the following reasons **(Box 7)**

Source: Modified from Chandalia HB. Acute metabolic complications. In: Chandalia HB, Shridhar GD, Das AK, Madhu SV, Mohan V, Rao PV (Eds). RSSDI Textbook of Diabetes, 3rd edition. New Delhi: Jaypee Brothers Medical Publishers Pvt. Ltd.; 2014. pp. 786-811.

BOX 7: Reasons for minimizing alkali therapy.

- Diabetic ketoacidosis is a reversible metabolic acidosis. Hence with hydration and insulin infusion, body carbonate is regenerated
- Rapid correction of peripheral acidosis can aggravate intracerebral acidosis
- Oxygen delivery and renal ketone excretion is better in acidotic than alkalotic state.
- Rapid alkali therapy aggravates hypokalemia

BOX 8: Management of complications secondary to correction of DKA.

- *Hypokalemia:* If initial K^+ is low, replenishment must be started before insulin infusion. If normal or high, it drops rapidly with glucose lowering as K migrates from extracellular to intracellular compartment. Hence K^+ should be estimated hourly for the first 4–6 hours and 1–2 times a day thereafter and replacement undertaken. Starting of oral feeds restores serum potassium easily as most foods are good sources of potassium
- Magnesium deficiency can present as profound weakness and muscle cramps. It should be replaced by 50% magnesium sulfate, 2 mL added to 100 mL saline infused over 1 hour. Oral feeds obviates this problem considerably. If there is difficulty in restoring K^+ levels from low to normal, concomitant magnesium deficiency is likely
- *Hypoglycemia:* To avoid hypoglycemia, glucose-containing fluids must be infused when the BG drops to 200 mg/dL. Insulin infusion must be scaled down at this stage
- *Cerebral edema:* It is usually seen in children but occasionally in adults. To prevent the same, BG should not be lowered by >100 mg/dL/h. Advent of cerebral edema is heralded by headache and stupor suddenly appearing at 4–12 hours post-treatment preceded by a period of initial improvement in the mental status. There is bradycardia and papilledema and occasionally seizures. Sodium is low due to administration of excess fluids. It accounts for >60% deaths seen in DKA. Treatment consists of IV mannitol, hypertonic saline, and corticosteroids
- Hypophosphatemia produces muscle weakness and respiratory depression. It can be corrected by replacing part of K with the use of potassium phosphate
- Avoid use of excess saline as it can lead to hyperchloremic acidosis. Use 5% dextrose once the BG has come down to around 200 mg/dL

BOX 9: Special scenarios.

Use of antibiotics in DKA: There is some degree of leukocytosis seen in acidosis without any infection. It can be treated by a single antibiotic. If there is clear evidence of infection (usually urinary tract, lungs or skin or foot infection), appropriate antibiotics must be given

Sodium-glucose cotransporter-2 inhibitor (SGLT2i)-induced ketoacidosis: This group of drugs are widely used in type 2 DM at present. In patients with relative insulinopenia and in many critical illnesses, these drugs lead to increased ketones (β-hydroxybutyrate, acetone, and acetoacetic acid) and produce acidosis. The BG is moderately high but occasionally only around 150 mg/dL, producing a condition of euglycemic ketoacidosis. This should be treated by prompt omission of SGLT2i and treating DKA as per usual guidelines. For planned surgery and wherever possible, these drugs should be omitted about 3–7 days prior to the procedure as their ketogenic action can continue for 3–7 days after omission

BOX 10: Hyperglycemic hyperosmolar state.

Clinical features:

- Box shows a comparison of DKA and HHS. HHS occurs in elderly subjects and occasionally in infants and children
- It is characterized by poor access to water, mental obtundation, absence of acidosis (or minimal acidosis), colossal water deficit (about 150 mL/kg body weight), hypernatremia, and azotemia
- Many drugs may contribute toward its genesis **(Box 11)**

BOX 11: Precipitation of HHS by drugs.

Drugs	*Effect*
Cortisone	• Decreased insulin secretion • Increased insulin resistance
Thiazides	Decreased insulin secretion
Furosemide	Increased water loss
Beta-blockers	Decreased insulin secretion
Calcium channel blockers	Decreased insulin secretion
Alcohol	Subclinical pancreatitis

BOX 12: Management.

- It differs from DKA regarding the fluids and electrolyte replacement strategy and insulin dosage
- Initial hydration by 1–2 liters fluid is crucial before starting insulin therapy. In case of hemodynamic instability, initial fluid can be saline, but soon it should be ½ normal saline or dextrose infusion or if possible, plain water orally
- The insulin infusion strategy is same as in DKA. It is important to start SC insulin a couple of hours before discontinuation of insulin infusion. The dosage of insulin required is rather low, compared to the requirement in DKA
- A majority of these elderly patients may have a concomitant problem such as myocardial infarction, stroke, renal failure, or sepsis. These have to be identified and treated. Osmolarity of <320 mOsm/L is against the diagnosis of HHS and points toward other etiologies of mental obtundation

SUGGESTED READING

1. Chandalia HB. Acute metabolic complications. In: Chandalia HB, Shridhar GD, Das AK, Madhu SV, Mohan V, Rao PV (Eds). RSSDI Textbook of Diabetes, 3rd edition. New Delhi: Jaypee Brothers Medical Publishers Pvt. Ltd.; 2014. pp. 786-811.
2. Diabetic ketoacidosis and hyperosmolar hyperglycemic state. In: Kolief MH, Isakow W, Buris AC, Despotovic V. (Eds). Washington Manual of Critical Care (Asian Edition). Wolters Kluwer Publishers; 2022. pp. 281-87.
3. Kitabchi AE, Umpierrez GE, Fisher JN, Fisher JN. Thirty years of personal experience in hyperglycemic crises: diabetic ketoacidosis and hyperglycemic hyperosmolar state. J Clin Endocrinol Metab. 2008;93:1541-52.
4. Usher-Smith JA, Thompson MJ, Sharp SJ, Walter FM. Factors associated with the presence of diabetic ketoacidosis at diagnosis of diabetes in children and young adults: a systemic review. BMJ. 2011;343:d4092.

8.1.2 Hyperglycemia in Emergency Room

Shaival H Chandalia

BOX 1: Introduction.

Actionable level in emergency room (ER), random blood glucose >180 mg/dL

BOX 2: Evaluation.

- Arterial blood gas (ABG)/serum ketones to rule out diabetic ketoacidosis (DKA)
- Serum osmolarity—to rule out hyperosmolar hyperglycemic state (HHS)
- Electrolytes, creatinine, and assessment of volume status

BOX 3: Treatment.

- DKA/HHS treatment as per algorithm of DKA/HHS
- *Isolated hyperglycemia:*
  - Intravenous (IV) fluids and IV insulin and correction of electrolytes
  - *Treatment of underlying cause of hyperglycemia:* Sepsis and critical illness (stroke and myocardial infarction)
  - *IV fluids:* Normal saline bolus of 250–500 cc, especially if volume depleted. Smaller bolus with cardiac and renal impairment

BOX 4: Intravenous insulin.

- Bolus IV regular insulin 10–20 units depending on blood glucose
- Insulin infusion via syringe pump 50/50, i.e., 50 units of regular insulin in 50 cc of normal saline
- Capillary blood glucose 1 hourly
- Concentration of insulin infusion can be increased after 3–4 hours if blood glucose remains high
- Overlap with subcutaneous insulin and oral hypoglycemic agents (OHAs) if plan for discharge
- Correction of electrolytes during ER stay

BOX 5: Insulin infusion protocol.

- Start with 50/50 insulin infusion in syringe pump
- Rate as per blood glucose algorithm

For example:

Blood glucose	*Rate*
120–160	0.5 mL/h
161–200 ↓ >400	1 mL/h 10 mL/h

- If blood glucose remains high, increase concentration to 75/50 or 100/50
- After increasing concentration, algorithm remains the same (above scale)
- In effect, insulin dose increased by increasing concentration, algorithm (rate) remains the same

BOX 6: Tips for insulin infusion via syringe pump.

- Flush the tubing with 10 mL of infusion outside the patient to saturate adsorption sites
- Increasing concentration rather than rate results in uniform single algorithm throughout the hospital (multiple algorithms not required)
- Reduce insulin infusion rate to half from 12 midnight to 4 am (to avoid hypoglycemia) as it is the period of maximum insulin sensitivity
- Check electrolytes, especially potassium as mentioned earlier

SUGGESTED READING

1. Chandalia S. Glycemic management in hospitalized patients. In: Mohan V, Chandalia HB, Sridhar GR, Das AK, Madhu SV, Rao PV (Ed). RSSDI Textbook of Diabetes Mellitus, 3rd edition. New Delhi: Jaypee Brothers Medical Publishers; 2014. pp. 612-21.
2. Mehta A, Emmett M. (2023). Fasting ketosis and alcoholic ketoacidosis. [online] Available from https://www.uptodate.com/contents/fasting-ketosis-and-alcoholic-ketoacidosis [Last accessed September, 2024].

8.1.3 Alcoholic Ketoacidosis

Hemraj B Chandalia

BOX 1: Definition.

Ketoacidosis in the appropriate clinical setting, i.e., usually in malnourished patients with moderate or severe alcohol use disorder who have a recent history of binge alcohol ingestion

Clinical features:

- Nausea, vomiting, and abdominal pain in 60–70% of patients
- Generalized abdominal tenderness, and/or hepatomegaly and/or laboratory evidence of alcoholic hepatitis and/or pancreatitis
- Hypovolemia and/or electrolyte disturbances like potassium deficiency
- Tachycardia, hypertension, and tachypnea
- Alert, absence of mental obtundation

BOX 2: Laboratory findings.

- Plasma ethanol levels may be normal
- Normoglycemia, sometimes hypoglycemia or mild hyperglycemia
- Hypokalemia, hypophosphatemia, and hypomagnesemia
- Elevated serum osmolal gap (>10 mOsm/kg greater than calculated osmolality)
- High anion gap metabolic acidosis—ketoacidosis

BOX 3: Differential diagnosis.

	Fasting ketoacidosis	***Alcoholic ketoacidosis***	***Diabetic ketoacidosis***
Blood glucose	Normal	Normal, low or rarely high If high, hemoglobin A1c (HbA1c) may help to distinguish from DKA	Elevated, rarely normal in euglycemic DKA, e.g., with sodium-glucose cotransporter-2 (SGLT2) inhibitors
Severity of acidosis (bicarbonate)	Mild, bicarbonate rarely <17 mEq/L	Moderate to severe also seen	Moderate to severe also seen
Ratio of beta-hydroxybutyrate to acetoacetate	1:1	3:1	Close to 10:1

BOX 4: Treatment.

- Thiamine and dextrose/normal saline infusions
- Avoid dextrose infusion before hypokalemia is treated
- Correct potassium, phosphate, and magnesium deficiency
- Correction of ketoacidosis—reversible acidosis by treating underlying disease and above measures

SUGGESTED READING

1. Chandalia HB. Acute metabolic complications. In: Chandalia HB, Shridhar GD, Das AK, Madhu SV, Mohan V, Rao PV (Eds). RSSDI Textbook of Diabetes, 3rd edition. New Delhi: Jaypee Brothers Medical Publishers Pvt. Ltd.; 2014. pp. 786-811.
2. Mehta A, Emmett M. (2023). Fasting ketosis and alcoholic ketoacidosis. [online] Available from https://www.uptodate.com/contents/fasting-ketosis-and-alcoholic-ketoacidosis [Last accessed September, 2024].

8.1.4 Hypoglycemia in Emergency Room

Shaival H Chandalia

BOX 1: Definition.

- Blood glucose <3.5 mmol/L (<63 mg/dL); range 50–70 mg/dL
  - Symptoms and signs of low blood glucose
  - Relief with ingestion of glucose (Whipple's triad)
- Range is variable due to variation in threshold of counter-regulatory hormone release
- With sustained or recurrent hyperglycemia, threshold is higher
- With sustained or recurrent hypoglycemia, threshold is lower

BOX 2: Pathophysiology of hypoglycemia: Counter-regulatory responses.

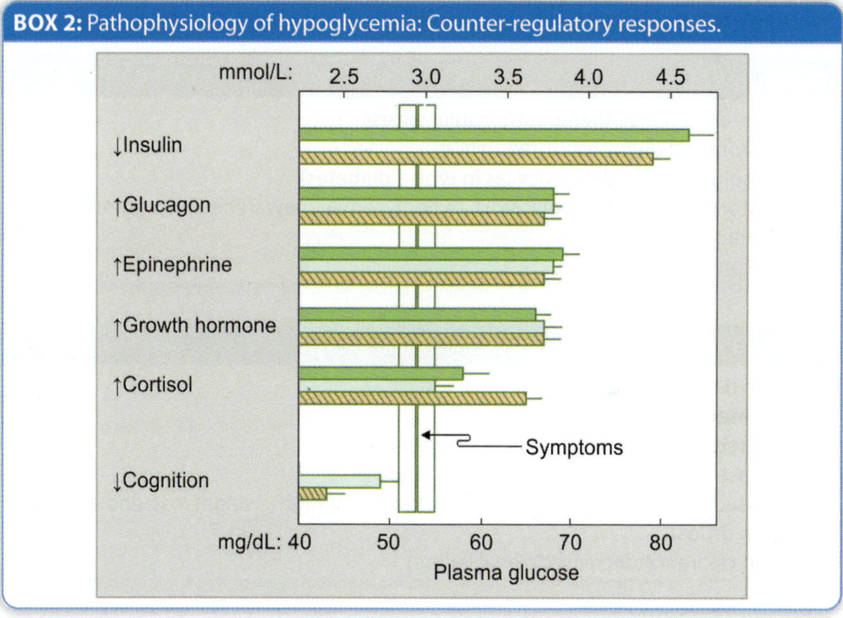

BOX 3: Symptoms of hypoglycemia are the result of central nervous system (CNS) neuronal glucose deprivation.

Indirect	***Direct***
Autonomic	Neuroglycopenic
Adrenergic and cholinergic	Cognitive
Sweaty, hungry, tingling, shaky (tremulous), heart pounding, and nervous/anxious	Warm, weak, difficulty thinking/ confused, tired/drowsy, faint, dizzy, difficulty speaking, and blurred vision

BOX 4: Causes of hypoglycemia in diabetics and nondiabetics (drugs and intercurrent causes).

Drugs:
- Insulin, sulfonylureas, and other secretagogues
- Metformin, thiazolidinediones, and acarbose (including in isolation)
- Alcohol, angiotensin-converting enzyme (ACE) inhibitors, and propranolol
- Quinine, quinidine, and disopyramide
- Salicylates (in children)
- Sulfonamides including cotrimoxazole and quinolones
- Pentamidine

Intercurrent causes: Gastroenteritis, severe malnutrition, hepatic disease, renal failure, adrenal insufficiency, and sepsis

BOX 5: Risk factors.

- Absolute or relative therapeutic insulin excess
- Compromised glucose autoregulation:
  - Absolute insulin deficiency (as in type 1 diabetes)
  - History of severe hypoglycemia, hypoglycemia unawareness, or aggressive therapy (lower HbA1c)
  - Autonomic neuropathy

BOX 6: Absolute or relative therapeutic insulin excess.

- Insulin dose excessive, ill timed
- Decreased food intake
- Increased glucose utilization (e.g., exercise)
- Decreased glucose production (e.g., alcohol)
- Increased insulin sensitivity (e.g., after exercise, at night, weight loss, and with certain drugs)
- Insulin clearance decreased (renal failure)

BOX 7: Investigations and diagnosis of causes of hypoglycemia.

- Assessment of nutritional status
- Assessment of possible medications causing hypoglycemia
- Liver function tests
- Renal function tests
- 8 am cortisol (for adrenal insufficiency)
- Assessment for sepsis
- Fasting blood glucose (during/post-termination of 72 hours fast), C peptide, insulin (all three from same collection):
  - If fasting blood sugar (FBS) is low and C peptide and/or insulin is high—inappropriate hyperinsulinism due to:
    - Insulinoma or nesidioblastosis
    - More commonly—autoimmune hypoglycemia (due to antibody to insulin or insulin receptor)
    - Clue to diagnosis—insulin levels are astronomically high due to assay interference
    - Sulfonylurea over dose—diagnosed by sulfonylurea screen

BOX 8: Treatment of hypoglycemia.

- Oral sugar (glucose for acarbose-induced hypoglycemia)
- Intramuscular or subcutaneous glucagon (except in sulfonylurea-induced hypoglycemia)
- Intravenous (IV) glucose for severe hypoglycemia
- Should be followed by a mixed meal (containing carbs, protein, and fat to sustain the blood glucose)
- Sulfonylurea—admit to hospital for at least 24 hours

SUGGESTED READING

1. Cryer PE. Hypoglycemia. In: Melmed S, Polonsky KS, Larsen PR, Kronenberg HM (Eds). Williams Textbook of Endocrinology, 13th edition. Elsevier; 2015. pp. 1582-607.

8.2 THYROID ABNORMALITIES RELATED EMERGENCIES

Sachna P Shetty, Shaival H Chandalia

BOX 1: Thyroid function test interpretation.

TSH	*Free T3*	*Free T4*	*Disease*
Normal	Normal	Normal	None
Low	Normal	Normal	Hyperthyroid subclinical
Low	High	High	Hyperthyroid
Low	High	Normal	Triiodothyronine (T3) toxicosis
Low	Normal	High	Thyroiditis, thyroxine (T4) ingestion, in older adults or with comorbidities
Low	Low	Low	Euthyroid, sick thyroid, central hypothyroid
High	Normal	Normal	Subclinical *hypothyroid*
High	Low	Low	Clinical hypothyroid

BOX 2: Clinical picture of hypothyroid and hyperthyroid.

System	*Hypothyroid*	*Hyperthyroid*
Constitutional	• Fatigue and lethargy • Cold intolerance • Weight gain, but decreased appetite	• Lethargy and weakness • Heat intolerance, diaphoresis • Fever (in subacute thyroiditis) • Hyperphagia–yet weight loss
Neuropsychiatric	Cognitive slowing, delayed reflexes, agitation, psychosis, seizures, coordination problems, carpal tunnel syndrome, sensorineural hearing loss, neuropathy, and tingling sensations	Emotional instability, anxiety, confusion, psychosis, coma, fine tremor, muscle wasting, increased reflexes, and periodic paralysis
Ophthalmic	Periorbital swelling	Double vision, eyelid retraction, bulging eyes, eye muscle weakness, periorbital swelling, and difficulty looking upward
Cardiac	• Dyspnea on exertion, chest pain • Sinus bradycardia • Long QT with increased chances of ventricular arrhythmia • Diastolic heart failure • Pericardial effusion (asymptomatic) • Peripheral edema	• Chest pain • Palpitations • Sinus tachycardia • Widened pulse pressure, bounding pulses • Systolic hypertension • Atrial fibrillation or flutter • High output heart failure, systolic rub (Means–Lerman scratch)
Respiratory	• Shortness of breath during physical activity • Obstructive sleep apnea • Primary pulmonary hypertension might be secondary to hypothyroid	Breathlessness
Gastrointestinal	• Constipation • Ileus or decreased gastric motility	• Diarrhea or increased gastric motility • Yellowish sclera/jaundice
Reproductive	• Menstrual disturbances (infrequent, absent, or heavy periods) • Early abortions • Decreased libido, erectile dysfunction, and infertility in both genders	• Menstrual disturbances (infrequent, absent, or heavy periods) • Decreased libido, erectile dysfunction infertility, and breast enlargement in males • Telangiectasia • Sparse pubic hair

Contd...

Contd...

System	***Hypothyroid***	***Hyperthyroid***
Dermatology	• Thinned and coarse hair • Pale and dry skin, decreased perspiration • Thickened skin and nails • Orange discoloration of skin and feet • Yellow tints in skin folds • Brittle nails with ridges • Delayed wound healing • Lateral thinning of the eyebrow	• Hair loss • Warm, moist skin, and diaphoresis • Onycholysis (separation of nails from its bed) • Pretibial myxedema • Hyperpigmented pretibial plaques, nodule or induration • Palmar erythema
General/others	• Hypothermia prone • Voice changes • Hearing loss • Goiter • Proximal myopathy • Pseudohypertrophy • Polyarthralgias • Joint effusions • Acute gout or pseudogout *Caveat:* Macroglossia (enlarged tongue, broad nose, and swollen lips)	• Hyperthermia prone • Neck fullness • Tenderness • Voice changes • Dysphagia mainly due to thyroid enlargement (goiter) • Venous prominence with arm elevation—Pemberton's sign • Pale skin • Anemia • Leukocytosis

BOX 3: Recognition of myxedema coma.	
Risk factors	• Known hypothyroidism; thyroidectomy scar • Evidence of severe chronic hypothyroidism • Acute precipitating illness • Drug toxicity
Presenting features	• Severe hypothyroidism symptoms with notable facial features (puffy eyelids and lips, large tongue, and broad nose) known as "myxedema face" • Altered mental state (myxedema madness) • Labored breathing with low oxygen and high carbon dioxide levels • Hypotension unresponsive to fluids and pressors without thyroid hormone therapy • Slow heart rate • Prolonged QT interval and ventricular arrhythmias • Hypothermia (check core rectal temperature) • Low sodium, low blood sugar
	Caveat: • *Diagnostic criteria:* A scoring system aids in diagnosing myxedema coma, with higher scores indicating a higher likelihood

BOX 4: Diagnostic scoring system for myxedema coma.

	Points
Thermoregulatory dysfunction (Temperature °F/°C)	
>95/35	0
89.6—95/32–35	10
<89.6/32	20
Central nervous system (CNS) effects	
• Absent	0
• Somnolent/lethargy	10
• Obtunded	15
• Stupor	20
• Coma/seizures	30
Gastrointestinal findings:	
• Anorexia/abdominal pain/constipation	5
• Decreased intestinal motility	15
• Paralytic ileus	20
Precipitating event	
• Absent	0
• Present	10
Cardiovascular dysfunction	
Bradycardia/heart rate:	
• Absent	0
• 50–59	10
• 40–49	20
• <40	30
Other EKG changes	10
Pericardial/pleural effusion	10
Pulmonary edema	15
Cardiomegaly	15
Hypotension	20
Metabolic disturbances:	
• Hyponatremia	10
• Hypoglycemia	10
• Hypoxemia	10
• Hypercarbia	10
Decrease in glomerular filtration rate (GFR)	10

Other EKG changes: QT prolongation, or low voltage complex, or bundle branch blocks, or nonspecific ST-T changes, or heart blocks.

Total score:
- >60: Highly suggestive/diagnostic of myxedema coma
- 25–59: Supportive of diagnosis of myxedema coma
- <25: Myxedema coma unlikely

Source: Adapted from Popoveniuc G, Chandra T, Sud A, Sharma M, Blackman MR, Burman KD, et al. A diagnostic scoring system for myxedema coma. Endocr Pract. 2014;20(8):808-17.

BOX 5: Management of myxedema.

Supportive care:
- Address airway, breathing, and circulation
- Treat hypoglycemia and low sodium
- *Vasopressors:* Effective after thyroid replacement
- Treat hypothermia (refer to Chapter 15.2.1)
- *Steroids:* Hydrocortisone [100–200 mg intravenous (IV)]

Thyroid replacement therapy:
- IV thyroxine (levothyroxine) at 4 μg/kg (typically 200–400 μg initially), followed by 100 μg IV in 24 hours, then 50 μg IV until oral medication can be taken. For elderly patients, start with 100 μg IV
- IV triiodothyronine (liothyronine) at 20 μg IV, followed by 10 μg IV every 8 hours until the patient regains consciousness. For elderly or coronary artery disease patients, start with no more than 10 μg IV. (T3 is less preferred for cardiac patients due to its potency)

Caveat:
- Begin with IV levothyroxine. IV liothyronine can be added if IV levothyroxine alone is insufficient or if the patient remains hemodynamically unstable or has poor respiratory effort
- Identify and treat precipitating and coexisting factors

Note: Hypothermia is a crucial indicator of myxedema (core rectal temperature is key)

BOX 6: Thyroid storm.

Definition and precipitants:
- Thyroid storm is a rare, life-threatening exacerbation of hyperthyroidism
- Triggers include infections, trauma, surgery, severe illness, eclampsia with preexisting hyperthyroidism, diabetic ketoacidosis, withdrawal of thyroid-suppressing drugs, iodine administration, or thyroid hormone ingestion

Clinical features:
- Exaggerated symptoms of hyperthyroidism including fever and prominent cardiovascular and neurological symptoms.
- The Burch and Wartofsky point scale aids in identifying thyroid storm

BOX 7: Burch and Wartofsky point scale.

Thermoregulatory Dysfunction [Temperature °C (°F)]	***Score/Points***
37.2–37.7 (99–99.9) 37.7–38.3 (100–100.9) 38.3–38.8 (101–101.9) 38.9–39.4 (102–102.9) 39.4–39.9 (103–103.9) ≥40 (≥104.0)	5 10 15 20 25 30
CNS effects: • Absent • Mild (agitation) • Moderate (delirium, psychosis, and extreme lethargy) • Severe (seizures and coma)	 0 10 20 30
Gastrointestinal (GI) hepatic dysfunction: • Absent • Moderate (diarrhea, nausea/vomiting, and abdominal pain) • Severe (unexplained jaundice)	 0 10 20
Cardiovascular dysfunction	
Tachycardia (beats/min) 90–109 110–119 120–129 ≥140	 5 10 15 25
Congestive heart failure: • Absent • Mild (pedal edema) • Moderate (bibasilar rales) • Severe (pulmonary edema)	 0 5 10 15
Atrial fibrillation: • Absent • Present	 0 10
Precipitating event: • Absent • Present	 0 10
Scoring system: Score of ≥45: Highly suggestive of thyroid storm, 23–44 impending storm	

BOX 8: Differential diagnosis.

- Infection and sepsis
- Sympathomimetic drug use (e.g., cocaine, amphetamines, and ketamine)
- Heat-related conditions, such as heat exhaustion or stroke, as well as malignant hyperthermia or neuroleptic malignant syndrome
- Withdrawal from substances like cocaine or opioids
- Psychiatric conditions or stress-induced disorders
- Anticholinergic toxicity

BOX 9: Management.

Initial management: (Treatment and pharmacopoeia)
- Evaluate airway, breathing, and circulation
- Provide IV fluids for dehydration
- Use external cooling measures for fever; paracetamol may be administered
- **Adrenergic blockade:**
  - *Propranolol:* Administer 0.5–1 mg IV over 10 minutes, then 1–2 mg every few hours, adjusting based on vital signs. For less severe cases, use oral doses. For patients with reactive airway disease, opt for cardioselective beta-blockers

Inhibition of thyroid hormone synthesis:
- *Methimazole:* Administer 20 mg orally every 6 hours. Avoid during the first trimester of pregnancy due to teratogenic risks
- *Propylthiouracil (PTU):* Start with an initial dose of 500–1,000 mg orally, followed by 250 mg every 4 hours. This is preferred during the first trimester of pregnancy
- *ESMOLOL:* 50–100 μ/kg/min to be given in acute severe thyrotoxicosis

Inhibition of thyroid hormone release:
- *Lugol's solution:* Administer 8–10 drops orally every 6–8 hours
- *Potassium iodide (SSKI):* Administer 5 drops (0.25 mL or 250 mg) orally every 6 hours

Inhibition of peripheral conversion of T4 to T3:
- *Hydrocortisone:* Administer 300 mg IV initially, then 100 mg every 8 hours until stable
- *Dexamethasone:* Administer 2 mg IV every 6 hours

Treat precipitating events and definitive therapy:
- Radioactive iodine ablation or surgery may be necessary
- Consider dialysis or plasmapheresis as last resort treatments for unresponsive patients

Caveats in thyroid storm:
- *Congestive heart failure:*
  - Beta-blockers for rate-related high output failure
  - Use diuretics as needed
  - Reduce beta-blocker dose if ejection fraction decreases
  - Provide oxygen and sildenafil for pulmonary hypertension
- *Atrial fibrillation:*
  - Beta-blockers are preferred for rate control
  - Avoid amiodarone due to its iodine content

SUGGESTED READING

1. Burch HB, Wartofsky L. Life-threatening thyrotoxicosis: thyroid storm. Endocrinol Metab Clin North Am. 1993;22(2):263-77.
2. Klein I, Levey GS. The cardiovascular system in thyrotoxicosis and myxedema. The Endocrinologist. 2002;12(3):227-39.
4. Popoveniuc G, Chandra T, Sud A, Sharma M, Blackman MR, Burman KD, et al. A Diagnostic Scoring System for Myxedema Coma. Endocr Pract. 2014;20(8):808-17.
5. Tintinalli JE, John MaO, Yealy DM, Meckler GD, Stephan Stapczynski J, Cline DM, et al. Tintinalli's Emergency Medicine: A Comprehensive Study Guide, 9th edition. McGraw Hill Professional; 2019.

8.3 ACUTE ADRENAL INSUFFICIENCY

Pinank Pandya

BOX 1: Introduction.

- The adrenal glands secrete five types of hormones, out of which two are mainly important in ER setting
- Mineralocorticoids (primarily aldosterone) regulate electrolyte balance and glucocorticoids (primarily cortisol) promote gluconeogenesis
- An aptitude toward the diagnosis is usually needed for patients who fail to respond to primary stabilizing therapies
- The uncertainty of biochemical diagnosis of adrenal hypofunction invokes the use of clinical judgement for starting therapy

BOX 2: Etiology

- Addison's disease is an Hashimoto thyroiditis
- Sepsis, anticoagulant therapy, adrenal infarction, hemorrhage, amyloidosis, tuberculosis (TB), fungi, acquired immune deficiency syndrome (AIDS), antiphospholipid antibodies (APLA), irradiation, metastatic disease, and drugs.
- Waterhouse–Friderichsen syndrome is one of adrenal hemorrhage and is associated with meningococcemia
- Other infectious etiologies

BOX 3: Definitions of an adrenal crisis.

Study	***Definition and grading of adrenal crisis***
Allolio et al.	• Major impairment of general health with at least two of the following signs/symptoms: – Hypotension [systolic blood pressure (BP) <100 mm Hg] – Nausea or vomiting – Severe fatigue – Fever – Somnolence – Hyponatremia (≤132 mmol/L) or hyperkalemia – Hypoglycemia • Parenteral glucocorticoid (hydrocortisone) administration followed by clinical improvement • *Grading:* – Grade 1: Outpatient care only – Grade 2: Hospital care (general ward) – Grade 3: Admission to intensive care unit – Grade 4: Death from adrenal crisis (with or without parenteral glucocorticoid administration)

Contd...

Contd...

Study	***Definition and grading of adrenal crisis***
Bornstein et al.	A medical emergency with hypotension, marked acute abdominal symptoms, and marked laboratory abnormalities, requiring immediate treatment
Puar et al.	An acute deterioration in a patient with adrenal insufficiency
Smans et al.	An acute impairment of general health requiring hospital admission and administration of intravenous (IV) saline and glucocorticoids in patients with adrenal insufficiency
Rushworth et al.	An acute deterioration in health that is associated with absolute (systolic BP <100 mm Hg) or relative (systolic BP <20 mm Hg lower than the patients usual BP) hypotension, the features of which resolve following parenteral glucocorticoid administration (demonstrated by a marked resolution of hypotension within 1 hour and improvement of clinical symptoms over 2 hours)

BOX 4: Clinical features and diagnoses.

- Severe hypotension that is unresponsive to IV fluids and vasopressors is a characteristic feature, occurring in almost all the cases
- Patients may present with symptoms such as dehydration, weakness, fatigue, altered mental state, confusion, pain in the flank or back, and discomfort in the chest
- Additionally, other common symptoms include abdominal pain, anorexia, nausea, vomiting, and diarrhea
- Assessing random cortisol levels in acutely ill patients can be challenging, but certain studies have evaluated this parameter
- Typically, cortisol levels >34 µg/dL rule out adrenal crisis, while levels <15 µg/dL strongly suggest the diagnosis
- This interpretation is affected by fluctuations in corticosteroid-binding globulin levels, which can vary under physiological stress, potentially rendering free cortisol measurements unreliable. Although not typically performed in the emergency room, a rapid adrenocorticotropic hormone (ACTH) stimulation test can be conducted
- The test begins with measuring a baseline cortisol level, then administering 0.25 mg of IV Cosyntropin (synthetic ACTH)
- Cortisol levels are subsequently checked at 30 minutes and 1 hour after the Cosyntropin injection
- An increase of at least 7 µg/dL, with levels exceeding 18 µg/dL, suggests that adrenal insufficiency is unlikely
- If adrenal insufficiency is confirmed, ACTH levels can be assessed to determine whether the condition is primary or secondary
- Imaging is generally not required for patients with a confirmed history of adrenal insufficiency and often produces unremarkable results
- However, if the diagnosis is unclear, a computed tomography (CT) scan of the head or a magnetic resonance imaging (MRI) of the brain may identify pituitary damage or tumors in cases of secondary adrenal insufficiency
- For primary adrenal insufficiency (PAI), an abdominal CT scan might reveal adrenal calcifications, tumors, or hemorrhages

BOX 5: Clinical features and routine laboratory findings in adrenal crisis.

	1° Adrenal insufficiency	*2°/3° Adrenal insufficiency*
K^+	High	Normal or low
Na^+	Low	High or low
Cl^-	Low	Normal
Blood urea nitrogen (BUN)	High or normal	Normal
Glucose	Normal or low	Low

BOX 6: Common signs and symptoms and routine laboratory findings in adrenal crisis.

Symptoms	*Signs*	*Routine laboratory tests*
Severe weakness	Hypotension	Hyponatremia
Syncope	Abdominal tenderness/guarding	Hypoglycemia
Nausea and vomiting	Fever	Hypercalcemia
Abdominal pain	Hyperpigmentation (PAI)	Normocytic anemia
Back pain	Altered Glasgow Coma Scale (GCS), delirium	Acute renal failure
Confusion		Hyperkalemia (PAI)

BOX 7: Management.

- Steroids should be administered promptly when adrenal crisis is suspected
- Hydrocortisone is the preferred steroid due to its combined glucocorticoid and mineralocorticoid effects. For adults and older children (over 12 years), the initial dose is 100 mg IV, followed by 100 mg IV every 8 hours while the acute condition persists
- Children aged 3–12 years receive 50 mg IV, and infants under 3 years get 25 mg IV
- Some physicians prefer dexamethasone 4 mg IV as an alternative, because it has less impact on the rapid ACTH stimulation test
- Fluid resuscitation should start with IV fluid boluses to address dehydration, with up to 2–3 liters potentially required. Maintenance IV hydration with D5 or normal saline should follow to correct the common issues, such as hypoglycemia and hyponatremia
- If BP remains difficult to maintain, vasopressors might be needed, though hypotension in these patients can be challenging to manage with fluids and vasopressors alone. Steroids are crucial for maintaining vascular tone
- Additionally, the underlying cause of the adrenal crisis must be identified and treated
- Fludrocortisone is often required with dexamethasone because dexamethasone lacks mineralocorticoid activity
- Based on data from three small trials and **the French** trial, patients in septic shock who got IV hydrocortisone had a 10% absolute decrease in mortality compared to others

Contd...

Contd...

- Nevertheless, in the trials **Corticus** and **Hypress**, there was not a noteworthy decrease in mortality in those patients who received hydrocortisone
- A meta-analysis of all the trials determines that there is improvement in shock reversal with glucocorticoids. This is although a weak recommendation
- **Intravenous hydrocortisone (50 mg q6h)** has been advocated for patients with **septic shock**
- Of note, those patients with secondary adrenal insufficiency should have evaluation and replacement of other pituitary hormone deficiencies
- Replacement of thyroid hormone without replacement of glucocorticoids can bring about acute adrenal crisis
- Almost all patients will need **ICU admission** for close monitoring and shock reversal

SUGGESTED READING

1. Adrenal insufficiency and adrenal crisis. In: Tintinalli JE, Ma OJ, Yealy DM, Meckler GD, Stapczynski JS, Cline DM, et al. (Eds). Tintinalli's Emergency Medicine: A Comprehensive Study Guide, 7th edition. Mc Graw Hill; 2011.
2. Allolio B. Extensive expertise in endocrinology. Adrenal crisis. Eur J Endocrinol. 2015;172(3):115-24.
3. Bornstein SR, Allolio B, Arlt W, Barthel A, Don-Wauchope A, Hammer GD, et al. Diagnosis and Treatment of Primary Adrenal Insufficiency: An Endocrine Society Clinical Practice Guideline. J Clin Endocrinol Metab. 2016;101(2):364-89.
4. Cooper M, Stewart P. Corticosteroid insufficiency in acutely ill patients. N Eng J Med. 2003;348(8):727-34.
5. Gupta P, Bhalla A, Sharma R. Bilateral adrenal lesions. J Med Imaging Radiat Oncol. 2012;56(6):636-45.
6. Hahner S, Loeffler M, Bleicken B, Drechsler C, Milovanovic D, Fassnacht M, et al. Epidemiology of adrenal crisis in chronic adrenal insufficiency: the need for new prevention strategies. Eur J Endocrinol. 2010;162(3):597-602.
7. Irwin RS, Lilly CM, Mayo PH, Rippe JM (Eds). Irwin & Rippe's Intensive Care Medicine, 8th edition. Wolters Kluwer; 2018.
8. Levasseur KA, Tigchelaar H, Kannikeswaran N. Persistent hypoglycemia. Pediatr Emerg Care. 2013;29(7):838-41.
9. Papierska L, Rabijewski M. Delay in diagnosis of adrenal insufficiency is a frequent cause of adrenal crisis. Int J Endocrinol. 2013;2013:482370.
10. Puar TH, Stikkelbroeck NM, Smans LC, Zelissen PM, Hermus AR. Adrenal crisis: still a deadly event in the 21st century. Am J Med. 2016;129(3):339.e331-9.
11. Rushworth RL, Torpy DJ. A descriptive study of adrenal crises in adults with adrenal insufficiency: increased risk with age and in those with bacterial infections. BMC Endocr Disord. 2014;14:79.
12. Smans LC, Van der Valk ES, Hermus AR, Zelissen PM. Incidence of adrenal crisis in patients with adrenal insufficiency. Clin Endocrinol (Oxf). 2016;84:17-22.
13. Tucci V, Sokari T. The clinical manifestations, diagnosis, and treatment of adrenal emergencies. Emerg Med Clin North Am. 2014;32(2):465-84.
14. Vattoth S, DeLappe RS Jr, Chapman PR. Endocranial lesions. Semin Ultrasound CT MR. 2013;34(5):393-411.

8.4 ACUTE ELECTROLYTE IMBALANCES

Rushi V Deshpande, Ashwin Patil, Ashitosh R Patil

SODIUM DISORDERS

BOX 1: Introduction.

- Disorders of serum Na^+ concentration are caused by abnormalities in water homeostasis, leading to changes in the relative ratio of Na^+ to body water
- Water intake and circulating arginine-vasopressin (AVP) constitute the two key effectors in the defense of serum osmolality; defects in one or both of these two defense mechanisms cause most cases of hyponatremia and hypernatremia

BOX 2: Hyponatremia.

It is defined as a plasma Na^+ concentration <135 mEq/L

Classification based on serum sodium levels:

Mild (130–134 mEq/L)	Only gastrointestinal (GI) symptoms anorexia, vomiting, nausea, lethargy, and apathy
Moderate (120–129 mEq/L)	Predominant GI symptoms, mild headache, lethargy as neurological symptoms
Severe (100–119 mEq/L)	Predominantly neurological symptoms affecting gait, ataxia, confusion, disorientation, agitation, and psychosis intracranial pressure
Very severe (<100 mEq/L)	Features of raised intracranial pressure, stupor coma, Cheyne–Stokes respiration, and death

Classification based on volume status:

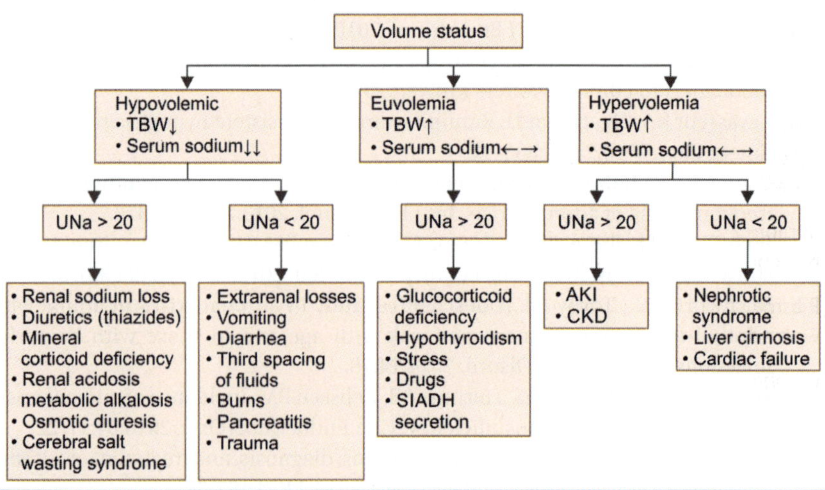

(AKI: acute kidney injury; CKD: chronic kidney disease; SIADH: syndrome of inappropriate antidiuresis hormone; TBW: total body water; UNa: urinary sodium)

BOX 3: Pseudohyponatremia.

It is a laboratory artifact that rarely occurs in patients with marked hypertriglyceridemia or hypergammaglobulinemia

Symptoms: Nausea, headache, confusion, and seizures

Diagnosis:
- *Laboratory tests:*
  - *Serum sodium levels:* Levels <135 mEq/L are considered hyponatremic
  - Serum osmolality
  - *Urinalysis:* Evaluate urinary sodium and osmolality to help distinguish between various causes, such as SIADH (low urinary sodium) and renal causes (high urinary sodium)
- *Volume status assessment:*
  - Assess signs of dehydration (hypovolemia), fluid overload (hypervolemia), or normal fluid status (euvolemia)
  - *Blood urea nitrogen (BUN) and creatinine:* Evaluate renal function, especially in cases of hypervolemic hyponatremia, where renal failure may be a contributing factor
- *Hormonal assessment:*
  - *Serum antidiuretic hormone (ADH):* Measure ADH levels to identify conditions like SIADH, where inappropriate secretion of ADH leads to water retention
  - *Thyroid function tests:* Evaluate thyroid function, as thyroid disorders can contribute to hyponatremia

Treatment:
- Pseudohyponatremia from hypertriglyceridemia or hyperproteinemia requires no therapy
- Translational hyponatremia from glucose or mannitol can be managed by correcting glucose levels or discontinuing mannitol if possible

Acute: Symptomatic with <48 hours
- Use hypertonic 3% saline (513 mM) to increase plasma Na^+ concentration by 1–2 mM/h, targeting a total increase of 4–6 mM (rule of 6)
- This modest rise is usually sufficient to alleviate severe symptoms
- A 100 mL bolus of hypertonic saline is more effective than an infusion for rapid improvement
- For ongoing infusions, equations can estimate the required rate based on the Na^+ deficit

Sodium deficit = 0.6 × TBW × (target plasma Na^+ concentration starting plasma Na^+ concentration)

Plasma Na^+ concentration should be monitored every 2–4 hours during treatment, with adjustments made as needed

Chronic: >48 hours

BOX 4: Hypovolemic hyponatremia.

- Use of normal saline to slowly increase the sodium concentration by 4–5 mEq/L
- Patients with chronic hyponatremia are at risk for osmotic demyelination if plasma Na^+ concentration is corrected by >8–10 mEq/L within the first 24 hours and/or by >18 mEq/L within the first 48 hours
- *Osmotic demyelination syndrome:*
  - Results from overly rapid correction of serum sodium in chronic hyponatremia patients
  - It typically occurs 2–6 days after inappropriate sodium correction and presents with severe, often irreversible, neurological deficits. Risk factors include severe hyponatremia (serum sodium <120 mEq/L), alcoholism, liver disease, malnutrition, and concurrent hypokalemia
  - The ideal rate of correction for hyponatremia is 4–6 mEq/L/day for patients at high risk, and it should not go over 8 mEq/L in a 24-hour period
  - Water diuresis may be avoided in patients at risk of abrupt cessation of vasopressin action by administering prophylactic intravenous (IV) desmopressin acetate (DDAVP)
  - When there is overcorrection, free water should be infused, either with or without DDAVP, to bring the serum sodium down to a manageable level

BOX 5: Euvolemic hyponatremia.

- The focus should be on treatment or withdrawal of the underlying cause
- Initial treatment of syndrome of inappropriate antidiuresis (SIAD) includes combined oral furosemide (20 mg twice daily, higher doses for renal insufficiency) and oral salt tablets. Furosemide inhibits the renal countercurrent mechanism and reduces urinary concentrating ability, while salt tablets counteract diuretic-associated natriuresis. However, this approach risks hypokalemia and renal dysfunction, requiring careful titration
- AVP antagonists (vaptans) are highly due to their aquaretic effects. Oral tolvaptan is suitable for persistent SIAD cases (e.g., small cell lung carcinoma) unresponsive to water restriction and/or furosemide and salt tablets

BOX 6: Hypervolemic hyponatremia.

- Water deprivation is the key treatment, but patients excreting minimal electrolyte-free water need aggressive fluid restriction

$$\text{The urine to plasma electrolyte ratio} = \text{urinary } [Na^+] + [K^+]/\text{plasma } [Na^+]$$

- Patients with a ratio >1 should restrict fluids to <500 mL/day, those with a ratio ~1 to 500–700 mL/day, and those with a ratio <1 to <1 L/day
- In hypokalemic patients, potassium replacement can increase plasma Na^+ concentration
- AVP antagonists (vaptans) are highly effective in hypervolemic hyponatremia due to heart failure or cirrhosis, reliably increasing plasma Na^+ concentration due to their "aquaretic" effects (augmentation of free water clearance)

BOX 7: Key points.

- Lower the sodium and the faster the fall, more symptomatic a patient will become
- *Rule of 6:* "Six in six hours for severe symptoms and then stop" implies that if you need to rapidly increase serum sodium due to a neurologic emergency do not correct >6 mmol
- For hypovolemic hyponatremia, the priority is to restore adequate circulating volume
- For hypervolemic hyponatremia, the priority is sodium restriction, water restriction, and diuretics
- For euvolemic, management should concentrate on preventing worsening hyponatremia
- *Rule of 100:* During correction if urine output >100 cc/h, send STAT urine osmolarity and sodium, if urine osmolarity <100, consider 1 µg DDAVP IV. This is to prevent overcorrection and prevent demyelination
- Ascertain the cause of hyponatremia
- Correcting hypokalemia helps improve hyponatremia

BOX 8: Hypernatremia.

Hypernatremia is defined as an increase in the plasma Na + concentration to >145 mEq/L

Causes of hypernatremia:
- *Inadequate water intake:* Decreased thirst perception
- *Excessive water loss:* Renal losses, extrarenal losses
- *Hypertonic sodium gain:* Sodium ingestion
- *Redistribution of water:* Shift of water out of cells
- *Endocrine disorders:* Primary hyperaldosteronism
- *Medications:* Diuretics, lithium, and anticholinergic medications

Symptoms:
- Intense thirst (polydipsia)
- *Neurological manifestations:* Restlessness, irritability, confusion, agitation, and seizure
- Decreased urination
- Dry mucus membranes
- Orthostatic hypotension
- Weakness and fatigue
- Nausea and vomiting
- Hyperthermia

Diagnosis:
- Obtain a detailed history to identify potential risk factors
- Assess the patient's fluid intake, including oral and IV sources
- Evaluate for signs and symptoms, such as increased thirst, altered mental status, weakness, lethargy, or seizures
- *Measurement of serum sodium levels:* >145 mEq/L
- *Assessment of volume status:* Hypovolemic, euvolemic, and hypervolemic hypernatremia
- Laboratory tests, including BUN and creatinine, can aid in evaluating renal function
- *Urine osmolality and urine sodium:*
  - Urine osmolality and urine sodium levels are crucial for further differentiation
  - High urine osmolality (>600 mOsm/kg) suggests that the kidneys are conserving water, indicating appropriate response to hypernatremia
  - Low urine osmolality suggests impaired urinary concentrating ability, which can occur in diabetes insipidus (DI) or certain renal disorders
  - Urine sodium levels can help differentiate between renal and extrarenal causes of water loss

Water deficit calculation: Estimate the TBW deficit to determine the amount of water needed for correction

$$\text{Water deficit (L)} = \text{TBW} \times [1 - 140/\text{serum Na}]$$

$$\text{Total body water} = 0.6 \times \text{Weight}$$

BOX 9: Identification of underlying causes.

- *Hypovolemic hypernatremia:* Often due to water loss from the body (e.g., diarrhea, excessive sweating). Replace water deficits and address ongoing losses
- *Euvolemic hypernatremia:* It can be seen in DI or primary polydipsia. Distinguish between these conditions using water deprivation tests, urine osmolality, and response to desmopressin
- *Hypervolemic hypernatremia:* Typically due to sodium gain, often associated with underlying renal or endocrine disorders. Treat the underlying condition and restrict sodium intake

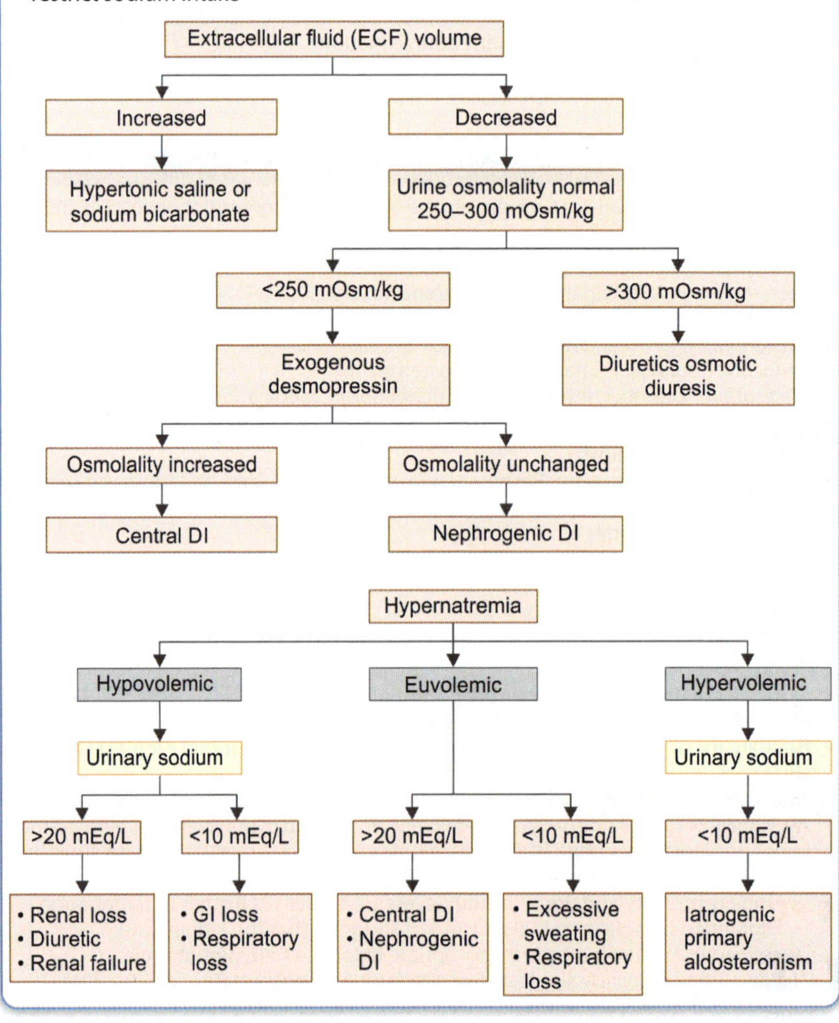

BOX 10: Treatment.

- *Estimate TBW:* 50% of body weight in women and 60% in men

$$\text{Calculate free water deficit: } [(Na^+ - 140)/140] \times TBW$$

- Administer deficit over 48–72 hours, without decrease in plasma Na^+ concentration by >10 mM/24 h
- Ideally, water should be given orally or through a nasogastric tube without electrolytes
- Alternatively, patients can receive free water via IV solutions containing dextrose, such as 5% dextrose; blood glucose levels should be monitored to avoid hyperglycemia
- It is necessary to calculate the urinary electrolyte free water clearance to estimate and replenish the daily loss of free water in patients with nephrogenic diabetes insipidus (NDI) or central DI

Free water clearance = Urine volume × [1(urine sodium + urine potassium)/plasma sodium]

Hypovolemic hypernatremia: Fluid replacement with hypotonic saline and free water by mouth

Euvolemic hypernatremia: Free water replacement by mouth with IV 5% dextrose with vasopressin for central DI

Hypervolemic hypernatremia: Diuresis, dialysis if required

BOX 11: Key points.

- Hypernatremia is a disorder of water metabolism, not sodium homeostasis. As such, the high Na^+ (>145 mEq/L) is secondary to a free water deficit
- The organ that is most adversely affected is the brain, because as its volume shrinks, vessels coming from the inner surface of the skull become stretched and thus they may rupture, leading to focal intracerebral and subarachnoid hemorrhages
- In acute cases, correction should not exceed more rapidly than 1–2 mEq/L/h
- 50% of the water deficit in the first 12–24 hours and the rest over the next 24 hours
- Measure electrolytes every 2 hours during correction to adjust the rate of correction to avoid cerebral edema
- In patients with chronic hypernatremia, one should not permit the plasma sodium (PNa) to fall by >8 mmol/L/24 h
- In asymptomatic chronic hypernatremia, the correction should not exceed 0.5 mEq/L/h, and not >10 mEq/L over 24 hours

POTASSIUM DISORDERS

BOX 12: Introduction.

Homeostatic mechanisms maintain plasma K^+ concentration between 3.5 and 5.0 mM, despite marked variation in dietary K^+ intake

BOX 13: Hypokalemia.

Serum potassium concentration of <3.5 mEq/L

Causes of hypokalemia	***Details***
Abnormal losses	Medications: Diuretics, laxatives, corticosteroids Gastrointestinal losses Renal losses: Osmotic diuresis, mineralocorticoid excess, renal tubular acidosis, polydipsia, intrinsic renal transport defects, hypomagnesemia, and dialysis/plasmapheresis
Transcellular shifts	Medications: Insulin overdose, beta-2 sympathomimetics, decongestants Alkalosis, refeeding syndrome, increased beta-2 adrenergic stimulation, etc.
Inadequate intake	Anorexia, dementia, starvation, total parenteral nutrition
Pseudohypokalemia	Delayed sample analysis, significant leukocytosis
Laboratory analysis	***Details***
Serum potassium Measurement	Diagnosis confirmation with repeat serum potassium measurement
Other laboratory tests	Includes serum glucose and magnesium levels, urine electrolyte and creatinine levels, and assessment of acid–base balance
Evaluation of urinary Potassium excretion	*24-hour timed urine potassium collection:* Normal excretion is 15–30 mEq/L (15–30 mmol/L) per day. *Urine potassium to creatinine ratio from a spot urine specimen:* Ratio >1.5 mEq/mmol (13 mEq/g) indicates renal potassium wasting
Assessment of thyroid and adrenal function	Consideration if initial workup does not identify a cause
Electrocardiogram findings	***Details***
Manifestations on electrocardiogram (ECG)	• Decreased T-wave amplitude is typical • Progression to ST interval depression, T wave inversions, PR interval prolongation, and U waves **(Fig. 1)**
Arrhythmias associated with hypokalemia	• Sinus bradycardia, ventricular tachycardia or fibrillation, and torsade de pointes
Reliability of ECG findings	• ECG changes and arrhythmias are not always present, even in severe hypokalemia

Contd...

Contd...

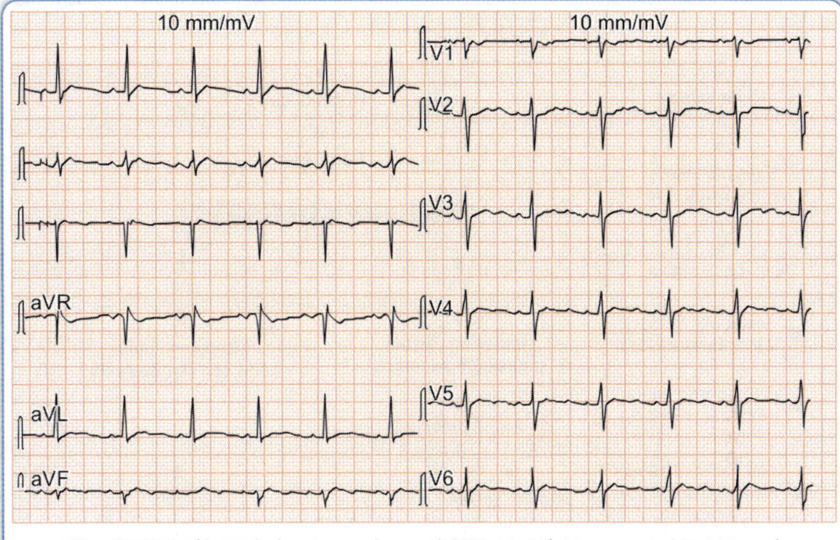

Fig. 1: ECG of hypokalemia; prolonged QT interval, U waves in V1–V6, and flattened t waves.

BOX 14: Evaluation of hypokalemia.

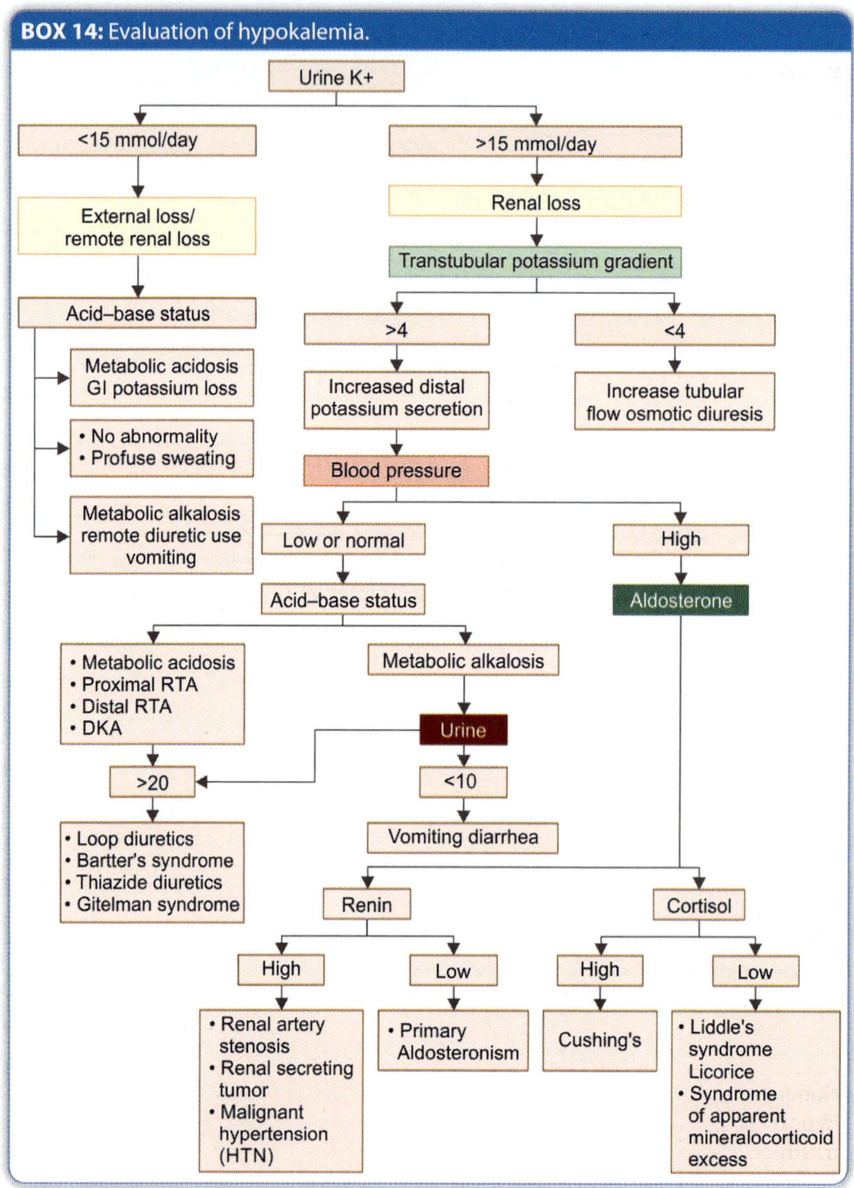

BOX 15: Treatment of hypokalemia.

Treatment approach	*Details*
Immediate goal	Prevention of potentially life-threatening cardiac conduction disturbances and neuromuscular dysfunction by raising serum potassium to a safe level
Target serum potassium level	Patients with a history of congestive heart failure or myocardial infarction should maintain a serum potassium concentration of at least 4 mEq/L (4 mmol/L)
Monitoring during treatment	Careful monitoring due to the risk of hyperkalemia from supplemental potassium, especially in hospitalized patients. Risk of rebound hyperkalemia is higher in redistributive hypokalemia
Estimation of potassium deficit	Serum potassium drops approximately 0.3 mEq/L (0.3 mmol/L) for every 100 mEq (100 mmol) reduction in total body potassium
Treatment strategies	Stopping or reducing the dosage of diuretics. Use of angiotensin-converting enzyme (ACE) inhibitors, angiotensin II receptor blockers (ARBs), beta blockers, or potassium-sparing diuretics if indicated to treat a comorbid condition. Dietary potassium increases, although effectiveness is limited due to coupling with phosphate in food; supplemental potassium chloride is preferred
Intravenous potassium administration	Reserved for severe hypokalemia, hypokalemic ECG changes, physical signs or symptoms of hypokalemia, or for those unable to tolerate oral form. Rapid correction is possible with oral potassium; combining oral and IV administration for fastest results
Standard intravenous administration	20–40 mmol of potassium in 1 L of normal saline. Correction should not exceed 20 mmol/h, continuous cardiac monitoring if rate exceeds 10 mmol/h. Dosing in children is 0.5–1.0 mmol/L/kg over 1 hour (maximum of 40 mmol). Avoid potassium in dextrose-containing solutions due to potential exacerbation of hypokalemia
Nonurgent hypokalemia treatment	40–100 mmol of oral potassium per day over days to weeks. For prevention in patients with persistent losses, 20 mmol/day is usually sufficient

BOX 16: Key points.

- Major components for the diagnostic evaluation of hypokalemia:
  - Assessment of urinary potassium excretion to distinguish renal potassium losses from other causes of hypokalemia (e.g., gastrointestinal losses, transcellular potassium shifts)
  - Assessment of acid–base status as majority cases of hypokalemia are associated with metabolic alkalosis or metabolic acidosis
- Every 1 mEq/L decrease in serum potassium represents a potassium deficit of approximately 200–400 mEq
- In patients with renal impairment, potassium should be very cautiously replaced
- 0.9% sodium chloride is the preferred infusion fluid, as 5% glucose may cause transcellular shift of potassium into cells
- It is essential to correct the levels of serum magnesium, to achieve an adequate treatment of hypokalemia

BOX 17: Hyperkalemia.

Serum potassium concentration above 5.0 mEq/L.

Clinical presentation:

The symptoms of hyperkalemia can vary depending on the severity and rate of rise in serum potassium levels. They can include:

- Muscle weakness or paralysis
- Fatigue
- Paresthesia
- Cardiac arrhythmias (e.g., bradycardia, ventricular fibrillation, and asystole)
- Nausea and vomiting

BOX 18: Diagnosis.

- Serum potassium measurement
- *Electrocardiogram findings:*
  - Characteristic changes may include peaked T waves
  - Prolonged PR interval
  - Widened QRS complex, and in severe cases
  - Sine wave pattern leading to cardiac arrest **(Figs. 2 and 3)**
- Assessing underlying causes through history, physical examination, additional tests
- For example, renal function tests, blood gas analysis, and hormone levels

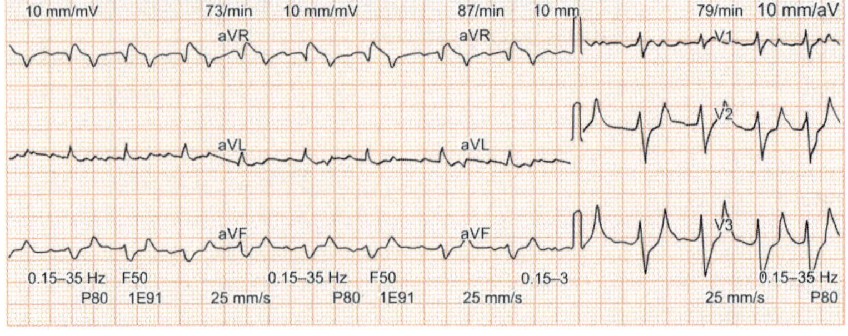

Fig. 2: ECG hyperkalemia, prolonged PR, short QT, and peaked T waves.

Contd...

Contd...

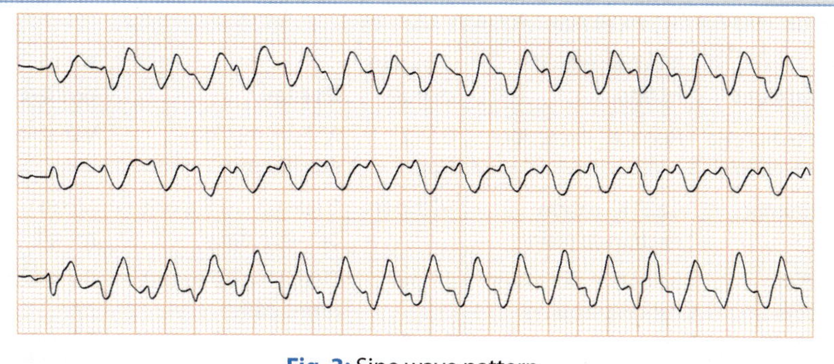

Fig. 3: Sine wave pattern.

BOX 19: Causes.

Causes of hyperkalemia	*Details*
Impaired excretion	Acute/chronic kidney disease: Medications like ACE inhibitors, nonsteroidal anti-inflammatory drugs (NSAIDs), potassium-sparing diuretics, etc.
Transcellular shifts	Insulin deficiency/resistance, acidosis, hypertonicity, hyperglycemia, etc.
Increased intake	Potassium supplementation, high potassium foods, salt substitutes, penicillin G potassium, etc.
Pseudohyperkalemia	Hemolysis, tourniquet use, fist clenching, blood sample cooling, etc.

BOX 20: Treatment in emergency cases.

Treatment	*Mechanism of action*	*Onset of action*	*Duration*	*Dosage*	*K^+ removed*
Calcium gluconate	Antagonizes cardiac conduction abnormalities	0–5 minutes	1 hour	IV: Calcium gluconate 10%, 5–30 mL or calcium chloride 5%, 5–30 mL	None
Sodium bicarbonate	Distributes K^+ into cells	15–30 minutes	1–2 hours	IV: $NaHCO_3$, 50–100 mEq	None
Insulin	Distributes K^+ into cells	15–60 minutes	4–6 hours	IV: Regular insulin, 5–10 units, plus glucose 50%, 25 g	None
Salbutamol	Distributes K^+ into cells	15–30 minutes	2–4 hours	Nebulized Salbutamol, 10–20 mg in 4 mL normal saline, inhaled over 10 minutes	None

Contd...

Contd...

Treatment for maintenance/excretory therapy:				
Treatment	***Mechanism of action***	***Onset of action***	***Dosage***	***K^+ removed***
Loop diuretic (furosemide)	Renal K^+ excretion	0.5–2 hours	IV: Furosemide, 40–160 mg	Variable
Patiromer	$Ca2^+$ K^+ cation exchange resin	~7 hours	Oral: 4.2–16.8 g once or twice daily	Mean 0.75 mEq/L
Sodium zirconium cyclosilicate	Selective potassium cation trapping agent	1 hour	Oral: 10 g up to three times daily	0.7 mEq/L per 10 g dose
Sodium polystyrene sulfonate (Kayexalate)	Ion exchange resin binds K^+	1–3 hours	Oral: 15–60 g in 20% sorbitol (60–240 mL) Rectal: 30–60 g in 20% sorbitol	0.5–1 mEq/g resin
Hemodialysis	Extracorporeal K^+ removal	1–8 hours	As per requirement	25–50 mEq/h

BOX 21: Key points.

- Hyperkalemia is a potentially life-threatening illness that can be difficult to diagnose because of a paucity of distinctive signs and symptoms
- Hyperkalemia is suggested in any patient with a predisposition toward elevated potassium level such as renal diseases, trauma, and postoperative patients
- The aggressiveness of therapy for hyperkalemia is directly related to the rapidity with which the condition has developed, the absolute level of serum potassium, and the evidence of toxicity
- Continuous ECG monitoring with frequent vital sign checks is the key
- Definitive therapy is dialysis in patients with renal failure or when pharmacologic therapy is not sufficient
- Any patient with significantly elevated potassium levels should undergo dialysis, as pharmacologic therapy alone is not likely to adequately bring down the potassium levels in a timely fashion

CALCIUM DISORDERS

BOX 22: Introduction.

Extracellular calcium concentrations are maintained within an exquisitely narrow range through a series of feedback mechanisms that involve parathyroid hormone (PTH) and the active vitamin D metabolite 1,25-dihydroxyvitamin D [1,25(OH)2D]

BOX 23: Hypocalcemia.

Serum calcium concentrations <8.5 mg/dL (2.12 mmol/L)

Causes:

Low PTH levels (hypoparathyroidism):
- Parathyroid agenesis
- DiGeorge syndrome
- Parathyroid destruction Surgical Radiation
- Infiltration by metastases or systemic diseases
- Autoimmune
- Reduced parathyroid function Hypomagnesemia Autosomal dominant hypocalcemia

High PTH levels (secondary hyperparathyroidism):
- Vitamin D deficiency
- Vitamin D resistance
- PTH resistance syndromes
- Calcium chelators
- Inhibitors of bone resorption (bisphosphonates and plicamycin)
- Altered vitamin D metabolism (phenytoin, ketoconazole)

Miscellaneous causes:
- Acute pancreatitis
- Hungry bone syndrome after parathyroidectomy

Clinical presentation:

The clinical manifestations of hypocalcemia vary depending on the severity and rapidity of onset. Symptoms may include:
- *Neuromuscular:* Tetany, muscle cramps, paresthesia, seizures, and Chvostek's and Trousseau's signs
- *Cardiac:* Arrhythmias, prolongation of QT interval, and heart failure **(Fig. 4)**
- *Neurological:* Confusion, depression, and hallucinations
- *Dermatological:* Dry skin, brittle nails, and hair

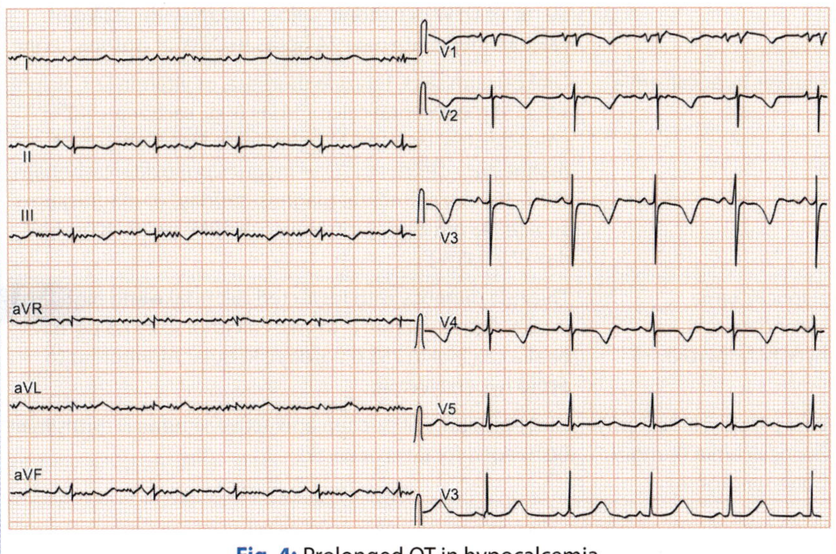

Fig. 4: Prolonged QT in hypocalcemia.

BOX 24: Diagnostic approach.

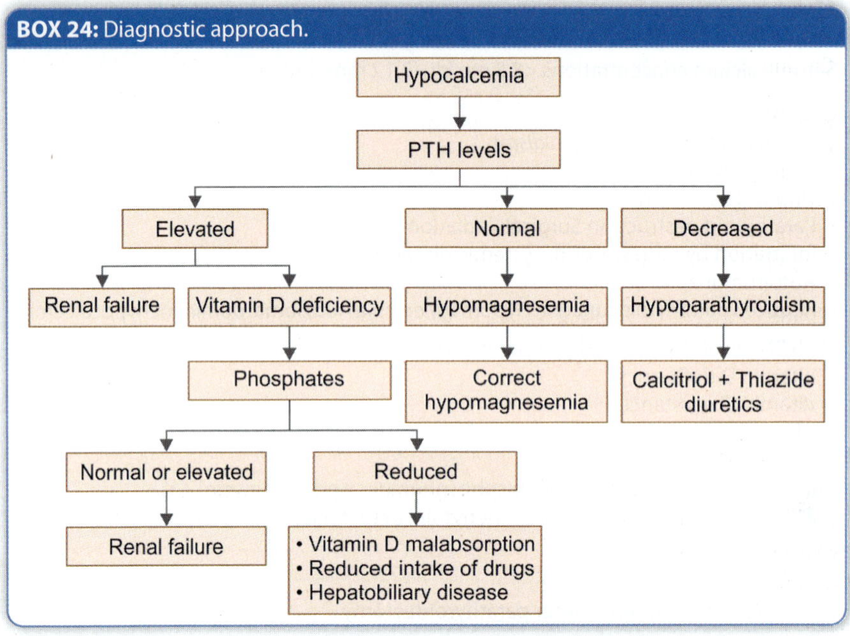

BOX 25: Management.

Condition	***Treatment***
Severe and symptomatic hypocalcemia	Correct acute respiratory alkalosis (if possible). Functional cause: CO_2 retention (e.g., breathing into a paper bag). Intravenous bolus: Calcium gluconate (10 mL of 10% weight/volume solution, 2.2 mmol) in 50 mL of D5W or isotonic saline. Follow with 1224 g of calcium gluconate over 24 hours in D5W or isotonic saline
Chronic hypocalcemia	Oral calcium salts, thiazide diuretics, or vitamin D. Calcium salts: 14 g elemental calcium/day (e.g., carbonate 40%, chloride 36%, lactate 12%, gluconate 8%). Concurrent magnesium deficiency: Oral magnesium oxide/carbonate (100–300 mg elemental magnesium/day) or magnesium sulfate [48 mmol/day intramuscular (IM) or 20–40 mmol/day IV in D5W]
Hypocalcemia secondary to hypoparathyroidism	Thiazide diuretics with restricted salt intake and high fluid intake. Active vitamin D forms: Calcitriol (0.251.5 µg/day) or alfa calcidol (0.253.0 µg/day). Regular monitoring to avoid hypercalcemia
Post parathyroidectomy hypocalcemia (hungry bone syndrome)	Large amounts of calcium and active vitamin D forms may be needed for days or weeks

BOX 26: Key points.

- Calcium gluconate is generally preferred over calcium chloride as it is less likely to cause tissue necrosis if extravasation occurs. Alkaline solutions like bicarbonate and phosphorus-containing solutions should be avoided through the same IV to prevent the precipitation of calcium salts
- Checking an ECG and aggressively correcting calcium levels in these situations is imperative
- The first part of the evaluation should focus on confirming the hypocalcemia by checking a serum albumin level to correct the total calcium or directly measuring the ionized calcium level. For each 1 g/dL decrease in albumin <4 g/dL, 0.8 mg/dL should be added to the total serum calcium level
- Serum magnesium should be corrected before correcting hypocalcemia when hypomagnesemia suspected
- Hypocalcemia due to vitamin D deficiency cannot be corrected unless vitamin D is repleted first

BOX 27: Hypercalcemia.

Hypercalcemia is typically defined as a serum calcium concentration above 10.5 mg/dL

Causes:

Excessive PTH production:

- Primary hyperparathyroidism (adenoma, hyperplasia, rarely carcinoma)
- Tertiary hyperparathyroidism (long-term stimulation of PTH secretion in renal insufficiency)
- Ectopic PTH secretion (very rare)
- Alterations in CaSR function (lithium therapy)
- Overproduction of parathyroid hormone-related protein (PTHrP) (many solid tumors)

Excessive 1,25(OH)2D production:

- Granulomatous diseases (sarcoidosis, tuberculosis, and silicosis)
- Lymphomas
- Vitamin D intoxication
- Hyperthyroidism
- Immobilization

Excessive calcium intake:

- Milk alkali syndrome

Others:

- Familial hypocalciuric hypercalcemia (FHH)

Symptoms of hypercalcemia: Symptoms can vary depending on the severity and the rate at which calcium levels increase. They are often remembered by the mnemonic "stones, bones, abdominal groans, thrones, and psychiatric overtones":

- *Stones:* Kidney stones due to high levels of calcium in the urine
- *Bones:* Bone pain and fragility fractures due to calcium being leached from bones
- *Abdominal groans:* Gastrointestinal symptoms such as nausea, vomiting, constipation, and abdominal pain
- *Thrones:* Polyuria and polydipsia due to the nephrogenic DI effect
- *Psychiatric overtones:* Cognitive dysfunction, including confusion, lethargy, depression, and, in severe cases, coma

BOX 28: Diagnosis.

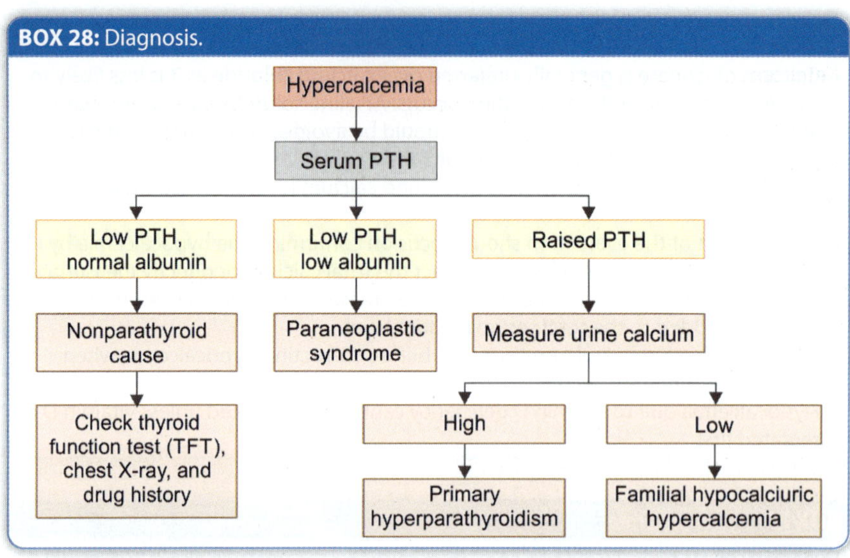

BOX 29: Treatment.

Therapeutic approach	***Details***
Hydration to restore euvolemia	• Hydration with normal saline to correct ECF deficit due to nausea, vomiting, and polyuria. Bolus infusion of 0.9% sodium chloride, followed by 34 L over 24–48 hours • *Initial rate:* 200–300 mL/h, adjusted to maintain urine output at 100–150 mL/h. Caution in patients with compromised cardiovascular or renal function
Inhibition of bone resorption	• *Preferred treatment:* Denosumab 120 mg SC, repeated 1, 2, and 4 weeks later, then monthly • *Alternative:* Nitrogen-containing bisphosphonates (e.g., zoledronic acid 4 mg IV over 15 minutes, repeatable every 7 days and then every 34 weeks; Pamidronate 60–90 mg IV over 24 hours). Salmon calcitonin for rapid effect (IM or SC, 48 IU/kg, repeat every 6–12 hours for 48–72 hours)
Calciuresis	If PTHrP or PTH is suspected: Loop diuretic (e.g., furosemide 20–40 mg IV) after rehydration Monitor for low potassium or worsening kidney function
Glucocorticoids	Decrease GI calcium absorption and increase urine calcium excretion. • *Initial:* Hydrocortisone 200–400 mg IV over 24 hours for 35 days. Chronic: Oral prednisone 20–40 mg/day or higher, if necessary • *Caution:* Hyperglycemia, altered mental status, hypertension, myopathy, infection, bone loss, and avascular necrosis

Contd...

Contd...

Ketoconazole	Inhibits 1,25(OH)2D production in granulomatous diseases and inactivating CYP24A1 variants. May be used alone or with lower doses of glucocorticoids
CaSR agonism (calcimimetics)	Cinacalcet to increase CaSR sensitivity and reduce PTH secretion (30 mg twice daily, up to 90 mg four times daily). Can be combined with bisphosphonates or denosumab
Dialysis	• Reserved for severely hypercalcemic patients refractory to other therapies or with renal insufficiency • Effective in removing ionized calcium from ECF (peritoneal or hemodialysis)
Mobilization	Rapid mobilization advised. Continued antiresorptive treatment if mobilization is not possible
Address underlying disorder	After managing the acute episode, focus on treating the underlying hypercalcemic disorder

BOX 30: Key points.

- The key in management of hypercalcemia is to determine the etiology
- Treatment of hypercalcemia not only involves practicing evidence-based medicine but also completing a targeted diagnostic approach to practice cost-effective patient-centered care
- Patients need to alter their lifestyle and diet to prevent the worsening of hypercalcemia, and this may involve some education on the part of the physician or possibly a dietician
- In addition to treatment, follow-up is equally as important to allow for long-term management of the patient's condition

MAGNESIUM DISORDERS

BOX 31: Introduction.

Magnesium is an essential mineral involved in numerous biochemical processes, including muscle and nerve function, protein synthesis, and the regulation of blood pressure and glucose levels. Magnesium disorders primarily manifest as either hypomagnesemia (low serum magnesium) or hypermagnesemia (high serum magnesium)

BOX 32: Hypomagnesemia

Hypomagnesemia is defined as a serum magnesium concentration <1.7 mg/dL (0.7 mmol/L)

Causes:
Inadequate intake:
- Poor dietary intake
- Chronic alcoholism

Increased losses:
- *Gastrointestinal losses:*
  - Diarrhea
  - *Malabsorption:* Conditions like celiac disease, Crohn's disease, and ulcerative colitis
  - Bowel resection
- *Renal losses:*
  - Diuretics: Certain diuretics, especially loop and thiazide diuretics, can increase renal excretion of magnesium
  - Hyperaldosteronism
  - Bartter syndrome
  - Gitelman syndrome
- *Shift into cells:*
  - Refeeding syndrome
  - Acute pancreatitis
  - *Medications:*
    - Proton pump inhibitors (PPIs)
    - Aminoglycosides
    - Cisplatin

BOX 33: Clinical presentation.

- *Neuromuscular symptoms:*
  - Muscle weakness
  - Cramps and spasms
- *Tremors:*
  - Tetany (severe, sustained muscle contraction)
  - Seizures
  - Paresthesia (tingling or numbness)
- *Cardiovascular symptoms:*
  - Arrhythmias (e.g., atrial fibrillation, ventricular tachycardia, torsades de pointes)
  - Hypertension
- *Metabolic symptoms:*
  - Hypokalemia (low potassium levels)
  - Hypocalcemia (low calcium levels)

Diagnosis:
- *Serum magnesium measurement:* Low magnesium levels with serum concentrations <1.7 mg/dL
- *Additional tests:*
  - Serum calcium and potassium levels to assess associated electrolyte disturbances
  - Renal function tests to evaluate kidney function
  - ECG to detect arrhythmias

BOX 34: Management.

Treatment of hypomagnesemia depends on the severity and underlying cause

- *Mild hypomagnesemia:*
  - *Oral magnesium supplements:* Magnesium oxide, magnesium gluconate, or magnesium chloride
- *Severe or symptomatic hypomagnesemia:*
  - *Intravenous magnesium sulfate:* Used in cases of severe deficiency or when rapid correction is necessary
- *Addressing underlying causes:*
  - *Dietary modification:* Increase intake of magnesium-rich foods
  - Adjusting medications
  - *Treating associated conditions:* Managing chronic diarrhea, malabsorption syndromes, or correcting other electrolyte imbalances

Prevention:

- Adequate dietary intake of magnesium
- Avoiding excessive alcohol consumption
- Careful use of diuretics and other medications that can cause magnesium loss
- Regular monitoring of serum magnesium in patients with chronic conditions or on long-term medications that affect magnesium level

BOX 35: Hypermagnesemia.

Serum magnesium concentrations exceeding 2.5 mg/dL (1.05 mmol/L)

Causes:

- *Excessive magnesium intake*
- *Decreased excretion:*
  - Impaired renal function
  - *Addison's disease:* Impaired magnesium excretion
  - *Certain medications:* Drugs like ACE inhibitors, ARBs, and potassium-sparing diuretics can interfere with renal magnesium excretion
- *Other causes:* Tumor lysis syndrome

Clinical presentation:

- Mild to moderate hypermagnesemia may present with symptoms such as nausea, vomiting, flushing, lethargy, and weakness
- Severe hypermagnesemia can lead to loss of deep tendon reflexes, muscle paralysis, respiratory depression, hypotension, bradycardia, and cardiac arrest

BOX 36: Diagnosis of hypermagnesemia.

- *Serum magnesium measurement:* Confirm elevated serum magnesium levels (>2.5 mg/dL)
- *Additional tests:* ECG to detect cardiac effects, renal function tests to assess kidney function

BOX 37: Management of hypermagnesemia.

- Discontinue magnesium sources
- *Enhance elimination:*
  - Administer IV fluids to increase urine output and promote renal magnesium excretion
  - Consider loop diuretics (e.g., furosemide) to enhance magnesium excretion
- *Antagonize magnesium effects:*
  - Intravenous calcium gluconate: It counteracts the effects of magnesium on neuromuscular and cardiac function
- *Hemodialysis:*
  - In severe cases or when renal function is compromised, hemodialysis may be necessary to remove excess magnesium from the bloodstream

SUGGESTED READING

1. Johnson RJ, Floege J, Tonelli M (Eds). Comprehensive Clinical Nephrology. Elsevier Health Sciences; 2023.
2. Loscalzoj J, Fauci A, Kasper D, Hauser S, Longo D, Jameson JL (Eds). Harrison's Principles of Internal Medicine 21st edition. McGraw Hill; 2022.
3. UpToDate. Fluid and electrolytes. [online] Available from https://www.uptodate.com/contents/table-of-contents/endocrinology-and-diabetes/fluid-and-electrolytes [Last accessed September, 2024].

CHAPTER 9

Hematological Emergencies

Balkrishna P Padate

BOX 1: Massive hemorrhage and massive blood transfusion: bleeding patient presenting to emergency.

- *Massive bleeding:* Defined as the loss of more than one blood volume within 24 hours, 50% of the patient's total blood volume in <3 hours, or bleeding exceeding 150 mL/min
- *Massive blood transfusion:* Involves replacing one blood volume or more within 24 hours, administering 10 or more units of packed red blood cells (PRBCs) in 24 hours or replacing over 50% blood volume in 4 hours
- Hemorrhage necessitating massive transfusion due to trauma is discussed in the trauma section
- Secure intravenous (IV) access and initiate resuscitation in the casualty room
- Minimize the use of crystalloids in treating massive hemorrhage
- Begin packed red cell transfusions early to prevent pulmonary edema, coagulopathy, acidosis, and poor tissue perfusion in patients with ongoing hemorrhage
- Quickly identify the cause of bleeding
- Administer tranexamic acid promptly
- Utilize damage control surgery and interventional radiology to manage bleeding
- Implement the massive hemorrhage protocol (MHP), which ensures rapid delivery of predetermined, fixed ratio blood components and products at the bedside. Modern MHPs aim to mimic whole blood by providing a ratio of one unit of plasma: one unit of platelets: one unit of red blood cells
- Plasma, platelets, and fibrinogen supplementation should be based on early and frequent assessment of coagulation parameters, including fibrinogen concentration and platelet count. Frequency of these measurements should correspond to the rate of bleeding and resource availability, with hourly checks being a reasonable starting point
- Check for a history of anticoagulant and antiplatelet consumption
- Early administration of tranexamic acid (TXA) improves outcomes in traumatically injured patients
- In massively bleeding trauma patients, fibrinogen levels drop to critically low levels shortly after injury
- Ensure adequate fibrinogen replacement using cryoprecipitate or fibrinogen concentrate to maintain levels of at least 150–200 mg/dL
- Perform baseline laboratory tests [completed blood count (CBC), prothrombin time (PT), international normalized ratio (INR), partial thromboplastin time (PTT), fibrinogen, arterial or venous blood gas, lactate, electrolytes, and ionized calcium] upon presentation and at least hourly to guide transfusion decisions and monitor metabolic abnormalities

Contd...

Contd...

- Clinical urgency will determine whether red blood cell transfusion is done using uncrossmatched emergency type O red blood cells, group-specific red blood cells, or fully crossmatched units. Always obtain and send a pretransfusion blood sample to the blood bank for typing and compatibility testing
- The risk of ABO transfusion errors is high in urgent clinical situations, so patient's identification procedures must be meticulously followed
- Use type O uncrossmatched red blood cells if the patient's blood type is unknown and immediate transfusion is necessary
- Transfuse type O Rh-positive red blood cells to males with no prior history of Rh-positive blood transfusion
- Reserve type O Rh-negative red blood cells for females of child-bearing age, children, and individuals suspected or known to be alloimmunized to the D antigen
- Type-specific uncrossmatched blood can usually be provided within 15 minutes; however, completing an antibody screen and crossmatch can take 30–60 minutes
- In emergency, transfusions started with type O blood, switch to group-specific blood as soon as the patient's blood type is confirmed, and ABO verification is complete
- Use thromboelastography (TEG) guidance in emergencies to determine the administration of blood products

BOX 2: Acute thrombosis (deep vein thrombosis) and pulmonary embolism (Chapter 3.5).

- Thrombosis can result from local obstruction of circulation, embolization of the clot, or consumption of coagulation factors
- Most patients presenting with symptomatic pulmonary embolism (PE) have asymptomatic deep vein thrombosis (DVT) and most patients with symptomatic DVT have asymptomatic PE
- Common symptoms of DVT are leg swelling and pain

Investigations:
- *D-dimer:* Not specific
- Use Wells's score which determines risk of presence of DVT, high Wells's score is associated with >75% risk of DVT or PE
- Review past history of thrombosis, bleeding history and family history of thrombosis
- Check if patient is already on antiplatelets or anticoagulants
- Perform complete blood count (CBC), creatinine, prothrombin time (PT), international normalized ratio (INR), activated partial thromboplastin time (APTT), and D-dimer
- Do ultrasonography (USG) of venous Doppler of both legs
- If creatinine is normal, administer therapeutic dose of low-molecular weight heparin (LMWH)
- Do not wait for thrombophilia tests for treatment of DVT
- Patients with acute DVT need hospital admission

BOX 3: Bleeding on oral anticoagulant therapy.

- In addition to vitamin K antagonists, currently physicians and patients have access to many new oral anticoagulants (NOAC) and antiplatelet agents. Several of these medicines have multiple trade names
- When patients come to emergency with bleeding, it is important to check what medicines they are taking regularly including checking the contents of all medicines
- Check vitals and stabilize as discussed in patient with hemorrhage
- Assess neurology to make sure that there is no intracranial (IC) bleed
- If there is suspicion of IC bleed, get an urgent CT head and neurosurgical review (details in the chapter)
- If there is history of intake of warfarin or acitrom, stop anticoagulant and administer prothrombin complex concentrate (PCC) (Octaplex) 15 units/kg before sending patient for imaging in a suspected case of IC bleed
- If PCC is not available, administer fresh frozen plasmas (FFPs) (15 mL/kg) if volume is acceptable
- Give one dose of 10 mg vitamin K for all patients on warfarin who are bleeding
- Incidence of IC bleed is very high in patients who are on antiplatelet
- If patient presents with bleeding while on new antiplatelet medicine like ticagrelor, prasugrel, administration of platelets even in patients with normal platelet count to arrest the bleeding
- Early administration of tranexamic acid in patients with bleeding while on antiplatelet agents will reduce the blood loss.

Caveat:

- Avoid tranexamic acid in patients with urinary tract bleeding because of potential chances of obstruction
- Based on the symptoms, perform imaging to rule out internal bleeding, e.g., abdominal pain, etc.
- While on warfarin if no clinical bleeding and INR >8, reverse with only vitamin K2 mg one dose
- If no bleeding and international normalized ratio (INR) is <8, just stop warfarin and repeat INR the next day

BOX 4: Thrombocytopenia in emergency.

- Severe thrombocytopenia is a medical emergency
- Severe bleeding is a rare but serious complication of immune thrombocytopenia (ITP)
- Emergency management of thrombocytopenia is similar irrespective the cause of thrombocytopenia
- Severe bleeding like intracranial (IC) bleed in patients with severe thrombocytopenia can be fatal
- As soon as the patient presents, check vitals to make sure that patient is not actively bleeding, not hypotensive, or tachycardic
- Stabilize patient's vital parameters
- Refer this patient to hematologist immediately
- Transfuse platelets [six random donor platelets (RDPs) or one single donor platelets (SDP)] as soon as possible, repeat complete blood count (CBC) after 1 hour to check the increment, increment suggests the possible diagnosis. Patients with no increment after 1 hour are likely suffering from immune thrombocytopenia (ITP) patients
- Check remaining parameters in CBC such as hemoglobin (Hb) and white cell counts (WCCs) to understand the possible diagnosis such as aplastic anemia, leukemia as well as to understand the transfusion needs
- Urgently assess clotting tests such as prothrombin time (PT), international normalized ratio (INR) and activated partial thromboplastin time (APTT). Fibrinogen to make sure that the patient is not in disseminated intravascular coagulation (DIC) or coagulopathy
- Correct clotting of abnormalities with fresh frozen plasma (FFP), cryoprecipitates, and prothrombin complex concentrate (PCC) in a bleeding patient
- In a patient with severe pancytopenia and coagulopathy, we must rule out M3 acute myeloid leukemia (AML) [acute promyelocytic leukemia (APML)] as it has high risk of severe internal bleeding if not treated and DIC not corrected promptly
- Send following investigations: CBC with peripheral smear, PT, INR, APTT, fibrinogen, liver function test, creatinine, phospholipid antibodies, antinuclear antibody (ANA), and idiopathic pulmonary fibrosis (IPF)
- Advise admission
- If ITP is a possible diagnosis, consider intravenously immunoglobulin (IVIG) infusion and methylprednisolone (after consultation with a hematologist)
- Based on the CBC findings, patient might need a bone marrow assessment and treatment in addition to treatment offered to increase platelet number

BOX 5: Anemia in emergency.

- Anemia is a widespread issue globally, often presenting with nonspecific symptoms
- The primary focus during the emergency assessment of anemia is to determine if the condition is acute or chronic. Acute anemia is typically linked to blood loss, and patients usually exhibit symptoms. Conversely, chronic anemia is generally well-tolerated and often found incidentally, even when hemoglobin levels are significantly low
- The severity of anemia influences clinical outcomes, especially in critically ill patients; however, the precise transfusion threshold remains uncertain. It is crucial to check for active bleeding and stabilize the patient's vital signs if bleeding is present
- If a drop in hemoglobin is due to acute bleeding, consult a gastroenterologist and an interventional radiologist to manage the bleeding. Adhere to the severe bleeding protocol in cases of bleeding secondary to acute hemorrhage. Additionally, take a thorough medical history to determine if the patient is using anticoagulants or antiplatelets
  - Order investigations such as complete blood count (CBC) with peripheral smear, lactate dehydrogenase (LDH), reticulocyte count, direct Coomb's test (DCT), iron studies, ferritin, B12 level, red cell folate level, liver function test, creatinine, stool occult blood, abdominal and pelvic sonography
  - Some patients may need a bone marrow examination when suitable to understand the cause of anemia
  - In an emergency, transfuse packed red blood cells (PRBCs) as per massive hemorrhage protocol.
- *Caveat:* Crossmatched PRBCs can be transfused safely in an emergency in case of hemolytic anemia

BOX 6: Admission criteria for nonemergent anemia.

- Developing cardiac symptoms, such as shortness of breath or chest pain or neurological symptoms
- Initial unexplained hemoglobin values <8–10 g/dL (also these values further depend on associated comorbidities and symptoms)
- Hematocrit <25–35%

SUGGESTED READING

1. Provan D, Baglin TP, Dokal I, De Vos J. Oxford Handbook of Clinical Haematology. 4th ed. Oxford University Press; 2015.
2. Wilkinson IB, Kelly D, Wiles K, McGurgan I, Raine T, Hateley P. Oxford Handbook of Clinical Medicine. 11th ed. Oxford University Press; 2024.

SUGGESTED READING

SECTION 2

Trauma

CHAPTER 10

Trauma Overview

Sachna P Shetty, Sandeep A Seth

BOX 1: General approach to trauma.

The correct sequence of priorities for assessment of a multiply injured patient in an emergency room is:

- Preparation before arrival:
  - To check the availability of resuscitation material for trauma
  - Ready the laboratory, radiology, and appropriate medical personnel
- Triaging of the patient
- Primary survey **(Box 2)**
- Adjuncts to primary survey and resuscitation **(Box 3)**
- Secondary survey **(Box 4)**
- Adjuncts to secondary survey **(Box 5)**
- Reevaluation and definitive care
- Mechanism of injury is important to identify injuries **(Box 6)**
- Reassessment is important
- Records and legalities (*See* Chapter 47: Medico-legal Queries with the Expert)

BOX 2: Primary survey.

(Rapid identification and management of immediate life-threatening injuries) and adjuncts	
A. *Airway and cervical spine stabilization*	• Assess, clear, and protect the airway: Perform a jaw thrust and chin lift (if a cervical spine fracture is not suspected), and suction as needed **(Figs. 1 and 2)**. Always maintain cervical spine alignment throughout these procedures (refer to Chapter 12.4) • If the airway is compromised: – Interventions include: - Perform endotracheal intubation with inline stabilization for patients with a low Glasgow Coma Scale (GCS) • If endotracheal intubation is difficult, perform a surgical airway *Caveat:* • Any patient with a head injury and low GCS, or those with a mechanism of injury indicating potential spinal injury, requires cervical neck stabilization techniques (as shown in **Figure 1**)

Contd...

Contd...

(Rapid identification and management of immediate life-threatening injuries) and adjuncts	
B. *Breathing*	*Monitor:* Track oxygen saturation and respiratory rate • *Inspect the neck and thorax:* Check for indicators such as a deviated trachea, open chest wounds, unusual chest wall movement, and crepitus in the neck or chest regions • Auscultate for breath sounds, paying close attention to the presence or absence of breath sounds on one side of the chest Interventions at this level include: • Provide appropriate oxygen or perform intubation/surgical airway as necessary • Consider immediate needle thoracostomy, if tension pneumothorax suspected • If hemopneumothorax is suspected, consider tube thoracostomy
C. *Circulation (Chapter 11: Trauma part B)*	• Assess blood volume status by checking: – Radial, femoral, and carotid pulses – Blood pressure – Skin color and capillary refill • Interventions for blood volume assessment include: – Place two large bore peripheral IV catheters – If peripheral sites are unavailable, consider external jugular vein, central venous, or intraosseous access – Rapidly administer warm crystalloid solution unless contraindicated – Apply direct pressure to control external bleeding – For suspected pericardial tamponade, consider pericardiocentesis – For abdominal or pelvic trauma, consider EFAST (*See* Chapter 12.3) (Extended Focused Assessment with Sonography in Trauma) and possibly laparotomy – Administer blood products according to the class of shock (*See* Chapter 9)
Caveat	In late trimester pregnancy consider lateral decubitus position (left side)
D. *Disability*	• Perform a neurological and mental status examination, assessing: – Pupil size and reactivity – Lateralizing signs and spinal cord level injury – Limb power assessment – Glasgow Coma Scale score (refer Chapter 6.6) – Measure blood glucose levels in patients with altered mental status
E. *Exposure*	• Expose the patient fully for a thorough inspection • Log roll the patient, maintaining a neutral position and inline neck stabilization, to inspect and palpate the thoracic spine, flank, back, and buttocks

Contd...

Contd...

(Rapid identification and management of immediate life-threatening injuries) and adjuncts	
Adjuncts	Monitor: • Pulse oximetry and blood pressure • Urinary output (checking for hematuria) and gastric catheter (for distension/bleeding) • Arterial blood gas (ABG) levels, lactate, base deficit, and CO_2 levels • Use X-ray examinations (e.g., chest and pelvis), EFAST, and whole body CT with or without contrast as necessary
Caveat	• Airway management in trauma: – There are no definitive guidelines for tracheal intubation in trauma. Early intubation is generally recommended for patients with significant facial or neck injuries to prevent airway obstruction. Clinical judgment is crucial for identifying a threatened airway – For patients with hemodynamic instability, stabilize hemodynamics before intubating, as rapid sequence induction drugs can cause collapse – Temporarily remove the anterior portion of the cervical collar while maintaining manual inline stabilization for all patients with blunt traumatic injuries during airway management • Prevent hypothermia: – After removing the patient's clothing and completing the assessment, cover the patient with warm blankets or use an external warming device in the trauma receiving area – Administer warmed intravenous fluids and ensure the environment is warm (i.e., maintain room temperature) • Care of pediatric patients: – Similar to adults in early resuscitation, except for differences in size and drug dosages (use the Broselow scale for guidance) • Care of pregnant females: – As with nonpregnant females, early recognition of pregnancy is crucial. This involves palpating the abdomen for a gravid uterus, conducting laboratory tests such as human chorionic gonadotropin (hCG), and performing early fetal assessments to ensure the survival of both the mother and the fetus

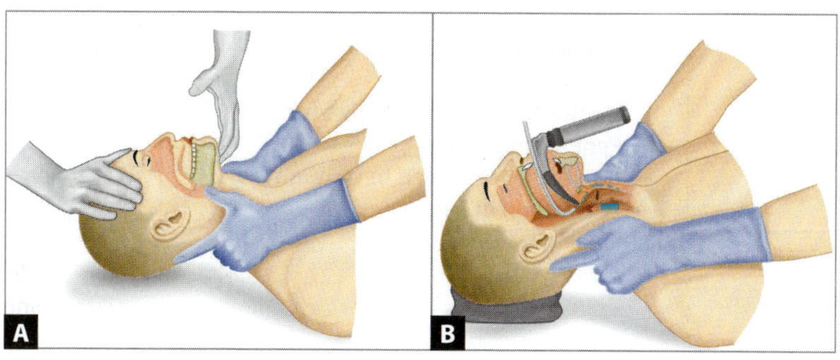

Figs. 1A and B: Airway and c-spine stabilization.

BOX 3: Secondary survey.

- The secondary survey begins only after the primary survey (ABCDEs) is completed, resuscitation is done, and the normalization of vital functions has been achieved
- The secondary survey is a head-to-toe evaluation **(Box 4)** of the trauma patient, with a complete history and physical examination as mentioned below *(AMPLE)*
  - *A*llergy
  - *M*edication currently used
  - *P*ast illness/pregnancy
  - *L*ast meal
  - *E*vents/environment related to injury (mechanism box)
  - General level of consciousness Glasgow Coma Scale (GCS) ≤8
  - Glasgow Coma Scale score: Focal motor deficit

BOX 4: Head-to-toe examination-secondary survey.

Specific complaints "head-to-toe" Physical examination "Head-to-toe"		
Part of body to be examined	***Examination findings***	***Interventions***
1. *Head and face*	• Head: – Contusions – Lacerations • Evidence of skull fracture: – Hemotympanum (blood around middle ear, causing purple discoloration/ ecchymosis of tympanic membrane) – Battle's sign – Raccoon eyes – Palpable defects – Cerebrospinal fluid leak • Identify epistaxis or septal hematoma • Identify avulsed teeth or jaw instability • Mid-face instability: – Airway obstruction due to bleeding – Facial fractures • Malocclusion: Mandible fracture • Eyes: – Visual acuity – Pupillary size – Hemorrhage of conjunctiva/fundus – Penetrating injury – Contact lenses (need to be removed) – Dislocation of lens	• Control bleeding from scalp wounds by applying direct pressure, using sutures, or utilizing surgical clips • Imaging and details in individual chapter

Contd...

Contd...

Part of body to be examined	*Examination findings*	*Interventions*
	– Ocular entrapment noted by movement of eyes – Diplopia – Enophthalmos – Exophthalmos – Excessive tearing	
2. *Neck*	*(Maintain cervical immobilization)* • Penetrating injury and lacerations • Tracheal deviation • Jugular venous distention – Pericardial tamponade • Subcutaneous emphysema – Tracheal and laryngeal fracture • Hematoma – Vascular injury • Midline cervical tenderness – Cervical fracture and dislocation	Computed tomography angiography (CTA)/ Exploratory Surgery (details in the Chapter 12.5)
3. *Chest*	• Contusions/lacerations – Cardiopulmonary injury • Focal tenderness/crepitus – Rib fractures • Subcutaneous emphysema – Flail chest/Pneumothorax • Heart tones (muffled) – Cardiac tamponade • Breath sounds (asymmetric) – Tension pneumothorax/Pneumothorax/ Hemothorax	Details in the chapter
4. *Abdomen*	• Evaluate for abdominal distension and tenderness • Lacerations and contusions: – Penetrating injury – Solid hollow viscous injury • Peritoneal signs: – Intra-abdominal hemorrhage – Solid and hollow viscous injury	Details in the chapter

Contd...

Contd...

Part of body to be examined	***Examination findings***	***Interventions***
5. *Pelvis*	• Assess for pelvic: – Stability – Symphyseal tenderness - Unstable pelvic fracture • Blood (urethral meatus, vaginal bleeding, and hematuria) – Unstable pelvic fracture and urethral injury • Inspect perineum for laceration or hematoma • Consider rectal examination for sphincter tone and gross blood	• Consider pelvic sling • Imaging
6. *Extremity*	• Identify extremity deformities • Palpation of bones and joints • Mobility/movements of range of motion of every joint • Excruciating pain for compartment syndrome • Assess peripheral pulses for vascular compromise • Paresthesia for nerve root involvement	• Consider imaging • Slings/slabs if required • Immobilize fractures and dislocations • Pain management • Tetanus • Intravenous antibiotics for open compound fractures
7. *Spinal cord/ vertebral column*	• Verbal response to pain • Lateralizing signs • Palpate for tenderness • Deformity • Motor response • Pain response • Quadriplegia • Paraplegia • Vertebral instability • Fracture versus dislocation	• Imaging • Maintain stability • Details in Chapter 12.4: Acute Spinal Injuries

BOX 5: Secondary survey adjuncts.

- Depending on secondary assessment and mechanism of injury, can ask for EFAST (Extended Focused Assessment with Sonography in Trauma), X-ray of extremity (according to Ottawa rules), CT head/CT spine (according to NEXUS/Canadian head rule or C-pine rule) CT chest (according to NEXUS)
- Whole body CT is done if polytrauma patients in the available centers as per the latest norms, contrast is not needed but repeat CT with contrast can be done if patient has no primary diagnosis and has worsening hemodynamics

BOX 6: Resuscitation and reassessment.

- Every injury needs to be evaluated, diagnosed, and treated as per severity (details in Chapter 12)
- Reassessment is a very important step in every trauma to avoid missing any diagnosis, for example, musculoskeletal injuries might be overwhelming if there is an excruciating pain where an abdominal injury might be missed
- Similarly in the setting of a patient with poor Glasgow Coma Scale (GCS), a musculoskeletal injury might be missed
- After finishing the resuscitation and before transfer, every institution should have a checklist to avoid missing anything. WHO checklist for trauma is a standard checklist meant for the same

World Health Organization

Trauma Care Checklist

Immediately after primary & secondary surveys:

IS FURTHER AIRWAY INTERVENTION NEEDED? May be needed if: • GCS 8 or below • Hypoxaemia or hypercarbia • Face, neck, chest or any severe trauma	☐ YES, DONE ☐ NO
IS THERE A *TENSION* PNEUMO-HAEMOTHORAX?	☐ YES, CHEST DRAIN PLACED ☐ NO
IS THE PULSE OXIMETER PLACED AND FUNCTIONING?	☐ YES ☐ NOT AVAILABLE
LARGE-BORE IV PLACED AND FLUIDS STARTED?	☐ YES ☐ NOT INDICATED ☐ NOT AVAILABLE
FULL SURVEY FOR (AND CONTROL OF) EXTERNAL BLEEDING, INCLUDING:	☐ SCALP ☐ PERINEUM ☐ BACK
ASSESSED FOR PELVIC FRACTURE BY:	☐ EXAM ☐ X-RAY ☐ CT
ASSESSED FOR INTERNAL BLEEDING BY:	☐ EXAM ☐ ULTRASOUND ☐ CT ☐ DIAGNOSTIC PERITONEAL LAVAGE
IS SPINAL IMMOBILIZATION NEEDED?	☐ YES, DONE ☐ NOT INDICATED
NEUROVASCULAR STATUS OF ALL 4 LIMBS CHECKED?	☐ YES
IS THE PATIENT HYPOTHERMIC?	☐ YES, WARMING ☐ NO
DOES THE PATIENT NEED (IF NO CONTRAINDICATION):	☐ URINARY CATHETER ☐ NASOGASTRIC TUBE ☐ CHEST DRAIN ☐ NONE INDICATED

Before team leaves patient:

HAS THE PATIENT BEEN GIVEN:	☐ TETANUS VACCINE ☐ ANALGESICS ☐ ANTIBIOTICS ☐ NONE INDICATED
HAVE ALL TESTS AND IMAGING BEEN REVIEWED?	☐ YES ☐ NO, FOLLOW-UP PLAN IN PLACE
WHICH SERIAL EXAMINATIONS ARE NEEDED?	☐ NEUROLOGICAL ☐ ABDOMINAL ☐ VASCULAR ☐ NONE
PLAN OF CARE DISCUSSED WITH:	☐ PATIENT/FAMILY ☐ RECEIVING UNIT ☐ PRIMARY TEAM ☐ OTHER SPECIALISTS
RELEVANT TRAUMA CHART OR FORM COMPLETED?	☐ YES ☐ NOT AVAILABLE

WWW.WHO.INT/EMERGENCYCARE

BOX 7: Mechanisms of injury and suspected injury patterns.

Blunt Injury:

- *Frontal impact (automobile collision):* Cervical spine fracture, thoracic injuries, traumatic aortic disruption, cardiac contusions, abdominal spleen/liver injuries, hip and/or knee fracture/dislocation, head injury, and facial injury
- *Rear impact (automobile collision):* Cervical spine injury and head injury
- *Side impact (automobile collision):* Contralateral neck sprain or cervical injury, head injury, lateral chest injury, diaphragmatic rupture, spleen/liver and/or kidney injury, and fractured pelvis or acetabulum
- *Vehicle impact with pedestrian:* Head injury, traumatic aortic disruption, abdominal visceral injuries, and fractures of lower extremities/pelvis
- *Ejection from vehicle:* Life-threatening injuries to major organs
- *Fall from height:* Head injury, spinal injury, abdominal injuries, fractured pelvis or acetabulum, and bilateral lower extremity fractures

Penetrating injury:

- *Stab wounds:* Cardiac tamponade, hemothorax, pneumothorax, hemopneumothorax, left diaphragm injury, spleen injury, and abdominal visceral injury
- *Gunshot wounds (GSW):* High likelihood of injury, neurovascular injury, fractures, and compartment syndrome

Restraint injuries:

- *Lap belt/Shoulder belt:* Sternal and rib fractures, pulmonary contusions, chance fractures, abdominal injuries, and head/cervical spine/facial injuries and fractures

Air bag deployment:

- Mild-to-moderate head and upper torso injuries in frontend collisions; severe injuries in children

Source: Table 8 from Advanced Trauma Life Support (ATLS) 10

SUGGESTED READING

1. American College of Surgeons. Advanced Trauma Life Support (ATLS) Student Course Manual (10th edition). Chicago, IL: American College of Surgeons; 2018.
2. Inaba K, Byerly S, Bush LD, Martin MJ, Martin DT, Peck KA, et al.; WTA C-Spine Study Group. The Western Trauma Association (WTA). J Trauma Acute Care Surg. 2016;81(6):1122-30.
3. Kerwin AJ, Haut ER, Burns JB, Como JJ, Haider A, Stassen N, et al.; Eastern Association for the Surgery of Trauma Practice Management Guidelines Ad Hoc Committee. The Eastern Association for the Surgery of Trauma (EAST) approach to practice management guideline development using Grading of Recommendations, Assessment, Development, and Evaluation (GRADE) methodology. J Trauma Acute Care Surg. 2012;73(5 Suppl 4):S283-7.
4. Tintinalli JE, Ma OJ, Yealy DM, Meckler GD, Stapczynski JS, Cline DM, et al. Tintinalli's Emergency Medicine: A Comprehensive Study Guide, 9th edition. New York, NY: McGraw-Hill Education; 2019.
5. Walls RM, Hockberger RS, Gausche-Hill M (Eds). Rosen's Emergency Medicine: Concepts and Clinical Practice, 9th edition. Amsterdam, Netherlands: Elsevier; 2018.

CHAPTER 11

Medical Management for Post-traumatic Hemorrhage after Trauma

Jamshed D Sunavala

BOX 1: Understanding post-traumatic hemorrhage.

- Most commonly associated with road traffic accidents, homicidal injuries, mass injuries following bombing, mob violence, riots, and terrorist attacks
- At least one-third of patients with uncontrolled hemorrhage will manifest with signs of coagulopathy and may continue to bleed and have higher mortality than those without coagulopathy
- Initial coagulopathy is a result of tissue injury, hypoperfusion, loss of platelets, and clotting factors through hemorrhage
- Coagulopathy is further accelerated by combination of hypothermia and acidosis. Hypothermia is caused by transfusion of cold saline and blood given in an emergency. Heat loss may also occur with the body exposed to low room temperature
- Immediate trauma care and minimum delay between the time of injury and bleeding control decreases overall mortality significantly **(Fig. 1)**

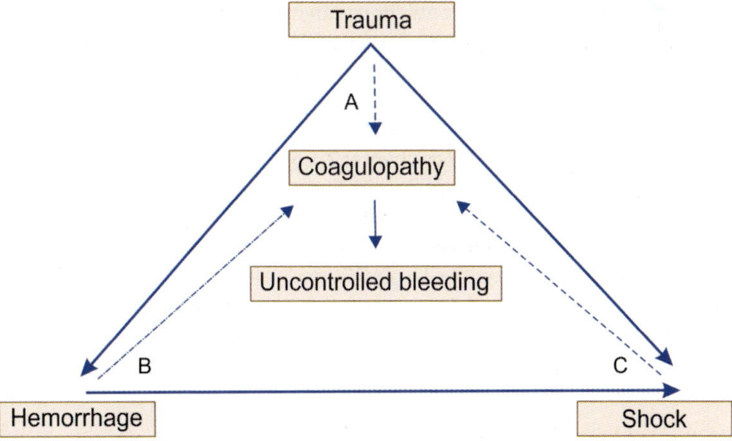

Fig. 1: Fatal triad. *Path A:* Trauma causes coagulopathy by inflammation and tissue injury. *Path B:* Hemorrhage leads to coagulopathy secondary to hypoperfusion and loss of platelets. Coagulopathy is further accentuated by the combination of acidosis and hypothermia secondary to volumes of cold normal saline leading to hyperchloremic acidosis and dilutional coagulopathy. *Path C:* Trauma and shock also cause the acute coagulation of trauma shock (ACoTS) associated with factor consumption and fibrinolysis.

MANAGEMENT

BOX 2: Initial resuscitation.

- This is usually given at the site of accident or at the nearest health care facility
- Serious attempts to limit the source of bleeding by applying local compression or use of tourniquets in case of injury to the limbs and should be fastened proximal to the site of injury
- Application of cervical collar for head and neck injuries
- Cleansing of the oral cavity and securing airways with oropharyngeal tubes and oxygen to be delivered whenever necessary through nasal cannula or mask (*see* Chapter 30: Airway Management)
- Pelvic fracture injuries, head injuries, and intrathoracic or intra-abdominal injuries have high mortality as hemorrhage at these sites are not easily compressible nor manageable. These groups of patients require to be shifted immediately to a major hospital if the health care facility does not have the expertise to deal with severe polytrauma needing complex surgeries
- However, correcting hypoxemia and deranged hemodynamics with whatever means available should be attempted before transfer with continuing resuscitation during transport

BOX 3: Advanced resuscitation.

- *Intubation, oxygenation, and ventilation:* Intubation becomes necessary for a secure and patent airway mainly in patients with poor sensorium, obstructed airways, facial injury, severe hemoptysis, lung injury, shock, and respiratory failure. Also, for immediate ventilator support. PaO_2 levels should be maintained between 90 and 96 mm Hg. Hypoxia and hyperventilation with hypocapnia should be avoided
- *Life-threatening hypotension* is initially managed with fluid challenge and vasopressors till replacement with blood transfusions are available
- *Empirical broad spectrum antibiotics* (after collection of appropriate cultures) and further management according to septic bundle protocol to be initiated for patients with septic shock (refer to chapter 7.1 on "Septic Shock")
- *Caveat:* Latest recommendation as per the European Guidelines (Critical Care 2019) is to target systolic BP at 80–90 mm Hg and mean arterial pressure (MAP) at 50–60 mm Hg until major bleeding has ceased. However, in patients with severe traumatic brain injury (TBI) with Glasgow Coma Scale (GCS) ≤8, the MAP should be maintained at 80 mm Hg. After resuscitation and stabilization, restricted use of crystalloids and avoidance of excessive normal saline is recommended

BOX 4: Rapid assessment of blood loss at the bedside.

- *Clinical assessment:* Visual observation, appraisal of vitals may fail to estimate the extent of bleeding. However, knowing the anatomical site and type of injury can predict the magnitude of hemorrhage (e.g., retroperitoneal hemorrhage in pelvic ring fractures)
- *Advanced trauma life support (ATLS) classification:* This gives a rough guide during initial presentation. Spectrum of tachycardia, tachypnea, hypotension, decreased pulse pressure, oliguria, decreased Glasgow Coma Scale (GCS), and base deficit of <-10 mEq/L is suggestive of severe blood loss
- *Initial hemoglobin* <8 g/dL (before resuscitation) is an indication for substantial bleeding and rapid transfusion **(see Box 6)**
- *Bedside imaging: Focused assessment with sonography for trauma (FAST)* assessing free fluid in thoracoabdominal and pelvic cavities is a rapid noninvasive technique now accepted as first line of imaging in emergency room (ER). Ultrasound can also assess volume status noninvasively by evaluating the inferior vena cava (IVC) collapsibility index

TABLE 1: Clinical estimation of estimated blood loss and immediate measures.

Parameters	*Very mild*	*Mild*	*Moderate*	*Severe*
Approximate blood loss	<15%	15–30%	30–40%	>40%
Heart rate (HR)	WNL	↑	↑	↑↑
Respiratory rate (RR)	WNL	WNL	↑	↑↑
Blood pressure (BP)	WNL	WNL	↓	↓↓
Sensorium	C/A	C/A	C/D	Poor
Base deficit	0 to –2	–2 to –6	–6 to –10	Less than –10
Blood transfusion	Observe	Physician's discretion	Yes	Massive transfusion

(C/A: conscious and awake; C/D: conscious but drowsy; Poor: semi-conscious (Glasgow Coma Scale (GCS) = 9 to 12; WNL: within normal limits)

Source: Adapted with modification from advanced trauma life support (ATLS) classification.

BOX 5: Detecting source of bleeding for blunt trauma.

- *Focused assessment with sonography for trauma (FAST):* Ultrasound can readily assess injuries and bleeding in pleural, thoracoabdominal, and pelvic cavities and also evaluate inferior vena cava (IVC) collapsibility index
- *Multiple computed tomography (MSCT):* MSCT has a superior diagnostic accuracy and higher sensitivity than FAST. It is now considered a "Gold Standard" particularly for intra-abdominal blunt trauma injuries and identification of retroperitoneal hemorrhage
- *Delay phase CT:* This is often used to detect an active bleed within solid organs which could be missed otherwise. For example, pooling of contrast in peritoneal cavity in blunt liver injury indicates massive bleeding and can be responsible for rapid hemodynamic collapse and requires urgent surgery, whereas intraparenchymal pooling of contrast in an unruptured liver capsule mainly indicates limited hemorrhage and these patients may respond to nonoperative treatment

BOX 6: Standard laboratory tests.

Hemoglobin: Though the initial low hemoglobin (Hb) level of <8 gm% is indicator of substantial bleed, its main limitation here is the influence of fluids and blood products transfused during the initial resuscitation

Serum lactate and base deficit: It is useful measurement as a prognostic marker of hemodynamic shock. Lactate clearing time provides an early sign of positive response to therapy. Lactate level returning to normal levels (<2 mmol/L) within 24 hours have good chances of survival whereas levels remaining high for >24 hours have increased probability of developing organ failure. *Lactate determination may not be reliable after alcohol consumption* as it may result in increased level of lactate in the blood as ethanol metabolism is known to convert pyruvate to lactate by lactate dehydrogenase. Monitoring of base deficit may be a better predictor of prognosis in such cases

Prothrombin time (PT) and activated partial thromboplastin time (aPTT), platelet count, and fibrinogen levels: These are standard coagulation parameters to be monitored

Viscoelastic method (VEM): Assessment of the above-mentioned coagulation parameters has a prolonged turnover time and further, coagulation assays such as PT, PTT, and thrombin have been shown as insufficient to correlate with bleed in acute trauma setting. VEM such as thromboelastography (TEG) and the newer rotational thromboelastography (ROTEM) devices have a faster turnover time of around 10 minutes which becomes a major asset while dealing with life-threatening hemorrhage from severe trauma and hence helps in early decision making

Platelet dysfunction: Early detection of platelet dysfunction associated with traumatic injury is an important parameter to be measured by platelet aggregometry. This is useful to identify traumatic brain injury (TBI) patients who are on aspirin

BOX 7: Antidotes for reversing the effects of anticoagulants and antiplatelets agents.

Anticoagulant agents	***Reversing agents***	***Monitoring the anticoagulant effect***
VKA (warfarin)	• Vitamin K IV • PCC for immediate reversal	Prothrombin time
New oral factor Xa inhibitors (rivaroxaban and apixaban)	No validated antidote available	Antifactor Xa assay
Dabigatran	Idarucizumab	Thrombin time
Fondaparinux (factor Xa inhibitor)	rVIIa*	—
LMWH	Protamine sulfate (25–50 mg stat)	—
Antiplatelets (aspirin, clopidogrel, prasugrel, or ticagrelor)	Platelet concentrate DDAVP (0.3–0.4 μg/kg in 100 mL normal saline over 30 minutes)*	Platelet aggregation test

(DDAVP: de-amino d-arginine vasopressin; LMWH: low molecular weight heparin; PCC: prothrombin complex concentrate; VKA: vitamin K antagonist)

*Adapted from Levi M. Annual update in intensive care and emergency medicine. Berlin, Germany: Springer; 2016.

BOX 8: Transfusion management.

- *Massive blood transfusion:* Involves replacing one blood volume or more within 24 hours, administering 10 or more units of packed red blood cells (PRBCs) in 24 hours, or replacing over 50% blood volume in 4 hours
- Management of acute coagulopathy associated with trauma involves massive transfusions with red blood cells, plasma, and platelets. Today with the availability of viscoelastic method (VEM) more accurate assessment of the requirement of these blood components can be made
- *Packed red cells (RBCs)* transfusion are given to achieve a hemoglobin (Hb) level of 8 gm%. Stored RBC can add on to the trauma related hyperkalemia, hence administration of calcium gluconate 1,000 mg over 2–3 minutes rapidly averts hyperkalemia
- *Fresh frozen plasma (FFP)* contains all the coagulation factors present in blood and is an ideal replacement for factors lost during major bleeding. ABO compatible units should be transfused as plasma contains antibodies to RBC antigen. The European guidelines for major traumatic bleed recommend FFP at a dose of 10–15 mL/kg; further doses will depend on coagulation monitoring. Overdosing of FFP can lead to serious circulatory overload
- *Platelet* count of at least 50,000/uL should be maintained. However, if disseminated intravascular coagulation (DIC) or hyperfibrinolysis is suspected or in case of massive bleeding the platelet count should be maintained above 1,00,000. ABO compatible platelets should be given, one random donor unit per 10 kg of body-weight. Five to six random donor platelets or one single donor platelet provides about 3 to 4 x 10^{11} platelets and this raises the platelets count by about 30,000/uL within 10 minutes of infusion
- *Cryoprecipitate* is derived from FFP and contains a major factor of fibrinogens, factor VIII, factor XIII, and Von Willebrand factor. Plasma fibrinogen levels are routinely used to assess cryoprecipitate transfusion requirements. Dose of 50 ug/kg is recommended for massive hemorrhage and if plasma fibrinogen level is <1.5–2 g/L or if thromboelastometry facility is available and if it shows signs of functional fibrinogen deficit
- *Massive transfusion* may lead to transfusion related lung injury (TRALI), multiple organ dysfunction syndrome (MODS) and increased risk of infection, hence a proactive transfusion strategy should be adopted
- *Tranexamic acid:* It is an antifibrinolytic agent and can be used when hyperfibrinolysis is an established concern. An empirical bolus of 10–15 mg/kg followed by infusion of 1–5 mg/kg/hour is the standard recommended dose. Antifibrinolytic therapy is best guided by thromboelastometric assessment, if available
- *Recombinant Factor VIIa* is a salvage therapy. It should be used only as an option in cases where major life-threatening bleed persists despite standard attempts to control the bleeding fails. This is also applicable where antidote to ongoing anticoagulant is not available. There is no established dose, however, a dose of 15 ug/kg has been effective

SUGGESTED READING

1. American College of Surgeons. ATLS® Student Course Manual, 10th edition. Chicago: American College of Surgeons; 2018.
2. Briggs A, Gates JD, Kaufman RM, Calahan C, Gormley WB, Havens JM. Platelet dysfunction and platelet transfusion in traumatic brain injury. J Surg Res. 2015;193(2):802-6.
3. Caspers M, Maegele M, Frohlich M. Current strategies for hemostatic control in acute trauma hemorrhage and trauma-induced coagulopathy. Expert Rev Hematol. 2018;11(12):987-95.
4. Foster JC, Sappenfield JW, Smith RS, Kiley SP. Initiation and termination of massive transfusion protocols: current strategies and future prospects. Anesth Analg. 2017;125(6):2045-55.
5. Gonzalez E, Moore EE, Moore HB, Chapman MP, Chin TL, Ghasabyan A, et al. Goal-directed hemostatic resuscitation of trauma-induced coagulopathy: a pragmatic randomized clinical trial comparing a viscoelastic assay to conventional coagulation assays. Ann Surg. 2016;263(6):1051-9.
6. Hagemo JS, Christiaans SC, Stanworth SJ, Brohi K, Johansson PI, Goslings JC, et al. Detection of acute traumatic coagulopathy and massive transfusion requirements by means of rotational thromboelastometry: an international prospective validation study. Crit Care. 2015;19:97.
7. Holcomb JB, Tilley BC, Baraniuk S, Fox EE, Wade CE, Podbielski JM, et al. Transfusion of plasma, platelets, and red blood cells in a 1:1:1 vs a 1:1:2 ratio and mortality in patients with severe trauma: the PROPPR randomized clinical trial. JAMA. 2015;313(5):471-82.
8. Skitch S, Engels PT. Acute management of the traumatically injured pelvis. Emerg Med Clin North Am. 2018;36(1):161-79.
9. Spahn DR, Bouillon B, Cerny V, Duranteau J, Filipescu D, Hunt BJ, et al. The European guideline on management of major bleeding and coagulopathy following trauma: 5th edition. Crit Care. 2019;23(1):98.
10. Sunvala JD, Kriplani Suvarna D. Medical Management of Post-traumatic Hemorrhage. In: Sunvala JD (Ed). Essentials of Critical Care Medicine for the Physician. New Delhi: Jaypee Brothers Medical Publishers, 2022.

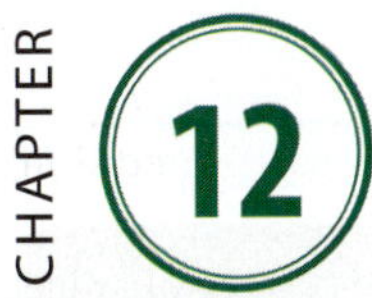

Trauma in Sections

12.1 TRAUMATIC BRAIN INJURY

Nikhil S Chamankar, Sudheer Ambekar

BOX 1: Introduction.

- "Traumatic brain injury (TBI)" is injury to the brain and spinal cord due to external forces causing direct or indirect impact to them leading to bleeding or fractures causing varying degrees of damage from minor concussion to death
- Common causes of TBI are motor vehicular accidents, fall from height and assault
- Motor vehicular accidents are the most common cause of TBI followed by fall from height

BOX 2: Classification.

"Traumatic brain injury (TBI)" can be classified by the following ways:

- Clinical
- Radiological
- Mechanism of injury

Clinical Classification of Traumatic Brain Injury

Mild:

Glasgow Coma Scale score = 14

Or,

Glasgow Coma Scale score = 15 + *either* brief loss of consciousness (<5 minutes) *or* amnesia

Moderate:

Glasgow Coma Scale score = 8–13

Or,

Loss of consciousness ≥5 minutes

Or,

Focal neurologic deficit

Severe:

Glasgow Coma Scale score = 3–8

Contd...

Contd...

Radiographic Classification of Traumatic Brain Injury

TABLE 1: Marshall CT classification scale for "traumatic brain injury".

Category	*Definition*	*Mortality*
Diffuse injury I	No visible intracranial pathology	10%
Diffuse injury II	Cisterns patent; shift 0–5 mm and/or lesions present; no lesion >25 cm^3	13%
Diffuse injury III	Cisterns compressed or absent; shift 0–5 mm; no lesion >25 cm^3	33%
Diffuse injury IV	Midline shift >5 mm; no lesion >25 cm^3	56%
Evacuated mass lesion V	Any lesion surgically evacuated	35%
Non-evacuated mass lesion VI	High- or mixed-density lesion >25 cm^3; not surgically evacuated	91%

Rotterdam CT Classification Score

Score element	*Points*
Basal cisterns • Normal • Compressed • Absent	 0 1 2
Midline shift • No shift or shift ≤5 mm • Shift >5 mm	 0 1
Epidural mass lesion • Present • Absent	 0 1
Intraventricular blood or traumatic subarachnoid hemorrhage • Absent • Present	 0 1
Sum score: Calculate the sum of all variables and add 1 point to the total +1	

Mechanism of injury:
- Closed head injury
- Penetrating head injury
- Motor vehicular or crash injury
- Blast injury

BOX 3: Pathology.

Brain suffers from two types of pathologic injuries at the time of impact:

1. Direct injury
2. Indirect injury

Direct injury:

- Skull and spine fracture
- Intracerebral hemorrhage
  - Epidural hematoma
  - Subdural hematoma
  - Intracerebral hematoma
  - Subarachnoid hemorrhage
    - Concussion
    - Diffuse axonal injury

Indirect injury:

- Oxidative stress
- Free radical formation
- Hypoxia
- Cell apoptosis
- Hypercarbia
- Seizures
- Calcium-mediated damage
- Proapoptotic expression
- Astrocytic inflammation
- Cerebral edema

BOX 4: Assessment.

- In the emergency room (ER) a patient presenting with traumatic brain injury (TBI) has to be assessed clinically and radiologically
- The presenting Glasgow Coma Scale (GCS) is noted
- Hard cervical collar is applied and patient is mobilized by the log roll technique
- Airway secured. If GCS is <8 then patient is intubated
  - Lung protective ventilation
  - Target PaO_2 >13 kPa
  - Target $PaCO_2$ 4.7–5.3 kPa
  - Avoid routinely decreasing $PaCO_2$ <4.0 kPa except in critical situations when hyperventilation may be needed to "buy time" (e.g., prior to theater or CT scan)
  - The decision to reduce $PaCO_2$ to <4.0 kPa must be made by a consultant intensivist and neurosurgeon, ideally with partial pressure of brain tissue oxygen ($PbtO_2$) monitoring in situ
- Broad gauge intravenous access is secured and fluid resuscitation is started
- Chest, abdomen, and long extremities are examined to rule out other injuries

BOX 5: Investigation.

Blood investigation: Complete hemogram, liver function test, renal function test, arterial blood gas analysis, coagulation prolife, and blood grouping for cross matching

X-ray: Chest X-ray to see for hemothorax or pneumothorax. Cervical spine X-ray to see for cervical fractures. Abdomen X-ray to see for pneumoperitoneum. Extremity X-ray to see for long bone fracture

CT scan: Easily available and short duration for image procurement makes it the investigation of choice in the emergency room to rule out intracerebral hemorrhage. Additionally, it also gives details regarding skull bone and facial fractures

Canadian CT Head Rule (CCTHR) for mild traumatic brain injury (TBI)
[Glasgow Coma Scale (GCS) = 13–15]
Head CT is indicated for patients ≥16 years of age with GCS = 13–15 from witnessed TBI, only if one or more of any of the following are present

High-risk criteria ("CT is mandatory") (presence of any one often requires neurosurgical intervention):
- Glasgow Coma Scale <15 at 2 hours post injury
- Suspected open or depressed skull fracture
- Signs of basal skull fracture (includes hemotympanum, "raccoon's eyes", cerebrospinal fluid (CSF) rhinorrhea or otorrhea, and Battle's sign)
- Two or more episodes of vomiting
- Age ≥65 years

Medium risk criteria (presence of any two often has clinically important findings on CT):
- Amnesia before injury >30 minutes
- *Dangerous mechanism of injury:* Pedestrian hit by motor vehicle, ejection from automobile, and fall from height >3 feet or >5 stairs

New Orleans Criteria (NOC) for Head CT
Head CT scan is indicated for patients with TBI and GCS = 15 only if one or more of the following are present:
- Headache
- Vomiting
- Age ≥60 years
- Drug or alcohol intoxication
- Persistent anterograde amnesia (short-term memory deficits)
- Visible trauma above the clavicle
- Seizure

Magnetic resonance imaging (MRI): Useful in diagnosing diffuse axonal injury especially in patients who have a normal CT scan with poor neurology

Ultrasonography (USG): To rule out intra-abdominal injury

BOX 6: Monitoring.

In patients with moderate-to-severe traumatic brain injury, intracranial pressure (ICP) monitoring helps to reduce mortality

The aim of ICP monitoring is to keep a normal cerebral perfusion pressure (CPP) which is normally 60–65 mm Hg

Cerebral perfusion pressure is calculated by the equation:

$$CPP = MAP - ICP$$

where, MAP is the mean arterial pressure and ICP is the intracranial pressure. Normal ICP is 10–12 mm Hg

Various techniques of ICP monitoring have been introduced but "external ventricular drain" remains gold standard. Other methods include subarachnoid bolts, subdural transducers cerebral microdialysis, jugular bulb arteriovenous oxygen content difference, and pressure-reactivity index

Clinical standardization guidelines for moderate-to-severe traumatic brain injury

Tier 0:

- Maintain euvolemia
- Cerebral perfusion pressure >60 mm Hg
- PCO_2 = 35–40 mm Hg
- SaO_2 >90%
- Serum sodium >135 mmol/L
- Serum glucose >60 mg/dL and <180 mg/dL
- Hemoglobin >7 g/dL
- Normothermia
- Evacuate intracranial mass lesions
- Head of bed 30°

Tier 1:

- Adjust head of bed
- Ensure normothermia
- Titrate sedation to ICP
- Standard-dose hyperosmolar therapies
- Cerebrospinal fluid (CSF) drainage if external ventricular drain available
- Consider electroencephalogram (EEG) to rule out nonconvulsive seizures
- If ICP is persistently >25 mm Hg, consider to repeat CT

Tier 2:

- High-dose hyperosmolar therapy
- Adjust PCO_2 to 30–35 mm Hg
- Increased sedation to ICP target
- Vasopressor trial for increased cerebral perfusion pressure (70 mm Hg)
- Neuromuscular paralysis
- Consider EEG to rule out nonconvulsive seizures
- If ICP is persistently >25 mm Hg, consider to repeat CT

Tier 3:

- Adjust temperature to 35–37°C (95–98.6°F)
- Sedative bolus dosing
- Decompressive craniectomy
- Barbiturate coma
- Consider EEG to rule out nonconvulsive seizures
- If ICP is persistently >25 mm Hg, consider to repeat CT

Tier 0 in the algorithm is aimed at primary prevention and prophylaxis of secondary injury and is applied to all patients treated for traumatic brain injury (TBI). Tiers 1 through 3 are aimed at interventions based on abnormalities in ICP, CPP, cerebral blood flow (CBF), cerebral metabolic rate of oxygen ($CMRO_2$), and cerebral autoregulation

BOX 7: Treatment.

Medical management:
- Patient is started on antiedema measures like 20% mannitol or 3% hypertonic saline
- Analgesics are given to reduce pain. Fentanyl infusion may be started for those on ventilatory support
- No role of steroids in management of traumatic brain and spine injury
- Patients presenting with seizures are started on antiepileptics like leveteracetam or phenytoin. Prophylactic antiseizure medication is indicated in patients with severe traumatic brain injury (TBI) for a duration of 7 days
- Intravenous fluids in the form of crystalloids and if needed colloids are started

Surgical management:

Extradural hematoma (EDH): Indications for surgery are as follows:
- Extradural hematoma volume* >30 cm^3 should be evacuated regardless of Glasgow Coma Scale (GCS)
- Extradural hematoma with all of the following characteristics can be managed nonsurgically with serial CT scans and close neurological observation in a neurosurgical center:
  - Volume* <30 cm^3
  - And thickness <15 mm
  - And midline shift (MLS) <5 mm
  - And Glasgow Coma Scale (GCS) >8
  - And no focal neurologic deficit

Subdural hematoma (SDH): Indications of surgery are as follows:
- Subdural hematoma with thickness >10 mm or midline shift (MLS) >5 mm (on CT) should be evacuated regardless of GCS
- Subdural hematoma with thickness <10 mm and MLS <5 mm [see text regarding the evacuation of acute subdural hematoma (ASDH) <10 mm thick] should undergo surgical evacuation if:
  - Glasgow Coma Scale drops by ≥2 points from injury to admission
  - And/or the pupils are asymmetric or fixed and dilated
  - And/or intracranial pressure (ICP) is >20 mm Hg
- Monitor ICP in all patients with SDH and GCS <9

SUGGESTED READING

1. Bullock MR, Chesnut R, Ghajar J, Gordon D, Hartl R, Newell DW, et al. Surgical management of posterior fossa mass lesions. Neurosurgery. 2006;58:S47-S55; discussion Si-iv.
2. Bullock MR, Chesnut R, Ghajar J, Gordon D, Hartl R, Newell DW, et al. Surgical management of acute subdural hematomas. Neurosurgery. 2006;58:S16-S24.
3. Bullock MR, Chesnut R, Ghajar J, Gordon D, Hartl R, Newell DW, et al. Surgical management of acute epidural hematomas. Neurosurgery. 2006; 58(3 suppl):S7-S15.
4. Maas AI, Hukkelhoven CW, Marshall LF, Steyerberg EW. Prediction of outcome in traumatic brain injury with computed tomographic characteristics: a comparison between the computed tomographic classification and combinations of computed tomographic predictors. Neurosurgery. 2005;57:1173-82; discussion 117382.
5. The Brain Trauma Foundation. The American Association of Neurological Surgeons. The Joint Section on Neurotrauma and Critical Care. Initial management. J Neurotrauma. 2000;17(6-7):463-9.
6. The Brain Trauma Foundation. The American Association of Neurological Surgeons. The Joint Section on Neurotrauma and Critical Care. Resuscitation of blood pressure and oxygenation. J Neurotrauma. 2000;17(6-7):471-8.

12.2 THORACIC INJURIES

Sachna P Shetty

BOX 1: General approach.

The most common symptoms of thoracic trauma are:
- Localized chest pain
- Shortness of breath
- Dyspnea and tachypnea but can be nonspecific if no other relevant symptoms or signs:
  - Primary survey includes management of:
    - Airway obstruction (Chapter 30 on Airway)
    - Tension pneumothorax **(Table 1)**
    - Open pneumothorax **(Table 1)**
    - Massive hemothorax **(Table 1)**
    - Cardiac tamponade (Chapter 3.10)
  - Secondary survey includes management of:
    - Simple pneumothorax
    - Hemothorax
    - Pulmonary contusion
    - Tracheobronchial tree injury
    - Blunt cardiac injury
    - Traumatic aortic disruption
    - Diaphragmatic injury
    - Blunt esophageal rupture
  - Manifestation hinting to greater injury are:
    - Subcutaneous emphysema
    - Crush injuries of chest
    - Injury to upper rib 1–3, scapula
    - Injury to sternum

BOX 2: Rib fracture.

*Rib fracture is often diagnosed clinically **(Fig. 1)***

Symptoms include:
- Focal chest pain
- Ecchymosis over the rib
- Severe point tenderness
- Bony crepitus
- Pain upon bimanual compression of the chest remote from the injury site can be used as a bedside diagnostic tool

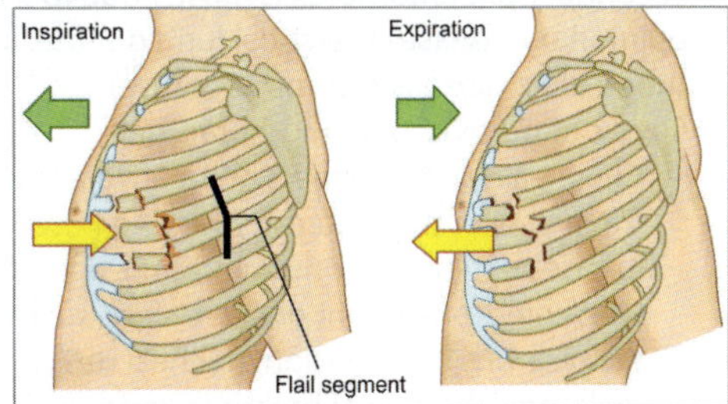

Fig. 1: Flail chest with a segment displacement.

Caveat:
- Flail chest is characterized by paradoxical motion of a portion/segment of the chest wall portion during respiration
- Caused by fractures of 3 or more ribs anteriorly and posteriorly within each rib

BOX 3: Management.

- Treatment of acute rib fractures focuses on:
  - Adequate pain relief
  - Maintenance of lung function
- Stable patients with single rib fractures are managed with opioid and nonopioid analgesia
- Intercostal nerve blocks may relieve symptoms (see part on procedure)
- Stabilization of the flail segment is outdated
- Continuing daily activities and deep breathing exercises should be advised to ensure ventilation and prevent lung collapse
- Flail segments may require consultation with a trauma or thoracic surgeons
- Open fixation for flail chest is indicated for patients with:
  - Persistent pain
  - Severe chest wall instability
  - Progressive decline in lung function
  - Difficult to wean off the mechanical ventilation secondary to the mechanics of flail chest

BOX 4: Disposition.

- Hospitalization is advised for patients with:
  - Three or more fractured ribs
- Elderly patients with six or more fractured ribs should be treated in intensive care units
- Most rib fractures heal uneventfully within 3–6 weeks

BOX 5: Pneumothorax.

- Pneumothorax, which is the accumulation of air in the pleura space between visceral and parietal
- Primary pneumothorax is mainly due to a chest trauma
- Secondary pneumothorax is mostly due to a lung pathology. (Chronic obstructive pulmonary disease, interstitial lung disease, lung abscesses, and pulmonary tuberculosis are a few common cause)
- Classic features of pneumothorax are:
  - Chest pain and shortness of breath are the most prevalent symptoms of thoracic trauma, with their intensity varying based on the specific type of injury
  - In cases of tension, communicating, or a simple pneumothorax that is worsening, one might observe signs such as tachypnea, respiratory distress, tachycardia, hypotension, tracheal deviation away from the injury side, unilateral absence of breath sounds, neck vein distention, and cyanosis (a late sign) **(Table 1)**

TABLE 1: Classic features of pneumothorax.

	Simple	*Communicating/open*	*Tension*	*Occult*
Definition	A simple pneumothorax (see Chapter 40: Imaging) is characterized by the absence of communication with the atmosphere. It is nonexpanding, meaning there is no shift of the mediastinum or hemidiaphragm	A communicating pneumothorax (see Chapter 40: Imaging), also known as a sucking chest wound, occurs when there is a defect in the chest wall, creating a connection between the pleural space and atmospheric pressure	Tension pneumothorax involves the accumulation of inhaled air under pressure within the pleural cavity due to a one-way valve effect, resulting in a shift of the mediastinum to the opposite side and compression of the contralateral lung	An occult pneumothorax is one that is not visible on the initial chest radiograph but is identified on subsequent chest imaging
Etiology	Rib fractures, some bullet injury	Combat injuries and gunshot wounds	One way injury, leading to no escape for air	
Clinical presentation	• Might be asymptomatic depending on the size • Can cause pleuritic chest pain, if increase in size dyspnea and hemodynamic instability might start showing up	Pain mainly pleuritic can be associated with shortness of breath, tachypnea, decreased breath sounds on the affected area	• Deteriorates rapidly with cardio-vascular compromise and respiratory distress • Experiences severe breathlessness, hypoxic agitated, restless, cyanotic, tachycardic, and hypotensive and some might develop altered mental sensorium • The look out signs of a tension pneumothorax are tachycardia, hypotension, desaturation, absent breath sounds on the affected side • In some jugular venous distention (JVD) and tracheal deviation may be observed	Asymptomatic

Contd...

Contd...

	Simple	***Communicating/open***	***Tension***	***Occult***
Management	• Mainly observation • Nonrebreather mask (NRBM) might help in most situations	• A sterile dressing large enough to overlap the wound and close the opening (plastic wrap or petroleum gauze), tape it on three sides to provide flutter valve effect aim is to prevents outside air to enter but allows inside air to exit **(Fig. 2)** • Place a chest tube later (procedures), followed by surgical closure of wound	Needle decompression followed by tube thoracostomy (procedure)	Observation, but if mechanical ventilation or positive pressure is needed to keep chest tube ready if hemodynamic instability noted

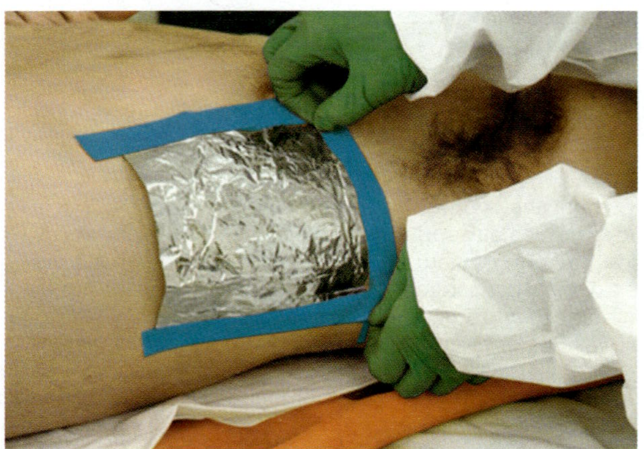

Fig. 2: Open pneumothorax.

BOX 6: Investigation.

- An erect posteroanterior chest X-ray is the usual initial test in relatively stable patients
- In unstable patients, *extended focused assessment with sonography in trauma* (E-FAST) can help in diagnosis (refer Chapter 40)

Caveat:

- The British Thoracic Society classifies a small pneumothorax as having a rim of <2 cm between the lung edge and the chest wall, while a large pneumothorax is defined by a rim of 2 cm or greater

CT chest imaging is essential for diagnosing pneumothorax that may have been missed on X-ray, as well as for distinguishing blebs in patients with chronic obstructive pulmonary disease (COPD)

BOX 7: Criteria for stable patients with pneumothorax.

- Respiratory rate <24 breaths/min
- No breathlessness or distress at rest
- Pulse <100 beats/min
- Normal blood pressure for the patient
- Room air oxygen saturation >90%

Treatment of pneumothorax:

- *Small primary pneumothorax or asymptomatic:*
  - Observation for >3 hours
  - Repeat chest X-ray to monitor size; discharge if asymptomatic and reassess in 2 weeks or if symptoms recur
  - Option for small-size catheter aspiration with immediate removal, followed by observation; discharge if asymptomatic and monitor for recurrence of symptoms in 2 weeks
  - Alternatively, consider small-size catheter aspiration or insertion of a small-size chest tube with a Heimlich valve or water seal, with admission if needed

Caveat: Catheter aspiration for small pneumothorax is primarily indicated in patients requiring intubation, mechanical ventilation, long-distance transport, or when close observation for clinical deterioration is challenging

- *Small secondary pneumothorax:*
  - Consider small-size catheter or small-size chest tube insertion with a Heimlich valve or water seal, and admission
- *Large pneumothorax (primary or secondary) or bilateral pneumothoraces:*
  - Insertion of a moderate-size chest tube and admission
  - Consider a large-size chest tube if there is fluid or hemothorax present, with water seal drainage and admission
- *Tension pneumothorax:*
  - Immediate needle decompression followed by insertion of a moderate- or large-size chest tube, water seal drainage, and admission; ideally, perform immediate chest tube placement

Contd...

Contd...

Caveat:
- Sizes of needles and chest tubes:
  - Needle aspiration: 18-gauge needle
  - Small-size catheter: ≤14 F
  - Small-size chest tube: 10–14 F
  - Pigtail catheter: 14 F, placed using the Seldinger technique
  - Moderate-size chest tube: 16–22 F
  - Large-size chest tube: 24–36 F
- If pneumothorax is suspected despite normal initial chest radiography, obtaining serial films, performing point-of-care ultrasound (POCUS), or CT imaging may be beneficial
- Pneumothorax following a stab wound may present delayed symptoms for up to 6 hours
- Causes of failure of lung expansion post chest tube include improper connections or leaks in external tubing or water-seal collection apparatus, improper positioning of the chest tube, occlusion by secretions or foreign bodies, or tear of a large bronchus or lung parenchyma

BOX 8: Hemothorax.

- Hemothorax, which is the accumulation of blood in the pleural space after blunt or penetrating chest trauma, if large causes hemodynamic compromise
- It is commonly associated with pneumothorax or extrathoracic injuries
- Massive hemothorax is when accumulation of >1,500 mL blood in one side of chest is noted
- To insert chest tube FR 28–32
- If >200 mL/hour massive simultaneous blood transfusion, or persisting hemodynamic instability thoracic team to be addressed, for thoracotomy

Caveat:
- Difference between tension pneumothorax and massive hemothorax:

Condition	***Tension pneumothorax***	***Massive hemothorax***
Breath sounds	Decreased or absent	Decreased
Percussion	Hyperresonant	Dull
Trachea	Deviated away	Midline
Neck veins	Distended	Collapsed
Chest movement	Expanded immobile	Mobile

NEXUS: Chest computed tomography criteria for chest computed tomography after blunt trauma
- Abnormal chest X-ray
- Rapid deceleration mechanism (defined as fall >20 feet or motor vehicle collision >40 mph)
- Distracting painful injury
- Chest wall tenderness
- Sternal tenderness
- Thoracic spine tenderness
- Scapular tenderness

BOX 9: Traumatic circulatory arrest (Flowchart 1).

Flowchart 1: Traumatic circulatory arrest (penetrating or blunt) with no pulse.

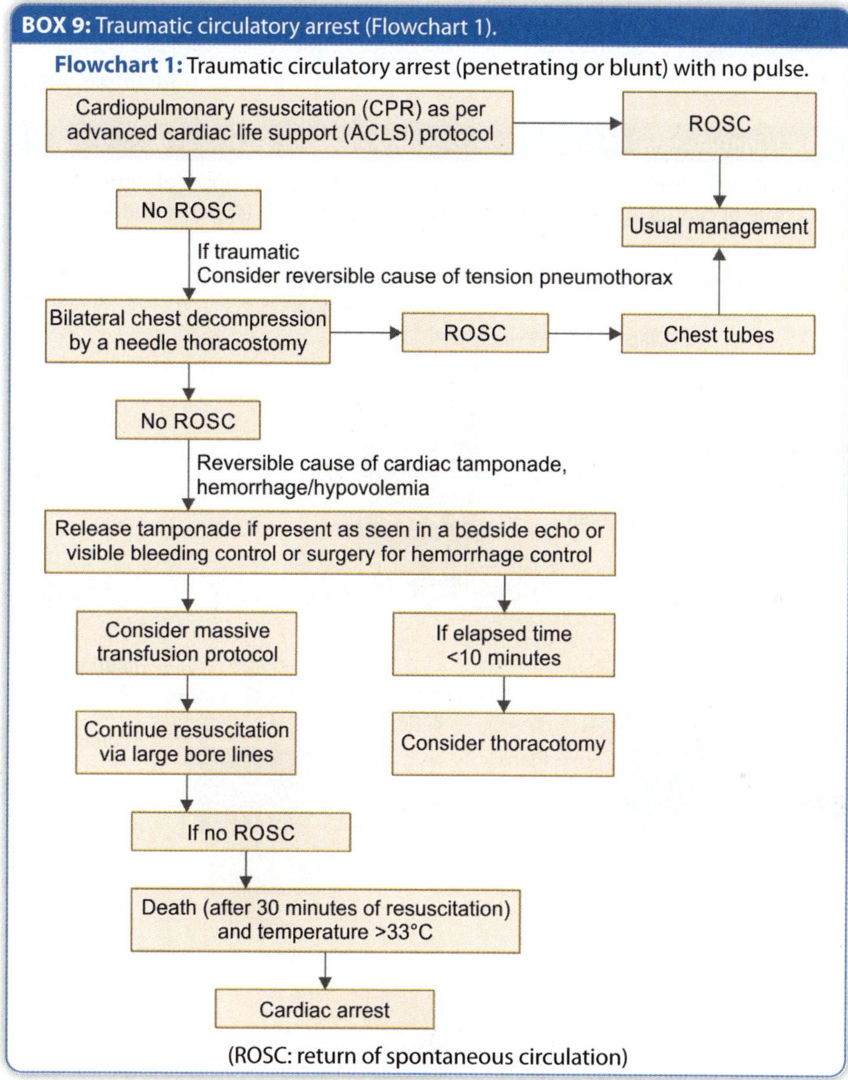

(ROSC: return of spontaneous circulation)

SUGGESTED READING

1. American College of Surgeons. Advanced Trauma Life Support: Student Course Manual. 10th ed. Chicago, Il: American College of Surgeons; 2018.
2. Tintinalli JE, Ma OJ, Yealy DM, Meckler GD, Stapczynski JS, Cline DM, et al. Tintinalli's Emergency Medicine: A Comprehensive Study Guide, 9th edition. New York, NY: McGraw- Hill Education; 2019.
3. Walls RM, Hockberger RS, Gausche-Hill M. Rosen's Emergency Medicine: Concepts and Clinical Practice. Philadelphia, PA: Elsevier; 2018.

12.3 ABDOMINAL AND PELVIC INJURIES

Sachna P Shetty

BOX 1: Introduction.

- Abdomen is divided into 4 components: (1) intrathoracic or upper abdomen, (2) true or central abdomen, (3) retroperitoneal abdomen, (4) pelvic abdomen

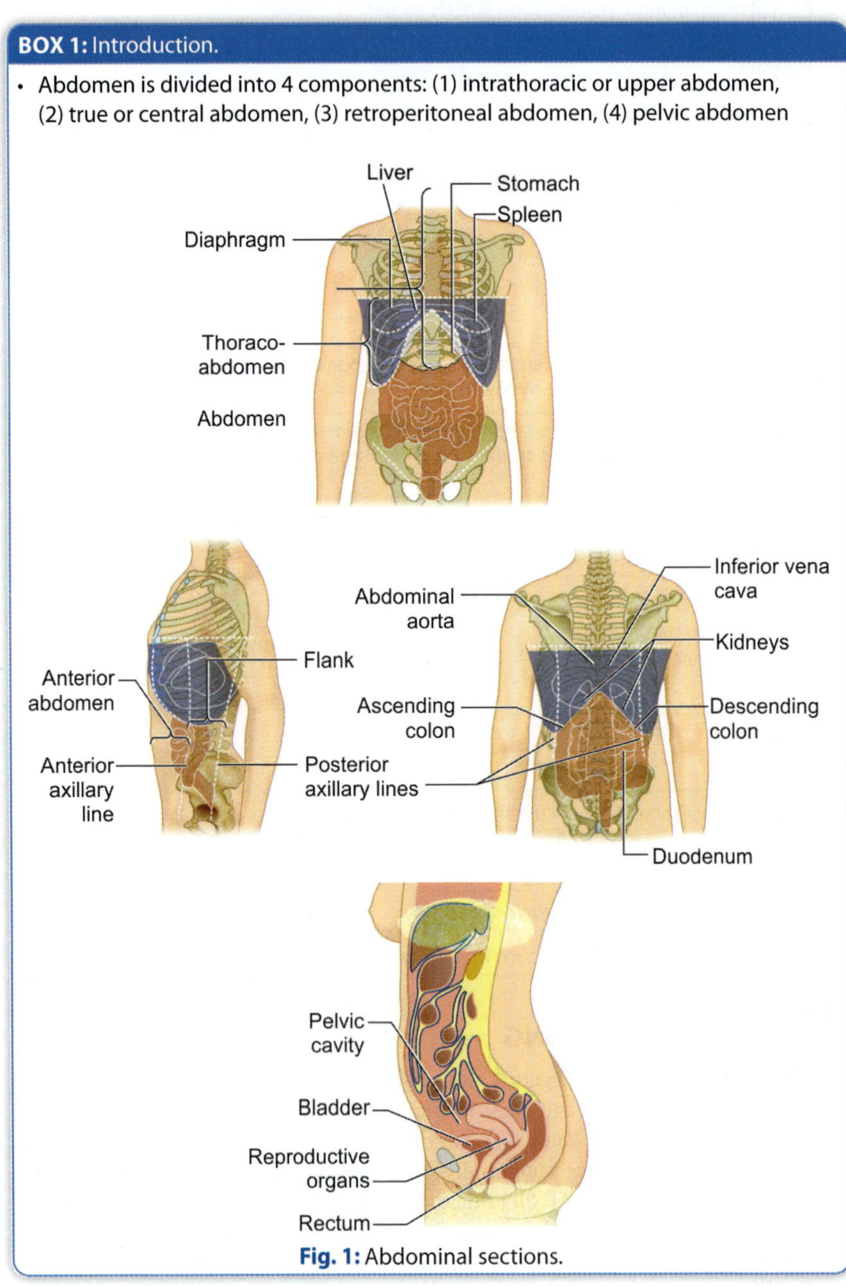

Fig. 1: Abdominal sections.

BOX 2: Clinical presentation.

Clinical presentation:
- Mechanism of injury gives a clue to type of injury (Trauma Part A—refer Chapter 10)
- Pain abdomen and tenderness are the main clinical feature
- Evisceration
- Hypotension
- Abdominal assessment (Trauma Part A—refer Chapter 10) consists of-inspection, palpation, percussion of abdomen, and perineum with flanks

Pelvic assessment:
- Unexplained hypotension can be the only presenting complaint
- Inspection of the scrotum, meatus, vagina, and perineum (Trauma Part A—refer Chapter 10)
- Without an obvious deformity, discrepancy in limb length and external rotation of leg can give clues to pelvic injury
- Gentle palpation of bony pelvis for tenderness

Caveat:
- Factors making the diagnosis of an abdominal injury challenging include concomitant injuries (particularly significant head injuries), referred pain, intoxication with alcohol, or other toxicologic substances
- Elderly patients may be on anticoagulation medications or on medications limiting physiologic response like tachycardia, such as antihypertensives (β-blockers or calcium-channel blockers)
- Gastric catheters—help in decompressing and prognostic for gastric bleed avoided in signs of facial injuries
- Urinary catheter—helps to relieve distention, look for hematuria, and allows monitoring. *Avoided,* if known complex urethral injury

BOX 3: Comparison of focused assessment sonograph trauma (FAST)/CT.

	FAST (More details in Chapter 4)	***CT***
Advantages	• Early operative decision • Noninvasive • Rapid • Repeatable • No need for transport	• Anatomical diagnosis • Noninvasive • Repeatable • Visualizes retroperitoneal, bony, soft-tissue extraluminal air
Disadvantages	• Subjective to the operator and their efficiency • Bowel gas and subcutaneous air distorts imaging • Diaphragm, bowel, pancreatic injuries, retroperitoneal structure, and extraluminal air are generally missed • Body habitus can limit	• Higher cost and time consuming • Radiation and IV contrast can be an issue • Chances of missing diaphragmatic injuries, some bowel injuries, and pancreatic injuries • Mobilization in hemodynamically unstable patient might be an issue
Indication	Abnormal hemodynamics with blunt trauma, penetrating injuries	Normal hemodynamics Penetrating and back or flank trauma

BOX 4: Management.

- Airway, breathing, and circulation (ABC) stabilization as per (Part A/B—refer Chapters 10 and 11)
- Identification of abdominal/pelvic injuries in primary/secondary assessment
- When in doubt patient should be transferred to the operation theater (OT) for laparotomy
  - Laparotomy indications:
    - Blunt abdominal trauma with hemodynamic instability
    - Positive focused assessment sonograph trauma (FAST)
    - Clinical evidence of intraperitoneal bleed
    - Penetrating wound
    - Gunshot through peritoneal cavity
    - Evisceration
    - Peritonitis
    - Free air, retroperitoneal air, and rupture of hemidiaphragm

Nonoperative management of blunt trauma:

- Nonoperative management of trauma patients has been greatly advanced by the evolution of CT. Solid visceral injuries are graded according to their severity
- Both the Eastern Association for the Surgery of Trauma and the Western Trauma Association have published guidance on nonoperative management of blunt abdominal trauma
- Nonoperative management is now the treatment of choice in hemodynamically stable blunt hepatic and splenic injured patients "irrespective of the grade of injury, patient's age, or the presence of associated injuries"

Caveat:

- Medication-induced coagulopathy is a management challenge in abdominal trauma patients (Trauma Part B—refer Chapter 11)
- Consider tranexamic acid in all patients with traumatic abdominal hemorrhage
- Based on the CRASH-2 (Clinical Randomization of an Antifibrinolytic in Significant Hemorrhage 2) trial, the risk of death was most reduced with tranexamic acid administration within 1 hour and in those with the most severe hemorrhagic shock, whereas treatment beyond 3 hours implicated an increased risk of death

BOX 5: Pelvic fractures.

- Pelvic fractures and associated injury types
  - Lateral
  - Anterior/open book
  - Vertical
  - Mixed

Management

- Airway, breathing, and circulation (ABC) stabilization is the priority (Chapter 30)
- Additionally, mechanical stabilization of the pelvic ring and external counter pressure through internal rotation of pelvis—sheet pelvic binder when applied at greater trochanter **(Figs. 2A and B)**
- Unstable with intraperitoneal bleed laparotomy is the choice
- Angiographic embolization for arterial hemorrhage related to pelvis is employed. If delay in this, preperitoneal packing can be done to temporarily stabilize the patient

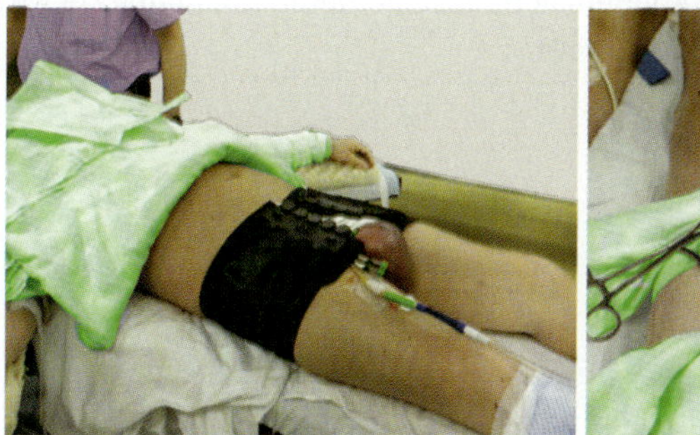

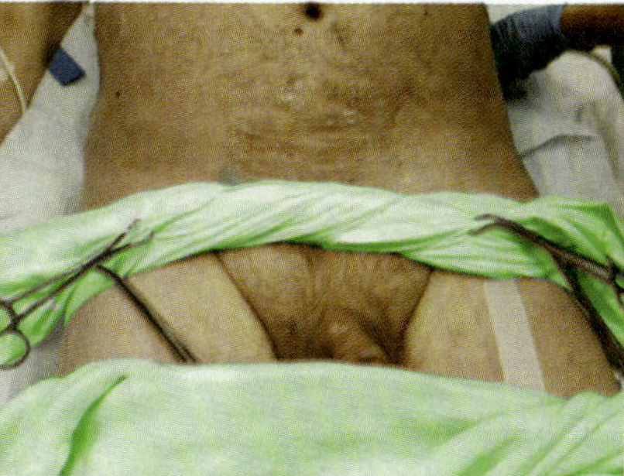

Figs. 2A and B: Pelvic binder post pelvic injury.

BOX 6: Disposition.

- Most of the trauma with abdominal injuries needs admission
- Reassessment is the most important to avoid delayed morbidity and mortality
- *Isolated pelvic injuries in adults* who are stable need no admission, just rest for 3 weeks with a stabilizer
- Pelvic injuries in trauma with hemodynamic instability need to be admitted

SUGGESTED READING

1. American College of Surgeons. Advanced Trauma Life Support (ATLS) Student Course Manual, 10th edition. Chicago, IL: American College of Surgeons; 2018.
2. CRASH-2 collaborators; Roberts I, Shakur H, Afolabi A, Brohi K, Coats T, et al. The importance of early treatment with tranexamic acid in bleeding trauma patients: An exploratory analysis of the CRASH-2 randomized controlled trial. Lancet. 2011;377(9771):1096-101, 1101.e1-2.
3. Kerwin AJ, Haut ER, Burns JB, Como JJ, Haider A, Stassen N, et al. The Eastern Association of the Surgery of Trauma approach to practice management guideline development using Grading of Recommendations, Assessment, Development, and Evaluation (GRADE) methodology. J Trauma Acute Care Surg. 2012;73(5 Suppl 4):S283-7.
4. The Western Trauma Association (WTA). California, 2016.
5. Tintinalli JE, Ma OJ, Yealy DM, Meckler GD, Stapczynski JS, Cline DM, et al. Tintinalli's Emergency Medicine: A Comprehensive Study Guide,9th edition. New York, NY: McGraw-Hill Education; 2020.
6. Trauma.org. (n.d.). Trauma: Abdominal trauma. Retrieved from https://www.trauma.org/index.php/main/article/384/

12.4 ACUTE SPINAL INJURIES

Manish Kothari

BOX 1: Definition of terms.

- *AIS: ASIA (American Spinal Injury Association) Impairment Scale*—Globally accepted classification system for level of injury
- *Neurogenic shock:* Hypotension due to bradycardia and vasodilation due to loss of sympathetic tone. Most effects noted in the first few days with most patients stabilizing in the first week to 10 days
- *Paraplegia:* Dysfunction of lower body with/without bowel and bladder due to spinal cord injuries (SCI)
- *Quadriplegia (also referred to as tetraplegia):* Dysfunction of arms, legs, bowel, and bladder
- *Spinal shock:* Transient areflexic state with loss of autonomic control, and muscle tone below the level of the injury. Functional recovery may improve after spinal shock resolves. Return of bulbocavernous reflex marks end of spinal shock

BOX 2: Principles of management in the emergency room (ER).

Spinal cord injuries can be devastating and has high morbidity and mortality

The most important aspect of management in acute care setting is:
- Diagnosis (Missed diagnosis is common)
- Prevention of secondary spinal cord injury due to repeated movements of the patient while shifting and turning. This needs knowledge of external stabilization of spine and restriction of spinal movements during turning and shifting
- Early surgery and prevention of complications

BOX 3: Diagnosis.

Always elicit history and mechanism of acute spinal injures
- Fall from height
- Road traffic accident (RTA)
- Blunt trauma

Diagnosis: Conscious aware patient
- Pain localizing to spine and/or flanks. However, absence of pain does not rule out an injury if the mechanism of injury is high-velocity trauma
- Neurological deficit and/pain/paresthesias radiating toward arm/leg

Diagnosis: Unconscious/drowsy unaware patient—not verbalizing
- Head injury patients have high prevalence of concurrent cervical spine injury. Always head CT should include cervical spine by default as protocol
- High-velocity trauma (RTA and fall from height) should include the entire spine, chest and abdomen, and pelvis. Patient to be assumed to have spinal injury until spine is cleared on CT. Radiologist to see the scan in reformatted images of sagittal and coronal planes (CT images acquired and read in axials often). Certain fractures like chance fractures are easily missed on axial plane only
- Direct bruise injuries on the back during inspection of *A*irway, *B*reathing, *C*irculation, *D*isability, and *E*xposure (ABCDE) in emergency room (ER)
- Asymmetric movement of limbs suggestive of neurological injury
- Hypotension/shock with bradycardia not responding to fluid resuscitation may be suggestive of neurogenic shock in cervical or high thoracic spinal cord injury

BOX 4: Methods of stabilization of spine to prevent secondary spinal cord injury due to movement.

- Always shift the patient on the same bed/stretcher for investigation. *Avoid shifting to bed and trolley repeatedly*
- Application of two pieces

Philadelphia collar ***(Figs. 1A and B):***

- Not to lift head/neck during application. Posterior piece to flatten out and passed through the gap between neck and bed. Front piece to give adequate chin support with causing extension of the neck. If needed, the collar can be trimmed to size using large scissors **(Figs. 2A to C)**
- *If collar is not available, then use sand bags/bolsters on the side of the neck and strap the neck on the bed before shifting*

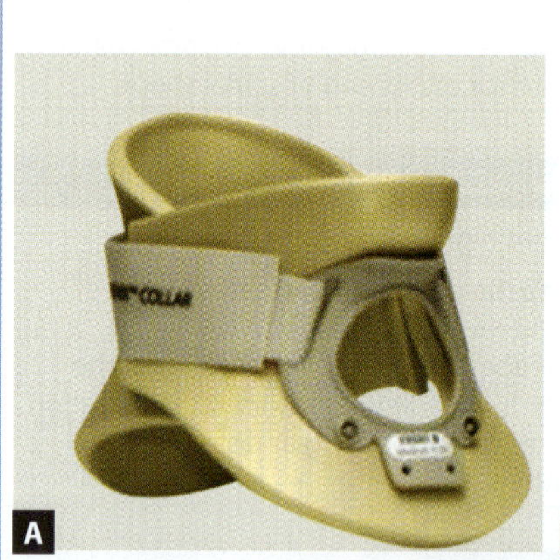

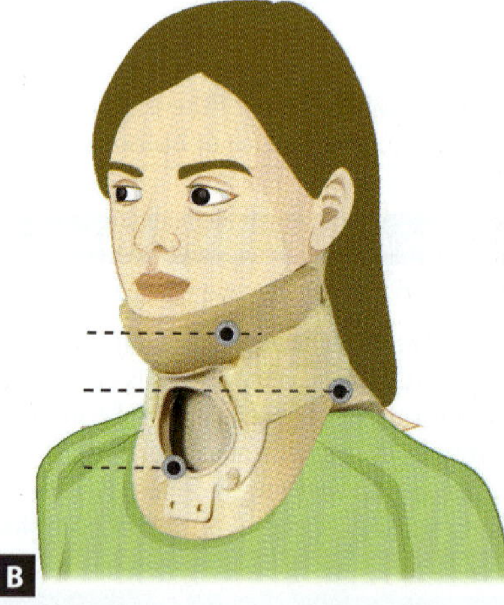

Figs. 1A and B: Philadelphia collar.

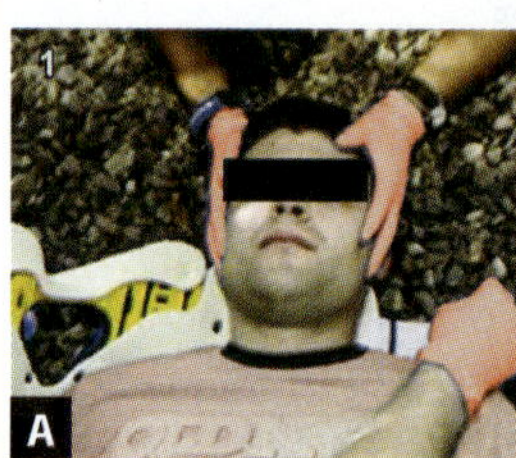

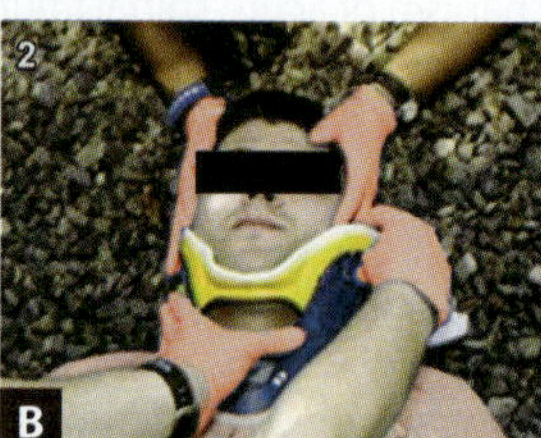

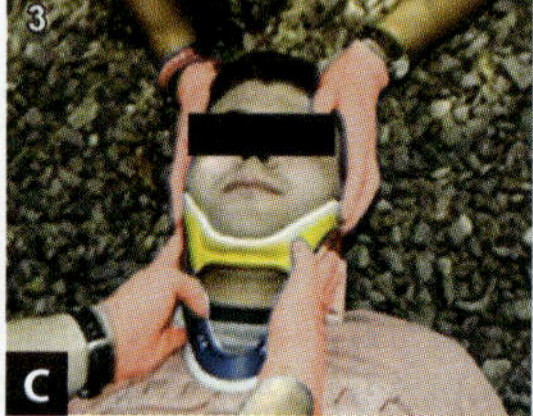

Figs. 2A to C: Placement of cervical collar with manual in line stabilization (in this posterior is placed first).

Contd...

Contd...

- Use *spinal board* for shifting. In pediatric patient, place the head in the head cut-out
- Spinal boards are hard and can cause pressure sore if kept for too long. Once the patient is shifted to definitive bed/spine is "cleared", the board should be removed
- There is no role of Taylors Brace [thoraco-lumbo-sacral orthoses (TLSO)] in acute care setting
- *Log rolling the patient:* In suspect cervical spine injuries, use four-person technique with one for head and neck, two for torso and one for legs. The aim of the technique is to allow patient's mobility without movement of the spine in neck and thoracolumbar region **(Figs. 3A and B)**

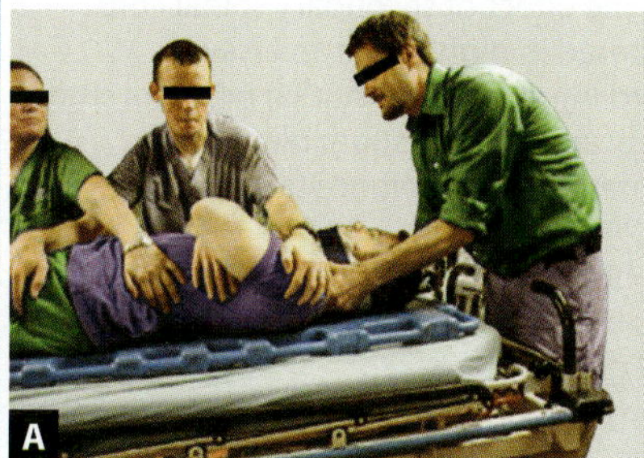

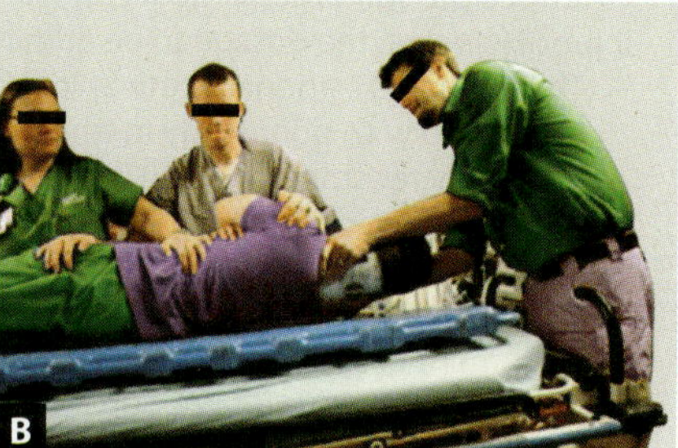

Figs. 3A and B: Log rolling a patient.

BOX 5: Investigations.

- *Low suspicion/low velocity injury:*
  - X-rays are first-line investigations. Always ask for anteroposterior (AP) and lateral views. Mention the area of pain for the radiologist to see the images carefully
  - Cervical spine X-rays should be able to show cranium to C7 vertebra minimum
  - In upper thoracic injuries/low cervical injuries, ask for swimmers' view lateral
- *High suspicion/high-velocity injury:*
  - CT scan is the FIRST investigation of choice. In head injury, ask for cervical by default. In polytrauma, ask for "trauma scan" which is head-neck-chest-abdomen-pelvis. MRI is not advisable as first investigation in adults. In children there can be spinal cord injuries without radiographic abnormality (SCIWORA) fracture where MRI is the investigation of choice (though not urgent)

BOX 6: Acute medical management in emergency room (ER).

- *Airway management* in the setting of spinal cord injury (SCI) with a cervical spine injury is complex and difficult
  - The cervical spine must be maintained in neutral alignment at all times
  - Clear oral secretions and/or debris and to prevent aspiration
  - Awake fiber optic intubation when patient's conditions and logistics allow
- *Spinal shock:* Due to loss of sympathetic tone. Fluid resuscitation fails to respond
  - Apply deep vein thrombosis (DVT) pumps.
  - Sympathomimetic drugs will improve venous tone and stabilize shock.
  - Norepinephrine is the recommended first-line vasopressor in SCI.
  - Overzealous crystalloid administration may cause pulmonary edema
- *Role of steroids (always after adequate external stabilization of injury):* Steroids help to reduce the spinal cord edema and limit the effect of secondary spinal cord injury. However, the dosage to be administered in highly controversial.
  - The infamous National Acute Spinal Cord Injury Study (NASCIS) protocol study is plagued with poor study methodology and has questionable results.
  - The study recommended 30 mg/kg IV methylprednisolone stat dose over 1 hour followed by 5.4 mg/kg/hour for 24 hours.
  - This dosage has been reported to have high morbidity and mortality.
  - The author personally does not use this high dose
- Management of spinal cord perfusion and general care
- Ensure optimal perfusion pressure and oxygenation for the spinal cord. Administer vasopressors as necessary to maintain a mean arterial pressure (MAP) above 85 mm Hg
- Keep a stable sinus heart rate within normal range
- Position the spine at the level of the heart, avoiding an elevated position to preserve cord perfusion
- Secure a Foley catheter and an enteral feeding tube to ensure proper urinary and nutritional management

BOX 7: Charting the neurological level and hourly neurological charting thereafter.

- Utilize the American Spinal Injury Association (ASIA) scale to document baseline neurological status, repeating the assessment every hour until the patient is transferred to specialty care. Any deterioration in neurological status should be addressed urgently
- In the emergency room (ER), conduct and document a comprehensive neurological assessment, including sensory level, motor function, and bowel and bladder involvement. Perform these assessments hourly for the first 24 hours, then reduce to every 4 hours if the patient stabilizes
- The *extent of injury is defined by the American Spinal Injury Association (ASIA) Impairment Scale* (modified from the Frankel classification), using the following categories:

A = Complete: No sensory or motor function is preserved in sacral segments S4–S5

B = Incomplete: Sensory, but not motor, function is preserved below the neurologic level and extends through sacral segments S4–S5

C = Incomplete: Motor function is preserved below the neurologic level, and most key muscles below the neurologic level have a muscle grade of <3

D = Incomplete: Motor function is preserved below the neurologic level, and most key muscles below the neurologic level have a muscle grade that is ≥3

E = Normal: Sensory and motor functions are normal

Contd...

Contd...

Definitions of complete and incomplete spinal cord injury ***(Fig. 4)****,* as based on the above ASIA definition, with sacral-sparing, are as follows:

- *Complete:* Absence of sensory and motor functions in the lowest sacral segments
- *Incomplete:* Preservation of sensory or motor function below the level of injury, including the lowest sacral segments

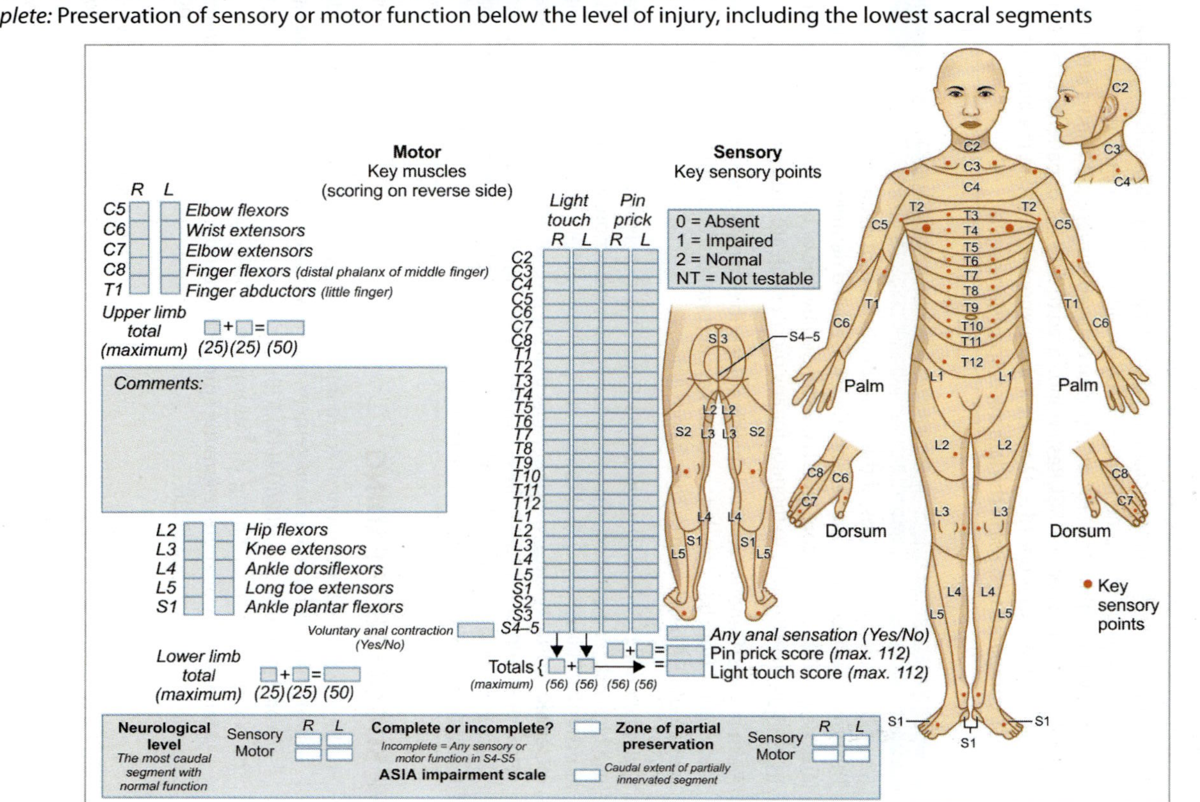

Fig. 4: Measurement of the extent of spinal injuries.

BOX 8: Surgical intervention.

- Emergency decompression of the spinal cord is recommended for acute spinal cord injury (SCI) with progressive neurological deterioration, facet dislocation, or bilateral locked facets. It is also advised for spinal nerve impingement with progressive radiculopathy and for patients with extradural lesions such as epidural hematomas or abscesses, as well as in cases of cauda equina syndrome
- The Surgical Treatment for Acute Spinal Cord Injury Study (STASCIS), a prospective surgical study by the Spine Trauma Study Group, compared early surgical intervention (within 24 hours of injury) to delayed surgery (>24 hours after injury) for patients with cervical SCI. Results indicated that 19.8% of patients undergoing early surgery experienced a ≥2 grade improvement in the ASIA Impairment Scale (AIS), compared to 8.8% in the late decompression group

BOX 9: Complications.

Neurologic deterioration: One of the earliest indicators of neurological decline is the upward extension of the sensory deficit. Detailed neurological examinations may detect that the sensory level has ascended by one or two segments. Regular neurologic assessments to monitor for any progression are crucial

Pressure sores: Denervated skin is highly susceptible to pressure sores. Remove belts and objects from back pockets, such as keys and wallets, and aim to transfer the patient off the backboard as soon as possible

Aspiration and pulmonary complications: Patients with spinal cord injuries (SCI) are at a high risk for aspiration; therefore, nasogastric decompression of the stomach is essential. Pulmonary complications are common and are directly associated with increased mortality rates, which are linked to the level of neurological injury. Severe sepsis or pneumonia often follows treatment with high-dose methylprednisolone, which is commonly administered in SCI cases. Prevent hypothermia using external warming techniques and/or warm humidified oxygen

SUGGESTED READING

1. Sandean D. Management of acute spinal cord injury: a summary of the evidence pertaining to the acute management, operative and non-operative management. World j orthopedics. 2020;11(12):573.
2. Wang TY, Park C, Zhang H, Rahimpour S, Murphy KR, Goodwin CR, et al. Management of acute traumatic spinal cord injury: a review of the literature. Front surg. 2021;8:698736.

12.5 FACE AND NECK INJURIES

Sachna P Shetty

BOX 1: Facial fractures.

- For the emergency clinician, the key to managing facial fractures and neck injuries is accurate diagnosis through head-to-toe examination followed by recognizing emergent signs and managing them followed by appropriate referral
- Forehead in skull fractures rather than facial fractures should be addressed with special attention to risk of injury to the underlying brain
- Cerebrospinal fluid (CSF) leak to be identified and the underlying fracture needs to be repaired
- Broad-spectrum antibiotics against the typical sinus and nasal pathogens are indicated for open fractures and fractures that violate a sinus
- Admit patient for depressed fractures for intravenous antibiotics and surgery for repair

BOX 2: Orbital fractures.

Orbital fracture complication that needs attention by an emergency physician are as follows:

- Enophthalmos—caused by increased intraorbital pressure leading to herniation
- Diplopia—restricted upward gaze due to inferior rectus entrapment—mostly self-resolving
- Exophthalmos: Injury to the orbit can cause a hematoma or orbital emphysema to form within the orbit, behind the globe, mostly associated with fractures
- Further causing ocular compartment syndrome of the retro-orbital space, resulting into decreased visual acuity or blindness—urgent lateral canthotomy/cantholysis by ophthalmologist

BOX 3: Face fractures.

- Mid-face fractures are classified as per LeFort—might need surgery as per complication
- Temporo-mandibular joint (TMJ): Significant trauma is more likely to cause a fracture-dislocation
- The patient may report being unable to close the mouth or causes significant protrusion of the jaw, associated with drooling and some might present with speech difficulties
- There is a depression in the area of the affected TMJ on inspection of the patient's face
- The area should be imaged with plain X-ray or Panorex examination before reduction is attempted, if there is a suspected fracture

BOX 4: Neck injuries.

- For evaluation of penetrating neck trauma, the neck has been divided into Zones I, II, and III **(Fig. 2/Box 5)**, and the location of an injury within one of these zones guided the management approach
- Now most institutions have abandoned the zone system of nomenclature, instead use hard and soft signs **(Box 6)** to identify the severity of neck injury and need for further investigation and aggressive management

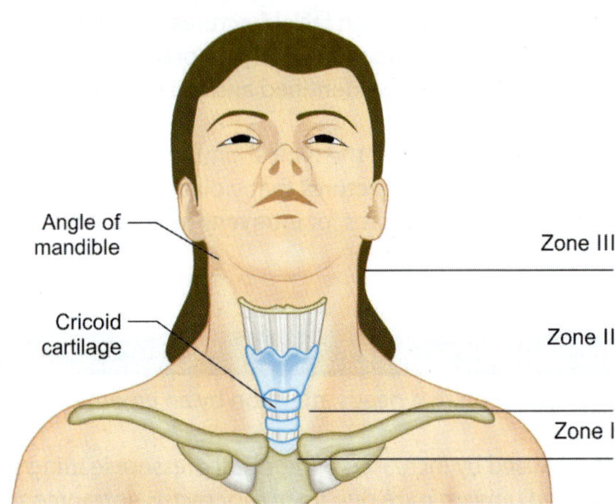

Fig. 2: Anatomical division of the neck.

BOX 5: Features of the different zones of the neck.

Neck zone	***Anatomic boundaries***	***Structures***
Zone I	Clavicles to the cricoid cartilage	• Proximal carotid vertebral arteries • Major thoracic vessels • Superior mediastinum • Lungs • Esophagus • Trachea • Thoracic duct • Spinal cord
Zone II	Cricoid cartilage to the angle of the mandible	• Carotid and vertebral arteries • Jugular veins • Esophagus • Trachea • Larynx • Spinal cord
Zone III	Angle of the mandible and the base of the skull	• Distal carotid and vertebral arteries • Pharynx • Spinal cord

BOX 6: Symptoms and signs.

Clinical:

Symptoms and signs of particular importance in neck trauma are:

- "Soft" and "Hard" Signs of Penetrating Neck Trauma
  - Soft signs:
    - Minor hemoptysis and oral bleed
    - Hematemesis
    - Dysphonia and dysphagia
    - Nonexpanding hematoma
    - Subtle neurological findings
    - Wound with proximity to the vital organs
  - Hard signs:
    - Rapidly expanding/pulsatile hematoma
    - Massive hemoptysis
    - Air bubbling from wound
    - Severe hemorrhage and shock
    - Vascular or nerve damage
    - Vascular bruit or thrill
    - Stridor/hoarseness or airway compromise
    - Cerebral ischemia
    - ± Massive subcutaneous emphysema

All the above signs need to be evaluated further with head and neck CT angiography (CTA) and some especially the hard signs urgently need to be taken to the operation room (OR) for surgery or endovascular intervention after stabilizing the airway, breathing, and circulation (ABC), which involves mainly securing airway, and managing exsanguinations

Caveat:

- Venous/air embolism can occur which needs to be dealt

BOX 7: Disposition.

- Many nondisplaced or minimally displaced facial fractures can be discharged only to be posted for a definitive repair or fixation
- Patients with limitation in the visual field and discharge instructions with acute diplopia should include patching for comfort and a request not to drive until the diplopia is resolved

SUGGESTED READING

1. American College of Surgeons. Advanced Trauma Life Support (ATLS) Student Course Manual, 10th edition. Chicago, IL: American College of Surgeons; 2018.
2. Tintinalli JE, Ma OJ, Yealy DM, Meckler GD, Stapczynski JS, Cline DM, et al. Tintinalli's Emergency Medicine: A Comprehensive Study Guide, 9th edition. New York, NY: McGraw-Hill Education; 2020.
3. Walls RM, Hockberger RS, Gausche-Hill M (Eds). Rosen's Emergency Medicine: Concepts and Clinical Practice, 9th edition. Amsterdam: Elsevier; 2018.

SECTION 3

Miscellaneous Emergencies

CHAPTER 13

Obstetric and Gynecological Emergencies

13.1 ACUTE PELVIC PAIN

GN Mansukhani, Sachna P Shetty

The causes and differential diagnosis of pelvic pain in women are extensively covered in Part 1 of this book. Below, some critical causes are discussed in detail.

BOX 1: Ovarian torsion.

- **Overview:**
  - Ovarian torsion is a surgical emergency requiring prompt intervention to preserve ovarian function
  - It typically results from ischemia, often due to enlarged ovaries or ovarian cysts
- **Risk factors:**
  - Large ovarian cysts or tumors
  - Polycystic ovaries
  - Ovulation induction (ovarian hyperstimulation syndrome)
  - Tubal ligation
- **Differential diagnosis:**
  - Appendicitis
  - Ruptured ovarian cyst
  - Urinary tract infection
  - Nephrolithiasis
  - Pelvic inflammatory disease
  - Uterine leiomyoma
  - Diverticulitis
  - Bowel obstruction
  - Ectopic pregnancy
- **Clinical features:**
  - Patients often present with severe, sharp, unilateral lower abdominal pain that can be gradual, intermittent, or sudden
  - Nausea and vomiting are common
  - Unilateral tenderness is typical, though bilateral tenderness with a palpable mass may also occur
- **Caveat:**
  - Diagnosing ovarian torsion can be challenging as symptoms may be absent.
  - Torsion can occur at any age
  - An elongated ovarian ligament, often observed during laparoscopy, is a significant risk factor for bilateral ovarian torsion

Contd...

Contd...

- **Investigation:**
  - Transvaginal ultrasound with Doppler is preferred
  - Key findings include abnormal blood flow, free fluid, and ovarian enlargement
  - The venous supply is typically the first to be compromised
- **Treatment:**
  - Immediate surgical intervention is required
  - If ovarian torsion is suspected, laparoscopy should be performed to attempt to salvage the ovary
  - The ovarian arterial blood flow often remains intact even if the ovaries appear dusky or discolored
  - Only gangrenous parts of the ovary should be removed

BOX 2: Ectopic pregnancy.

- **Overview:**
  - Ectopic pregnancy occurs when a fertilized egg implants outside the uterine cavity
- **Risk factors:**
  - Pelvic inflammatory disease
  - History of sexually transmitted infections
  - Previous tubal surgery or sterilization
  - Intrauterine device use
  - Maternal age (35–44 years)
  - Assisted reproduction techniques
  - Previous ectopic pregnancy
  - Cigarette smoking
  - Pharmacologically induced abortion
- **Clinical presentation:**
  - Ectopic pregnancy is often indicated by delayed, scanty, or irregular menses, severe, and constant abdominal pain
  - Sudden, sharp, and lateralized pain suggests rupture
  - Shoulder pain may indicate significant hemorrhage
  - Physical findings can include mild vaginal bleeding, tachycardia, normal hemoglobin levels, hypotension, peritoneal signs, and adnexal tenderness
- **Caveat:**
  - Vaginal spotting or bleeding in the absence of pain does not rule out ectopic pregnancy
  - Be cautious during pelvic examinations to avoid rupturing the ectopic pregnancy
- **Diagnosis:**
  - *Hormonal assays:* Beta-human chorionic gonadotropin (β-hCG) levels decline in nonviable or ectopic pregnancies but may overlap; hence, serial measurements are necessary
  - Progesterone levels are lower in nonviable pregnancies
  - *Ultrasonography:* Transvaginal ultrasound is more sensitive and can show moderate to large cul-de-sac fluid, an adnexal mass without intrauterine pregnancy, or direct evidence of ectopic pregnancy (e.g., fetal heart activity in the Fallopian tube)
  - *Laparoscopy:* Indicated for unstable patients or when ultrasound results are indeterminate

Contd...

Contd...

- **Caveat:**
  - Ultrasound findings of a definitive intrauterine pregnancy usually exclude ectopic pregnancy unless the patient is at high risk for heterotopic pregnancy
  - Ring of fire in ultrasound is highly diagnostic
- **Treatment:**
  - *Medical:* Methotrexate is suitable for hemodynamically stable patients with minimal abdominal pain and normal liver and renal function tests
  - Absolute contraindications include intrauterine pregnancy, immunodeficiency, severe anemia, and others
- **Unstable patients:**
  - Stabilize airway, breathing, and circulation
  - Rapid volume resuscitation with intravenous (IV) fluids and blood products as needed
  - Salpingectomy is preferred if the patient is relatively stable
  - Laparoscopy is indicated for stabilized patients or those with significant peritoneal signs but stable hemodynamics
- **Caveats:**
  - In medical management, β-hCG should be rechecked on day 4; if no decline, repeat methotrexate may be necessary
  - Target β-hCG levels should be <5 mIU to ensure resolution
  - Identification of free fluid in Morison's pouch on bedside ultrasound predicts the need for operative intervention in suspected ectopic pregnancies
  - Rh-negative patients with ectopic pregnancy should receive Rh immunoglobulin

BOX 2A: Disposition for medically managed ectopic pregnancy.

Disposition:
- Assess for treatment failure, requiring elective or emergency surgical intervention in case of medical therapy failure or tubal rupture
- Symptoms such as vaginal bleeding, abdominal pain, weakness, dizziness, or syncope post-treatment should prompt immediate evaluation for tubal rupture
- Patients should abstain from sexual intercourse for 14–21 days posttreatment (until β-hCG levels are undetectable) to minimize the risk of tubal rupture

BOX 3: Pelvic inflammatory disease (PID).

- **Overview:** PID is an ascending infection starting at the endocervix and progressing to the upper reproductive tract, causing endometriosis, salpingitis, and peritonitis
- **Clinical features**
  - Common symptoms include lower abdominal pain, dyspareunia, abnormal vaginal discharge or bleeding, dysuria, and fever
  - Physical findings may include lower abdominal tenderness, cervical friability, mucopurulent discharge, and adnexal tenderness
  - Systemic signs such as fever and tachycardia may also be present
- **Diagnosis**
  - Diagnosis is primarily clinical, supported by risk factors and a history of sexually active females

Contd...

Contd...

  - Minimum criteria include cervical motion tenderness, adnexal tenderness, and uterine tenderness
  - Additional criteria can include mucopurulent cervical discharge, elevated temperature, elevated erythrocyte sedimentation rate, and elevated C-reactive protein
- **Treatment:**
  - Immediate commencement of antibiotics is crucial
  - Treatment regimens vary based on inpatient or outpatient status
  - For inpatients, options include cefotetan plus doxycycline or cefoxitin plus doxycycline, or clindamycin plus gentamicin
  - Outpatient treatment typically involves ceftriaxone single IM dose plus doxycycline, with or without metronidazole
- **Disposition:**
  - Most women with PID are treated as outpatients
  - Hospitalization is reserved for severe cases, pregnancy, tubo-ovarian abscess, or failure to respond to outpatient therapy
  - Follow-up within 72 hours is recommended to ensure an appropriate response to treatment

SUGGESTED READING

Ovarian Torsion

1. American College of Obstetricians and Gynecologists. Practice Bulletin No. 193: Acute pelvic pain. Obstet Gynecol. 132(5):e208-e218.
2. Memon S, Zubair H. Ovarian torsion: a review of the literature. J Ovarian Res. 2020;13(1):51.
3. Mettler L, Zieman M. Gynaecology and Obstetrics: Clinical Practice and Procedures. Berlin, Germany: Springer Nature; 2021.

Ectopic Pregnancy

4. Eubanks TR, Miller R. Gynecology: Evidence-Based Clinical Practice. United States: Wiley Blackwell.
5. Lichtenberg DA, Riviello M. Management of ectopic pregnancy: A review. J Maternal Fetal Neonat Med. 2019;32(3):361-8.
6. Royal College of Obstetricians and Gynaecologists. (2016). Greentop Guideline No. 21: Early Pregnancy Loss. [online] Available from https://www.rcog.org.uk/en/guidelinesresearchservices/guidelines/gtg21/ [Last accessed September, 2024].

Pelvic Inflammatory Disease

7. Centers for Disease Control and Prevention. (2021). Sexually Transmitted Infections Treatment Guidelines. [online] Available from https://www.cdc.gov/std/treatmentguidelines/ [Last accessed September, 2024]
8. Ghanem KG, Paltiel O. Pelvic inflammatory disease: diagnosis and management. Clin Infect Dis. 2018;67(1):115-23.
9. Kohn LS. Infectious Diseases in Obstetrics and Gynecology. Amsterdam, Netherlands: Elsevier; 2020.

13.2 ABNORMAL UTERINE BLEEDING

Sudeshna Ray

BOX 1: Obstetric emergencies.

- Differential point is that one has to deal with two patients:
  - The mother
  - The fetus
- Most of the obstetric emergency management should aim for salvaging both the mother and the fetus. Of course, saving the mother comes first
- The first principle of securing airway, breathing, and circulation (ABC) remains the same for all obstetric emergencies
- While resuscitation, remember to put a wedge behind her back for giving a 15° tilt with either a hard pillow or even a saline bottle

BOX 2: Placental abruption.

- A condition where a normally situated placenta prematurely separates from the uterine wall
- Bleeding is almost always maternal
- More common in smokers, advanced aged mothers, poorly nourished, and low socioeconomic conditioned mothers and multiparas
- Predisposing factors are preeclampsia/hypertension in pregnancy and gestational diabetes
- Often caused by blunt trauma on abdominal wall or sudden uterine decompression followed by premature rupture of membranes especially if polyhydramnios
- Previous abruption increases the risk of abruption by up to 15%

Symptoms and signs:
- Shock is often disproportionate to the visible bleeding per vaginal (PV)
- Bleeding PV is usually dark colored, continuous or blood-stained serous discharge
- Pain of abdomen which is often constant (vs. labor pain which is intermittent at regular intervals)
- Hard tense abdomen; may be discolored; corresponding or more than gestational age
- Fetal movements or FHS present or absent

Emergency treatment:
- Call for help
- Quick assessment of vitals for shock
- Start high-flow oxygen
- Secure an 18- or 20-intravenous (IV) line and send bloods for complete blood count (CBC), coagulation profile, grouping, and cross match six units of bloods
- Start IV fluids preferably Ringer lactate as per her shock features. If not in shock and is hypertensive, the rate should not be >80 mL/hour; start bloods, if necessary
- Enquire about allergies and document them
- Put a urinary indwelling catheter under aseptic conditions and check the urinary volume
- Analgesics like 1 g paracetamol or diclofenac
- Order for ultrasonography (USG) and inform the obstetrician and gynecologist on call

Contd...

Contd...

- Order for ultrasonography (USG) and inform the obstetrician and gynecologist on call
- Definitive management depends on her general condition, predisposing factors, and fetal viability, and is usually termination of pregnancy either by allowing a normal delivery or performing a cesarean section
- Check for her previous notes for pregnancy so far for a thorough handover to the obstetrician and gynecologist (Check for hypertension, diabetes, polyhydramnios, previous abruption, trauma or tobacco, and substance abuse)
- Assign someone to communicate with the patient's relatives about status and take necessary consents
- If there are facilities of ICU, blood bank, and efficient obstetric and anesthetist team available for 24 hours. If operating team is not available, please transfer the patient to a tertiary center as quickly as possible

BOX 3: Placenta previa.

- Placenta situated either partially or completely over the lower uterine segment
- More seen in multiparous women
- Usually severe in third trimester. Second trimester hemorrhage due to placenta previa usually is big enough to cause shock
- Blood is almost always maternal

Symptoms and signs:

- Vaginal bleeding is almost always sudden onset, fresh red, painless, and often recurrent
- At times, the woman might be having labor pains, inform of intermittent pains at regular intervals with tightening of abdomen
- General condition of the mother is mostly proportionate to the amount of blood loss
- Size of the uterus is corresponding to her gestational age
- Abdomen is soft and relaxed without any area of tenderness
- Often the head is floating or presenting part is breech or transverse
- Avoid any vaginal digital examination

Emergency treatment:

- Call for help
- Quick assessment of her vitals
- Secure an 18- or 20-IV line and send bloods for complete blood count (CBC), coagulation profile, grouping, and cross match 6 units of bloods
- Start IV fluids preferably Ringer lactate/Normal saline
- If excessive hemorrhage leading to shock, along with airway, breathing, and circulation (ABC), put in a urinary indwelling catheter, and check for urinary volume
- Start blood transfusion, if necessary
- Call for obstetrician and gynecologist
- Call for ultrasonography (USG) assessment
- Check her previous notes for placental localization in the most recent scan and presenting part and any history of previous bleed. Bleeding from placenta previa is often progressively increased in volumes with each episode of bleeding
- Expectant treatment can continue, if the mother is hemodynamically stable, bleeding stops, gestational age (GA) <37 weeks and FHS is present. Definitive management is delivery with a multidisciplinary team of senior obstetricians, anesthetists, interventional radiologists, hematologists and neonatologist
- Assign someone to communicate with the patient's relatives about status and take necessary consents

BOX 4: Postpartum hemorrhage.

Any amount of bleeding from or into the genital tract following the birth of the baby up to the end of puerperium (42 days after birth) which adversely affects the general condition of the mother leading to tachycardia and hypotension

- Minor postpartum hemorrhage (PPH) is up to 1 L; major is >1 L and severe is >2 L
- Primary PPH occurs at or within 24 hours of birth
- Secondary PPH occurs beyond 24 hours and within puerperium
- *Third stage of hemorrhage* occurs when there is bleeding before the expulsion of placenta
- *True PPH* happens when bleeding happens after the expulsion of placenta

Causes can be:

- Atonic (80%) seen mostly in multifetal pregnancies, polyhydramnios, grand multipara and poor nutrition, antepartum hemorrhage, induction or augmentation of labor, uterine fibroid in pregnancy, adherent placenta, and prolonged labor
- Traumatic due to extension of episiotomy or vaginal and cervical tears, uterine artery injury at cesarean section (CS) and rarely ruptured uterus
- Retained tissues in form of bits of placenta
- Blood coagulation disorders (least common) seen in abruption placentae, jaundice in pregnancy, thrombotic thrombocytopenic purpura (TTP), hemolysis, elevated liver enzymes, and low platelets (HELLP) or intrauterine fetal death

Signs and symptoms:

- Usually revealed bleeding in form of continuous trickle and big clots; rarely concealed in form of vulvovaginal or broad ligament hematoma
- It is a life-threatening emergency. All PPH cases should be taken up on war footing as death can occur if corrective steps are not taken at the right time
- In atonic hemorrhage, uterus is found to be flabby which often becomes hard intermittently on messaging
- If the uterus seems to be well contracted, a traumatic cause in the genital tract should be looked for

Management

Principles:

1. Ensure effective sustained contraction of the uterus
2. Replace the lost volume and blood
3. To stop traumatic bleeding

Caveat: Please remember that traumatic and atonic cause of hemorrhage can coexist

Steps:

1. Call for help from all colleagues present there and also call for the obstetrician and gynecologist on call
2. Quick assessment of her vitals
3. Ensure airway and breathing; start oxygen 10 L/min
4. Secure an 18- or 20-IV line and send bloods for complete blood count (CBC), coagulation profile, grouping, and crossmatch 6 units of bloods
5. Keep patient flat and warm
6. Rapidly infuse IV fluids preferably Ringer lactate/Normal saline preferably with 20 units of oxytocin in 1 L of fluids

Contd...

Contd...

7. Catheterize the bladder
8. Assign someone to communicate with the patient relatives about status and take necessary consents
9. Call for USG assessment
10. In a confirmed postpartum hemorrhage (PPH) secondary to uterine atony, which is the most common cause, the first temporary step is to do a bimanual uterine massage by placing the fist in the anterior fornix against the suprapubic area compressing the uterine fundus **(Fig. 1)**
11. This is to buy time before doing a definitive step which is surgical exploration

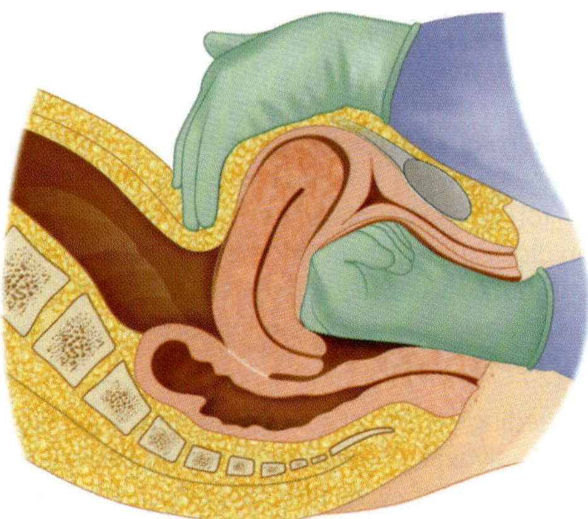

Fig. 1: Intrauterine massage for uterine atony.

SUGGESTED READING

1. Arias F, Bhide AG, S A, Damania K, Daftary SN. Arias' Practical Guide to High-Risk Pregnancy and Delivery: A South Asian Perspective. 5th ed. Elsevier India; 2019.
2. Cunningham FG, Leveno KJ, Dashe JS, Hoffman BL, Spong CY, Casey BM. Williams Obstetrics. 26th ed. New York: McGraw Hill Medical; 2022.
3. James D, Steer PJ, Weiner CP, Gonik B, Robson SC. High-risk pregnancy: Management options Volume 1. 5th ed. Cambridge: Cambridge University Press; 2017.
4. Konar H. DC Dutta's Textbook of Obstetrics. 10th ed. Jaypee Brothers Medical Publishers; 2022.

13.3 COMMONEST MATERNAL EMERGENCIES

Shilpa P Agarwal

BOX 1: Hypertensive disorders in pregnancy.

Gestational hypertension:
- Onset of hypertension after 20 weeks of gestation without proteinuria

Preeclampsia:
- Hypertension that occurs after 20 weeks of pregnancy with accompanying proteinuria:
  - **Blood pressure criteria:**
    - Persistent blood pressure readings above 140/90 mm Hg on at least two separate occasions, with a minimum of 6 hours but no >7 days between measurements
    - If the systolic pressure surpasses 160/110 mm Hg, a single confirmation within minutes is sufficient
  - **Proteinuria criteria:**
    - Protein excretion >300 mg within a 24-hour period, or a protein to creatinine ratio exceeding 0.3
    - In cases where quantitative measurement is not available, a dipstick reading of 1+ can be used as an alternative indicator

BOX 2: Preeclampsia with severe features.

Preeclampsia with severe features:
- Blood pressure (BP) >160/110 mm Hg
- Thrombocytopenia (platelets <100,000/mm^3) and/or evidence of microangiopathic hemolytic anemia (MAHA)
- Elevated alanine transaminase (ALT) and/or aspartate transaminase (AST), at least twice the upper limit of normal
- Progressive renal insufficiency, indicated by creatinine levels >1.1 mg/dL, a doubling of serum creatinine, or oliguria (<500 mL of urine in 24 hours)
- Persistent headache or ongoing cerebral or visual disturbances
- Persistent epigastric pain
- Pulmonary edema or cyanosis

Investigations:
- Complete blood count (CBC) including platelet count
- Complete urine examination
- Total direct and indirect bilirubin
- Serum glutamic-oxaloacetic transaminase (SGOT) and serum glutamic-pyruvic transaminase (SGPT)
- Serum creatinine
- 24-hour urine protein
- Urine protein creatinine clearance
- Fundoscopy when indicated
- Ultrasound for maternal kidneys

Contd...

Contd...

Management:
- Initial airway breathing circulation to be stabilized
- Admission in high-dependency unit (HDU)/intensive care unit (ICU)
- Start antihypertensive medications according to BP
- Magnesium sulfate, if indicated
- Maternal vitals monitoring (Maternal Obstetric Early Warning Chart)
- Maternal stabilization and evaluation
- Assess end-organ damage
- Confirm gestational age
- Confirm fetal well-being

Watch for premonitory symptoms:
- Headache
- Oliguria
- Epigastric pain
- Blurring of vision
- Nausea/vomiting
- Steroids for fetal lung maturity (26–34 weeks)
- Delivery criteria
  - Severe pulmonary embolism (PE) >34 weeks
  - Severe PE and previable pregnancy

Maternal indications:
- Uncontrolled severe hypertension
- Eclampsia
- Hemolysis, elevated liver enzymes, and low platelets (HELLP)
- Abruption placenta
- Disseminated intravascular coagulation (DIC)
- Hepatic rupture
- Renal function compromised
- Cerebral hemorrhage

Fetal indications:
- Nonreactive nonstress test (NST)
- Doppler abnormalities [reversed end-diastolic flow (REDF)]
- An estimated fetal weight (EBW) <5th percentile
- Oligohydramnios
- Physician's counseling
- Anesthesia check up
- Neonatal counseling

Expectant management:
- Vitals and BP monitoring every 4 hourly
- Urine output monitoring (Foleys catheter, if required)
- Investigations every 34 days
- Ultrasonography (USG) obstetrics and Doppler
- Nonstress test

BOX 3: Magnesium sulfate regimen.

Loading dose:
- 4 g IV 20% solution

Maintenance dose:
- 12 g/hour IV infusion

Dose in renal failure:
- Loading same as above
- Maintenance reduce to half

IV fluids:
- If required
- 75 mL/hour
- Medication protocol

Labetalol:
- 20 mg IV bolus
- Further 40 mg 10 minutes later, if needed
- Further 80 mg every 10 minutes if needed for two doses
- Maximum dose 220 mg

Nifedipine:
- 10 g oral to start
- Repeat 10 mg in 30 minutes, if needed

Hydralazine:
- 5 mg or 10 mg intramuscularly (IM)
- Repeat 510 mg at 20 minutes intervals as needed
- If no response after 20 mg IV or 30 mg IM, consider other drug

Nitroglycerine:
- 5 µg/min continuous IV infusion
- Increase by 5 µg/min every 35 minutes as needed up to 20 µg/min
- Increase by 1,020 µg/min, if needed

BOX 4: Eclampsia.

Eclampsia:
- Patient in left lateral position
- Protection with railings to prevent self-injury
- Oral secretion gentle suction
- Oxygen via face mask
- Magnesium sulfate
- Antihypertensive as discussed above
- Steroids
- 26–34 weeks

Maternal monitoring:
- BP monitoring
- Neurological status
- Foley catheter strict input-output charting
- Fundoscopy
- Laboratory evaluation

Fetal evaluation:
- USG
- Nonstress test (NST)
- Rule out abruption

Planning delivery

Mode of delivery depending on:
- Maternal condition
- Fetal condition
- Gestational age
- Cervix status
- Obstetric-associated factors
- Vaginal delivery is preferable but within a time frame
- Induction of labor after maternal evaluation
- Adequate pain relief

BOX 5: Hemolysis, elevated liver enzymes, and low platelets (HELLP) syndrome.

HELLP syndrome

Triad of

- Hemolysis
- Elevated liver enzymes
- Low platelet count
- Life-threatening condition
- Hypertension may be absent in 20% of cases
- Can present antenatally of early postpartum
- Usually presents in the late second and third trimester of pregnancy

Clinical features:

- Nausea vomiting
- Right upper quadrant pain
- Headache
- Blurring of vision
- High BP (20% of cases may be absent)

Investigations:

- Microangiopathic hemolytic anemia
- Thrombocytopenia
- Elevated transaminases
- Urinary protein

Differential diagnosis:

- Acute fatty liver of pregnancy (AFLP)
- Twin-to-twin transfusion syndrome (TTTS)
- Hemolytic uremic syndrome (HUS)
- Acute hepatitis

Autoimmune thrombocytopenic purpura:

- Complications
- Hepatic rupture, hepatic infarction, and periportal liver dysfunction
- Acute renal failure
- Pulmonary edema/pleural effusions
- Acute respiratory distress syndrome (ARDS)
- Placental abruption
- Disseminated intravascular coagulation (DIC)

Management:

- Delivery is the only way to stop progress
- *Timing of delivery depends on:*
  - Maternal condition
  - Fetal condition
  - Gestational age
  - $MgSO_4$ for neuroprotection and seizure prophylaxis
  - Antihypertensive medications
  - Corticosteroids for fetal lung maturity
  - Platelet transfusions, if indicated
  - Supportive care

SUGGESTED READING

1. Cunningham FG, Leveno KJ, Dashe JS, Hoffman BL, Spong CY, Casey BM. Williams Obstetrics. 26th ed. New York: McGraw Hill Medical; 2022.
2. James D, Steer PJ, Weiner CP, Gonik B, Robson SC. High-risk Pregnancy: Management Options, Volume 1. 5th ed. Cambridge: Cambridge University Press; 2017.
3. Landon MB, Galan HL, Jauniaux ERM. Gabbe's obstetrics: Normal and Problem Pregnancies, 9th edition. Amsterdam, Netherlands: Elsevier; 2024.
4. NICE. Hypertension in pregnancy: Diagnosis and Management | Guidance | NICE [Internet]. Nice.org.uk. NICE; 2023. Available from: https://www.nice.org.uk/guidance/ng133

CHAPTER

14 Orthopedic Emergency

14.1 INITIAL EVALUATION AND MANAGEMENT OF ORTHOPEDIC EMERGENCIES

Ameet P Pispati, Sana Aamir

BOX 1: Approach to orthopedic patients in emergency room.

- *Chief complaint including:*
  - Mechanism of injury
  - Constitutional symptoms
  - Referred symptoms
- *Physical examination:*
  - Observe—bleeding, erythema, swelling, atrophy, deformity, and skin changes
  - Range of movements—first check active then passive movement for affected joint(s) and joints proximal and distal
  - Check neurovascular status—sensation, power, and reflexes should be checked
- *Investigations:*
  - *X rays:* Anteroposterior (AP), lateral and oblique views, and special views where necessary
  - Complete blood count, triple H, blood grouping, and crossmatching
  - Joint fluid aspiration for analysis is done where septic arthritis is suspected
  - Ultrasound evaluation is done where indicated

BOX 2: Principles of management of musculoskeletal injuries.

- Relevant history taking
- Perform "Rapid Trauma Survey"
- If spine injury is suspected, apply a hard cervical collar immediately
- Perform splintage of swollen or deformed extremities after addressing life-threatening conditions
- Manage the airways, breathing, and circulation, immobilize the body on a spine board, and splint the inured parts
- Start intravenous (IV) antibiotics as soon as possible
- Open wounds should be irrigated with normal saline or even copious tap water to decrease the contamination, followed by a sterile wound dressing
- Do not suture dirty or complex wounds
- Tetanus prophylaxis should be given in all cases
- Gas gangrene prophylaxis if wound is contaminated with soil

BOX 3: Basic fracture evaluation and management.

- Start with airway, breathing, and circulation followed by primary and secondary surveys
- Fracture location should be thoroughly examined especially location and associated dislocation
- Assess the type of fracture—closed versus open, and the amount of contamination, if open
- Thorough neurovascular assessment should be done
- All relevant imaging studies should be carried out
- Chest, abdomen, pelvic, and other associated injuries should be ruled out
- Analgesics to be given as required
- Appropriate splinting of injured limbs should be carried out before shifting the patient
- If reduction has been performed, then assessment of neurovascular status is must prior to and after reduction
- If necessary, then refer the patient to other relevant specialities

BOX 4: Complications of fractures.

- *Early local:*
  - Compartment syndrome
  - Neurovascular injury
  - Infection
  - Fracture blisters
- *Late local:*
  - Reflex sympathetic dystrophy
  - Osteomyelitis
  - Malunion/nonunion
  - Avascular necrosis
  - Posttraumatic arthritis
- *Systemic:*
  - Sepsis
  - Deep vein thrombosis
  - Pulmonary embolism
  - Acute respiratory distress syndrome
  - Hemorrhagic shock

BOX 5: X-rays in orthopedic injuries.

- All relevant views must be included in X-ray imaging. The proper diagnosis is greatly dependent on getting correct views
- How orthopedic X-rays are described:
  - *Anatomic location:* Which bone and the location of the fracture within the bone
  - *Fracture pattern:* Whether oblique/spiral/comminuted/transverse
  - Are the fragments shifted in relation to each other?—Displacement
  - Is there an angle between longitudinal axis of fragments? Angulated
  - If fracture extends into the joint—Intra-articular
- Pediatric X-rays are unique:
  - Pediatric X-rays because of the on-going growth look different
  - Growth centers appear as gaps between bones which are normal finding
  - Compare with the opposite side of X-ray in case of doubt

BOX 6: Acute orthopedic emergencies.

- Open fracture **(Box 7)**
- Fractures or dislocations associated with neurovascular compromise
- Osteomyelitis **(Box 9)**
- Septic arthritis
- Compartment syndrome **(Box 8)**
- Polytrauma
- Cauda equina syndrome **(Box 10)**

Prompt diagnosis and timely intervention are mandatory to preserve limb and save life

BOX 7: Open fracture management.

Presentation: High-velocity injuries in areas of the body with relatively less soft-tissue coverage or with fracture fragments with more extreme angulation

Examination: Gross contamination, devitalized tissue, and lacerations should be assessed

Management:
- Urgent irrigation and debridement in the operating room for all open fractures
- Surgical debridement 6–8 hours after time of injury is preferred
- Irrigation in emergency room with low pressure normal saline for grossly contaminated wounds and debridement of contaminants and dead tissue should be done
- The key to reducing infection is early antibiotic administration
- After operative debridement, the full extent of wound is assessed and then only classification of grade of open injury by Gustillo–Anderson classification should be determined
- Send culture swab from the wound and from fracture ends
- Irrigate with copious amounts of normal saline or even tap water to reduce contamination
- Antiseptic sterile dressing to be applied
- Immobilization with appropriate splint should be done
- Administration of tetanus vaccine and gas gangrene serum when necessary
- Start IV antibiotics
- Keep nil orally and make urgent referral, if needed

BOX 8: Management of compartment syndrome.

Causes: Fractures, burns, tight casts or wraps, bleeding, intravenous (IV) extravasation; reperfusion injury

- Earliest finding is pain out of proportion to the injury which should be alarming
- Pain not relieved by analgesia or increased with passive stretch (most specific)
- Early findings are pallor and paresthesia whereas pulselessness and paralysis are late findings)

Treatment:

- Primarily, it is a clinical diagnosis but direct compartment measurements should be measured whenever feasible
- All constrictive dressings (casts and splints) should be removed
- Limb elevation to be maintained
- To decompress compartmental pressure patient should be referred for urgent fasciotomy
- To release all affected compartments and to prevent further tissue ischemia emergency fasciotomies to be done

Complications: Volkmann's ischemic contracture, rhabdomyolysis, myoglobinuria leading to renal failure

BOX 9: Management of septic arthritis and bone infection (Osteomyelitis).

Septic joint is defined as infection within joint space and presents as localized joint pain with warmth, swelling, and restriction of active and passive range of motion (ROM), along with fever

Osteomyelitis presents as pain, fever along with localized extremity swelling and redness, with difficulty in weightbearing

Investigations:

- Complete blood count (CBC), erythrocyte sedimentation rate (ESR), C-reactive protein (CRP), and blood culture should be sent before starting antibiotics
- Frank pus or turbid fluid from joint aspirate can be sent for cell count and culture-sensitivity
- It takes 10–14 days for X-rays changes to appear

Treatment:

- Arthrotomy for septic arthritis; drilling, and decompression of bone for osteomyelitis, along with IV antibiotics, followed by oral antibiotics for minimum 6 weeks

BOX 10: Cauda equina syndrome.

It is a compression of the lumbosacral nerve roots below the conus medullaris, and may be due to a large central disk prolapse (L4-5 or L5-S1) with or without lumbar canal stenosis, or an extrinsic mass like a tumor or a burst fracture

It presents with progressive neurological deficit. The patient has:
- Pain
- Motor signs include weakness/paraparesis in multiple root distribution, diminished deep tendon reflexes, urinary retention, and fecal incontinence due to loss of anal sphincter tone)
- Sensory signs include saddle anesthesia, low back pain with lower limb radiation, bilateral sensory loss or pain involving multiple dermatomes, and sexual dysfunction at times though this is then a late finding

Treatment:
- This is a surgical emergency
- MRI scans of spine for diagnosis and surgical planning
- Emergency surgical decompression should be done

BOX 11: General principles to be kept in mind.

- X-ray findings along with detailed history and physical examination will increase the diagnostic accuracy
- In cases of suspected fracture clinically but negative X-ray films, treat for a fracture
- Do not accept inadequate studies where proper X-ray views are not taken
- Always perform X-ray examinations before reductions, unless it is associated with neurovascular compromise
- Neurovascular status assessment should always be done prior to reduction and after all reductions
- Full circumferential casting in plaster soon after injury is usually not advised in emergency room; slabs are preferred
- The patient should be able to ambulate safely before being discharged from the emergency room
- Detailed after-care instructions should be explained before leaving the room especially regarding monitoring signs of neurovascular compromise, splint care, and follow-up
- In the multiple trauma patient, airway, head, and intracavitary injuries are addressed first and then noncritical orthopedic injuries can be diagnosed and treated later on

BOX 12: Common pitfalls.

- Airways, breathing, and circulation are to be addressed first and then address orthopedic injuries during your resuscitation
- Neurovascular status should always be assessed distal to the injury during the initial assessment and after application of a splint
- Orthopedic injuries distract an examiner from potentially life-threatening injuries as they can be quite dramatic
- A common issue in fracture care is that it is associated with missed fracture. Always look for a second fracture after finding one fracture on a radiograph not to miss on second occult/missed fracture
- Many anatomic variants may be mistaken for fractures on radiographs
- Comparison of radiographs of the other side may be helpful in cases of doubt
- Additionally, clinical correlation should be sought in case of doubt

SUGGESTED READING

1. Adams JC, Hamblen D. Outline of Fractures: Including Joint Injuries. 12th ed. Livingstone; 2007.
2. Adams JC, Hamblen DL. Outline of orthopaedics. 13th ed. Edinburgh: Churchill Livingstone; 2001.
3. Blom A, Warwick D, Whitehouse M, Solomon L. Apley & Solomon's System of Orthopaedics and Trauma. 10th ed. CRC Press; 2018.
4. Buchholz RW, Court-Brown CM, Heckman JD, Torne P. Rockwood and Green's fractures in adults, 7th edition. Philadelphia: Lippincott Williams and Wilkins; 2010. p. 2174.
5. Greene WB. Essentials of Musculoskeletal Care. 6th ed. American Academy of Orthopaedic Surgeons; 2003.

14.2 MUSCULOSKELETAL PAIN IN EMERGENCY

14.2.1 Acute Back and Neck Pain

Gautam Zaveri, Siddharth Shah

BOX 1: Introduction.

- Back and neck pain are among the top 10 reasons for a visit to the "emergency room (ER)"
- Back pain accounts for approximately 5% of all ER presentations
- Nonspecific back pain (nonserious causes) contributed 60.8% of all back pain presentations in the emergency room (ER)
- Diagnosis and further management of acute episodes of back and neck pain can be challenging for ER physicians leading to inappropriate imaging referrals, potentially avoidable hospital admissions and unnecessary surgical procedures

BOX 2: Classification.

Classification of low back pain (LBP)	*Classification of neck pain*
• Acute LBP 0–6 weeks • Subacute LBP 6–12 weeks • Chronic LBP >12 weeks	• Acute (transitory) neck pain <1 week • Subacute (short duration) 1–12 weeks • Chronic (long duration) >12 weeks

BOX 3: Etiology of back and neck pain.

Group A (nonspecific pain): 80–90%

- *Degenerative:* Wear and tear of intervertebral disk, vertebral endplates, facet joints, ligaments, and muscles
- *Metabolic:* Osteoporosis, osteomalacia, and hyperparathyroidism
- *Functional:* Nonorganic causes—stress, anxiety, depression, overwork, fatigue, and secondary gain

Group B (Sinister pain): <10%

- *Inflammatory:* Rheumatoid arthritis, seronegative spondyloarthropathies—psoriasis, and ankylosing spondylitis
- *Traumatic: Ligament injury, muscle sprains, vertebral fractures, intervertebral disk injuries—herniation and annular tear*
- *Infective:* Tubercular, pyogenic, and brucellosis
- *Neoplastic:* Metastases, primary tumors—benign or malignant
- *Connective tissue disorders:* Systemic lupus erythematosus (SLE)

Group C (Secondary pain): 10%

- *Back pain secondary to nonspinal conditions:* Urinary infections, renal stones, pelvic inflammatory disease, gallstones, gastritis, pancreatitis, chest infections, cardiac, aortic aneurysm, ectopic pregnancy, etc.
- *Neck pain secondary to nonspinal conditions*—periarthritis shoulder, cardiac (angina/infarct), migraine, and herpes zoster

BOX 4: Triage of acute pain in emergency room (ER).

- **Sinister pain:**
  - Sinister causes account for <10% cases of acute back/neck pain
  - Early diagnosis of sinister causes is based on identification of red flags on history and examination supplemented with appropriate investigations
  - The presence of red flags on the history and examination should supplement, not replace, and clinical judgment regarding further work-up in the ER
  - Avoid focusing on a single feature in isolation, and instead combine red flags with additional clinical and examination findings to more accurately determine the likelihood of serious underlying disease
  - Based on pathology identified, specific treatment must be instituted

TABLE 1: The red flags.

- *Neurological signs that signify significant neurologic dysfunction involving the nerve roots, the cauda equina or the spinal cord:*
  - Unilateral/bilateral numbness or weakness in the lower limbs
  - Gait disturbance
  - Ataxia (imbalance on walking)
  - Loss of bladder/bowel function (urinary retention, incontinence, absent anal sphincter tone, patulous anus, and reduced/absent bulbocavernosus reflex), sexual dysfunction, and saddle anesthesia
- *Back/Neck pain associated with structural spinal deformity such as scoliosis, kyphosis, and torticollis*
- *Risk factors or signs of infection, fracture, or malignancy:*
  - Patient <20 years or >50 years of age suffering from back/neck pain for first time
  - Night pain, rest pain, continuous pain, and thoracic back pain
  - Back/neck pain associated with fever, weight loss, and anorexia
  - Past history of tuberculosis or tuberculosis contact
  - History of trauma with any focal spinal tenderness on palpation, contusion or abrasion, altered consciousness or distracting injury
  - Past history of cancer or currently being treated for cancer
  - Immunocompromised status—chronic illnesses, posttransplant patient, and immunosuppressive therapy
  - Intravenous (IV) drug abusers
  - Patients on long-term steroids and anticoagulants
- Intractable pain or pain persistent for >4–6 weeks

- **Nonspecific pain:**
  - In 80–90% of back/neck pain patients, the precise cause cannot be identified
  - Primarily due to degenerative pathology, muscle pulls, fatigued muscles, and ligament injuries
  - Degenerative acute pain is a self-limiting condition. It resolves with minimal intervention within 4–8 weeks in 90% patients. 60% return to work within 1 month and 90% within 3 months
  - Treatment is primarily nonoperative
  - For all nonoperative treatments, precise diagnosis does not matter
  - Hence, investigations are unnecessary

Contd...

Contd...

TABLE 2: Patterns of degenerative back pain.

Type	*Description*
I	Predominantly back pain. Worse on lumbar spine flexion. Better on extension
II	Predominantly back pain. Worse on lumbar spine extension. Better on flexion
III	Predominantly radicular leg pain. Worse on lumbar spine flexion. Better on extension. Straight leg raising test/Femoral stretch test may be positive
IV	Predominantly buttock, thigh, leg pain/paresthesia/numbness. Worse on lumbar extension, standing, and walking. Better on lumbar flexion, sitting, or bending forward

Flowchart 1: Flowchart for triage of back/neck pain patients presenting in the emergency room (ER).

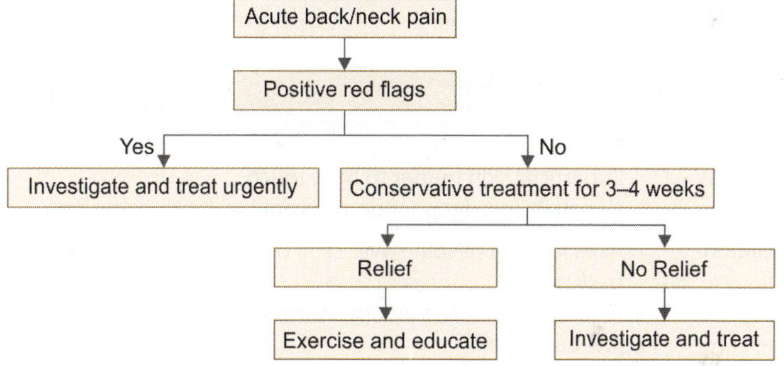

- **Illness behavior:**
  - Back/neck pain should be viewed within a psychosocial context
  - Psychological, emotional, and social factors can play a significant role in the production, severity, and persistence of acute and chronic back/neck pain. They can also determine how much the pain impacts one's life
- The diagnosis of illness behavior is facilitated by identification of the yellow flags on history and examination
- The Waddell signs were developed to evaluate nonorganic components of acute back pain complaints. The overall test is considered positive when a patient scores positively in three or more categories
- Early diagnosis of illness behavior enables institution of appropriate behavioral therapy and drugs that may alter the chronicity of the problem

Contd...

Contd...

TABLE 3: The yellow flags.

- Unremitting pain—diffuse pain, whole body pain, hemibody pain, migraine, and vertigo
- Location of pain varies, and symptoms expand
- Pain present for months without a clear supporting diagnosis
- Belief that back/neck pain is harmful or disabling
- Fearing or avoiding activity due to back/neck pain
- Strong expectation that passive rather than active treatment would help
- Tendency toward low mood and isolation
- Abnormal behavior pattern
- Depression, anxiety—past history of disorder, and mental health affection
- Problems at work, poor job satisfaction, unemployment, and litigation
- Sleep disturbances, loss of libido, family problems, and physical abuse
- Positive Waddell's signs

TABLE 4: Waddell (Nonorganic signs).

Category	***Signs***
Tenderness	• Superficial skin tender to light touch • Nonanatomic deep tenderness not localized to one area
Simulation	• Axial loading of spine over skull of standing patient elicits low back pain • *Rotation:* Shoulders and pelvis rotated in the same plane elicit low back pain
Distraction	• Differences in supine straight-leg-raising and seated straight-leg-raising
Regional	• *Weakness:* Many muscle groups give away weakness (patient does not give full effort on minor muscle testing) • *Sensory:* Sensory loss in stocking or glove distribution; nondermatomal
Overreaction	• Disproportionate facial or verbal expression (i.e., pain behavior)

BOX 5: Investigations—When and what?

- Neurologic deficit
- Positive red flags
- Trauma—suspicion of fracture
- Polytrauma
- Persistent symptoms >4 weeks
- Recurrent symptoms

TABLE 5: Investigation and rationale for the pain.

Investigation	*Rationale*
Radiographs	• Plain films (anteroposterior and lateral) are helpful for suspected structural abnormalities such as fractures, spondylolisthesis, and dislocations
CT scan	• Superior to plain radiographs for the detection of vertebral fractures, other bony disorders, bone fragments within the spinal canal, or spinal sagittal deformities or dislocations • For atraumatic neck/back pain, CT should be performed only when MRI is not available or contraindicated (e.g., metallic implants)
MRI	• The modality of choice for evaluation of acute neck and back pain in the emergency room (ER) • MRI is highly sensitive and specific in delineating the exact bony or soft-tissue spinal pathology such as spinal infections, malignancy, disk herniation, and epidural compression syndrome • Obtain an MRI scan with contrast when there is suspicion for metastatic disease, osteomyelitis, abscess, and inflammatory conditions
Laboratory investigations	• Rarely needed for the initial evaluation of acute low back pain (LBP) • White blood cell count, erythrocyte sedimentation rate (ESR), and C-reactive protein (CRP) can be considered in cases of suspected infection, malignancy, or nonspinal causes
Angiography	• To ascertain vascular injury especially in cases of polytrauma with systemic decompensation, hyperextension ankylosing spondylitis fractures with aortic injury, or vertebral artery injuries with cervical fractures/dislocations
Miscellaneous	• Further tests based on clinical assessment can be pursued to evaluate the suspicion of nonspinal causes of the back or neck pain such as CT abdomen, pelvic, cardiac markers, etc.

BOX 6: Limitations of magnetic resonance imaging (MRI) in diagnosis.

- MRI is a highly sensitive test but too nonspecific to differentiate patients with back/neck pain from those without pain
- The drawback of MRI as an investigation is that preexisting degenerative changes in the cervical and lumbar spine may confound the clinical management
- One-third of all asymptomatic patients will have degenerative changes on MRI and all patients >60 years have at least one degenerative disk or disk bulge
- In symptomatic patients, MRI findings of degeneration often do not correlate with the severity of patient's symptoms
- Patient's pain may worsen without any change on imaging or may improve despite radiographic progression
- Thus, careful protocol driven patient's selection and astute clinical assessment are vital in clinic-radiological decision making

BOX 7: Nonoperative treatment.

- Nonoperative treatment for patients with back/neck due to a sinister pathology may be continued in-hospital or at home, based on the recommendations of a spine specialist
- 90% of patients with degenerative back/neck/radicular pain can be treated nonoperatively at home
- The cornerstones of nonoperative treatment include:
  - Education about back/neck pain
  - Reassurance about the benign nature of the problem
  - Instituting appropriate nonoperative treatment
    - Local heat
    - Rest
    - Pharmacological treatment
    - Exercises
    - Pain blocks
    - Alternative treatments

Local heat:
- Offers symptomatic analgesia by allowing local vasodilatation and reducing muscle spasm
- Applied to the painful area for 15–20 minutes twice or thrice daily
- Alternatively, short-wave diathermy/local ultrasound/transcutaneous electrical nerve stimulation (TENS) can be administered by physiotherapists

Rest: For patients with low back pain, rest in supine position reduces focal axial diskal pressure and mechanical compression of neural elements besides relieving inflammation
- Short period (2–3 days) of rest may be advised
- However, activities within limits of pain are encouraged
- Exercises within limits of pain are encouraged
- Prolonged bed rest is not advisable because it results in stiffness of joints, deconditioning/wasting of muscles, and osteoporosis
- Prolonged bed rest also increases the risk of deep vein thrombosis, urinary tract infection (UTI), chest infection, and depression

Contd...

Contd...

Pharmacological treatment: Aims at pain relief by relieving inflammation or by direct analgesic action

- *Anti-inflammatory medications:* Nonsteroidal anti-inflammatory drugs (NSAIDS)—primary function is to relieve local inflammation which in turn alleviates pain and muscle spasm
- *Neuropathic analgesics:* Gabapentin, pregabalin—reduce neuronal irritation and reduce impulse transmission across peripheral nerves. Efficacy in neurogenic pain symptoms and paresthesia
- *Opioid analgesics:* Tramadol and morphine
- *Steroids:* Oral/IV—most potent anti-inflammatory. Breaks the neuroglial inflammatory cascade
- Generally, anti-inflammatory medications are combined with either opioid analgesics or neuropathic agents in order to provide adequate pain relief while limiting the adverse effects of either class of drugs
- Anti-inflammatories are prescribed for acute pain for a period of 5–7 days
- Neuropathic agents/opioid analgesics are continued for a longer period of time until adequate pain relief is obtained and then tapered off
- Topical application of creams/gels containing anti-inflammatory agents may also be used to obtain pain relief

Exercises—relieve pain by releasing endorphins, improve the local blood flow, prevent development of stiffness of muscles, and joints and prepare the patient for function

- Exercises are started early—preferably soon after onset of pain
- Do not wait for pain relief before instituting exercises
- Exercises must be performed within limits of pain under the supervision of physiotherapists
- Exercises are preferably performed for short duration of 5–10 minutes, four to five times a day during the acute stage
- McKenzie directional exercises (stretches) based on the pattern of degenerative pain are highly efficacious. They work on the principle of centralization of pain
- Strengthening exercises started only after relief of severe pain
- Manual therapy such as massage, manipulation, and mobilization is not recommended in the first few days
- Early mobilization and activity within limits of pain must be encouraged

Pain blocks—reduce inflammation and alleviate pain

- Injection of steroid + long-acting local anesthetic, administered locally at the site of pain
- Recommended for emergency room (ER) patients with severe, acute, or acute-on-chronic axial/radicular pain not responsive to IV analgesia where MRI scan has ruled out any sinister pathology
- Performed by either the pain physicians or a spine specialist
- Nerve root blocks or epidural injections are indicated for patients with severe radicular pain secondary to a prolapsed intervertebral disk/spinal canal stenosis
- Facet joint blocks are indicated for patients with severe lower back pain secondary to facet joint synovitis, and arthritis

BOX 8: When to admit?

- Persistent pain not settling with IV analgesia
- Recurrent episodes of presentation to emergency room (ER)
- Associated red flag symptoms
- Neurological dysfunction
- Trauma/Fracture
- Associated systemic disease

BOX 9: When to discharge from emergency room (ER)?

- Absence of red flags
- Patients with red flags in whom serious pathology has been ruled out by appropriate investigations (usually MRI scan) or by an expert consultation
- Adequate pain control
- Ability to mobilize safely and independently

BOX 10: Discharge advice.

- Educate patient regarding benign nature of problem and likelihood of significant recovery within 4–6 weeks
- Emphasize importance of staying mobile and performing easy stretches under supervision of physiotherapist
- To see a spine specialist in case of:
  - Development of any red flags symptoms or signs
  - Sudden deterioration in pain
  - Absence of improvement in symptoms
  - Persistence of symptoms for >4 weeks
- Provide appropriate prescriptions for medications—what, when, and for how long?
- Reference to psychologist/psychiatrist, if indicated

BOX 11: Role of emergency surgery.

- Emergency surgery is not required for a majority of patients referred to the emergency room (ER) for neck/back pain
- Indications for emergency spine surgery include:
  - Progressive neurologic deficit/major neurologic dysfunction involving spinal cord, cauda equina, and nerve roots
  - Significant spinal instability secondary to trauma or secondary spinal vertebral column destruction (metastasis and infection)

TABLE 6: Emergency surgery for pain: when and what.

When?	***What?***
Spinal fracture/dislocation with neurological deficit	Reduction of fracture/dislocation, neural decompression and spinal stabilization
Unstable spinal fracture without neurological deficit	Spinal stabilization
Acute prolapsed intervertebral disk resulting in cauda equina syndrome in lumbar spine or spinal cord compression with significant/progressive myelopathy in cervical/thoracic spine	Neural decompression ± Diskectomy
Metastatic epidural spinal cord compression	Spinal cord decompression ± Stabilization ± Biopsy
Spinal epidural hematoma/abscess with progressive/severe neurologic deficit	Hematoma/abscess evacuation + Biopsy + Neural decompression

SUGGESTED READING

1. Corwell BN, Davis NL. The Emergent Evaluation and Treatment of Neck and Back Pain. Emerg Med Clin North Am. 2020;38(1):167-91.
2. Edwards J, Hayden J, Asbridge M, Gregoire B, Magee K. Prevalence of low back pain in emergency settings: a systematic review and meta-analysis. BMC Musculoskelet Disord. 2017;18(1):143.
3. Martel JW, Potter SB. Evaluation and Management of Neck and Back Pain. Semin Neurol. 2019;39(1):41-52.

14.2.2 Acute Joint Pain

Kiran M Ladkat

BOX 1: Definition of terms.

- *Arthralgia:* Joint pain
- *Arthritis:* Joint inflammation
- *Monoarticular:* Single joint involvement
- *Polyarticular:* Multiple joint involvement
- *Septic:* Infective etiology
- *Osteoarthritis:* Degenerative etiology

BOX 2: Principles of management in emergency room (ER).

- Acute joint pain is a major cause of "*preventable*" disability, if diagnosed in emergency room (ER) early. Missed diagnosis is very common
- Eliciting pertinent history is of utmost importance!
- Investigating to come to diagnosis and provisional joint immobilization will aid in decreasing major morbidity and good functional outcome

BOX 3: Presentation.

Acute onset joint pain may be presented as:

- Traumatic or nontraumatic
- Monoarticular (single) or Oligoarticular (1–3)/Polyarticular (>3)
- Nontraumatic joint pain may be symmetric or asymmetric
- Fever, restricted range of motion (ROM), joint swelling (effusion) may be associated with presenting features

BOX 4: Diagnosis.

Posttraumatic joint pain:

Always elicit history for mechanism of injury:

- Road traffic accident (RTA)
- Fall from height
- Blunt trauma
- Injury sustained during sports

Nontraumatic joint pain:

- Single or multiple joints
- Symmetry in joint involvement
- History of recent travel
- Postoperative status
- History of any preceding or ongoing focus of infection, viz., respiratory tract/ urinary tract/gastrointestinal
- Ongoing treatment for any tumor pathology
- Associated fever/rash

BOX 5: Differential diagnosis acute joint pain in emergency room (ER).

Pathology	***Type***	***Salient clinical features***
Infective	Septic	• Fever • Immunocompromised state • Indwelling urinary catheter • Inflammatory arthritis, viz., RA • Postoperative arthroplasty status
	Viral	• Fever • Rash • Exposure to viral infection
Degenerative	Osteoarthritis Chondromalacia	• The most common type • Advanced age • Rigorous activity • Obesity
Autoimmune/ Systemic/ Rheumatoid	Autoimmune disease	• Acute-on-chronic presentation • Associated disease • Early morning onset, sudden flare of symptoms • Elevated markers like CRP/ESR
Crystal disease	Gout	Family history, thiazide use, consumption of red meat/alcohol
	Pseudogout	Prior joint surgery and hematological disorder
Reactive	Postinfective (Gastrointestinal or genitourinary)	History of prior infection, exposure, endemic location
Traumatic	Bony injury (fracture), soft tissue (hemarthrosis)	History of injury

(CRP: C-reactive protein; ESR: erythrocyte sedimentation rate; RA: rheumatoid arthritis)

BOX 6: Arthritis clinical presentation.

Type	***Joints involved***	***No. of affected joints***	***Distribution***
Osteoarthritis	Knees, hips, and hands	Mono- or oligoarticular	Asymmetric
Rheumatoid/Viral/ Reactive	Hands, feet, ankle, wrist knees, and hips	Oligoarticular	Symmetric
Septic arthritis	Knees, hips, wrists, and ankle	Mono- or oligoarticular	Asymmetric
Gout	Great toe, knee, and ankle	Mono- or oligoarticular	Asymmetric

- Monoarticular: Single joint
- Oligoarticular: 1–3 joints
- Polyarticular: >3 joints

BOX 7: Arthritis versus bursitis.

Condition	*Joint effusion*	*Erythema tenderness*	*Location*	*ROM*	*Synovial fluid*	*Patient demography*
Bursitis	Absent	Present	Olecranon/ Prepatellar Monoarticular	Pain on ROM	WBC high in bursa aspirate	Young and healthy
Arthritis	Present	May or may not be present	Knee/Hip/ Shoulder Mono/Poly	Unable to move	WBC high in joint aspirate	Chronic illness or joint pathology

(ROM: range of motion; WBC: white blood cells)

BOX 8: Factors indicating high suspicion for septic arthritis.

- Presence of fever along with joint pain
- Severe pain with range of motion
- Preexisting joint disease or surgery
- Immunocompromised state
- History of skin or soft-tissue infection
- History of indwelling catheter

BOX 9: Investigations.

Traumatic:
- X-ray/Radiograph: Anteroposterior (AP) and lateral/oblique plane
- Computed tomography (CT) in case major intra-articular or periarticular trauma

Nontraumatic:
- X-ray/Radiograph: Anteroposterior (AP) and lateral/oblique plane

Blood parameters:
- Complete blood count with differential count
- C-reactive protein (CRP)
- Erythrocyte sedimentation rate (ESR)
- Lactate
- Lactate dehydrogenase (LDH)
- Uric acid
- Arthritic profile: Rheumatoid arthritis (RA)/anticyclic citrullinated peptide (CCP)/ antinuclear antibody (ANA) joint
- Blood culture

Arthrocentesis/Joint tapping for synovial fluid sampling—white blood cells (WBC)/ polymorphonuclear leukocytes (PMN), crystals, culture, and antibiotic sensitivity

BOX 10: Principles of management in emergency room (ER).

- Assessment of causative factors of painful joint
- Joint immobilization in removable splint or rigid plaster support
- Anti-inflammatory medications—oral and parenteral
- Management of septic shock in case of possible septic arthritis:
  - Fluid electrolyte balance
  - Swift investigations: Arthrocentesis or joint tap for fluid sample and transient pain relief
  - Blood and radiological investigations
  - Preparation for urgent joint lavage and debridement

SUGGESTED READING

1. Carpenter CR, Schuur JD, Everett WW, Pines JM. Evidence-based diagnostics: adult septic arthritis. Acad Emerg Med. 2011;18(8):781-96.
2. Long B, Koyfman A, Gottlieb M. Evaluation and management of septic arthritis and its mimics in the emergency department. West J Emerg Med. 2019;20(2):331-41.
3. Sullivan R. Diagnosis and management of acute joint pain in the emergency department. Emerg Med Pract. 2022;24(1):1-28.

CHAPTER 15

General Emergencies

15.1 TOXICOLOGY

15.1.1 General Toxicology

Sachna P Shetty

BOX 1: Initial stabilization in poisonings.

- When a patient presents with a history or suspicion of poisoning, *the first priority is to resuscitate by addressing life-threatening conditions such as airway compromise, breathing difficulties, and circulatory issues such as hemodynamic instability and severe dysrhythmias*
- After ensuring the "ABCs" (airway, breathing, and circulation) are stable, *assess the patient's level of consciousness* as it will guide further management strategies
- If the patient arrives in *cardiac arrest*, follow cardiopulmonary resuscitation (CPR) according to advanced cardiovascular life support (ACLS) protocol, *addressing potential toxins by administering the appropriate antidote if the substance is known and available*
- In cases of arrhythmia, evaluate for hypoxia and metabolic abnormalities, and consider administering sodium bicarbonate if a sodium channel blocker overdose is suspected or if the ECG shows a wide QRS complex
- Perform a clinical evaluation, checking central nervous system function, blood glucose levels, and rectal temperature
- Administer dextrose, naloxone, and thiamine as indicated
- For patients presenting with seizures, use benzodiazepines, pyridoxine, barbiturates, or propofol as needed
- Toxidromes, which are groups of signs and symptoms primarily based on vital signs and neuropsychiatric functions, are characteristic of certain toxic exposures. Recognizing a toxidrome can help identify a potential toxin and guide early intervention and management strategies

Caveat:

- Avoid phenytoin in seizures secondary to overdose
- Address thermal dysregulation hyperthermia/hypothermia (Chapter 15.2)
- If patient is agitated, consider sedation with benzodiazepine
- If altered mental sensorium, look for toxidromes **(Box 4)**, check for blood sugars consider Wernicke's, if malnourished consider ethanol (EtOH) poisoning

BOX 2: History and examination in poisonings.

History:

- When a patient presents with suspected poisoning, gather a detailed history from relatives and assess the patient's *psychological state* to support the suspicion
- Poisoning most commonly occurs through *ingestion*, but other routes of exposure include inhalation, insufflation, cutaneous and mucous membrane contact, and injection
- Identify the substances involved, their doses, and the routes of exposure. Collect all prescription and over the counter medication bottles from the patient's home, perform a pill count, and thoroughly search the patient for any marks, hidden substances, or relevant items in their clothing

Examination:

- General mental state and appearances along with vital signs to be assessed
- Look for signs of injury, hesitation cuts
- Odour can be really helpful to identify the drug **(Box 3)**
- The vital signs also are a valuable parameter used to assess and monitor a patient's response to treatment and antidotal therapy
- Examination of every system can be a clue to all toxidromes
- Vital signs include heart rate (HR), blood pressure (BP), respiratory rate (RR), temperature, which are of utmost importance in case of poisoning
- Mofenson and Greensher coined the term toxidromes **(Box 4)** from the word's toxic syndromes to describe the groups of signs and symptoms that consistently result from particular toxins along with combination of the relevant abnormal vital signs
- Toxidromes is particularly helpful when relevant history is not available acting as a clue to diagnosing and managing toxicology

***Caveat:* Combination of history of information regarding what medications or substances were consumed/inhaled, timing of exposure, proper identification of the substance along with the toxidromes is the main stay in toxicology**

BOX 3: Agents with a characteristic odor.

Odor	***Possible source***
Bitter almonds	Cyanide
Fruity	Diabetic ketoacidosis and isopropanol
Garlic	Organophosphates, arsenic, dimethyl sulfoxide (DMSO), and selenium
Gasoline	Petroleum distillates
Mothballs	Naphthalene and camphor
Pears	Chloral hydrate
Rotten eggs	Sulphur dioxide, hydrogen sulfide

BOX 4: Common toxidromes.

Toxidrome	*Examples of agents*	*Vital signs*				*Examination findings (most common in bold)*
		BP	***HR***	***RR***	***T***	
Anticholinergic	Atropine, *Datura* spp., antihistamines, and antipsychotics	/↑	↑	+/	↑	• Altered mental status, mydriasis, dry flushed skin, urinary retention, decreased bowel sounds, hyperthermia, and dry mucous membranes • Seizures, arrhythmias, and rhabdomyolysis
Cholinergic	• Organophosphate and carbamate insecticides • Chemical warfare agents (sarin, VX)	+/	+/	/↑	↑	• Salivation, lacrimation, diaphoresis, vomiting, urination, defecation, bronchorrhea, muscle fasciculations, and weakness • Miosis/mydriasis, bradycardia, and seizures
Ethanolic	Ethanol	↓	↓	↓	/↓	• Central nervous system (CNS) depression, ataxia, dysarthria, odor of ethanol
Extrapyramidal	Risperidone, haloperidol, phenothiazines	VE	VE	VE	↑	• Dystonia, torticollis, and muscle rigidity • Choreoathetosis, hyperreflexia, and seizures
Hallucinogenic	• Phencyclidine • Psilocybin, mescaline • Lysergic acid diethylamide	VE	VE	VE	VE	• Hallucinations, dysphoria, and anxiety • Nausea and sympathomimetic signs
Hypoglycemic	Sulfonylureas, insulin	VE	VE	VE	VE	• Altered mental status, diaphoresis, tachycardia, and hypertension • Dysarthria, behavioral change, and seizures

Contd...

Contd...

Toxidrome	***Examples of agents***	***Vital signs***				***Examination findings (most common in bold)***
		BP	***HR***	***RR***	***T***	
Neuromuscular malignant	Antipsychotics	↓	↑		↑	• Lead pipe muscle rigidity, bradyreflexia, hyperpyrexia, and altered mental status • Autonomic instability, diaphoresis, mutism, and incontinence
Opioid	Codeine, heroin, and morphine	↓	↓	↓	↓	• Miosis, respiratory depression, and CNS depression • Hypothermia and bradycardia
Salicylate	Aspirin Oil of wintergreen (methyl salicylate)				↑	• Altered mental status, respiratory alkalosis, metabolic acidosis, tinnitus, tachypnea, tachycardia, diaphoresis, nausea, and vomiting • Hyperpyrexia (low grade)
Sedative/hypnotic	Benzodiazepines Barbiturates	↓	↓	↓	/↓	• CNS depression, ataxia, and dysarthria • Bradycardia and respiratory depression
Serotonin	• Selective serotonin reuptake inhibitors (SSRIs) • Monoamine oxidase inhibitors (MAOIs) • Tricyclic antidepressants • Amphetamines • Fentanyl • St John's wort	↓ [MAO ↑]	↑	VE	↑	• Altered mental status, hyperreflexia and hypertonia (more in lower limbs), clonus, tachycardia, and diaphoresis • Hypertension, flushing, and tremor
Sympathomimetic	Amphetamines Cocaine	↑	↑	↑	↑	• Agitation, tachycardia, hypertension, hyperpyrexia, and diaphoresis • Seizures and acute coronary syndrome

(VE: varied effects)

Source: Hoffman RS, Nelson LS, Lewin NA, Howland MA, Smith SW, editors. Goldfrank's Clinical Manual of Toxicologic Emergencies. 2nd ed. New York: McGraw-Hill Education; 2023.

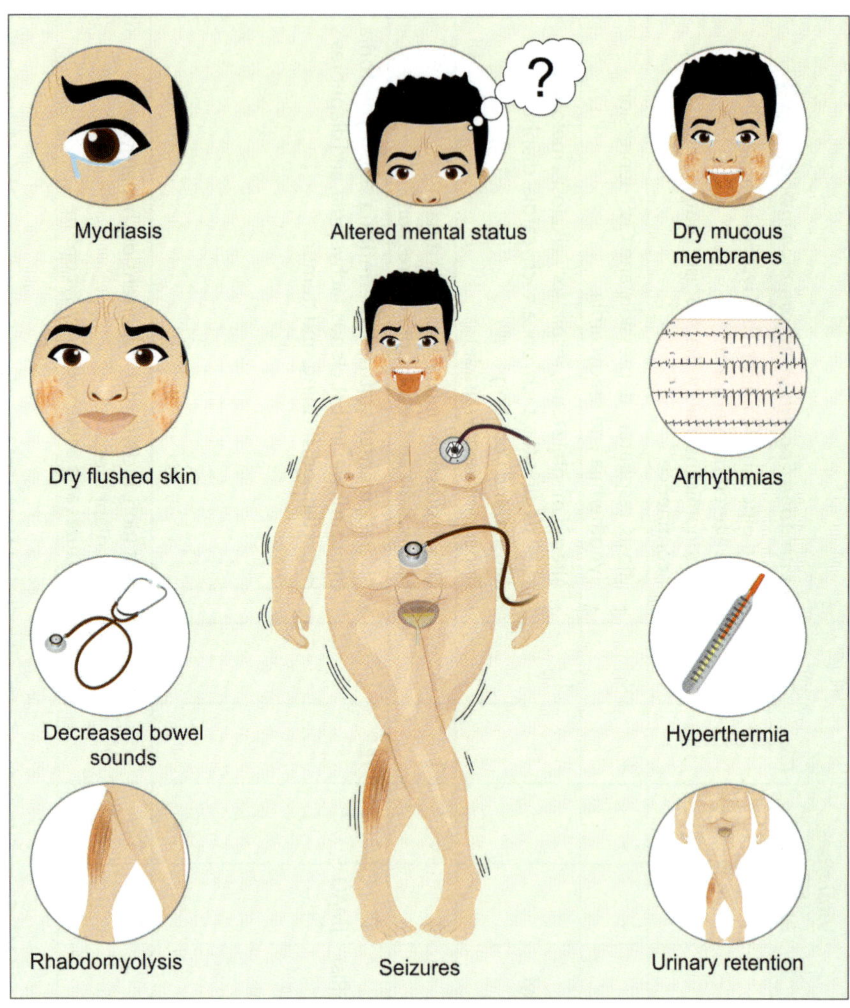

(A) Anticholinergic Toxidrome

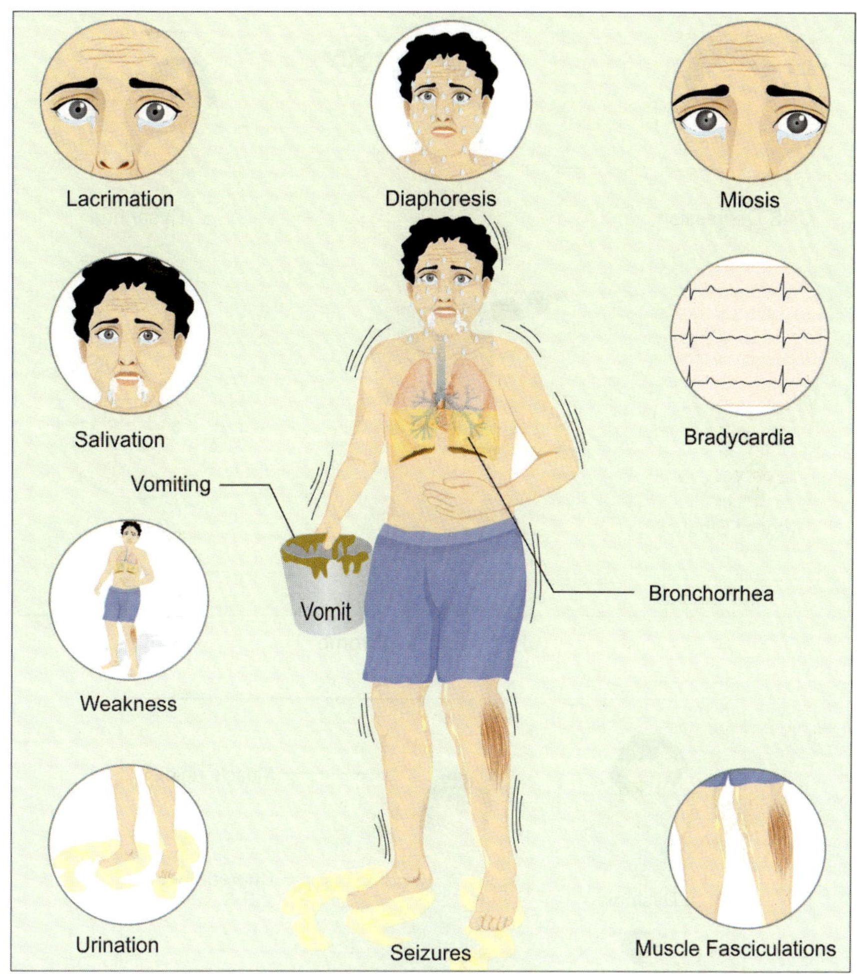

(B) Cholinergic Toxidrome

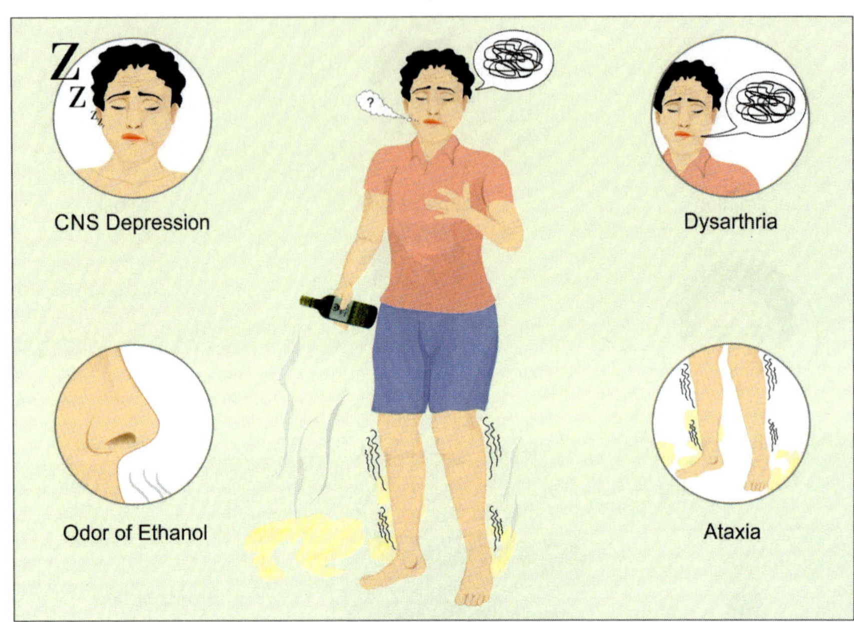

(C) Ethanolic Toxidrome

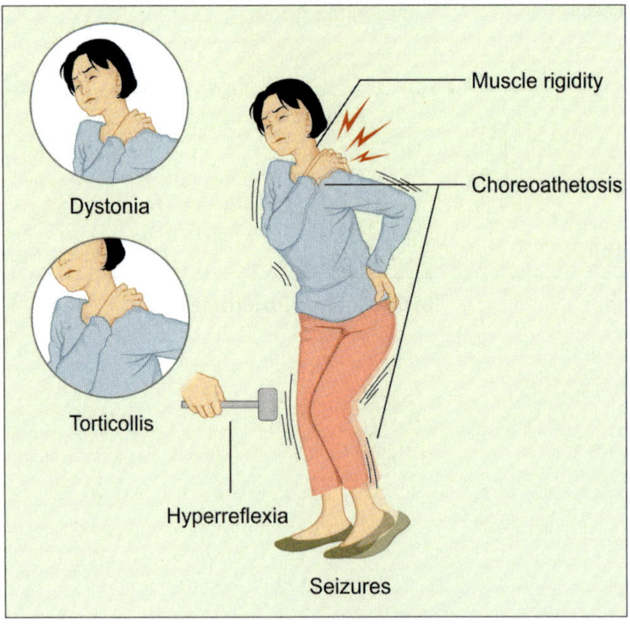

(D) Extrapyramidal Toxidrome

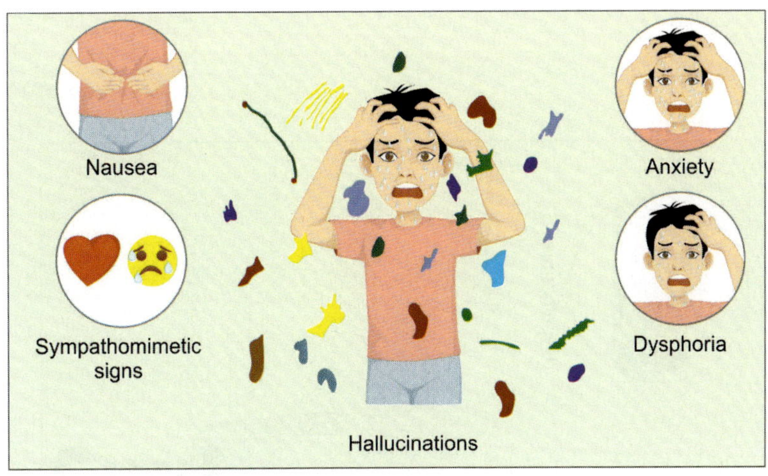

(E) Hallucinogenic Toxidrome

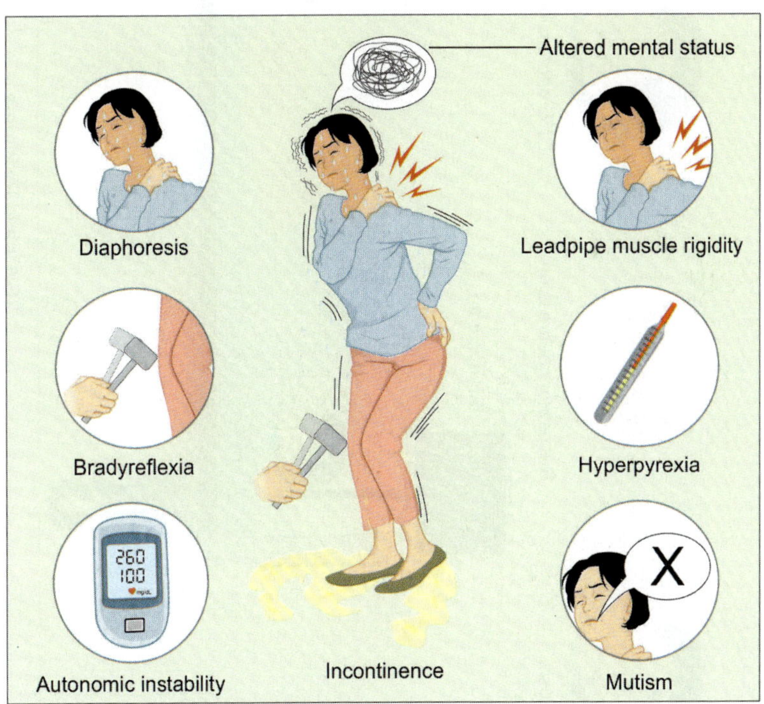

(F) Neuromuscular Malignant Toxidrome

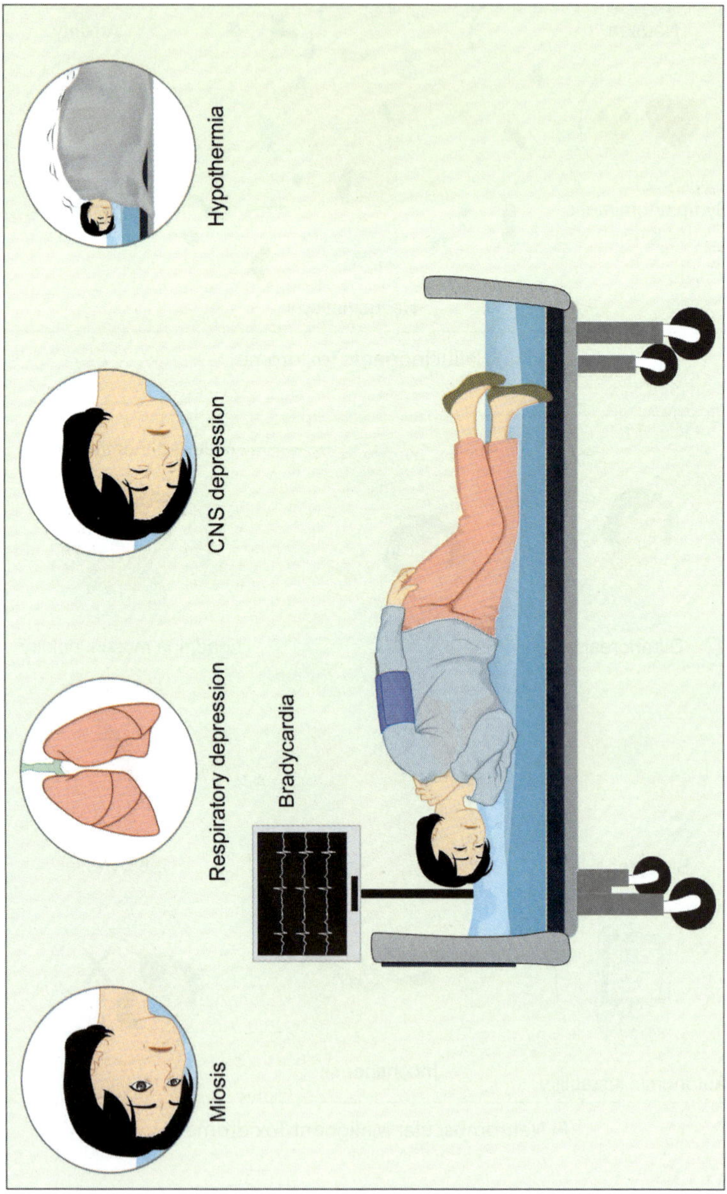

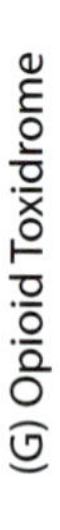

(G) Opioid Toxidrome

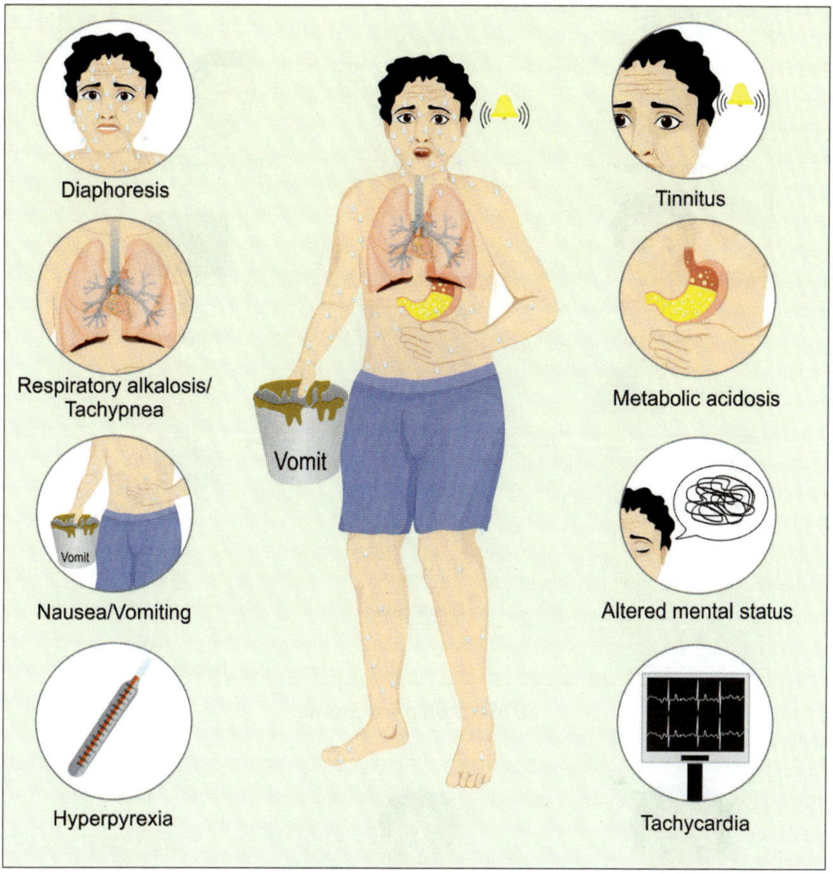

Diaphoresis
Tinnitus
Respiratory alkalosis/
Tachypnea
Metabolic acidosis
Vomit
Nausea/Vomiting
Vomit
Altered mental status
Hyperpyrexia
Tachycardia

(H) Salicylate Toxidrome

CNS depression
Dysarthria
Respiratory
depression
Bradycardia
Ataxia

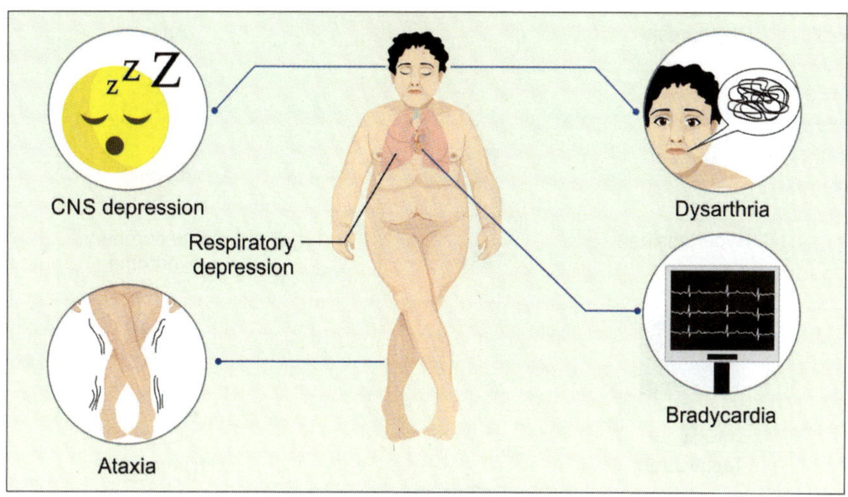

(I) Sedative-Hypnotic Toxidrome

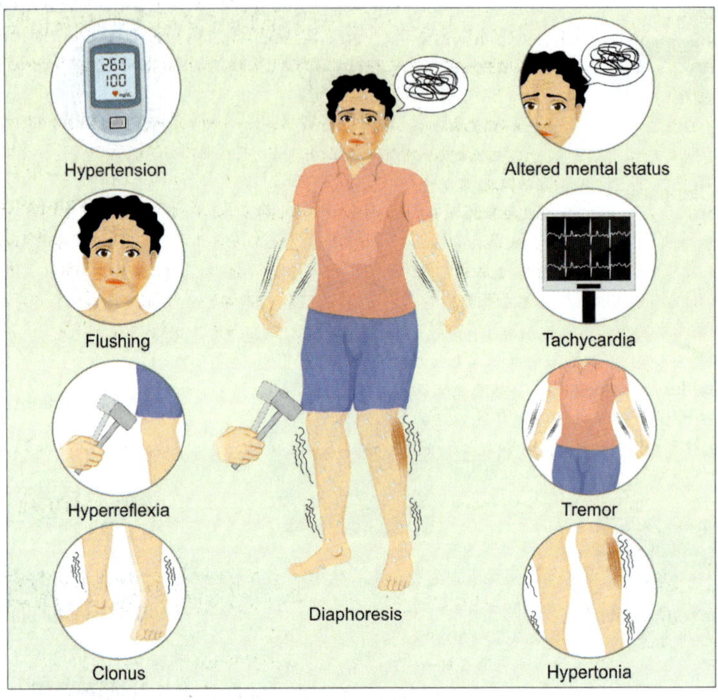

(J) Serotonin Toxidrome

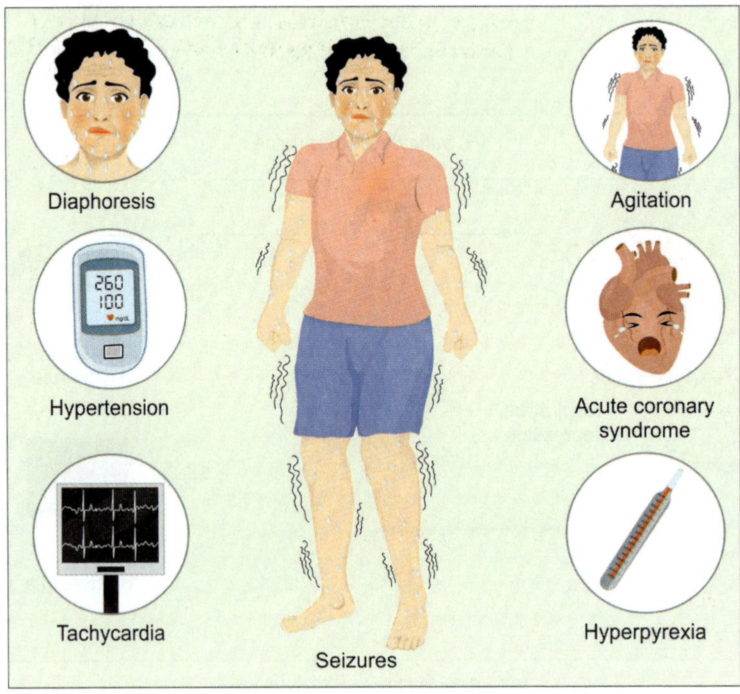

(K) Sympathomimetic Toxidrome

BOX 5: Diagnosis.

- Diagnosis is primarily based on the patient's history and the identification of toxidromes
- Measuring serum levels of certain drugs can be crucial for treatment decisions
- Urine drug screening is particularly important in cases of mixed drug poisoning and for medicolegal purposes
- **Important tests include ETCO$_2$ levels, arterial blood gas (ABG) analysis for bicarbonate and CO$_2$ levels, ECG to check for dysrhythmias and QRS duration, and electrolyte measurements.** Additional tests may include urine beta human chorionic gonadotropin (hCG), osmolality (especially in cases involving ethanol), X-rays for body packing, and evaluations for acute respiratory distress syndrome (ARDS) secondary to poisoning or heavy metal exposure
- *For acetaminophen (APAP) poisoning, check urine or serum ketones*
- *Assess hepatic function and coagulation profile*
- *Evaluate cardiac or skeletal muscle status by measuring troponin (Tn) and creatine phosphokinase (CPK)*
- Conduct studies to rule out nontoxicological causes of the patient's symptoms

BOX 6: Management.

- Main aim is to alter toxin pharmacokinetics
- Perform risk–benefit assessment to decide on the following
  - Dermal or ophthalmic decontamination (or both) **(Box 7)**
- Gastric emptying (orogastric lavage) **(Box 8)**
- Limit absorption [activated charcoal (AC) and whole bowel irrigation (WBI)] [Box]
- Enhance elimination [e.g., multiple-dose activated charcoal (MDAC), alkaline diuresis, hemodialysis (HD)/hemoperfusion (HP)] **(Box 6)**]
- Antidotes **(Box 11)**

BOX 7: Decontamination.

Ocular decontamination:

- For eye exposures, it may be necessary to use a local anesthetic
- Alkalis cause more severe damage than acids, because they penetrate deeper into tissues through liquefaction, necessitating extended irrigation, often for 1–2 hours.
- 10 minutes after irrigation, to allow the crystalloid and conjunctival sac pH to equilibrate, the pH of the conjunctival sac should be tested
- Irrigation should continue until the pH is between 7.2 and 7.4. All ocular alkali injuries require an ophthalmologic consultation

BOX 8: Indications, contraindications, and complications of gastrointestinal (GI) decontamination procedures.

Orogastric lavage:	
Indications	• Recommended for recent (<1 hour) ingestion
Contraindications	• Ingestion of corrosive/hydrocarbon • Lack of airway protection • Patient is unstable and needs additional resuscitation
Complications	• Risk of aspiration pneumonia and hypoxia • Potential for water intoxication • Risk of hypothermia • Possibility of laryngospasm • Potential for mechanical injury to the gastrointestinal tract • Can be time-consuming, which may delay other essential treatments
Activated charcoal: Adults 50 g orally, children 1 g/kg orally	
Indications	• Ingestion within the previous hour of a toxic substance known to be absorbed by activated charcoal
Contraindications	• Nontoxic ingestion • Nonabsorbed toxin by activated charcoal • Ingestion of corrosive substances • Risk of upper gastrointestinal perforation
Complications	• Vomiting • Risk of aspiration of the activated charcoal
Whole bowel irrigation: Polyethylene glycol 2 L/h in adults, children 25 mL/kg/h (maximum 2 L/h) via Ryles tube	
Indications (potential)	• Ingestion of iron exceeding 60 µg/kg with visible opacities on an abdominal X-ray • Life-threatening ingestion of diltiazem or verapamil • Individuals who have ingested or concealed drugs internally (body packers or stuffers) • Ingestion of slow-release potassium • Lead ingestion, including paint flakes containing lead • Symptomatic ingestion of arsenic trioxide • Life-threatening ingestion of lithium
Contraindications	• Unprotected airway • Gastrointestinal perforation, obstruction, ileus, or hemorrhage • Intractable vomiting • Cardiovascular instability
Complications	• Nausea and vomiting • Risk of pulmonary aspiration • Time-consuming, potentially delaying the implementation of other definitive treatments
Caveat: Charcoal is commonly available in the form of Flatuna tablets, which have a coating containing dimethicone that must be removed before administration. The recommended dose is 1 g/kg, meaning approximately 20–30 strips may be needed, as each tablet contains only 250 mg, with 10 tablets per strip.	

Contd...

Contd...

Indications, contraindications, and complications of enhanced elimination procedures	
Multidose activated charcoal: Initial dose: 50 g (1 g/kg), repeat dose of 25 g (0.5 g/kg) every 4–6 hours for 12–24 hours	
Indications	*ABCDQ:* • **A**minophylline/theophylline • **B**arbiturates • **C**arbamazepine/concretion forming drugs (e.g., salicylates) • **D**apsone • **Q**uinine
Contraindications	• Lack of protected airway • Bowel obstruction or reduction in GI motility
Complications	• Vomiting • Aspiration • Constipation • Charcoal bezoar, bowel obstruction/perforation
Urinary alkalinization	
Indications	• Moderate to severe salicylate toxicity • Phenobarbital • Chlorophenoxy herbicides (2,4-dichlorophenoxyacetic acid and mecoprop)
Contraindications	• Known case of fluid overload • Medical renal diseases • Hypokalemia
Complications	• Hypokalemia • Volume overload • Alkalemia • Hypocalcemia (usually mild)
Caveat protocol for urinary alkalinization in adults with normal renal function	
• Correct any existing hypokalemia • Administer a bolus of intravenous (IV) sodium bicarbonate at a dose of 1–2 mEq/kg • Infuse a solution of 100 mEq of sodium bicarbonate mixed in 1 liter of D_5W (5% dextrose in water) at a rate of 250 mL/h • To maintain normal potassium levels, 20 mEq of potassium chloride may be added to the infusion • Regularly monitor serum potassium and bicarbonate levels every 24 hours to check for hypokalemia or excessive serum alkalinization • Check urine pH frequently (every 15–30 minutes), aiming for a pH between 7.5 and 8.5 • If the urine is not sufficiently alkalinized, an additional IV bolus of 1 mEq/kg sodium bicarbonate may be required	

BOX 9: Indications, contraindications, and complications of extracorporeal removal techniques.

Hemodialysis:
- *Indications:* Life-threatening poisoning by dialyzable toxins, including:
  - **Stumbled:**
    - Salicylates
    - Theophylline
    - Uremia
    - Metformin/methanol
    - Barbiturates
    - Lithium
    - Ethylene glycol
    - Depakote (valproic acid in massive overdose)
- *Contraindications:*
  - Hemodynamic instability
  - Infants (generally)
  - Poor vascular access
  - Significant coagulopathy

Hemoperfusion:
- *Indications:* Life-threatening poisoning caused by:
  - Theophylline
  - Carbamazepine
  - Paraquat
- *Contraindications:*
  - Hemodynamic instability
  - Poor vascular access
  - Significant coagulopathy

Continuous renal replacement therapies:
- *Indications:* Life-threatening toxins require extracorporeal removal, but the patient is hemodynamically unstable for hemodialysis
- *Contraindications:* None

Complications of extracorporeal removal techniques:
- Fluid and metabolic disturbances
- Removal of antidotes
- Limited availability
- Limited by hypotension (excluding continuous renal replacement therapy)
- Infection or bleeding at catheter site
- Intracranial hemorrhage due to anticoagulation

BOX 10: Disposition.

The criteria used to determine whether the exposure is nontoxic are as follows:
- An unintentional exposure to a clearly identified single substance
- An estimate of the dose is known, and a recognized information source (poison control center) confirms the substance as nontoxic
- The drug according to literature is benign or self-limiting in the reported dose
- Adequate time postexposure to drug has occurred yet asymptomatic
- Asymptomatic patients with nontoxic exposures may be discharged after a short period of observation, providing they have access to further consultation and a safe discharge destination

Criteria for ICU admission:
- Patients with impaired airway, breathing, or circulation needing immediate intervention
- Lethal dose
- Substances known to cause delayed complications
- Cardiac dysrhythmia
- Patients with serious or needing supports
- Laboratory data suggesting severity
- High-risk patients prone to complication
- Drugs with known serious sequelae
- Continuous seizure
- Recurrent hypoglycemia
- If the patient is pregnant
- If the patient is suicidal
- If the nursing staff is not well trained to handle or identify complications in the ward

BOX 11: Common antidotes and their indications.

Antidote dose in individual chapter	***Dose***	***Indication***
Atropine	1–3 mg IV in adult or 0.01–0.04 mg/kg IV (never <.1 mg per dose) in children	Bradyarrhythmia and cholinesterase inhibitor toxicity
Acetylcysteine	• Oral 140 mg/kg PO • IV 150 mg/kg IV over 1 hour loading dose • Infusion and details given later	APAP and other causes of hepatotoxicity
Calcium chloride 10% 27.2 mg/mL elemental Ca	• 0.15 mL/kg/IV pediatrics • 10 mL adults	Calcium channel blockers (CCB)
Calcium gluconate 10%	• 0.5–0.45 mL/kg/IV pediatrics • 10–30 mL adults	Hypermagnesemia CCBs

Contd...

Contd...

Antidote dose in individual chapter	***Dose***	***Indication***
Cyanide antidote kit Sodium nitrite 3%	Nitrite 0.33 mL/kg IV pediatric 10 mL IV adults	Cyanide
Sodium thiosulfate 25%	1.65 mL/kg IV pediatric 15 mL IV adults	
Cyproheptadine	*Adults:* • Initial dose: 12 mg orally as a loading dose • Maintenance dose: 2 mg every 2 hours as needed until symptoms are controlled *Children:* • Initial dose (26 years): 2 mg orally • Initial dose (7–14 years): 4 mg orally • Maintenance dose: 0.25 mg/kg/day in divided doses every 6 hours as needed until symptoms are controlled	Serotonin
Dantrolene	• Initial dose: Adults and children: 2.5 mg/kg administered intravenously as quickly as possible • Maintenance dose: Continue administering additional doses of 1 mg/kg IV until the symptoms are controlled or the maximum cumulative dose of 10 mg/kg is reached • Postcrisis management: After the initial treatment and stabilization, administer 1 mg/kg IV every 4–6 hours for 24–48 hours to prevent recurrence	Malignant hyperthermia
Dimercaprol	*Adults:* • Arsenic, gold, mercury poisoning: 2.5–3 mg/kg intramuscularly (IM) every 4 hours for 2 days, then every 6 hours on the third day, and every 12 hours for up to 10 days	Arsenic, lead, and mercury

Contd...

Contd...

Antidote dose in individual chapter	***Dose***	***Indication***
	• Lead poisoning: 4 mg/kg intramuscular (IM) initially, followed by 3 mg/kg every 4 hours for 2 days, then every 4–6 hours for an additional 7 to 10 days in combination with EDTA (ethylenediaminetetraacetic acid) *Children:* • Arsenic, gold, mercury poisoning: 2.5–3 mg/kg IM every 4 hours for 2 days, then every 6 hours on the third day, and every 12 hours for up to 10 days • Lead poisoning: 4 mg/kg IM initially, followed by 3 mg/kg every 4 hours for 2 days, then every 4–6 hours for an additional 7 to 10 days in combination with EDTA	
Deferoxamine mesylate	• Adults and children: Initial dose of 1,000 mg IM. If needed, an additional 500 mg IM can be given in 4–12 hours. Maximum daily dose is 6,000 mg • IV administration (in severe cases): 15 mg/kg/h, reduced to 125 mg/h once the patient's condition stabilizes	Iron
Diphenhydramine	• Adults: 25–50 mg IM or IV initially, followed by 25–50 mg orally every 4–6 hours as needed • Children: 1 mg/kg/dose IM or IV (up to 50 mg/dose), followed by 1 mg/kg/dose orally every 6–8 hours as needed	Acute dystonia, histamine receptor blockade
Ethanol	10 mL/kg of 10% IV ethanol at 100 mg/kg/h to keep ethanol level 100–150 mg/dL (22–33 mmol/L) or PO or via nasogastric tube) using 80 proof liquor of 1.5–2 mL/kg	Ethylene glycol, methanol, and diethylene glycol
Fomepizole	15 mg/kg IV over 30 minutes a	Ethylene glycol, methanol, and diethylene glycol

Contd...

Contd...

Antidote dose in individual chapter	***Dose***	***Indication***
Idarucizumab	The recommended dose is 5 g given intravenously as two separate 2.5 g doses	Dabigatran
Leucovorin calcium/ folinic acid	Doses range from 15 mg to 100 mg every 6 hours until methotrexate levels are within safe limits	Methotrexate
L-carnitine	Loading dose is 100 mg/kg IV over 30 minutes (maximum 6 g)	Valproic acid (hyperammonemia)
Physostigmine	• 0.02 mg/kg IV not to exceed 0.5 mg/ kg IV over a minute in pediatrics • Adults: 0.5–2 mg IV slowly (rate not be exceed 1 mg/min). Repeat doses at intervals of 10–30	Anticholinergics
Phytonadione/ vitamin K1	• No active bleeding and international normalized ratio (INR) >4, post 48 hours. Ingestion—give vitamin K1, 10 mg slow IV (children: 250 µg/kg IV, maximum 10 mg): Alternatively oral dose: Adults: 15–25 mg; children: 510 mg, 2–4 times a day • Active bleeding or life-threatening hemorrhage—give vitamin K1 20–40 mg slow IV diluted in saline or glucose (rate not exceeding 5% of the total dose/minute) with further dosing guided by INR monitoring	Warfarin, rodenticide
Pralidoxime	12 g for adults or 20–40 mg/kg IV (up to 1 g in children), mixed with normal saline	Organophosphate
Protamine	For unfractionated heparin reversal: 1 mg protamine sulfate neutralizes approximately 100 units of unfractionated heparin	Heparin
Sugammadex	Typical doses range from 2 to 16 mg/ kg based on the degree of block and the specific agent	Reversal of neuromuscular blockade induced for rocuronium and vecuronium
Dextrose (glucose)	• 0.5–1 mg/kg IV pediatrics • 1 g/kg IV adults	Insulin oral hypoglycemics

Contd...

Contd...

Antidote dose in individual chapter	***Dose***	***Indication***
Digoxin Fab	• 5–10 vials pediatrics • 10 vials adults	Digoxin and other cardioactive steroids
Flumazenil	• 0.01 mg/kg IV pediatrics • 2 mg IV adults	Benzodiazepines
Glucagon	• 30 µg/kg IV over 1–2 minutes for CCB toxicity and • 30–150 µg/kg IV over 1–2 minutes for beta-blocker (BB) toxicity pediatric • 5 mg IV adults	CCBs BB
Hydroxocobalamin	• 70 mg/kg (maximum 5 g) IV over 15 minutes pediatric • 5 g IV over 15 minutes adults	Cyanide
IV lipid emulsion 20%	• 1.5 mL/kg IV bolus over 1 min (may be repeated 2 times at 5 minutes intervals), followed by 0.25 mL/kg per minute IV infusion for 20 minutes pediatrics • 100 mL IV bolus over 1 min (may be repeated 2 times at 5 minutes intervals), followed by 18 mL/min IV infusion for 20 minutes adults	Local anesthetic systemic toxicity rescue therapy for lipophilic cardiotoxins
Methylene blue	• 1 mg/kg IV • Neonates: 0.3–1.0 mg/kg IV	Oxidizing toxins (e.g., nitrites, benzocaine, and sulfonamides)
Naloxone	• Start: 0.01 mg IV pediatrics • As much as required • Start: 0.1–0.4 mg IV adults	Opioids Clonidine
Pyridoxine	Gram for gram if amount of isoniazid ingested is known, otherwise 70 mg/kg IV (maximum 5 g) 5 g IV	Isoniazid
Sodium bicarbonate	1–2 mEq/kg IV over 1–2 minutes, followed by 0.3 mEq/kg per hour IV infusion Sodium channel blockers Urinary alkalinization	
Thiamine	• 5–10 mg IV pediatrics • 100 mg IV adults	• Wernicke's syndrome • Wet beriberi

BOX 12: Caveat.

- Hemodialysis is indicated in certain drugs as mentioned above. It may be useful in cardiac arrest caused by some other drugs—the indications are unclear, but case reports record dramatic recovery from cardiac arrests due to a variety of drugs
- Consider lipid emulsion in drug-induced cardiac arrest unresponsive to standard treatment
- Although lipid emulsion is not licensed for use in drug overdose, and the safety of rapid infusion is unknown
- Poisoning with cardiac drugs, such as CCBs and beta-blockers may cause severe hypotension. If standard treatments are ineffective, consider using insulin therapy
- Qualitative urine drug screening are inferior to quantitative serum levels in terms of guiding specific therapy
- A pscyhchatriac consulation post stabilization is advisable
- **If any doubts while handling toxicology-related issues, one can always take assistance from the National Poison Center Helpline in AIIMS 1800116117**

SUGGESTED READING

1. Hoffman RS, Nelson LS, Lewin NA, Howland MA, Smith SW, editors. Goldfrank's Clinical Manual of Toxicologic Emergencies. 2nd ed. New York: McGraw-Hill Education; 2023.
2. Tintinalli JE, Ma OJ, Yealy DM, Meckler GD, Stapczynski JS, Cline DM, et al. Tintinalli's Emergency Medicine: A Comprehensive Study Guide, 9th edition. New York, NY: McGraw- Hill Education; 2019.
3. Walls RM, Hockberger RS, Gausche-Hill M. Rosen's Emergency Medicine: Concepts and Clinical Practice. Philadelphia, PA: Elsevier; 2018.

15.1.2 Most Common Poisonings in the Emergency Room

Sachna P Shetty

BOX 1: Anticholinergics.

Drugs and toxic dose:

- Atropine, hyoscyamine, antihistamine (especially diphenhydramine antitussive in children) hyoscine for colic, mydriatics for the eye, antipsychotic, cyclic depressants, plants like datura, mushrooms of amanita species, plant poisoning, and belladonna alkaloids
- Toxic dose is highly variable

Acute toxicity signs and symptoms:

As per anticholinergic toxidromes, the classic findings are:

- Dry as a bone (dry skin and mucous membranes)
- "Red as a beet" (flushing)
- "Hot as a hare" (hyperthermia)
- "Blind as a bat" (mydriasis with loss of accommodation)
- "Mad as a hatter" (delirium and hallucinations)

Mild to moderate:

- Flushing, mydriasis (might be delayed), dry mouth, hyperthermia, decreased bowel sounds, bladder retention tachycardia, hypertension, nausea, vomiting, agitation, confusion, and hallucinations

Severe:

- Agitated delirium, psychosis, hallucinations, seizures, hyperthermia, and coma
- QRS widening (thioridazine, chlorpromazine, haloperidol, and droperidol), prolonged QTc (diphenhydramine)
- Rhabdomyolysis and renal failure may rarely develop in patients with prolonged agitation, coma or seizures

Potential sequelae/delayed effects:

- Cognitive impairment may occur

General management

As outlined in the general toxicology chapter.

Specific management: Decontamination

For cases of large ingestion:

- *Gastric lavage:* Consider performing to reduce absorption
- *Activated charcoal:* Administer at 1–2 g/kg of body weight to limit absorption

Caveats:

- *Gastrointestinal (GI) decontamination:* May be beneficial for patients presenting later due to delayed GI motility
- *Sedation with benzodiazepines:* Helps reduce risks of hyperthermia, rhabdomyolysis, and traumatic injuries

Treatment for specific symptoms:

- For wide complex tachyarrhythmias, administer sodium bicarbonate to counteract sodium channel blockade
- Address other symptoms such as hyperthermia, seizures, tachycardia, psychomotor agitation, dysrhythmias, coma, and rhabdomyolysis as they arise

Monitoring (general toxicology parameters):

- *Creatinine phosphokinase (CPK):* Monitor in cases of prolonged agitation, seizures, or coma
- *Urine output:* Track in patients with rhabdomyolysis to assess renal function

Contd...

Contd...

Specific—antidote: Physostigmine

Physostigmine	
Indications	• Management of severe peripheral or central anticholinergic syndrome
Adults	• 0.5–2 mg intravenous (IV) slowly (rate not be exceed 1 mg/min). Repeat doses at intervals of 10–30 minutes, as needed • Consider continuous infusion of physostigmine at 2 mg/h in patients with prolonged anticholinergic delirium and titrate the dose based on clinical response
Children	• 0.02 mg/kg IV slowly (rate not to exceed 0.5 mg/min, maximum dose 0.5 mg). Repeat doses at intervals of 5–10 minutes and titrate to clinical effect. Maximum dose 2 mg
Contraindications	• Asthma, diabetes, intestinal or urogenital tract mechanical obstruction, cardiovascular disease, cardiac conduction defects, patients receiving depolarizing neuromuscular blocking agents, peripheral vascular disease, and gangrene. Do not use in patients with suspected or an ECG suggestive of tricyclic antidepressant overdose

Caveat:

- *Rapid administration of physostigmine can cause bradycardia and hypersalivation, which may lead to respiratory difficulties and seizures*
- Dryness of mouth and axilla is first noted
- Dysarthria, difficulty to comprehend speech common
- Dysphasia due to dry mucous membrane
- Jerky peripheries
- Visual/auditory (little people hallucinations may be noted)
- Repeated picking of bed clothes
- Disposition patient with moderate to severe symptoms and the ones received physostigmine needs admission

Important Dos √ and Don'ts ×	
Gastric decontamination early and late with charcoal √	**Extracorporeal elimination ×**
Enhanced eliminated ×	**Antidote √**

BOX 2: Caustics/corrosives.

Substances and toxic doses:

- Common caustic and corrosive agents are classified as either alkali or acidic substances
- These agents are typically found in household or industrial cleaners and preservatives, including:
  - *Alkali substances:* Sodium hydroxide, potassium hydroxide, calcium hydroxide, ammonium hydroxide, lithium hydroxide
  - *Additional alkali-containing items:* Photographic developers and batteries
  - *Other toxic chemicals:* Sodium tripolyphosphate, sodium hypochlorite
  - *Acidic substances:* Sulfuric acid, hydrochloric acid, hydrofluoric acid, formic acid, chromic acid, nitric acid, and phosphoric acid
- Toxic dose not determined:
- Less probability of serious burns in case pH >3 (acids) and pH <11.5 (alkalies)
- Greater injury with a large ingestion or highly concentrated products

Acute toxicity (signs and symptoms):

- Ingestion:
  - *Mild:* Burning in mouth/stomach, abdominal pain, vomiting, dyspnea, grade I burns (superficial hyperemia, edema) of oropharynx and esophagus or stomach
  - *Moderate:* Hematemesis, grade II burns (superficial blisters, erosions, and ulcerations). Risk for subsequent stricture formation (esophageal and gastric)
  - *Severe:* Upper airway edema, hypotension, tachycardia, hemorrhagic/hypovolemic shock, tachypnea, deep burns, and necrosis of GI mucosa. Complications often include esophageal, gastric, duodenal (rate) perforation, fistula formation (tracheoesophageal and aortoesophageal), and GI bleeding
  - *Rare complications:* Metabolic acidosis, hemolysis, renal failure, disseminated intravascular coagulation, elevated liver enzymes, and cardiovascular collapse
- Inhalation:
  - *Mild:* Dyspnea, pleuritic chest pain, cough, and bronchospasm
  - *Severe:* Upper airway edema, burns, hypoxia, stridor, pneumonitis, tracheobronchitis, and acute lung injury (rate)
  - *Ocular:* Conjunctival irritation, chemosis, corneal epithelial defects, limbal ischemia, and permanent vision loss
  - *Dermal:* Irritation and partial thickness burns

Potential sequelae/delayed effects:

- Stricture formation
- Esophageal carcinoma has been reported to occur after 10 years

Treatment:

- Initial management of all patients with caustic exposures begins with universal precautions in an effort to prevent further contamination of staff, other patients, and equipment
- Decontamination and irrigate with lots of water
- Irrigate mouth with lots of water
- **Do not do gastric lavage or administer activated charcoal**
- In case of small ingestion, can administer milk or water (adults: 100–200 mL, children: 2 mL/kg) if there is no respiratory compromise
- Irrigate eyes with lots of water or saline for at least 15 minutes and check pH of the eye
- Perform endotracheal intubation and provide assisted ventilation, tracheostomy might be required if extensive burns noted
- Consider endoscopy to rule out esophageal or gastric injury within 12 hours
- Obtain a surgical consultation in case of severe grade II or grade III burns on endoscopy
- Treat hypotension, metabolic acidosis, cardiac dysrhythmias, and coagulopathy, if present

Contd...

Contd...

Monitoring:
- Chest X-ray (CXR) in case of pulmonary signs or symptoms (upright CXR in case of suspected perforation and bleeding)

Specific: No specific antidote

Important Dos √ and Don'ts ×		
Emesis: ×	**Gastric lavage:** ×	**Activated charcoal:** ×
Enhanced elimination: ×	**Specific antidote:** ×	

Specific treatment:
- **Significant caustic injury should be suspected in all patients with intentional ingestions and in patients with unintentional ingestions presenting with stridor or 2 or more of the following: Vomiting, drooling, and pain in the oropharynx, chest, or abdomen. Thus endoscopy is recommended for all patients as above**
- Patients found to have minimal or no evidence of gastroesophageal injury can be discharged. In such patients, a nasogastric tube may be passed under direct visualization in appropriate patients to facilitate caloric intake
- Endoscopy is ideally performed within 12 hours and generally not later than 24 hours postingestion as might cause perforation
- Exceptions to the general rules of gastrointestinal decontamination of caustics exist in the management of zinc chloride ($ZnCl_2$) and mercuric chloride ($HgCl_2$). Both are caustics with severe systemic toxicity in the form of cationic metal injury
- Despite the imbalance of the quantity of studies demonstrating no benefit (or even harm) versus benefit for the use of steroids in the treatment of grade IIb lesions, the quality of the single prospective study supports our recommendation of a short course of methylprednisolone (1 g/1.73 m^2/day for 3 days) and ranitidine, ceftriaxone, and total parenteral nutrition in these patients
- Intraluminal stents/nasogastric tubes for 3 weeks postexposure prevents strictures

BOX 3: Barbiturates.

Substances and toxic dose:
- Phenobarbital and thiopental are commonly used
- The therapeutic level of phenobarbital is 15–40 μg/mL (65–172 μmol/L)

Acute toxicity:
- Sedative hypnotic in toxidrome
- Mild drowsiness, slurred speech, ataxia, unsteady gait, nystagmus, emotional ability, and impaired cognition
- Moderate to severe coma to respiratory depression, which is life-threatening, rapid, and shallow breaths
- Hypotension and noncardiogenic pulmonary edema
- Corneal and gag reflexes may be diminished or absent, and muscle tone flaccid and deep tendon reflexes may be diminished or absent

Caveat: Flexor (decorticate) and extensor (decerebrate) posturing can occur in patients comatose from barbiturate intoxication

Contd...

Contd...

Treatment:
- Airway protection is a must in severe to moderate
- Fluids should be carefully given
- Decontamination—gastric lavage is not contraindicated but multidrug charcoal might be more helpful
- Enhanced elimination with urinary alkalinization (Chapter 15.1) and hemodialysis is indicated in severe poisoning

Important Dos √ and Don'ts ×	
Gastric decontamination and charcoal √	**Antidote ×**
Enhanced elimination and extracorporeal elimination √	

BOX 4: Benzodiazepines.

Drugs and toxic dose:
- Diazepam, lorazepam, midazolam, clonazepam, and alprazolam are commonly used benzodiazepines
- Remarkably safe as single agent

Acute toxicity signs and symptoms: Sedative hypnotic toxidrome:

Mild to moderate	• CNS depression, lethargy, slurred speech, and ataxia • Respiratory depression may also occur (more common with coingestion of other CNS depressants)
Severe toxicity	• Respiratory depression/arrest (large overdoses or after rapid IV injection with short-acting benzodiazepines) • Coma, hypotension, hypothermia, and rhabdomyolysis (high doses)

Caveat:
- Propylene glycol, a diluent in parenteral preparations of diazepam and lorazepam, may cause severe metabolic acidosis (lactic acidosis), nephrotoxicity, and hyperosmolar states when infused at doses >1 mg/kg/day
- An osmolar gap >10 is predictive of elevated propylene glycol concentrations
- Treatment of propylene toxicity is generally supportive but may require hemodialysis

General treatment and monitoring
- In case of large ingestion:
  - Do gastric lavage
  - Administer activated charcoal (1–2 g/kg body weight)
- A negative screen does not rule out benzodiazepine ingestion as urine drug tests do not detect all benzodiazepines, particularly midazolam, chlordiazepoxide, and flunitrazepam

Contd...

Contd...

Specific—Antidote: ***Flumazenil***

Indication	• Only in cases of respiratory depression and/or coma
Adults	• 0.2 mg IV over 30 seconds, if no further response within 30 seconds, give further 0.3 mg over 30 seconds If further no response, give 0.5 mg at 1 minute interval up to a maximum of 3 mg. If partial response, may give up to 5 mg. If no response within 5 minutes, benzodiazepine poisoning is unlikely • If multiple repeated doses are required, consider continuous IV infusion at the rate of 0.2 mg/h • Because of short duration of action (15 hours) of flumazenil, monitor for resedation
Children	• Age >1 year: Bolus dose of 0.01 mg/kg (up to 0.2 mg); if no response, repeat dose at 60 seconds intervals, up to maximum total dose of 0.05 mg/kg or 1 mg, whichever is less
Drawbacks of flumazenil	• May induce withdrawal (including seizures and autonomic instability) in benzodiazepine addicts • May predispose to seizures in case of: – Concurrent tricyclic antidepressant overdose – Coingestion of epileptogenic agents – Epileptic subjects – Cardiac dysrhythmias (diluents) • Not useful in critical cases of mixed drug overdose • Repeat dosing or a continuous infusion may often be required because of its short duration of action

Important Dos √ and Don'ts ×	
Gastric decontamination and activated charcoal √	**Antidote √**
Enhanced elimination and extracorporeal elimination ×	

Nonbenzodiazepine sedative hypnotics toxidromes

Drugs and acute poisoning:

- ***Busiprone*** - sedation generalized seizures (rare), serotonin syndrome, and treat symptomatically
- **Melatonin** - sedation, disorientation, no toxicological side effect except exaggeration of side effects
- **Zolpidem** - sedation, coma possible, psychomotor side effects
- Treatment is symptomatic management

BOX 5: Household products.

Naphthalene

Toxic dose:

- Lethal dose: Children: 80–100 mg/kg. Adults: 5–15 g

Acute toxicity signs and symptoms:

Inhalation/Ingestion	• Vomiting, abdominal pain, diarrhea, restlessness confusion, and profuse sweating • Fever, tachycardia, tachypnea, convulsions, and coma • Methemoglobinemia, acute intravascular hemolysis
Dermal	• Irritation and dermatitis
Ocular	• Irritation, corneal damage, lens opacities, and cataracts

Treatment	• Decontamination gastric lavage indicated • Give IV hydration and urinary alkalinization in case of hemolysis and resulting hemoglobinuria
Monitoring	• Complete blood counts • Haptoglobin, free hemoglobin, urine dip stick for occult blood if hemolysis is suspected

Specific:

- No specific antidote
- Methemoglobinemia: Methylene blue **(Box 9)**

Important Dos √ and Don'ts ×		
Vomiting: ×	**Gastric lavage:** √	
Activated charcoal: √	**Enhanced elimination:** ×	**Specific antidote:** ×

Camphor:

Toxic dose: The lethal dose of camphor is often cited as 50–500 mg/kg in humans. Yet, as little as 1 g of camphor resulted in death in a 19-month-old infant

Oropharyngeal irritation:

- Inhalation injury causing dermatitis or mucositis
- Early seizures mostly self-resolving are noted
- CNS depression might be noted
- Treatment is stabilizing the airway, breathing, and circulation (ABCs)
- Gastric decontamination if done early
- No antidote, only symptomatic management by controlling seizures with benzodiazepines

BOX 6: Alcohol.

Drugs and toxin dose:

- Ethanol, methanol, ethylene glycol (EG), and isopropanol are commonly noted in the poisoning
- Ethanol beverages like beer, wines, spirits also seen in household products such as disinfectants and mouthwash
- The minimum lethal dose for an adult has been reported as approximately 2–4 mL/kg
- Methanol adulterated alcoholic beverages, windshield cleaner, etc.
- Lethal dose is 1 g/kg or 100 mL
- EG adulterated alcoholic beverages, glycerin substitute
- Lethal dose 1.11.7 g/kg or 100 mL

Acute poisoning sedative hypnotic toxidromes:

Ethanol	• CNS - initial inebriation, followed by ataxia, slurred speech and motor incoordination • Head, eyes, ears, nose, and throat (HEENT) - nystagmus • Respiratory depression in severe cases • Hypoglycemia *Caveat:* Altered mental sensorium can have other causes along with alcohol overuse
Methanol	• Delayed toxicological effect after ingestion • CNS - headache drowsiness, severe cases seizures, and coma • Abdominal—gastric irritation and transaminitis pancreatitis • Visual changes, blurring of vision, photophobia or blindness due to optic nerve damage • Metabolic acidosis, tachypnea and hypotension • Renal failure, rhabdomyolysis respiratory depression in severe cases
Ethylene glycol	• Initially neurological symptoms are similar to methanol, followed by cardiovascular stage in the form of tachycardia and hypertension • Renal stage is due to calcium oxalate deposition; hence, hypocalcemia is noted

Diagnosis

Ethanol	• Blood alcohol levels • Blood sugar, liver function tests, and amylase lipase • CT brain for any secondary insult due to trauma related to ethanol
Methanol	*As above:* • Arterial blood gases - metabolic acidosis (lactic acidosis) • **High osmolar gap appears first** • **High anion gap appears second** • **Sometimes double gap might exist**
Ethylene glycol	As above with calcium oxalate crystals and hypocalcemia

Contd...

Contd...

Treatment: A prescribed levels of methanol and ethylene glycol (EG) post-treatment to be achieved to monitor response to treatment and commence them

Ethanol	• Manage up to sobriety • IV fluids with multivitamins has no role
Methanol	• Fomepizole 15 mg/kg IV over 30 minutes and then 10 mg/kg IV over 30 minutes every 12 hours or • Ethanol 10 mL/kg of 10% IV ethanol at 100 mg/kg/h to keep ethanol level 100–150 mg/dL (22–33 mmol/L) or PO or via nasogastric tube) using 80 proof liquor of 1.5–2 mL/kg followed by maintenance dosing of 0.2–0.5 mL/kg/h. Do not use oral ethanol preparations via the IV route. For both the IV and PO routes, serum ethanol concentrations should be monitored every 1–2 hours. All maintenance doses need to be doubled for patients undergoing hemodialysis • Folinic or folic acid 1 mg/kg IV every 4–6 hours (up to 50 mg per dose), continue until toxicity resolved • IV sodium bicarbonate to maintain serum pH >7.30; IV sodium bicarbonate to maintain serum pH >7.20 • Hemodialysis, if indicated
Ethylene glycol	• All above, except folinic acid • Instead pyridoxine 50–100 mg IV every 6 hours for 24–48 hours • Thiamine 100 mg IV every 6 h for 24–48 hours • Magnesium sulfate 2 g IV (once)
Criteria for initiation of antidiuretic hormone (ADH) blockade by fomepizole/ethanol for methanol or EG poisoning	• Documented plasma methanol or EG concentration ≥20 mg/dL or • History of ingestion of methanol or EG and an osmolar gap >10 mOsm/L or • Strong clinical suspicion of ingestion of methanol or EG and at least two of the following: – Arterial pH <7.3 – Serum bicarbonate <20 mEq/L (mmol/L) – Osmolar gap >10 mOsm/L – Urinary oxalate crystals present (for EG ingestion)
Indications for hemodialysis after methanol or EG ingestion	• Refractory metabolic acidosis: pH <7.25 with anion gap >30 mEq/L and/or base deficit <–15 • Visual abnormalities • Renal insufficiency • Deteriorating vital signs despite aggressive supportive care • Electrolyte abnormalities refractory to conventional therapy • Serum methanol or ethylene glycol level of >50 mg/dL

Contd...

Contd...

Caveat: Alcohol withdrawal	• *Definition:* Alcohol withdrawal develops when a person known for heavy and prolonged consumption of alcohol who abruptly stop or reduce their drinking • Alcohol withdrawal symptoms exist on a continuum from uncomplicated to moderate and severe, **may begin as early as 2–6 hours after reduction in alcohol consumption, and can persist for up to 2 weeks in 6–24 hours** • **Minor symptoms like anxiety, insomnia, anorexia, nausea, vomiting, headache, palpitations, and tremor may not require medical care in 24–48 hours** • **Alcohol withdrawal: Hallucinations, tactile most common, and occasionally auditory or visual require no medical treatment in 36–60 hours** • **Withdrawal seizures, generalized tonic-clonic can be single or multiple status epilepticus uncommon (May occur as early as 6 h after alcohol cessation) in 60+ h Delirium Tremens Agitation, Disorientation, Hallucinations, Fever, Diaphoresis, Hypertension Tachycardia diagnosis and treatment the Clinical Institute Withdrawal** • Assessment for alcohol–revised (Scoring: Chapter 44) is the most commonly used instrument for guiding continuing treatment once a diagnosis of alcohol withdrawal is established as per the symptoms • *Treatment* is benzodiazepine • Uncomplicated alcohol withdrawal (no seizures, no delirium): – Lorazepam 2 mg PO or – Diazepam 10–20 mg PO If vomiting: – Diazepam 10–20 mg IV or – Lorazepam 2–4 mg IV and – Ondansetron 4 mg IV • Alcohol withdrawal seizures: Lorazepam 2 mg IV • Alcohol withdrawal delirium tremens – Lorazepam 2–4 mg IV; double the dose and repeat every 15–20 minutes until light somnolence or – Diazepam 10–20 mg IV over 2 minutes; double the dose and repeat every 5–10 minutes until light somnolence • If refractory to benzodiazepines: – Phenobarbital 65 mg IV every 15–30 minutes to maximum of 260 mg (respiratory depression more common than with benzodiazepines; typically requires intubation) or – Propofol 5 mg/kg/min (or 0.3 mg/kg/h) titrated to effect; typically requires intubation (unlabeled use, primarily case reports of effectiveness) *Caveat:* Antihistamines act like anticholinergic

Important Dos √ and Don'ts ×		
Decontamination ×	**Hemodialysis √**	**Antidote √**

BOX 7: Antiepileptic drugs.

Phenytoin/Fosphenytoin

Toxic dose:

- Phenytoin acute oral toxic dose: 20 mg/kg
- Fosphenytoin toxic dose is 1.5 times phenytoin

Acute toxicity:

- *Mild to moderate:* Nystagmus, ataxia, slurred speech, tremor, and mild CNS depression (common early after an overdose). Nausea, vomiting, agitation, diplopia, and irritability may develop
- *Severe:* Severe CNS depression, coma, rarely respiratory depression and seizures (large oral ingestions)
- *Rapid infusion of the parenteral formulation (>50 mg/min):* Hypotension, bradycardia, AV conduction delays, and ventricular dysrhythmias (may be fatal)
- The purple glove syndrome is a serious complication of IV administration mostly secondary to extravasation, initially causes edema later leading to necrosis leading to amputation of the same limb
- Toxicity may manifest at lower serum levels in patients with renal failure and hypoalbuminemia
- Abnormal laboratory findings may include hypoglycemia, hyperglycemia, and elevated serum transaminases
- Decreased appetite, poor feeding, diminished activity, abdominal distension, chorea, and opisthotonic posturing have been reported in children after oral overdose
- Hypersensitivity reactions may also occur

General treatment and monitoring

Decontamination:

- Do not induce vomiting
- In case of large ingestion:
  - Consider gastric lavage
  - Administer activated charcoal (12 g/kg body weight)
- Multiple-dose activated charcoal (weak evidence for improving outcome)

Treatment:

- Consider intermittent hemodialysis (acceptable alternative is intermittent hemoperfusion)
- Lipid resuscitation therapy may be considered in severe cardiovascular toxicity

Monitoring:

- Blood phenytoin concentrations every 4 hours until clearly declining
- Continuous cardiac status
- Serial neurological examinations

Important Dos √ and Don'ts ×		
Emesis: ×	**Gastric lavage:** ±	**Activated charcoal:** ±
Enhanced elimination: √	**Specific antidote:** ×	

Contd...

Contd...

Carbamazepine*—toxidrome similar to cyclic antidepressant:*
- **Clinical presentation and treatment is similar to phenytoin, except to treat the increase in QRS duration and therapy**

Topiramate:
- Clinical presentation: Lethargy, ataxia, nystagmus, myoclonus, hallucinations, coma, seizures, and status epilepticus are noted
- Hyperchloremic nonanion gap metabolic acidosis results along with hypocitraturia and high urine pH leading to formation of calcium phosphate stones treatment
- Sodium bicarbonate 1–2 mEq/kg bolus intravenously and an infusion and in severe refractory cases intermittent hemodialysis is helpful

Valproic acid:
- Clinical manifestation: Neurologic symptoms and metabolic disturbances are noted
- Severe cases might cause coma, respiratory depression, and hypotension. Hypernatremia, hypocalcemia, and hyperammonemia are the common metabolic abnormalities

Treatment:
- Gastric decontamination with multidose charcoal
- In severe cases, extracorporeal elimination can be done
- **For hyperammonemia L-carnitine loading dose is 100 mg/kg IV over 30 minutes (maximum, 6 g) followed by 15 mg/kg IV over 10–30 minutes every 4 hours until clinical improvement occurs**

BOX 8: Analgesic and anti-inflammatory.

Opioids:

Toxic dose:

- Widely variable

Acute toxicity (signs and symptoms) ***(opioid toxidromes)****:*

- *Mainly a triad; respiratory depression (reduced RR), coma (lethargy and miosis)*
- Euphoria, drowsiness, nausea, vomiting, constipation, miosis, mild bradycardia, or hypotension

Other symptoms and signs noted are:

- **Urticaria and pruritus are seen commonly with codeine**
- **Noncardiac pulmonary edema and rhabdomyolysis may occur after IV injection of opioid analgesics**
- ***Methadone*** **and** ***dextropropoxyphene*** **may cause QT prolongation**
- **Heroin abuse may cause hypoglycemia, leukocytosis, scleroderma (when mixed with talc), and wound botulism (with black tar)**
- **Seizures (*meperidine* and *propoxyphene*)**
- **Flushing and bronchospasm (histamine)**

Potential sequelae/delayed effects:

- Neuronal damage due to hypoxia

General treatment and monitoring

Treatment:

- In case of large ingestion:
  - Consider gastric lavage
  - Administer activated charcoal (12 g/kg body weight)
- Look for and remove any opioid containing transdermal patches

Specific—antidote: ***Naloxone***

Indications	• For reversal of acute opioid intoxication presenting as coma, respiratory depression, or hypotension • Empirical therapy for stupor or coma suspected to be caused by opioid overdose
Adults	• 0.4–2 mg IV. Repeat every 2–3 minutes up to a total dose of 10 mg. If clinical condition does not improve even at 10 mg, reconsider the diagnosis • In opioid dependent individuals, starting dose should be as low as 0.04–0.4 mg IV due to risk of opioid withdrawal
Children	• ≤12 years: 0.1 mg/kg IV or IM, may repeat every 25 minutes till response occurs (maximum 2 mg in <5 years). *In case of chronic opioid exposure:* 0.01 mg/kg IV or IM, if no response, may administer 0.1 mg/kg IV or IM • In case of ingestion of a long acting opioid, continuous infusion every hour may be given as two-third of the effective bolus dose for initial reversal and titrated as required • Also to stop the infusion temporarily if withdrawal develops

Contd...

Contd...

	• If patient has respiratory worsening on infusion repeat half bolus dose • Goal of naloxone administration is adequate ventilation and not to improve level of consciousness • It can be given nasally, subcutaneously or intramuscularly (2 mg) also, when IV access is not feasible • Duration of effect of naloxone is 12 hours. Awakened patients should be observed for at least 34 hours

Important Dos √ and Don'ts ×		
Gastric decontamination √	**Extracorporeal elimination ×**	**Antidote √**

Acetaminophen/Paracetamol:

Toxic dose and maximal therapeutic dose:

- *Adults:* Ingestion of 7.5–10 g is considered potentially toxic
- *Children:* Ingestion of >150 mg/kg is potentially toxic
- Maximum daily dose: Up to 4 g (adults) and 75 mg/kg (children)

Acute toxicity (signs and symptoms):

Chronology of appearance of symptoms are staged as I, II, III, and IV

- *0.5–24 hours (Stage I):* Nausea, vomiting, diaphoresis, pallor, lethargy, and malaise. Liver function test (LFT) is normal in most cases. Massive ingestion (>500 µg/mL) causes coma, metabolic acidosis, and hyperglycemia with normal serum transaminases
- *24–72 hours (Stage II):* Onset of liver toxicity occurs with right upper quadrant pain with liver enlargement and tenderness. Laboratory abnormalities include elevations of aminotransferases [aspartate transaminase (AST) being more sensitive and rises before alanine transaminase (ALT)], prothrombin time (PT), and total bilirubin. Oliguria may also occur
- *72–96 hours (Stage III):* Maximal hepatotoxicity occurs jaundice, confusion (hepatic encephalopathy), marked elevation in hepatic enzymes, hyperammonemia, and bleeding diathesis
- In severe toxicity, plasma ALT and AST levels often exceed 10,000 IU/L, prolongation of the PT or international normalized ratio (INR), hypoglycemia, lactic acidosis, and total bilirubin above 4 mg/dL (primarily indirect)
- *4 days to 2 weeks (Stage IV):* Patients who survive stage III enter a recovery phase that usually begins by 4th day and is complete by 7 days after overdose. Laboratory parameters get normalized over 1 month
- Renal failure may occur as a consequence of hepatorenal syndrome

Treatment:

- Treat hypotension, coagulopathy, acidosis, hepatic and renal failure, if present
- Hemodialysis is effective but not generally indicated and may be considered in massive ingestion

Contd...

Contd...

Monitoring:

- Blood glucose, electrolytes, renal function test (RFT), LFT, and PT/INR
- Plasma/serum paracetamol levels 4 hours postingestion (levels obtained 4–16 hours post ingestion are most predictive or potential hepatotoxicity and not useful in chronic or repeated ingestion) (Rumack–Matthew nomogram) to decide if antidote to be administered
- Recheck the INR, plasma creatinine, plasma bicarbonate and ALT every 8–16 hours to assess the course of liver injury

Specific—antidote: ***N-acetyl cysteine (NAC)***

Indications	• Suspected paracetamol dose >7.5 g or >150 mg/kg of total dose • 4 hours levels >150 µg/mL after acute ingestion and in patients with unknown time of ingestion: Serum acetaminophen >10 µg/mL • Any evidence of liver injury (INR >1.3 or ALT two times the upper limit of normal) or coexistent conditions (chronic alcoholism, intake of enzyme inducing drugs, and starvation)
Oral	
Loading dose	• 140 mg/kg as 5% solution (*diluted in soft drink, juice, or water to improve palatability*)
Maintenance dose	• 70 mg/kg every 4 hours for an additional 17 doses, for a total dose of 1330 mg/kg over approximately 72 hours • May administer through a nasogastric tube to prevent vomiting (*consider antiemetics 30 minutes before for prevention of NAC induced vomiting*)
Intravenous	
Loading dose	• 150 mg/kg infusion (maximum 15 g) in 200 mL of 5% dextrose in water (D5W) over 60 minutes
Maintenance dose	• 50 mg/kg infusion over 4 hours, i.e. 12.5 mg/kg/h (maximum 5 g) in 500 mL D5W followed by 100 mg/kg infusion (i.e., 6.25 mg/kg/h) over 16 hours (maximum 10 g) in 1,000 mL D5W, for 21 hours **(Fig. 1)** • In case of liver failure, continue 100 mg/kg infusion until resolution of encephalopathy, decreasing serum transaminases and improving coagulopathy

Important Dos √ and Don'ts ×		
Gastric decontamination √	**Antidote √**	**Hemodialysis (severe) √**

Contd...

Contd...

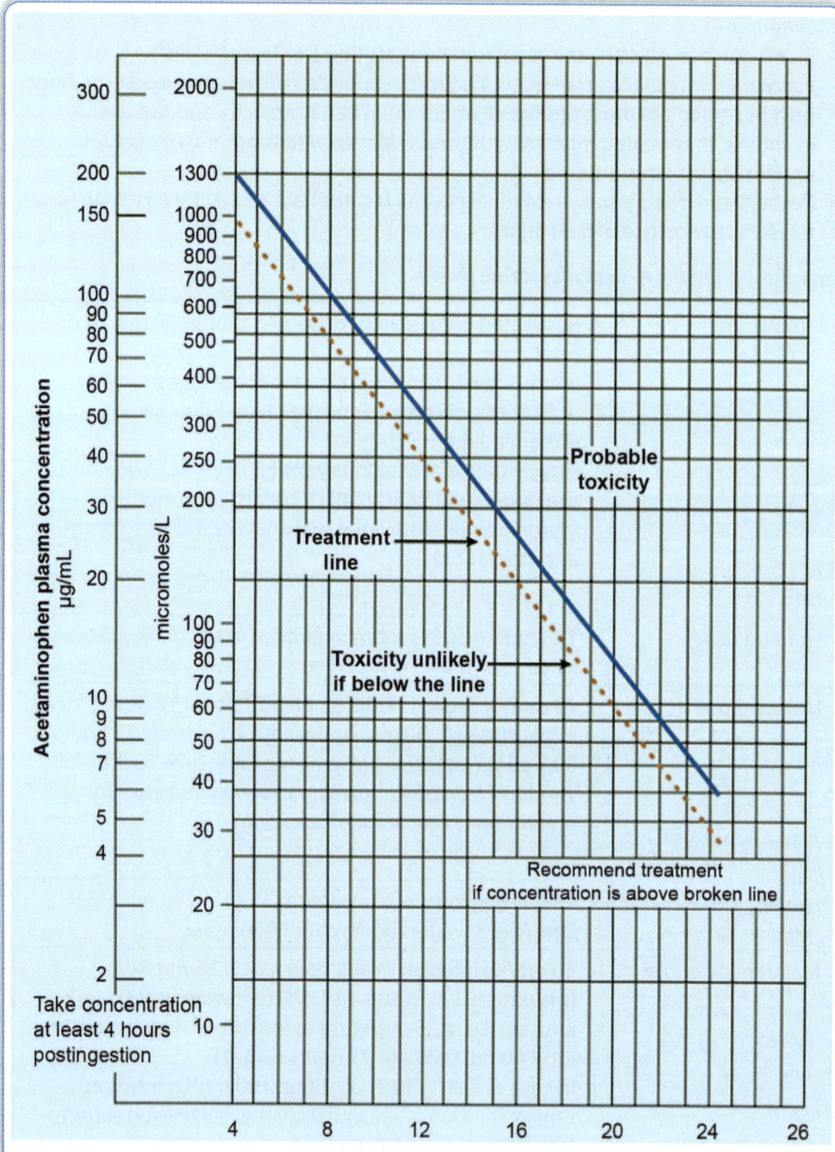

Fig. 1: Rumack curve to determine the concentration of acetaminophen and its potential for toxicity.

Nonsteroidal anti-inflammatory drugs (NSAIDs):

Toxic dose differs for each NSAIDs

- *Gastrointestinal:*
  - Acute: dyspepsia, ulceration, perforation, hemorrhage, and elevated hepatic aminotransferases

Contd...

Contd...

- *Renal:*
  - Acute: Acute kidney failure, fluid and electrolyte retention, hyperkalemia, hypertension interstitial nephritis, and azotemia
- *Hypersensitivity or pulmonary:*
  - Acute: Asthma exacerbation, anaphylactoid and anaphylactic reactions, urticaria, angioedema, and acute respiratory distress syndrome
- *Hematologic:*
  - Acute: Increased bleeding time, agranulocytosis, aplastic anemia, thrombocytopenia, neutropenia, and hemolytic anemia
- *Central nervous system:*
  - Acute: Headache, dizziness, lethargy, coma
- ***Mefenamic acid*** can cause seizures
- *Treatment:*
  - Stabilize ABC
  - Decontamination, charcoal multidose activated can be used
  - No antidote
- **Salicylate**
- Toxic dose 150–300 mg/kg

Clinical presentation:
- *Mild:* Starts with gastric presentation of nausea and vomiting, tinnitus, dizziness, and hearing loss
- *Moderate:* Tachypnea, hyperpyrexia, diaphoresis, and ataxia
- *Severe:* Abnormal mental status, seizures acute lung injury, renal failure, cardiac arrhythmias shock

Metabolic abnormalities; known to cause mixed acid–base disturbances
- Early: Respiratory alkalosis
- Intermediate: With respiratory alkalosis, AG metabolic acidosis starts to develop
- Late: Metabolic acidosis with either a respiratory alkalosis or respiratory acidosis [acute respiratory distress syndrome (ARDS) due to severe poisoning or secondary cause or mixed poisoning]
- Metabolic alkalosis secondary to severe vomiting might also be noticed in a few

Monitoring:
- Serum salicylate levels both for diagnosis and monitoring treatment
- Arterial blood gas/venous blood gas (ABG/VBG)
- Kidney function, CXR, and amongst others

Treatment:
- Decontamination with activated charcoal, multidose charcoal is helpful
- Urine alkalinization is helpful, especially in moderate to severe cases
- Extracorporeal elimination with hemodialysis is indicated in severe cases

Important Dos √ and Don'ts ×		
Decontamination with AC/MDAC √	**Extracorporeal elimination √**	**Antidote ×**

BOX 9: Methemoglobinemia.

- Medications: Amyl nitrite, local anesthetics (benzocaine, lidocaine, and prilocaine), dapsone, nitric oxide, nitroglycerin, nitroprusside, and quinones (chloroquine and primaquine)
- Sulfonamides (sulfanilamide, sulfathiazide, sulfapyridine, and sulfamethoxazole)
- Others: Aniline dye derivatives (shoe dyes, marking inks, chlorobenzene, copper sulfate fires (heat-induced denaturation), organic nitrites (e.g., isobutyl nitrite, butyl nitrite), naphthalene, nitrates (e.g., well water), and nitrites (e.g., foods)
- Pediatric reduced NADH (nicotinamide-adenine dinucleotide) methemoglobin (*Met Hb*) reductase activity in infants (<4 months)
- Associated with low birth weight, prematurity, dehydration, acidosis, diarrhea, and hyperchloremia

Acute toxicity signs and symptoms:

Met Hb levels (%)	***Met Hb concentration (g/dL)***	***Clinical symptoms***
13		Normal levels
<15	<2.2	Usually asymptomatic or slate gray skin coloration, pulse oximeter might show low oxygen
15–20	2.2–3.0	Cyanosis, chocolate brown-colored blood
20–50	37.5	Fatigue, weakness, headache, nausea, confusion, dizziness, dyspnea, and tachycardia
50–70	7.5–10.5	Lethargy, stupor, tachypnea, dysrhythmias, seizures, metabolic acidosis, and coma
>70	>10.5	Severe hypoxic symptoms, death

Normal range hemoglobin concentrations of 15 g/dL assumed. At lower hemoglobin concentrations and in patients with underlying cardiac, pulmonary or hematologic disease, symptoms may be more severe

General:
Diagnosis:
Clinical cyanosis along with low hemoglobin oxygen saturation on pulse oximetry (typically 85–89%), and normal PaO_2 on ABG is highly suggestive of methemoglobinemia

Bedside test: Place a drop of patient's blood on a filter paper and compare with normal drop of blood. Presence of chocolate brown blood shows Met Hb levels exceeding 15%

Contd...

Contd...

Monitoring:
- Complete blood counts and peripheral smear
- Serum electrolytes, glucose, blood urea nitrogen (BUN), CPK creatinine, and liver transaminases
- CXR
- Arterial blood gases (inhalation)
- Haptoglobin, urinalysis dipstick for occult blood

Treatment:
- Levels <15–20% do not require intervention and resolve spontaneously
- Maintain airway and assist ventilation if required
- Administer supplemental oxygen
- Provide symptomatic care
- Enhanced elimination
- Hyperbaric oxygen or exchange transfusion may be beneficial if methylene blue is not useful

Specific—antidote: Methylene blue
Methylene blue: 1–2 mg/kg, IV as a 1% solution (10 mg/mL) in saline over 3–5 minutes. It may be repeated at 1 mg/kg after every 30 minutes up to a total maximum dose of 7 mg/kg. However, if the patient dose not respond after second dose, suspect glucose-6-phosphate dehydrogenase (G6PD) deficiency. Patients with continued production of *Met Hb* may require repeated dosing every 6–8 hours for 3 days. Flush IV line with 15–30 mL of 5% dextrose every time to reduce pain

Important Do's √ and Don'ts ×		
Vomiting: ×	**Gastric Lavage: ±**	
Activated charcoal: ±	**Enhanced elimination: √**	**Specific antidote: √**

BOX 10: Antiseptics/disinfectants.

Formaldehyde:
Acute toxicity signs and symptoms

Ingestion	Abdominal pain, vomiting, diarrhea, mucosal ulceration, hemorrhage, necrosis, perforation of stomach, large anion gap metabolic acidosis, altered mental status, seizures, cyanosis, tachypnea, respiratory distress, hematuria, proteinuria, acute renal failure, hypotension, hypovolemic shock, and coma
Inhalation	Cough, dyspnea, wheeze, chemical pneumonitis, bronchospasm, laryngeal and pulmonary edema, weakness, headache, vomiting, CNS depression, convulsions, coma, and respiratory failure
Dermal	Irritation, rash, and burns
Ocular	Irritation and lacrimation may cause permanent vision impairment

Potential sequelae/delayed effects:
Corrosive gastritis, fibrosis of stomach, edema, and ulceration of esophagus

General treatment and monitoring
Monitoring:
- CXR
- Arterial blood gases
- Endoscopy

Treatment:
- Consider endoscopy to rule out esophageal or gastric injury
- Correct acidosis by administering sodium bicarbonate, IV
- Consider hemodialysis in refractory patients with severe acid–base disturbances or in patients with significant methanol levels

Enhanced elimination:
- Hemodialysis
- Urine alkalinization
- Folate 50 mg, IV, every 4 hours (1 mg/kg in children), may enhance elimination

Other common ones are briefly described with main clinical presentation and treatment

Boric acid:
- Bluegreen emesis and diarrhea
- Boiled lobster appearance of skin
- Hemodialysis (rare)
- CNS depression kidney failure
- Symptomatic management
- Only orogastric decontamination

Contd...

Chlorinated compounds	
Chlorhexidine	GI irritation symptomatic treatment
Chlorates	• Hemolysis, methemoglobinemia, and kidney failure • Treatment exchange transfusion, hemodialysis, methemoglobinemia treatment
Chlorine/sodium hypochlorite	• GI irritation • Treatment endoscopy
Iodinated compound [tincture/lugol/betadine]	GI irritation, orogastric lavage, activated charcoal electrolyte imbalance treatment and symptomatic management
Hydrogen peroxide	GI irritation, decontamination with lavage to manage oxygen emboli
Potassium permanganate	GI irritation, antiseptic-decontamination, endoscopy
Alcohol	Mentioned in **Box 6**

Important Do's √ and Don'ts ×		
Vomiting: ×	**Gastric Lavage: × (consider gastric aspiration in large ingestion)**	
Activated charcoal: ?	**Enhanced elimination: √**	**Specific antidote: ×**

Phenol:
Toxic dose 1 g

Clinical manifestation:
- Both local and systemic symptoms are noted
- Systemic symptoms include CNS and cardiac manifestations
- CNS effects include seizures, lethargy, and coma

Cardiac signs and symptoms:
- From phenol include tachycardia, bradycardia, and hypotension
- Local toxicity to the GI tract from the ingestion results in nausea, painful oral lesions, vomiting, severe abdominal pain, bloody diarrhea, and dark urine
- Dermal exposures to phenol usually result in a light brown staining of the skin

Treatment is symptomatic
- Endoscopy might be required in gastric burns
- Dermal exposure should be decontaminated with water, PEG wash might be useful for local dermal decontamination caveat; substitute phenol are less toxic
- GI decontamination not indicated

BOX 11: Pesticides.

Organophosphates/organocarbamates

WHO classification of pesticide toxicity:

		LD_{50} for the rat (mg/kg body weight)			
		Oral		***Dermal***	
	Class	***Solids***	***Liquids***	***Solids***	***Liquids***
Ia	Extremely hazardous	<5	<20	<10	<40
Ib	Highly hazardous	5–50	20–200	10–100	40–400
II	Moderately hazardous	50–500	200–2,000	100–1,000	400–4,000
III	Slightly hazardous	>500	>2,000	>1,000	>4,000

- Acute toxicity and symptoms
- **Cholinergic toxidromes**

In acute toxicity:
- *Mild* – light headedness, nausea, headache, dyspnea, lacrimation, rhinorrhea, salivation, and diaphoresis
- *Moderate* – Restless, confusion, vomiting, diarrhea, autonomic instability, muscle fasciculation, and bronchorrhea and spasm
- *Severe* – coma, seizure, flaccid paralysis, urinary, or fecal incontinence, and respiratory arrest
  - *Intermediate* – 15 days after exposure paralysis of neck flexor muscles, cranial nerve
  - Innervated muscles, proximal limb muscles, respiratory muscles
- No cholinergic excess symptoms though noted
- *Delayed/chronic*
  - Seen in farmers in daily exposure to pesticides in the form of symmetrical sensorimotor axonopathy is noted
  - Leg pain to weakness and paralysis, delayed neuropathy, and cognitive dysfunction

Management:
- Investigation/diagnosis: Cholinergic toxidrome is sufficient to diagnose
- Urine cholinesterase levels
- Red cell acetylcholinesterase—a more potent indicator, but butyrylcholinesterase is easy to assess
- Atropine challenge
- Routine tests may exclude other causes
- CXR to rule out pulmonary edema in severe cases
- ECG may show ventricular dysrhythmia, torsade de pointes, and idioventricular rhythm
- AV blocks prolongation of QT interval is common
- QTc corelates with severity
- EMG: For NM junction action

Contd...

Contd...

General:

Decontamination	• Protective clothing for healthcare workers • Handle and dispose all clothes as hazardous waste • Wash patient with soap and water • Handle and dispose of water runoff as hazardous waste
Monitoring	• Cardiac monitor, pulse oximeter, 100% oxygen
Gastric lavage	• No proven benefit, yet to be done especially if presented early
Activated charcoal	• No proven benefit
Urinary alkanization	• No proven benefit
Atropine	• 1–3 mg IV in adult or 0.01–0.04 mg/kg IV (never <.1 mg per dose) in children • Repeat every 5 minutes till tracheobronchial secretions attenuate • Followed by continuous infusion to maintain anticholinergic state • Dose varies from 0.4 to 0.04 mg /h IV infusion adults
Pralidoxime	• No proven benefit • 1–2 g for adults or 20–40 mg/kg IV (up to 1 g in children), mixed with NS and infused over 5–10 minutes • Followed by continuous infusion; 500 mg/h in adults • 5–10 mg/kg/h in children
Seizures	Benzodiazepine IV

Disposition:
- Every patient needs to be admitted
- Atropine dose depends on severity in acute cases
- In mild <2 mg IV is required, while moderate will need 2–10 mg IV
- Severe will need >10 mg IV of atropine
- Patient will mostly need intensive care for monitoring of symptoms
- Even in intermediate category early atropine and antidote will help in recovery

Caveat:
- **Atropine does not reverse nicotinic effects. Therefore, patients who improve after receiving atropine should be closely monitored in a critical care setting for impending respiratory failure from delayed neuromuscular junction (NMJ) dysfunction**
- **Patients should be clinically examined regularly for proximal muscle weakness (particularly neck flexor weakness); once recognized, tidal volume or negative inspiratory force measurements should be made at least every 4–6 hours to detect impending respiratory failure and allow early initiation of ventilatory support**

  When antimuscarinic CNS toxicity becomes evident yet peripheral cholinergic findings necessitate the administration of more atropine (e.g., bradycardia and bronchorrhea), some authors recommend substituting glycopyrrolate for atropine, because its quaternary ammonium structure limits CNS penetration

Contd...

Contd...

- **One randomized clinical trial (RCT) compared atropine with glycopyrrolate in ICU management of OP poisoning, but was too small to detect any difference between regimens. The initial IV dose of glycopyrrolate for adults and adolescents is 1–2 mg, repeated as needed, or in children 0.025 mg/kg up to adult doses. As with atropine, some patients with severe poisoning require higher doses of glycopyrrolate**
- **Although mostly titration of atropine is sufficient**
- **Oximes to be given as early as possible but should not be deferred if late diagnosis or in intermediate cases**
- **The duration of use is unclear. It is reasonable to stop oxime administration when atropine is no longer clinically required. Electrophysiological and clinical observation may allow the benefit of oxime administration to be assessed before atropine is stopped**
- **Transiently stopping the infusion after 2–3 days and carefully observing for clinical or electrophysiological deterioration is a reasonable approach to deciding whether to continue oxime therapy**
- **Titrated dose pralidoxime regimens have been recommended**
- **In carbamates oximes are contraindicated**

Pyrethroids:

Toxic dose:

- Acute oral toxic dose: 100-1,000 mg/kg
- Acute potentially lethal oral dose: 110 g
- Oral poisoning occurs in humans at dosages of 22–50 mg/kg, while ingestion of 100–250 mg/kg induces coma

Acute toxicity signs and symptoms:

Type II pyrethroids are more toxic than type I

Ingestion	• Nausea, vomiting, diarrhea, abdominal pain, burning sensation in mouth, sore throat, paresthesias, headache, hyperexcitability, dizziness, fatigue, hyperthermia, and coma. Large ingestion can cause abdominal pain, vomiting, coma, and seizures • Solvents and surfactants may cause corrosive GI effects and pneumonitis
Inhalation	• Headache, dizziness, burning or itching of face, rhinitis, cough, dyspnea, wheeze, chest pain, bronchospasm, and pulmonary edema • Respiratory paralysis and cardiopulmonary arrest (rare)
Dermal	• Tingling sensation or numbness (temporary paresthesia) in the area of contact, pruritus, and erythema on exposed areas
Ocular	• Eye irritation, burning, itching, pain, lacrimation, photophobia, conjunctivitis, corneal damage, and periorbital edema

Potential sequelae/delayed effects:

- Delayed weakness with upper motor neuron signs

General:

Decontamination:	• Remove patient from exposure • Remove contaminated clothing • Wash skin thoroughly with plenty of soap and water

Contd...

Contd...

	• Irrigate eyes with lots of water or saline • In case of large ingestion: – Consider gastric aspiration – Administer activated charcoal (12 g/kg body weight)
Treatment	• Administer humidified oxygen, if needed • Perform endotracheal intubation and provide assisted ventilation, if needed • Treat coma, seizures, hypotension, acute lung injury, bronchospasm, and anaphylaxis, if present
Monitoring	• ECG, ABG, and RFT • Pulse oximetry, CXR, and pulmonary functions in patients with respiratory symptom

Specific: No specific antidote

Important Dos √ and Don'ts ×		
Emesis: ×	**Gastric lavage:** × **(consider gastric aspiration in large ingestion)**	**Activated charcoal:** ±
Enhanced elimination: ×	**Specific antidote:** ×	

BOX 12: Rodenticides.

Rodenticides (super warf, strychnine, phosphorus yellow, aluminium/zinc phospide nicotinamide, barium salts)

Yellow phosphorus:

Common name	Ratol
Toxic dose	Acute oral dose of 1 mg/kg in adults
Acute toxicity (signs and symptoms)	• *Stage 1: Few minutes to 24 hours:* Nausea, vomiting, abdominal pain, hematemesis, garlic odor of breath and feces, photo luminescent, or smoky vomitus/faces. Irritability, lethargy, headache, delirium, stupor, seizures, and coma may occur • *State 2: 17 days (may extend up to 10 days):* Symptom free period showing apparent recovery • *Stage 3:* Hepatic failure, renal failure often followed by death. Recovery may occur usually over 12 weeks
Toxicity may not occur distinctly in stages	
Severe	Electrolyte abnormalities such as hypokalemia, hyperchloremia, hypocalcemia and either hyper/phosphatemia, hypoglycemia, encephalopathy, and cardiac dysrhythmias

Contd...

Contd...

Inhalation	Upper respiratory tract irritation, ocular, nasal, and throat irritation. Delayed onset of acute lung injury and hepatic injury may occur
Dermal	Yellowish color, severely painful, necrotic partial to full-thickness second- and third-degree burns (few minutes to hours). Acute systemic phosphorus poisoning may occur
Ocular	Eye irritation, lacrimation, blepharospasm, photophobia, and corneal damage

Management:
Monitoring
- Serial serum electrolytes, renal function test RFT, LFT, PT, ABG, CBC, urine output, and urine analysis
- Continuous cardiac status and pulse oximetry
- CXR

PFT in case of inhalational exposure

Decontamination
- Wash skin thoroughly with plenty of cold water for at least 15 minutes

Caveat: Avoid application of any lipid of oil-based ointments. (Immerse removed particles immediately in cool water to avoid ignition)
- Irrigate eyes with lots of water or saline
- *Do not induce vomiting and avoid giving milk or fatty substances, in case of large ingestion:*
  - *Consider gastric aspiration with a small, flexible nasogastric tube*
  - *Do not give activated charcoal*

Note: Keep contaminated clothing, vomitus, and gastric contents in a water-sealed bag to prevent secondary exposure
Symptomatic treatment as no antidote
Consider hemodialysis if renal failure

Barium carbonate:

Toxic dose	Barium salts: 200 mg; oral, lethal dose: 130 g of barium salts
Acute toxicity (signs and symptoms)	Nausea, vomiting, hypersalivation, colicky abdominal pain, diarrhea, paresthesias, chest pain, dyspnea (within 1 hour). Generalized muscle weakness due to profound hypokalemia, tremors, seizures, vertigo, mydriasis, hypertension, bradycardia, ventricular dysrhythmias, respiratory failure, shock, and cardiac arrest (23 hours). Rhabdomyolysis, pulmonary edema, and metabolic acidosis may also occur

Contd...

Contd...

Management:
Monitoring
- Vital signs
- Serum electrolytes, creatinine, urea, and ABG
- CXR, continuous cardiac status
- Serial neurologic examinations to evaluate for muscle weakness
- Serum potassium levels every 1–2 hours until stabilized
- Serum phosphorus, magnesium, and CK

Address the ABCs
Decontamination
- In case of large ingestion:
  - Consider gastric lavage or aspiration with a nasogastric tube
  - Give magnesium sulfate or sodium sulfate (adult: 30 g; children: 250 mg/kg) as a 5% solution by stomach tube to precipitate barium sulfate
- Treat hypokalemia with IV potassium chloride (up to 250 mEq administered over 24 hours has been used. High doses of 420 mEq over 24 hours have been used)

(Note: Rebound hyperkalemia may occur particularly in patients with renal dysfunction)

Symptomatic treatment
- Consider hemodialysis in case of severe poisoning
- No antidote

Zinc phosphide/aluminum phosphide

Common name (some examples)	Ratol, Norat, Zinphos, Ratil, Ratphos, Commando, Rat bite, Rat kill, Rat shoot, Ratox, and Rat seal
Toxic dose	Doses as low as 40 mg/kg may be fetal in humans
Acute toxicity (signs and symptoms)	• Nausea, vomiting, and abdominal pain are the early features • *Mild to moderate:* Tachycardia, fatigue, headache, dizziness, anxiety, restlessness, dyspnea, tachypnea, and hypoglycemia may develop • *Severe:* CNS excitation or depression, hypotension, dysrhythmias, metabolic and respiratory acidosis, jaundice, elevated liver enzymes, seizures, and acute lung injury. Hypoglycemia, hypokalemia, hypocalcemia, pancreatitis (rare), *shock, and cardiac failure are indicative of severe poisoning, and profound hypotension is the characteristic feature*
Potential sequelae/ delayed effects	Pulmonary edema may be delayed up to 48–72 hours subacute poisoning due to exposure for a few days may cause Reactive Airways Dysfunction Syndrome (RADS) after a few months

Contd...

Contd...

Management:

Monitoring

- Vital signs and mental status
- Continuous cardiac status and pulse oximetry
- Blood glucose, CBC, ABG, serum electrolytes, RFT, and LFT
- CXR in patients with respiratory symptoms

Decontamination

- Role of gastric lavage is not clear
- Water can react with stomach acid to produce phosphine gas. Hence to be avoided in orogastric decontamination
- *In case of large ingestion:*
  - Consider early gastric lavage with dilute potassium permanganate (1:10,000)/ sodium bicarbonate (3–5%)
  - Administer activated charcoal (1–2 g/kg body weight)
  - Symptomatic treatment
  - Consider acetylcysteine - very weak recommendations for hepatic injury
  - No antidote

Bromadiolone (anticoagulant super warfarins)

Common name (some examples)	Raton RB, Roban, Mortein Rat kill, Ratcon CB, and Kalrat RB
Toxic dose	Small ingestion is unlikely to cause toxic features. Inadvertent exposure to 1 mg or more of active ingredient of long acting anticoagulant rodenticides may cause coagulopathy 48–72 hours postingestion
Acute toxicity (signs and symptoms)	*Usually asymptomatic.* Clinical signs of bleeding may be delayed until 1–4 weeks after ingestion. Hemorrhage may manifest as mild features like spontaneous bruising, ecchymoses, epistaxis, gingival bleeding, hemoptysis to life-threatening complications such as hematuria, bilateral flank pain, gastrointestinal bleeding, intracranial bleeding, intra-abdominal or retroperitoneal bleeding. Onset of prolonged prothrombin time occurs generally within 48 hours. Normal PT after 48 hours indicates small or insignificant ingestion

Management:

Monitoring

- INR or PT after large or deliberate ingestions (at baseline, 48 hours postingestion; serial monitoring during therapy and 2 weeks after stopping the therapy)
- CBC, blood typing, and cross matching for patients with significant bleeding
- Stools and vomitus for occult blood

Treatment

- Address the ABCs
- Decontamination with activated charcoal

Contd...

Contd...

- No intervention is required in small ingestions
- Treat significant prolongation of the INR (>4.0) with vitamin K1 (phytonadione)
- Do not give vitamin K3 (Menadione)
- In case of active bleeding or life-threatening hemorrhage, give dried prothrombin complex (25–50 units/kg) or if this is unavailable, give fresh frozen plasma (15 mL/kg) in addition to fresh whole blood transfusion

Specific antidote

Vitamin K1 (Phytonadione)	• No active bleeding and INR <4, post 48 hours ingestion—no treatment required • No active bleeding and INR >4, post 48 hours ingestion—give vitamin K1, 10 mg slow IV (children: 250 µg/kg IV, maximum 10 mg): *Alternatively* oral dose—adults: 15–25 mg; children: 5–10 mg, 2–4 times a day • Active bleeding or life-threatening hemorrhage—give vitamin K1 20–40 mg slow IV diluted in saline or glucose, (rate not exceeding 5% of the total dose/min) with further dosing guided by INR monitoring • Initial IV dosses of up to 400 mg have been required in actively hemorrhaging patients • Switch to oral dosing once patient has stabilized. Oral daily maintenance doses of 500–1,000 mg have been required • Vitamin K1 may be required for weeks or months • Monitor INR, 2 weeks after stopping Vitamin K1 to ensure no recurrence of anticoagulation
Strychnine	• *Clinical manifestation:* – Restlessness, muscle twitching, and painful extensor – Spasms, awake seizures, opisthotonos, trismus, inability to swallow, and facial grimacing, hyperthermia rhabdomyolysis, medullary paralysis, and death can follow • *Treatment:* – Early lavage, activated charcoal can be done – Airway control, quiet environment (minimize sensory stimulation), and benzodiazepines, barbiturates, analgesia mainly to control seizures – If refractory seizures nondepolarizing neuromuscular blockage if necessary – No antidote

BOX 13: Cardiac group of drugs.

Digoxin:

Toxic dose: More than 2 mg in adults

Acute toxicity:
- Dysrythmia of all kinds varying from bradycardia to ventricular arrhythmia to AV blocks are noted
- Nausea, vomiting
- Headache, confusion, coma might be seen
- Hyperkalemia is noted

Difference between chronic and acute toxicity is that in chronic ventricular arrhythmia is noted whereas in acute bradyarrhythmia/AV blocks may be seen also in chronic potassium might be low.

Management:

Diagnosis: If chronic, generally elderly patients with history of cardiac disease

ECG:
- *The most common arrhythmias in digoxin toxicity are premature ventricular contractions and bradycardic rhythms*
- *The four findings are T-wave changes (such as flattening or inversion), QT interval shortening, "scooped" depression of the ST segment, and increased U-wave amplitude* **(Fig. 2)**

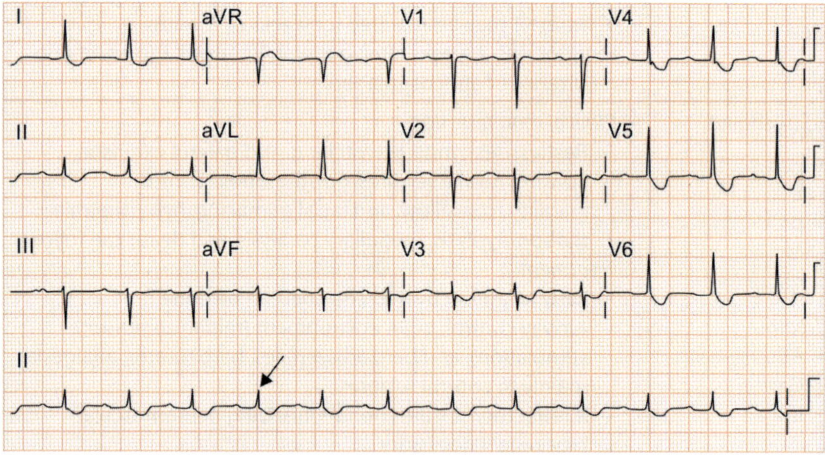

Fig. 2: ECG findings for arrhythmias in digoxin toxicity.

Treatment:
- Initial ABCs to be addressed
- Decontamination with charcoal
- Manage cardiac dysrhythmia
- Bradyarrhythmia/blocks by atropine, pacing might be needed but might not be useful unless antidote administered
- Tachydysrhythmia – phenytoin (although not routinely used) and lidocaine have most benefits

Contd...

Contd...

- Digoxin Fab antibodies is given in any life-threatening conditions irrespective of the digoxin concentration
- Calculation of digoxin-specific antibody fragment (Fab) full neutralizing dose:
- Based on suspected amount ingested:
  - Digoxin body load (mg) = 0.8 × suspected ingested amount (mg)
  - Digoxin body load (mg) = Serum digoxin concentration (nanograms/mL) × 5.6 L/kg × weight (kg)/1,000
  - One vial (about 40 mg) of digoxin Fab neutralizes
  - 0.5 mg of digoxin ingested
- Based on total serum digoxin concentration:

Number of vials = Serum concentration (nanograms/mL) × Patient weight (kg)/100

BOX 14: Beta-blocker toxicity: presentation and management.

Presentation:
- Primary sign: Wide complex bradycardia (QRS >120 ms) with associated shock
- Exception: Sotalol toxicity, as it acts as a potassium channel blocker, leading to QT interval prolongation
- Dysrhythmias: Potential for ventricular arrhythmias, including premature ventricular contractions, bigeminy, ventricular tachycardia, ventricular fibrillation, and torsades de pointes

Additional symptoms:
- Central Nervous System (CNS): Drowsiness, seizures, and coma
- Pulmonary: Bronchospasm

Diagnosis:
- Patient history: Often critical in identifying beta-blocker overdose
- ECG findings: Characterized by wide complex bradycardia, prolonged QRS, or prolonged QT interval in sotalol toxicity
- Monitoring: Regular assessment of electrolytes, acid–base balance, and blood glucose

Treatment approach:
- ABCs: Follow standard airway, breathing, and circulation procedures
- Gastric decontamination: Administer activated charcoal and consider whole bowel irrigation to reduce drug absorption

Hypotension and bradycardia:
- Start with IV fluids and atropine, though atropine may have limited effectiveness
- For QRS widening: If QRS duration exceeds 120 ms, administer sodium bicarbonate

Escalated therapies:
Begin with glucagon followed by calcium salts to counter both beta-blocker and calcium channel blocker effects (often seen in combination)

Contd...

Contd...

- Administer high-dose insulin therapy, ensuring euglycemia with dextrose infusions
- Initiate catecholamines/vasopressors as needed
- Critical cases: In severe toxicity, simultaneous administration of the above interventions may be required

Additional therapies:
- Lipid emulsion: Consider in refractory cases

Glucagon dosing:
- Adults: 3–5 mg IV, up to a maximum of 10 mg, followed by infusion at the response dose
- Pediatrics: 50 µg/kg, with a maximum dose of 10 mg

Calcium gluconate:
- Adults: 3 g of 10% solution IV; repeat every 10–20 minutes up to 9 g if hypotension persists
- Children: 60 mg/kg up to 3 g; may be repeated as needed up to 180 mg/kg

Insulin therapy:
- Start with a bolus of 1 unit/kg of regular insulin with 0.5 g/kg of dextrose (omit dextrose if blood glucose >300 mg/dL)
- Follow with an insulin infusion beginning at 1 unit/kg/h, titrated based on response (up to 10 units/kg/h if needed)
- Glucose monitoring: Every 15–30 minutes initially, then every 1–2 hours. Maintain blood glucose between 100–250 mg/dL

Calcium channel blocker toxicity:
Presentation and treatment are similar to beta-blocker toxicity, with hyperglycemia indicating severe overdose and poor prognosis

BOX 15: Antidiabetic medication overdose: hypoglycemic toxidromes.

Insulin overdose:
- Commonly intentional: Insulin overdose is often deliberate
- Presentation: Characterized by symptoms of hypoglycemia (see Chapter 8.1.3 for details)
- Treatment: In addition to routine hypoglycemia management, octreotide may be used
- Dosage: 50 µg subcutaneously every 6 hours until hypoglycemia resolves

Metformin overdose:
Severe toxicity: In extreme cases, metformin overdose can lead to MALA (metabolic acidosis with elevated lactate levels), which can be refractory to initial treatments

Management:
- Bicarbonate is administered to correct the acid–base imbalance, along with other supportive care
- Dialysis: Metformin is expected to be dialyzable due to its small size and limited protein binding, but its large volume of distribution complicates this
- Dialyzability: Literature suggests metformin is moderately dialyzable. Extracorporeal treatment is recommended if:
  - Blood lactate >20 mmol/L
  - pH ≤7.00

Standard treatments (including bicarbonate) are ineffective

Clinical improvement: Even if dialysis does not effectively remove metformin, clinical improvement may occur once acid–base status is corrected

BOX 16: Anesthetic drugs.

Toxic dose:
- Toxic IV doses of local anesthetics (mg/kg): Bupivacaine 1.6 m chloroprocaine 22.8, etidocaine 3.4, lidocaine 6.4, mepivacaine 9.8, procaine 19.2, and tetracaine 2.5
- Doses are mentioned in the Chapter 36 of Sedation and Anesthesia
- Significant direct neurotoxicity results from intrathecal injection or infusion of local anesthetics for spinal anesthesia
- Nerve damage often is attributed to the use of excessively concentrated solutions or inappropriate formulations
- Most episodes of systemic toxicity from local anesthetics, with the exception of methemoglobinemia from topical drug, occur secondary to unintentional intravascular injection rather than from over dosage, limiting the maximal dose will not prevent most toxic systemic reactions

Acute toxicity:
- Methemoglobinemia secondary to topical anesthesia (details in the **Box 9**)

Types of local anesthetic reactions	***Cause major clinical features***
Local anesthetic toxicity (intravascular injection)	Immediate seizure or dysrhythmias
Reaction to adjuvant catecholamine	Tachycardia, hypertension, and headache
Allergic reaction	Anaphylaxis
High spinal or epidural block	Bradycardia, hypotension, respiratory distress, and respiratory arrest

Treatment:
- Treat the ABCs
- Manage seizure with benzodiazepines, propofol is beneficial, especially in refractory seizures
- Treat dysrhythmia symptomatically, might need electrolyte/acidosis correction
- Cardioversion might be required
- In case of bradycardia, start with atropine, but atrioventricular (AV) pacing might be required
- Extracorporeal support might be helpful in refractory poisoning
- In case of arrest, standard advanced cardiac life support (ACLS) protocol to be followed

Role of an antidote in the form of lipid emulsion:
- In cardiac arrest, while continuing chest compressions, 1.5 mL/kg over 1 minutes, followed by continuous infusion of 0.25 mL/kg/min or 15 mL/kg/h to run for 30–60 minute
- Preferable is 20% lipid emulsion
- For persistent cardiovascular collapse, it is reasonable to repeat the bolus once or twice and double the infusion rate. If there is evidence of recovery, it is reasonable to continue the infusion for at least 10 minutes after stability

BOX 17: Psychiatric group of drugs: Cyclic antidepressants.

Mechanism of toxicity: Cyclic antidepressants exhibit antimuscarinic effects and sodium channel blockade

Toxic dose: Approximately 2.5 mg/kg

Acute toxicity symptoms:
Antimuscarinic/anticholinergic symptoms: Similar to the anticholinergic toxidrome, these include altered mental status

ECG findings:
- Sinus tachycardia, right axis deviation in the terminal 40 ms prolongation of the PR, QRS, and QT intervals
- Right axis deviation is identified by a positive terminal R wave in lead aVR and a negative S wave
- Also noted are right bundle branch block and high-degree AV blocks
- A Brugada pattern is present in about 10–15% of patients with cyclic antidepressant poisoning

Risk of seizures: Increased if QRS duration exceeds 100 ms

Risk of ventricular dysrhythmias: Increased if QRS duration exceeds 160 ms

Management:
Diagnosis:
- Clinical evaluation: Based on history and symptoms
- Urine toxicology screen: To identify substances
- Laboratory tests: Electrolytes and VBGs
- Serial ECGs: Changes typically start to appear within 6 hours postingestion

Routine management:
- Airway, breathing, circulation: Standard emergency procedures
- Decontamination: Administration of activated charcoal
- Sodium bicarbonate: Primary treatment to correct abnormalities or target a serum pH of ≤7.55, administered as 12 mEq/kg IV boluses every 35 minutes, followed by infusion

Indicated for:
- Sinus rhythm with a QRS complex >100 ms
- Wide complex tachycardia or ventricular tachycardia
- Refractory hypotension

Additional measures:
- Correction of hypoxia, acidemia, and hypotension: Essential supportive care
- Avoid certain drugs: Do not administer class I antiarrhythmics (e.g., procainamide, lidocaine, phenytoin, and flecainide), β-blockers, calcium channel blockers, or class III antiarrhythmics (e.g., amiodarone, sotalol, and ibutilide)

Alternative treatments:
- Hypertonic saline (3% sodium chloride): 12 mEq/kg bolus can be used if sodium bicarbonate is contraindicated
- Magnesium sulfate: 25–50 mg/kg (maximum 2 g) IV over 2 minutes, especially for torsades de pointes
- Torsades de pointes: DC cardioversion followed by magnesium sulfate or overdrive pacing (with caution due to rate dependence of cyclic antidepressants)

Seizure management:
- Benzodiazepines: For seizure control
- Refractory poisoning
- Advanced therapies: If standard treatments fail, consider extracorporeal membrane oxygenation (ECMO, cardiopulmonary bypass). Hemodialysis and hemoperfusion are not supported by evidence

Would you like further adjustments or additional details on any particular aspect?

BOX 18: Antipsychotics.

Clinical and toxicological manifestations of selected antipsychotics:

	a_1-adrenergic antagonism	***Muscarinic antagonism***	***Fast sodium channel (I_{Na}) blockade***	***Delayed rectifier (I_{kr}) blockade***
Clinical effect	***Hypotension***	***Central and peripheral anticholinergic effects***	***QRS complex widening; myocardial depression***	***QT interval prolongation; torsade de pointes***
Typical				
Chlorpromazine	+++	++	++	++
Fluphenazine	–	–	+	+
Haloperidol	–	–	+	++
Loxapine	+++	++	++	+
Mesoridazine	+++	+++	+++	++
Perphenazine	+	–	+	++
Pimozide	+	–	+	++
Thioridazine	+++	+++	+++	+++
Trifluoperazine	+	–	+	++
Atypical				
Amisulpride	–	–	–	++
Asenapine	++	–	–	–
Aripiprazole	++	–	–	–
Clozapine	+++	+++	–	+
Iloperidone	+++	–	–	++
Lurasidone	–	–	–	–
Olanzapine	++	+++	–	–
Paliperidone	++	–	–	+
Quetiapine	+++	+++	+	– to +
Remoxipride	–	–	–	–
Risperidone	++	–	–	–
Sertindole	+	–	–	++
Ziprasidone	++	–	–	+++

(+ to ++: effect present in increasing degree; –: effect is absent; – to +: presence of effect minimal or absent)
Source: Hoffman RS, Nelson LS, Lewin NA, Howland MA, Smith SW, editors. Goldfrank's Clinical Manual of Toxicologic Emergencies. 2nd ed. New York: McGraw-Hill Education; 2023.

- Other than the aforementioned symptoms, most antipsychotics have extrapyramidal symptoms noted in the adverse effect. Details in Chapter 6.5: Movement disorder.
- General management remains same as cyclic antidepressants

Contd...

Contd...

Selective serotonin reuptake inhibitor (SSRI)/atypical antidepressants

- Predictive analysis of the relative potential for seizures and abnormalities on electrocardiography of selective serotonin reuptake inhibitors and related antidepressants:

Drug	***Seizures***	***QT interval prolongation***	***QRS complex prolongation***
Classic SSRIs			
Citalopram	+++	+++	+
Escitalopram	+++	+++	+
Fluoxetine	+	0	0
Fluvoxamine	+	0	0
Paroxetine	+	0	0
Sertraline	+	0	0
Atypical Antidepressants			
Bupropion	++++	+	+
Desvenlafaxine	+++	+	+++
Duloxetine	++++	Unknown	Unknown
Levomilnacipran	Unknown	Unknown	Unknown
Milnacipran	Unknown	Unknown	Unknown
Mirtazapine	Unknown	Unknown	++
Nefazodone	0	0	0
Trazodone	+	+	0
Venlafaxine	+++	+	+++
Vilazodone	+	Unknown	Unknown
Vortioxetine	Unknown	Unknown	Unknown

(0: does not cause; +: very rarely causes; ++: rarely causes; +++: causes; ++++: commonly causes)

Source: Hoffman RS, Nelson LS, Lewin NA, Howland MA, Smith SW, editors. Goldfrank's Clinical Manual of Toxicologic Emergencies. 2nd ed. New York: McGraw-Hill Education; 2023

- Also known to cause syndrome of inappropriate antidiuretic hormone (SIADH)-induced hyponatremia
- Caused by certain common drug interaction such as linezolid, tramadol, fentanyl, cocaine, and other monoamine oxidase inhibitor (MAO) inhibitors

MAO inhibitors:

- These are rarely used now, unless refractory depression
- They can interact with any medications, hence an emergency physician should avoid any new drugs in a patient taking MAO inhibitors
- A biphasic response characterized by initial CNS excitation and peripheral sympathetic stimulation that terminates in coma and cardiovascular collapse, result from an initial adrenergic crisis, followed by inhibition of norepinephrine release
- Symptoms include early hypertensive crisis, neuropsychiatric effects, neuromuscular effects, headache, seizures, myoclonus, muscular rigidity, later develop hypotension, and cardiac dysrhythmia

BOX 19: Sympathomimetics.

- *Substances/toxic dose:* Cocaine and amphetamine toxicity
- *Routes of administration*: IV, inhalation, and ingestion

Acute toxicity:
Sympathomimetic toxidrome:
- Hyperthermia and hypertensive crisis
- Acute chest pain with ST elevation (particularly when cocaine is smoked), primarily due to vasospasm
- Cardiomyopathies and aortic dissection, more common in cocaine users
- Dysrhythmias, including QRS complex widening, Brugada pattern, and prolonged QTc interval
- Neurologic complications such as seizures, cerebral infarctions, and hemorrhages

Additional effects:
Other organ involvement:
- Mydriasis (dilated pupils)
- Nasal septum perforation
- Pneumothorax/mediastinum
- Bronchospasm (due to sympathomimetic effects)
- Limb and bowel ischemia
- Rhabdomyolysis (secondary to hyperthermia)

Management:
Monitoring and laboratory tests:
- *Drug screening:* To identify substances
- *Laboratory tests:* Electrolytes, acid–base status, creatinine, creatine phosphokinase (CPK) total, and myoglobins

Imaging and ECG: Serial ECGs and CXR to monitor for complications
Treatment:
- Sedation: Benzodiazepines to manage agitation and seizures
- Hyperthermia: Treat as indicated (refer to the relevant chapter)
- IV fluids: To manage and prevent rhabdomyolysis
- Hypertensive crisis: Manage with phentolamine
- Avoid beta-blockers: Due to potential exacerbation of vasospasm
- **Cocaine-induced myocardial infarction (MI):**
  - **Treat vasospasm with nitroglycerin**
  - **Use phentolamine for hypertensive crisis**
  - **Fibrinolysis offers no additional benefit but is not absolutely contraindicated unless other contraindications are present**
  - **Despite percutaneous intervention, there is a high risk of rethrombosis**
- Cocaine, amphetamine, can be taken via IV/inhalation/ingestion, which has varied effect on the body

BOX 20: Other substance abuse.

- Cannabinoids/hallucinogens have adverse effects such as tachycardia, hypertension, and hyperemesis
- Hallucinogen toxidrome is already mentioned
- Treatment is symptomatic
- Benzodiazepines is the treatment of choice for any agitation and fluid management for supportive care

BOX 21: Carbon monoxide (CO) poisoning.

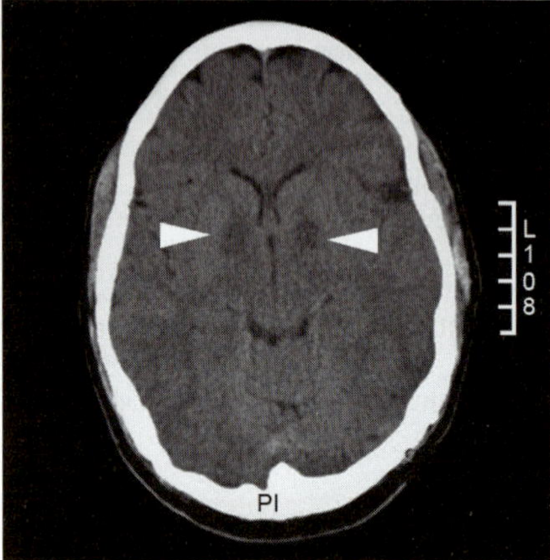

Fig. 3: Brain CT in CO poisoning.

Characteristics: CO is an odorless, colorless gas that constitutes about 1% of the atmosphere. It is produced by the incomplete combustion of carbon-containing compounds

Sources:
- Anesthetic absorbents
- Stored blood
- Camp stoves and lanterns
- Charcoal grills
- Coffee roasting
- Fires
- Formic acid decomposition in sulfuric acid
- Gasoline powered equipment (e.g., generators and power washers)
- Propane powered ice resurfacing machines
- Internal combustion engines (boats, cars, and trucks)
- Natural gas combustion appliances (water heaters, ranges, and ovens)
- Propane/methylene compositions
- Underground mine explosions

Toxic dose: Exposure to 250 ppm can cause minor symptoms

Acute toxicity: History of exposure followed by symptoms makes diagnosis straightforward. However, CO toxicity can also present with vague flu-like symptoms, some ECG changes, and episodes of syncope, which can complicate the diagnosis

Symptoms and signs:
- Headache
- Visual disturbances
- Nausea/vomiting

Contd...

Contd...

- Focal neurological deficits, ataxia, and seizures
- Dyspnea/tachypnea
- Metabolic acidosis with increased lactates
- Rare physical signs: Bullous skin lesions, cherry red oral mucosa
- Retinal hemorrhage
- Chest pain/shortness of breath, ECG changes/dysrhythmias, and syncope
- Confusion
- Cardiac arrest
- Delayed neurocognitive sequelae

Diagnosis:
- Pulse oximeter: It may falsely indicate normal oxygen saturation
- Best diagnostic tool: Co-oximeter to detect carboxyhemoglobin (COHb) levels, which should be around 05%
- VBG: Measures lactates and metabolic acidosis
- ECG: Nonspecific changes; global hypokinesia may be observed
- Imaging: CT scan can show bilateral globus pallidus lesions to rule out alternative diagnoses **(Fig. 3)**

Treatment and disposition:
Symptomatic treatment:
- Mild symptoms: Observe for 6 hours (8 hours for methylene chloride exposure) and administer 100% oxygen. Discharge if asymptomatic
- Hyperbaric oxygen therapy (HBOT): Recommended for all acute CO poisoning cases per the American College of Emergency Physicians. Some guidelines suggest HBOT for severe toxicity, pregnancy with COHb levels >15%, or COHb levels >25% in nonpregnant individuals. HBOT is most effective within 6 hours of exposure

BOX 22: Cyanide toxicity.

Sources and toxic dose:
- *Sources:*
  - Inhalation or ingestion of cyanide
  - Burning polyurethane foam
  - Sodium nitroprusside or ingestion of amygdalin (from apricot and cherry kernels)
  - Acetonitrile (methyl cyanide) in artificial fingernail removers
- *Toxic dose:* An adult lethal dose of potassium cyanide (KCN) is about 200 mg. An airborne concentration of 270 ppm of hydrogen cyanide (HCN) is immediately fatal, while exposure to over 110 ppm for more than 30 minutes is life-threatening. Occupational Safety and Health Administration (OSHA) permissible exposure limit (PEL) for HCN and cyanogen is 10 ppm over an 8 hour time-weighted average. The immediately dangerous to life or health value for HCN is 50 ppm

Acute toxicity:
- CNS effects: Hypoxia leads to headache, anxiety, agitation, confusion, lethargy, nonreactive dilated pupils, seizures, and coma. Initial tachypnea is followed by bradypnea and apnea
- CVS effects: Initial tachycardia and hypertension, followed by hypotension with reflex tachycardia. The terminal event is typically bradycardia and hypotension

Contd...

Contd...

Other symptoms:
- Severe metabolic acidosis
- Rare cherry red skin spots
- Nausea and vomiting
- Pulmonary edema in severe cases

Management:
Diagnosis:
- History and symptoms: Bitter almond odor (if detected) can help with diagnosis
- Blood tests: These may confirm diagnosis but could delay treatment

Treatment:
- Decontamination: Activated charcoal
- Supportive care: As needed

Antidotes:
- Hydroxocobalamin (preferred):
  - Initial adult dose: 5 g IV over 15 minutes; pediatric dose: 70 mg/kg up to 5 g. Repeat if necessary
- Cyanide antidote kit:
  - Amyl nitrite pearls: For prehospital use
  - Sodium nitrite ($NaNO_2$): 3% solution over 24 minutes IV. Adult dose is 10 mL (300 mg). Monitor blood pressure and treat hypotension with slower infusion rates and crystalloids or vasopressors. Check *Met Hb* levels 30 minutes after dose; excess *Met Hb* can worsen the condition. Withhold nitrites if COHb is suspected
  - Sodium thiosulfate (NaS_2O_3):
    - 25% solution IV: Adult dose is 50 mL (12.5 g); pediatric dose is 1.65 mL/kg up to 50 mL

SUGGESTED READING

1. Hoffman RS, Nelson LS, Lewin NA, Howland MA, Smith SW, editors. Goldfrank's Clinical Manual of Toxicologic Emergencies. 2nd ed. New York: McGraw-Hill Education; 2023.
2. Tintinalli JE, Ma OJ, Yealy DM, Meckler GD, Stapczynski JS, Cline DM, et al. Tintinalli's Emergency Medicine: A Comprehensive Study Guide, 9th edition. New York, NY: McGraw- Hill Education; 2019.
3. Walls RM, Hockberger RS, Gausche-Hill M. Rosen's Emergency Medicine: Concepts and Clinical Practice. Philadelphia, PA: Elsevier; 2018.

15.2 ENVIRONMENTAL EMERGENCY

15.2.1 Hypothermia

Sachna P Shetty

BOX 1: Introduction.

Definition	Accidental hypothermia is an unintentional decrease in core body temperature to below 35°C (95°F), which can lead to serious complications and increased risk of mortality
Classification and causes	• Accidental hypothermia can be categorized into two main types based on its cause: – *Primary accidental hypothermia:* This occurs due to exposure to cold environmental conditions – *Secondary accidental hypothermia:* This type is caused by impaired thermoregulation - It is not solely linked to cold climates but can happen under various circumstances where the body's ability to regulate its temperature is compromised - *It can be caused by:* ▪ Burns ▪ Iatrogenic (i.e., blood transfusions and other cold infusions, cooling blankets, and inadequate insulation) ▪ Recent birth ▪ Medications and toxins ▪ Alcohol, anesthetic agents ▪ Metabolic and endocrine disorders ▪ Diabetic ketoacidosis, hypoadrenalism, hypoglycemia, hypopituitarism, and hypothyroidism ▪ Neurologic stroke, spinal cord injury ▪ Sepsis (more common in the elderly or cachectic patient) ▪ Shock ▪ Trauma

BOX 2: Clinical presentation.

Head, eye, ear, nose, throat	Flushing, facial edema, epistaxis, rhinorrhea mydriasis, decreased corneal reflexes, extraocular muscle abnormalities
Cardiovascular	Initial tachycardia, subsequent bradycardia, dysrhythmias, and hypotension
Respiratory	Initial tachypnea, adventitious sounds, progressive hypoventilation, leading to apnea
Gastrointestinal	Abdominal distention or rigidity, ileus, and constipation
Genitourinary	Polyuria, oliguria, anuria, and testicular torsion
Neurologic	Initial hyperreflexia, hyporeflexia, areflexia, ataxia, hypoesthesia, anesthesia, dysarthria, amnesia, depressed level of consciousness, and central pontine myelinolysis
Psychiatric	Impaired judgment, perseveration, mood change, altered mental states, paradoxical undressing, neuroses or psychosis
Musculoskeletal	• Shivering or pseudo-rigor mortis • Rigidity, increased muscle tone, and compartment syndrome
Dermatologic	Pallor, frostnip, cyanosis, frostbite, erythema, pernio, icterus, cold urticaria, edema, ecchymosis, necrosis, and gangrene

BOX 3: General management in accidental hypothermia.

- Irrespective of the stage of hypothermia, the initial stabilization remains the management of Airway, Breathing, and Circulation, followed by Disability management. Lastly, Environmental factors to be managed, which are mentioned as per the stage of hypothermia
- *Cardiac monitoring:* Continuous cardiac monitoring is crucial
- *Core temperature monitoring:* Use esophageal, rectal, or bladder thermometers to monitor the patient's core body temperature closely
- *Large bore IV line*—14–16G: If sudden BP falls in hypothermic patient, rapid volume expansion can be lifesaving, especially in neonates. Adult patients with moderate or severe hypothermia should initially receive a 500 mL fluid challenge
- Vasopressors to be avoided initially
- *Airway management:* It is permissible and should not be deferred due to the patient's hypothermic state. Preoxygenation before intubation is superior in hypothermia
- **Rewarming methods:** Use gentle rewarming methods like warm intravenous fluids, heated normal saline, or warm water lavage for the bladder or thoracic cavity, avoiding direct heat application to the head. Additionally, minimize invasiveness by limiting invasive procedures to prevent further heat loss from the patient's body
- **Minimize invasiveness:** Limit invasive procedures to reduce additional heat loss from the patient's body **(Fig. 1)**

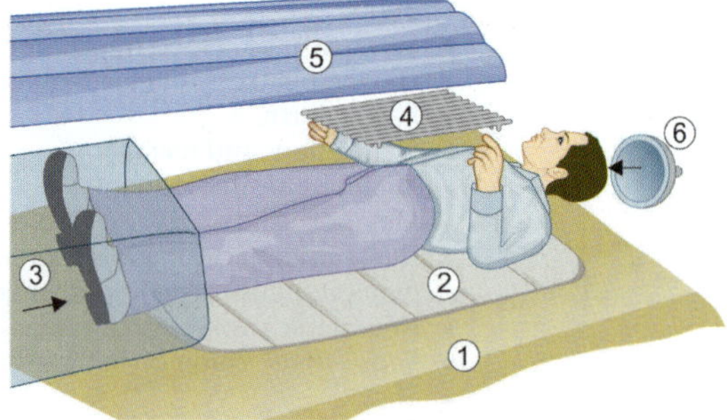

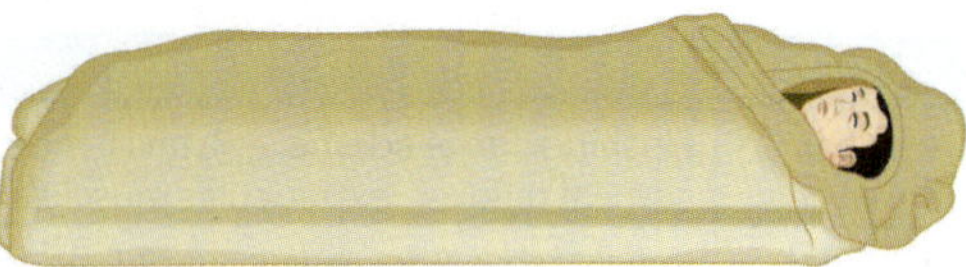

Fig. 1: Minimally invasive rewarming.

- *Active rewarming techniques* to be adopted only if needed
- **Continuation of resuscitation: Do not cease resuscitation efforts based solely on low core body temperature (<28°C); seek guidance from specialists**
- **Extracorporeal membrane oxygenation (ECMO) consideration:** For patients not responding to conventional resuscitation, especially if they have a good potential for recovery, consider transferring them to a facility equipped with ECMO
- *Investigation:* Complete blood count (CBC), renal profile, electrolytes, sugars, after arterial blood gases and coagulation profile are helpful to find the cause as well as manage a hypothermic patients during rewarming. ECG needs to be done **(Box 5)**

Laboratories and imaging should be ordered as per the etiology in cases of secondary hypothermia. To rule out trauma, CT head and USG fast can be done

A serum ethanol level and urine toxicology screening should be done when suspected. Thyroid function studies, cardiac markers, and serum cortisol levels may also be indicated

BOX 4: Staging and treatment as per stage of accidental hypothermia.

Mild (I)	• **Clinical symptoms:** This stage includes individuals who are conscious and shivering • With drop in temperature amnesia, dysarthria followed by ataxia might develop • *Typical core temperature:* The core temperature ranges from 33°C to 35°C • **Treatment:** Treatment involves creating a warm environment – Start by passive rewarming which is providing warm clothing – Offering warm drinks – Encouraging active movement if possible • Shivering usually generate enough heat to allow spontaneous rewarming (ineffective <32°C)
Moderate (II)	• **Clinical symptoms:** In this stage, individuals may have impaired consciousness, and they may or may not be shivering • With further drop in temperature patient might develop dysrhythmias, followed by drop in respiratory rate decreased pulse, and dilated pupils • *Typical core temperature:* 32–29°C • **Treatment:** Treatment includes: – Active external and minimally invasive rewarming techniques **(Box 4)** – Immobilize the patient, maintain a horizontal position, consider full-body insulation/heating pad – Monitoring cardiac and core temperature – Minimizing movements to avoid dysrhythmias
Severe (III)	• **Clinical symptoms:** Individuals in this stage are unconscious, with arrhythmias like ventricular fibrillation, acid–base disturbances, pulmonary edema, significant hypotension, loss of corneal and oculocephalic reflexes, but vital signs like a pulse and breathing are still present • *Typical core temperature:* 28–22°C • **Treatment:** – Airway management may be required – Anticipate and manage potential multiorgan failure and the need for ECMO for respiratory support (Chapter 34.1)
Hypothermic cardiac arrest (IV)	• **Clinical symptoms:** This stage represents a critical condition where vital signs are absent, and the person is in cardiac arrest • *Caveat:* – 14.2°C (57.6°F)—lowest accidental hypothermia survival in an infant – 13.7°C (56.7°F)—lowest accidental hypothermia survival in an adult – 9°C (48.2°F)—lowest therapeutic hypothermia survival • **Treatment:** In this critical stage, treatment includes cardiopulmonary resuscitation (CPR) • *Caveat:* – CPR in hypothermia is different as, airway management is also essential – If no return of spontaneous circulation (ROSC), do not stop CPR, prioritize transport to a facility with ECMO • *On-site rewarming:* If ECMO is not available quickly, use on-site rewarming methods by active external or internal rewarming • *Rewarm to 32°C:* Aim to increase the body temperature to this level

BOX 5: ECG findings.

- Bradycardia often present
- *Shifting of the ST Segment:* Hypothermia can cause changes in the ST segment, which can either be elevated or depressed
- *Prolonged intervals:* The PR, QRS, and QT intervals may be prolonged due to the slowed metabolic and electrical activity of the heart in the cold environment
- *Osborn waves (J waves):* These are positive deflections observed at the junction between the end of the QRS complex and the start of the ST segment, typically seen in leads II and V6 in the provided ECG. They are most commonly associated with hypothermia but can also be seen in other conditions **(Fig. 3)**

Caveat: The presence of Osborn waves is particularly significant as they are considered pathognomonic for hypothermia when found in conjunction with a history of exposure to cold temperatures or a core body temperature below normal. This ECG finding underscores the need for immediate rewarming and supportive measures in the management of hypothermia

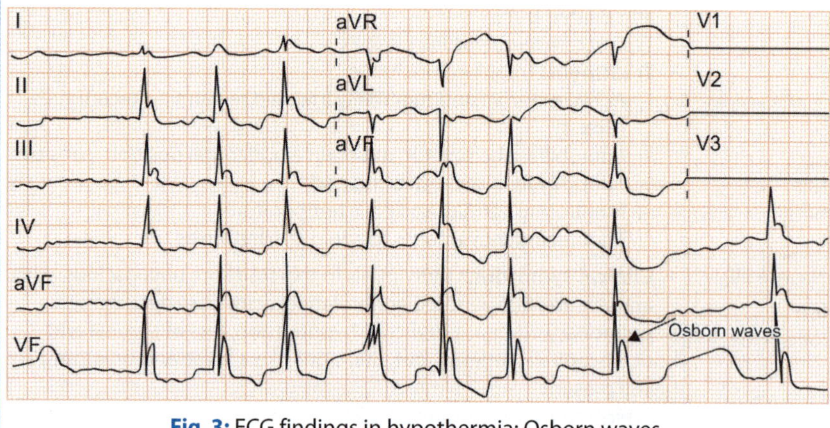

Fig. 3: ECG findings in hypothermia: Osborn waves.

BOX 6: Indications for active rewarming.

- Hemodynamic instability
- Moderate or severe hypothermia [≤32°C (89.6°F)]
- Failure to rewarm
- Endocrinologic insufficiency
- Traumatic or toxicological etiology
- Secondary hypothermia

BOX 7: Active external rewarming.

- A water bath at 41°C, but cannot be used during ongoing CPR
- A garment that circulates warm fluids, hot water bottles, and heating pads (be wary of thermal injuries)
- Forced air warming systems, which is hot air through a blanket (most efficient system)

BOX 8: Core/invasive rewarming.

- Airway rewarming with heated humidified oxygen is a simple and inexpensive method, should not exceed 41°C
- Peritoneal dialysis to deliver dialysate at 40–45°C (104–113°F)
- Heated irrigation-gastric and colonic, although might cause electrolyte imbalances
- In very severe cases, thoracostomy irrigation is considered
- *Extracorporeal rewarming:* Practical techniques are hemodialysis induced or ECMO induced (criteria are given further)

BOX 9: Resuscitation in the context of hypothermia and other related emergencies.

Assessment of irreversible death signs	• Before attempting resuscitation, it is critical to assess if there are any unmistakable signs of irreversible death, such as – Decapitation, decomposition, a frozen-solid body, or trunk transection or valued do-not-resuscitate (DNR) order – If yes to above, consider termination of resuscitation efforts – However, typical signs of death may not apply in cases of hypothermia, such as fixed and dilated pupils, areflexia, and stiffness resembling rigor mortis
Cardiac arrest from nonhypothermia causes	• If a patient experiences cardiac arrest from causes unrelated to hypothermia, such as major trauma or a medical condition, standard protocols for terminating resuscitation efforts should be followed
Special circumstances influencing resuscitation	• Situations like drowning, avalanche, or trauma necessitate specific considerations • For instance, drowning cases, particularly in the young who have experienced rapid cooling, may have a better prognosis consider shifting to ECMO center • Avalanches may offer a chance of survival if the individual has had access to air • Trauma, on the other hand, typically worsens prognosis, and standard termination of resuscitation guidelines might be applied
Tests to exclude need for ECMO/cardiopulmonary bypass (CPB)	• When core temperature is ≥32°C and serum potassium is dangerously high (>12 mmol/L) or >6 hours transport to ECMO center timing
Transport decisions	• The decision to transport a patient to an ECMO—capable facility depends on the expected duration of the transport. • If the transport time exceeds 6 hours, on-site rewarming should be considered
Post-resuscitation care	• Following successful resuscitation (ROSC), continued management should align with the patient's level of hypothermia, with tailored post-arrest care to ensure the best possible outcome

BOX 10: Caveats.

- Hypothermia enhances the cardiac toxicity of hyperkalemia and obscures premonitory electrocardiographic changes
- Failure to rewarm despite good technique should suggest infection, endocrine insufficiency, or a futile resuscitation
  - Warm fluids during resuscitation can be warmed in microwave
  - Ringer lactate to be avoided
  - Recommended rewarming rate is 0.5–2°C
  - Core temperature to be checked in areas such as rectal, bladder, tympanic membrane, and lower third esophagus
  - Intubation might be difficult due to trismus
  - Central line might precipitate arrhythmia if touches heart
  - Do not give per oral or intramuscular medication
  - Defibrillation to be used but efficacy not superior until core temperature rises
  - Internal pacing not much of value compared to external pacing
  - If failure to rewarm, consider hypothyroid or adrenal insufficiency
  - Consider hypoglycemia, hypovolemia, or an overdose if there is a tachycardia disproportionate to the temperature

BOX 11: Poor prognostic factors.

- Asphyxia (drowning and avalanche burial)
- Unwitnessed cardiac arrest
- Asystole
- Hyperkalemia
- Elevated serum lactate
- Hemodynamic instability
- Age >75 years
- Kidney injury (elevated creatinine)

While evidence is limited, the aforementioned factors are associated with worse outcomes following hypothermia due to environmental exposure

- Evidence about accidental hypothermia is limited. These factors are drawn primarily from retrospective, observational studies. They are not necessarily the independent risk factors. There are many potential confounders

SUGGESTED READING

1. Management of Accidental Hypothermia in Adults. In: UpToDate. Available from: https://www.uptodate.com/contents/accidental-hypothermia-in-adults-management [accessed on November, 2024].
2. Tintinalli JE, Ma OJ, Yealy DM, Meckler GD, Stapczynski JS, Cline DM, et al. (Eds). Tintinalli's Emergency Medicine: A Comprehensive Study Guide, 9th edition. Mc Graw Hill Education; 2020.
3. Walls RM, Hockberger RS, Gausche-Hill M. Rosen's Emergency Medicine: Concepts and Clinical Practice. Philadelphia, PA: Elsevier; 2018.

15.2.2 Heat Emergencies

Sachna P Shetty

BOX 1: Difference of terminology and the diagnosis.

Heat cramps	• Muscle cramps • Sweating • Normal to mildly elevated temperature • Oral salt solutions are helpful for the management
Heat stress (exhaustion)	Symptoms similar to heat cramps, plus: • Nausea • Vomiting • Headache • Malaise (general feeling of discomfort or unease) • Giddiness • Orthostatic hypotension (a form of low blood pressure that happens when you stand up from sitting or lying down) • Treat with intravenous (IV) hydration
Heat stroke	History of exposure to heat stress, endogenous, or exogenous symptoms of heat stress (exhaustion), plus: • Elevated body temperature >40°C (104°F) • Neurologic abnormalities, which may include: – Inappropriate behavior – Confusion – Delirium – Ataxia (lack of muscle control) – Coma – Seizures • Anhidrosis (absence of sweating) or sweating • Marked elevation of hepatic transaminases • Treatment discussed in details below.

BOX 2: Presentation of heat stroke.

- Elevated core body temperature >40.5°C
- Vital sign abnormalities such as sinus tachycardia, tachypnea, a widened pulse pressure, and hypotension
- Initial subtle symptoms may be weakness, lethargy, nausea, or dizziness
- Physical findings such as flushing, crackles due to pulmonary edema (noncardiogenic), and manifestation of coagulopathy in the form of bleeding tendencies, neurological dysfunction
- Complications (see **Box 3**)

BOX 3: Complications.

Vital signs	Hypotension
Muscular	Rhabdomyolysis
Neurologic	• Delirium/coma • Seizure
Cardiac	Heart failure
Pulmonary	Pulmonary edema
Renal	Oliguria progresses to renal failure
Metabolic	• Hypokalemia • Hypernatremia • Hyponatremia
Hematologic	Thrombocytopenia, progresses to disseminated intravascular coagulation (DIC)

BOX 4: Diagnosis.

- Diagnosis is based on elevated core body temperature, which is rectal (>40.5°C)
- Altered mental status and exposure to severe environmental heat
- Laboratory studies of importance are: Complete blood count (CBC), creatinine, electrolytes, blood urea nitrogen, hepatic transaminases, coagulation profile (with liver injury and DIC), arterial blood gas (ABG)/venous blood gas (VBG) as metabolic acidosis and respiratory alkalosis might be seen creatinine kinase, urine myoglobin for rhabdomyolysis
- Toxicology screening
- Imaging like CT brain to rule out neurological cause

BOX 5: Differential diagnosis of heatstroke.

Vascular	Cerebrovascular accident
Infectious	• Sepsis syndrome • Meningitis • Encephalitis • Malaria • Typhoid • Tetanus
Endocrine	• Thyroid storm • Pheochromocytoma • Diabetic ketoacidosis
Neurological	• Seizures • Status epilepticus • Neuroleptic malignant syndrome
Toxicologic	• Toxins; drugs • Anticholinergic toxidrome • Sympathomimetic overdose • Salicylate overdose • Serotonin syndrome • Malignant hyperthermia • Withdrawal syndromes—alcohol and benzodiazepine withdrawal
Other causes	• High fever • Sepsis

BOX 6: Management of heat stroke.

Initial stabilization	• Primary management in the emergency room (ER) remains airway, breathing, circulation assessment, and stabilization, followed by **early recognition, rapid cooling, correction of electrolyte abnormalities, and supportive care according to the organ involved** • Intravenous fluids as per point-of-care ultrasound (POCUS) • Avoid alpha adrenergic agonist for vasopressors • Agitation or shivering secondary to cooling techniques to be controlled with benzodiazepine or propofol or opioids, such as fentanyl, and for refractory cases neuromuscular blocking agents such as rocuronium can be used • Core temperature monitoring via rectal method to attain a target of 38–39°C after which aggressive cooling techniques needs to be stopped • But some studies proved a core temperature of 36°C improves neurological outcome

Contd...

Contd...

Evaporative cooling	**The patient is stripped of all clothing, and tepid tap water is sprayed while fans blow air continuously over the body, causing evaporative cooling** • *Advantages:* Effective in reducing body temperature; widely available and practical; integrates well into existing medical protocols • *Disadvantages:* Potential for inducing shivering which can counteract cooling efforts; reduced efficacy in humid environments; challenges in maintaining electrode contact due to moisture
Immersion cooling	**Immersion in ice water by placing supine on a porous stretcher placed on an ice water tub results in a rapid reduction of core temperature to below 39°C within 10–40 minutes** • *Advantages:* Provides rapid cooling; simple to administer • *Disadvantages:* It can induce shivering; may not be tolerated well by the patient; poses challenges in resuscitation settings due to water immersion
Ice packs on neck, axillae, and groin	• *Advantages:* Practical application; can complement other cooling strategies; facilitates fast and effective cooling • *Disadvantages:* Cooling may be slower than other methods; requires active management to maintain application • *Recommendations:* It can be utilized as an adjunctive cooling method, particularly when other resources are limited
Cardiopulmonary bypass	• *Advantages:* It provides rapid and sustained cooling • *Disadvantages:* Invasive nature; requires specialized equipment and personnel; the setup is intensive • *Recommendations:* Recommended in severe or refractory cases where available, given its invasive nature and resource requirements
Cold water gastric, urinary bladder, and peritoneal lavage	• *Advantages:* Directly cools core body temperature; can be implemented in the absence of more advanced cooling techniques • *Disadvantages:* Invasive and labor-intensive; may be less effective than other methods; human experience with these techniques is limited
Cooling blankets	• *Advantages:* Noninvasive, easily applied, and generally well-tolerated by patients. Allows for consistent application of cooling across a large body surface area • *Disadvantages:* May work slowly and cooling efficacy can be inconsistent. Requires monitoring to adjust settings and ensure effective temperature reduction

BOX 7: Caveats.

- Antipyretics are ineffective
- Heat stroke can cause right-sided cardiac dilation and elevated central venous pressure (CVP), and clinically resemble pulmonary edema, but still requires vigorous crystalloid resuscitation
- **Small case studies reveal cold compresses on smooth hairless skin surfaces like cheeks, palms soles cooling is faster**

SUGGESTED READING

1. Heat Stroke in Children. In: UpToDate, Ishimine P, editor. Available from: https://www.uptodate.com/contents/heat-stroke-in-children [accessed on November, 2024].
2. Tintinalli JE, Ma OJ, Yealy DM, Meckler GD, Stapczynski JS, Cline DM, et al. (Eds). Tintinalli's Emergency Medicine: A Comprehensive Study Guide, 9th edition. Mc Graw Hill Education; 2020.
3. Walls RM, Hockberger RS, Gausche-Hill M. Rosen's Emergency Medicine: Concepts and Clinical Practice. Philadelphia, PA: Elsevier; 2018.

15.2.3 Commonest Bites and Stings

Sachna P Shetty

BOX 1: Introduction.

- Insect and arthropod bites often result in minor itching but can also lead to significant medical issues, including insect-borne diseases and severe allergic reactions
- Mammal bites range from superficial wounds to serious infections, such as abscesses, septic arthritis, osteomyelitis, and tenosynovitis. Without appropriate treatment, these bites can escalate to life-threatening conditions like rabies or tetanus, particularly in unvaccinated individuals
- Stings deliver venom, causing reactions that vary from mild local irritation to critical, life-threatening situations
- This chapter provides an in-depth overview of common mammal bites, insect and arthropod bites, snake bites, and venomous stings from bees, and spiders

BOX 2: Mammalian bites assessment and management.

- General wound inspection and management are crucial (refer to Chapter 25)
- Check animal vaccination history
- Verify patient immunization status for tetanus and rabies, as all mammal bites can cause tetanus if the patient is not immunized (details in Chapter 15.3)
- Delay of 12–24 hours postbite increases infection risk
- Most wounds require delayed closure
- Primary closure is only indicated in specific cases **(Box 3)**
- Potential secondary infections include cellulitis, abscesses, flexor tenosynovitis, necrotizing soft tissue infections, septic arthritis, and osteomyelitis
- Conduct wound and blood cultures if immunocompromised
- Consider routine blood tests for sepsis
- Imaging may be necessary depending on infection type (e.g., USG for superficial abscess and MRI or contrast CT for deeper infections)
- Management includes postexposure vaccination (refer to Chapter 15.3)
- Antibiotics are recommended for specific bites (details in Chapter 7)
- Amoxicillin clavulanic acid is commonly used for dog and cat bites; trimethoprim–sulfamethoxazole (TMP–SMX) plus metronidazole is an alternative if beta-lactam intolerant; doxycycline/clindamycin may be used for anaerobic infections (details in Chapter 7)
- Intravenous antibiotics are considered for severe infections or immunocompromised patients
- Treat suspected methicillin-resistant *Staphylococcus aureus* (MRSA) accordingly with broad-spectrum beta-lactam IV antibiotics
- Mice and rat bites may require penicillin or ceftriaxone; rabbit bites may need fluoroquinolones or doxycycline
- Higher infection risk wounds include cat or human bites, livestock bites, monkey bites, puncture wounds, hand or foot wounds, bites in immunosuppressed patients, and wounds in fresh or saltwater or showing initial signs of local infection or with older, devitalized tissue

BOX 3: Indication for primary closure.

- Uninfected wound
- Immunocompetent patient
- Recent bite (<12 hours on extremity or <24 hours on face)
- No crush or puncture wound
- No prior cellulitis/lymphangitis on the affected extremity
- Primary closure is beneficial for healing and cosmetic purposes, but small puncture wounds have a higher risk of infection

BOX 4: Indications for antibiotics in mammal bites.

- Deep tissue or crush injury
- Puncture wound
- Closure by primary intention, surgical repair, or debridement
- Located on hand, face, or genitals
- Near a bone or vascular structure
- Immunocompromised patient
- Bites untreated for >8 days
- All cat bites
- Any injury undergoing surgical repair

BOX 5: Bee sting.

Clinical presentation:

- Local reaction: Mainly inflammatory response with itching, pain, erythema, and swelling
- Large reactions can increase in size over 1–2 days and may take 3–10 days to resolve; lymphangitis may develop even without infection
- Consider secondary cellulitis if edema persists at the sting site
- Anaphylaxis might develop (refer to Chapter 24: Anaphylaxis)
- Delayed allergic response or serum reaction might develop
- Possible organ involvement: AKI secondary to rhabdomyolysis
- Rarely, all major systems might be involved, with signs of encephalopathy, neuritis, vasculitis, and nephrosis; Guillain–Barré syndrome might develop

General management:

- Remove stinger immediately by any method to reduce venom injection; if delayed, removing the stinger is not as beneficial
- Wash the affected area thoroughly
- Apply cold compresses intermittently
- Use oral analgesics, including nonsteroidal anti-inflammatory drugs (NSAIDs) and antihistamines
- If edema is significant, elevation and rest of the affected limb may be beneficial
- Administer a single dose of oral steroids (prednisolone 40 mg)
- Large local reactions typically increase in size over 1–2 days and take 3–10 days to resolve
- Anaphylaxis treatment (refer to Chapter 24: Anaphylaxis)

BOX 6: Ants.

Presentation and management:
- Local inflammatory response: Reactions to the sting typically consist of a wheal and flare and characteristically exhibit a pustule at the sting site; intense pruritus may occur with local reactions
- Treatment consists of local wound care and antihistamines if needed
- In systemic reactions, treat for anaphylaxis

BOX 7: Other insect bites.

- *Centipedes:*
  - Extremities show two small puncture marks
  - Painful, localized erythema and edema
  - Treatment includes local wound management, antihistamines, and sometimes anaphylaxis management
- *Bed bugs:*
  - Bullous reaction is noted
  - Topical corticosteroids should be administered
- *Mosquitoes/flies:* Local reaction, pruritus, and possible systemic infection (refer Chapter 7)

BOX 8: Spiders.

Presentation:
- Local reaction: Depending on the type of spider, the bite can be painful or painless, with erythematous lesions, hemorrhagic blisters, or dermonecrosis
- Systemic symptoms: Muscle cramps extending to the trunk, back, and abdomen; hypertension; tachycardia; and anaphylaxis
- Some antivenoms are under trial
- Treatment is mainly symptomatic

SUGGESTED READING

1. Walls RM, Hockberger RS, Gausche-Hill M (Eds). Rosen's Emergency Medicine: Concepts and Clinical Practice, 9th edition. Elsevier; 2018.
2. Tintinalli JE, Ma OJ, Yealy DM, Meckler GD, Stapczynski JS, Cline DM, et al. (Eds). Tintinalli's Emergency Medicine: A Comprehensive Study Guide, 9th edition. McGraw-Hill Education; 2020.
3. Heat Stroke in Children. In: UpToDate, Ishimine P, editor. Available from: https://www.uptodate.com/contents/heat-stroke-in-children [accessed on November, 2024].
4. WHO GUIDELINES

15.2.4 Envenomation

Sachna P Shetty

BOX 1: Snake bites.

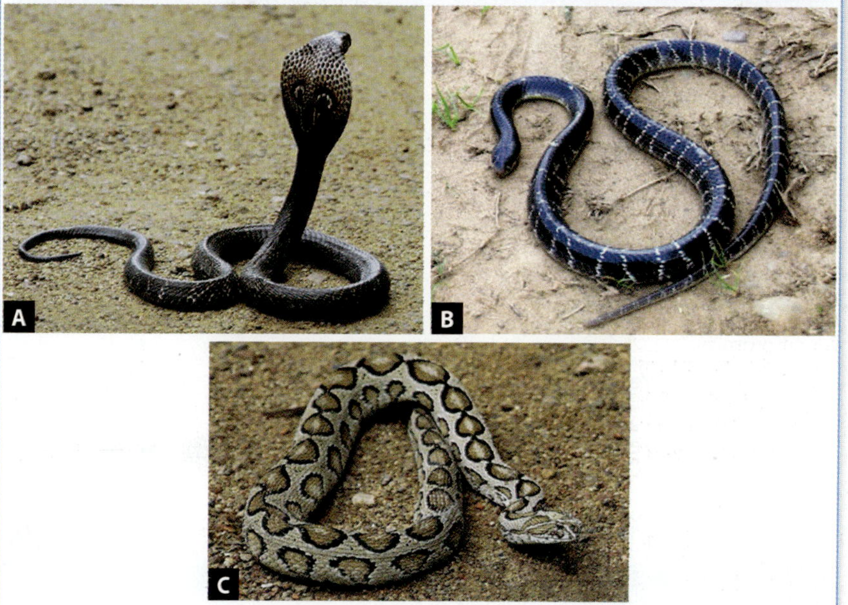

Figs. 1A to C: Identification of most common poisonous snakes. A. Cobra; B. Krait; C. Viper.

BOX 2: Early clues to diagnosis.

Identifying dangerous snakes:

Local symptoms:

- Rapid spread of local swelling from the bite site
- Early tender enlargement of local lymph nodes, indicating venom spread in the lymphatic system

Early systemic symptoms:

- Nausea, vomiting, and diarrhea
- Severe headache and a sensation of "heaviness" in the eyelids
- Drowsiness and early signs of ptosis/ophthalmoplegia
- Hemodynamic collapse
- Early onset of spontaneous systemic bleeding
- Passage of dark brown urine, progressing from oliguria to anuria, indicating kidney failure

Assessment must include:

- Time of the bite
- Activity at the time of the bite
- First aid actions taken

Contd...

Contd...

Observation period: All patients should be observed for a minimum of 24 hours
20-minute whole blood clotting test (20-min WBCT)

Features comparison:

Feature	*Cobra*	*Krait*	*Russell's viper*	*Saw scaled viper*	*Hump nosed viper*
Local pain/ tissue damage	Yes	No	Yes	Yes	Yes
Ptosis/ neurological signs	Yes	Yes	Yes	No	No
Hemostatic abnormality	No	No	Yes	Yes	Yes
Renal compromise	No	No	Yes	No	Yes
Response to neostigmine	Yes	No	No	No	No
Response to antisnake venom (ASV)	Yes	Yes	Yes	Yes	No

BOX 3: First aid.

- Scene safety
- Ensure that the patient is at a safe distance from the snake and further harm. And keep the patient warm
- Do not attempt to capture the snake. If possible, a photograph from a safe distance is often sufficient
- Do not cut or squeeze at the bite site
- Do not wash the wound [to prevent spreading the venom by stimulating lymphatic system]
- Do not attempt to suction the venom
- Do not use cryotherapy
- Do not administer electric shocks to the victim
- Do not tourniquet the extremity
- Remove any tight-fitting jewelry or clothing
- Immobilize the affected extremity at a functional position slightly below the level of the heart
- This is thought to decrease the risk of systemic venom absorption. While this is the most commonly recommended position, there is no data to support it
- Splint the affected extremity for pain relief and to reduce swelling and bleeding
- Administer analgesics
- Paracetamol and Opiates are recommended as compared to NSAIDs or Aspirin due to the adverse hematologic effects from crotaline bites
- Care should be taken when removing tight tourniquets applied by bystanders, as sudden removal can cause a massive surge of venom, leading to neurological paralysis and hypotension
- Pressure immobilization is recommended for neurotoxic elapid snake bites, including sea snakes, but not for viper bites due to the risk of increasing local effects of necrotic venom

BOX 4: Investigations.

Investigation includes: Complete hemogram, electrolytes, renal function test (RFT), liver function test (LFT), coagulation profile, creatine phosphokinase (CPK), urine routine, and arterial blood gas (ABG)

20-minute whole blood clotting test:
- Collect 2 mL of fresh blood in a glass container
- Leave it undisturbed for 20 minutes
- If the blood remains liquid and does not clot (incoagulable), this indicates hypofibrinogenemia
- Repeat the test; the normal WBCT range is 6–8 minutes **(Fig. 2)**

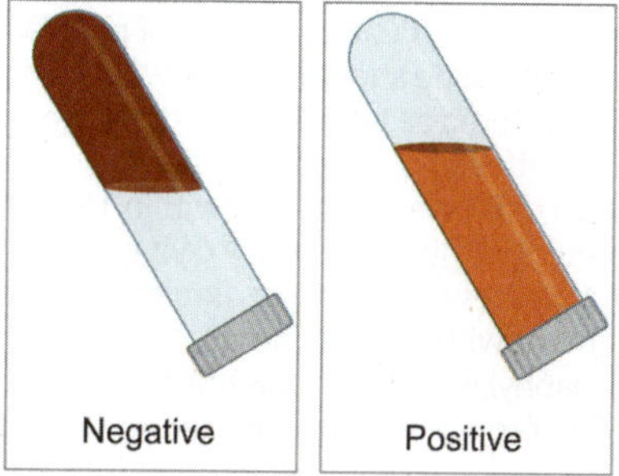

Fig. 2: Whole blood clotting test (WBCT)

Caveat:
- Performing a Tensilon (edrophonium) test and neostigmine dosing in snakebite victims.
- Administer the Tensilon (edrophonium) test and determine the appropriate dosing of neostigmine for snakebite victims with a positive result

Whole blood clotting test: The WBCT is a useful and quick bedside screening tool. If the blood fails to clot in a clean glass tube after 20 minutes, it indicates severe hypofibrinogenemia. Although WBCT has low sensitivity, it has high specificity, meaning a positive result signifies the need for antivenom administration. A negative result does not exclude the need for antivenom, particularly if clinical signs of coagulopathy are present, such as blood oozing from puncture sites, bleeding gums, or nosebleeds

BOX 5: Management.

Airway, breathing, circulation, disability, and exposure (ABCDE) is crucial in emergency room (ER) management

ASV administration:

- Polyvalent ASV*:* Neutralizes venoms of Indian cobra, Indian krait, Russell's viper, and saw-scaled viper
  - Indications: (Check **Box 2** for early diagnosis)
  - No test dose required: No predictive value
  - Prophylactic regimes: No statistical evidence supports prophylactic regimes in preventing ASV reactions
- Administration: No local administration or intramuscular (IM) injections. Available as lyophilized (freeze dried) powder, reconstituted in distilled water or saline (100 mL) just before use. Initial dosage is 100 mL (10 vials) of polyvalent ASV regardless of body weight and age. Adrenaline should be ready. Same dose for children can be given. ASV can be administered as long as evidence of coagulopathy persists, even more than 2 weeks. Best effect if used within 4 hours
- Response: Normalization of BP, bleeding stops within 15–30 minutes, normalization of coagulation parameters within 6 hours. Postsynaptic type (cobra) improvement within 30 minutes of ASV. Presynaptic toxins (kraits, sea snakes) will show neurological improvement within 30–48 hours
- Adverse effects: Early anaphylaxis (10–180 minutes) with angioedema, anaphylaxis, hypotension, shock, and bronchospasm. Late serum sickness (112 days)

Neurotoxin management:

- Anticholinesterase: IV atropine 0.6 mg for adults, 0.5 mg for children (0.02 mg/kg dose for both), or glycopyrrolate 0.2 mg for children (does not cross the blood–brain barrier). Neostigmine 0.02–0.04 mg/kg for adults/children (maximum dose 0.5 mg for children), repeated every 20 minutes until response is noted. Responding patients should be given 0.5–2.5 mg every 13 hours (maximum 10 mg/24 h). Mechanical ventilation if any airway compromise is noted

Criteria to repeat ASV:

- If blood remains incoagulable (PT, 20-min WBCT), as it takes 39 hours for the liver to restore coagulation factors
- If the patient continues to bleed or shows deteriorating neurotoxicity or cardiovascular signs

Local treatment:

- Keep the affected area slightly elevated
- Large and tense bullae should be aspirated only if likely to rupture
- Prophylactic antibiotics: Penicillin choice of drug unless is contraindicated
- Tetanus toxoid booster is recommended

Hematologic management:

- Heparin is ineffective against venom-induced thrombin and may cause bleeding. Antifibrinolytic agents are also ineffective
- Coagulation factor deficiency may require replacement with fresh frozen plasma (FFP) or cryoprecipitate (1.5 units/10 kg body weight for severe hypofibrinogenemia <100 mg/dL)
- Compartment syndrome (Chapter 5.2)

Dialysis considerations:

- If serum creatinine >4 mg/dL or rises >1 mg/day
- Urea >130 mg/dL
- Symptomatic acidosis
- Potassium >7 mmol/L with hyperkalemic ECG changes

BOX 6: Disposition.

- Bites from nonpoisonous snakes can be observed in the ER for a few hours and transferred to wards if no red flag signs are present
- Bites from unknown snakes require close observation for 8 hours for any red flags and WBCT monitoring, necessitating ICU admission

BOX 7: Scorpion sting.

- Scorpion venom contains many toxins, some of which cause the opening of neuronal sodium channels, leading to prolonged and excessive depolarization
- Motor hyperactivity is nearly universal, presenting as restlessness or uncontrollable jerking of the extremities that may appear seizure-like

Local effects:
- Pain at the sting site—**treat with acetaminophen, NSAIDs, or local lidocaine without epinephrine**
- Dermonecrosis may develop over hours or days

Systemic features:
- Tachycardia, hypertension, and mydriasis due to excess catecholamines
- Pulmonary edema, catecholamine-induced cardiac injury, myocardial depression, and cardiogenic shock
- Hypotension, bradycardia, salivation, and sweating
- Abdominal pain, diarrhea, and pancreatitis
- **Treat with antivenom and prazosin for cardiac symptoms, dobutamine for cardiogenic shock, and nitroglycerin for hypertension**

Neuromuscular agitation: Anxiety and agitation—**treat with benzodiazepines**

Cholinergic effects: Oculomotor abnormalities, uncoordinated neuromuscular activity, and muscle spasms

Multiorgan failure: Provide supportive care

Laboratory tests: Routine complete blood count (CBC), renal function test (RFT), liver function test (LFT), amylase, lipase, and cardiac enzymes; relevant patient history is crucial

Additional care:
- Administer tetanus prophylaxis
- Take antianaphylaxis measures if needed

Caveats:
- After envenomation, symptoms begin immediately and progress to maximum severity within 5 hours; in infants, symptoms take 15–30 minutes to appear. The dose of antivenom varies, taking approximately 4 hours to be effective, but pain can persist for up to 2 weeks
- **Centruroides Fab2 equine antivenom consists of three vials dissolved in 20–50 mL of normal saline and infused over 30 minutes. Administer two additional vials with a 30-minute gap, for a total of five vials**

BOX 8: Common marine bites/stings: Stingrays.

- Mostly found in warm waters, all stingrays' tails possess venomous spines
- **Stingray injuries cause immediate intense local pain that may radiate, laceration, and significant bleeding depending on the site of injury; the wound may be erythematous or dusky and can cause infections**

Treatment:

- Irrigate and remove the venomous object
- Obtain soft tissue imaging to confirm no retained foreign material near the wound
- Submerge the affected extremity in hot water between 110°F (43.3°C) and 114°F (45.6°C) to denature the venom protein and provide pain relief within 10–30 minutes
- Topical lidocaine can be applied for additional pain relief, and systemic analgesics can blunt the pain of hot water submersion
- Prophylactic tetanus and antibiotics should be given due to the high risk of infection with stingray injuries

SUGGESTED READING

1. Tintinalli JE, Ma OJ, Yealy DM, Meckler GD, Stapczynski JS, Cline DM, et al. (Eds). Tintinalli's Emergency Medicine: A Comprehensive Study Guide, 9th edition. McGraw-Hill Education; 2020.
2. Walls RM, Hockberger RS, Gausche-Hill M (Eds). Rosen's Emergency Medicine: Concepts and Clinical Practice, 9th edition. Elsevier; 2018.
3. WHO Guidelines.

15.2.5 Acute Burns

Dhimant Goleria, Rafat Ali Khan

BOX 1: Introduction.

Burn injury severely hampers the function of skin and creates systemic involvement. It should be managed in a specialized burn care unit, which has a multidisciplinary approach with plastic surgery department playing a key role in the management

BOX 2: Type of burns (etiology).

- *Thermal burns:* This is the most common type of burn. Fire and flame are the common type of thermal burns. It also includes scalds due to hot liquid spillage, contact burns, work related/industrial thermal burns, and friction burns
- *Chemical burns injury:* Prolonged exposure to acids, alkalies, solvents, usually in laboratories and industries
- *Electrical injury:* Low/high voltage, alternate/direct current
- *Acid burns:* Vitriolic attack
- *Radiation:* Prolonged exposure to ultraviolet (UV) radiation of Sun or other radiation source
- *Cold injury:* Frost bite

BOX 3: Burn wound assessment.

Depth of burns: Superficial (first degree), partial thickness (second degree—further classified as superficial, intermediate, and deep partial thickness), and full thickness (third degree)

- *First-degree burns:* These are characterized by erythema (localized redness). In appearance, they look like Sun burns. They are not included when calculating burn size. Usually heal by themselves
- *Second-degree burns:* Affected areas are mottled, red, painful with blisters; healing time is 14-21 days. Superficial second-degree burns heals with pigmentation. Deep second-degree burns heals with scarring and pigmentation, and sensation is present
- *Third-degree burns:* Affected areas are charred, parchment-like, painless, and insensitive with thrombosis of superficial vessels. Full-thickness burn is called as eschar. It may involve underlying tissues, muscles, and bones in depth

Burn size: It is calculated as a percentage of total body surface area (TBSA)

- Wallace's rule of nine and palm rule are some simple and easy methods for quick calculation **(Figs. 1A and B)**
- Miscalculation or overestimation may lead to inappropriate triage, transfer, and risk of overresuscitation
- Standard method is Lund and Browder method **(Fig. 2)**

Contd...

Contd...

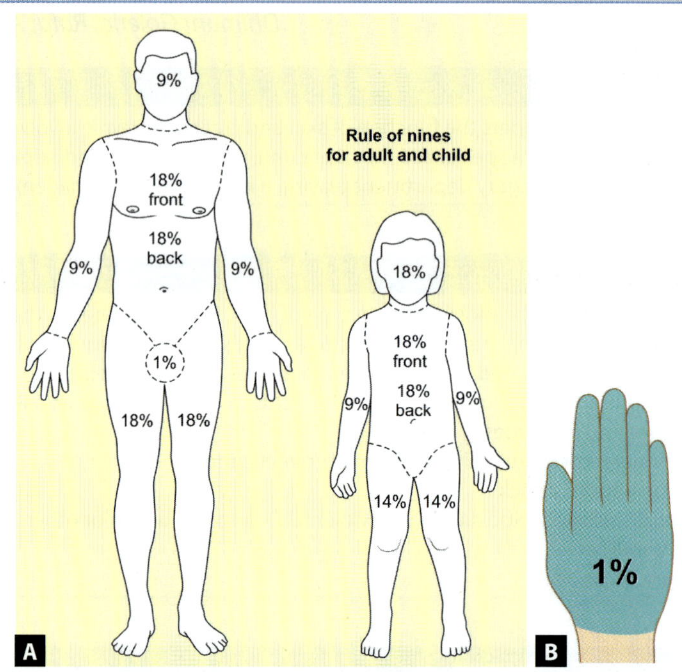

Figs. 1A and B: Wallace's rule of nine and palm rule.

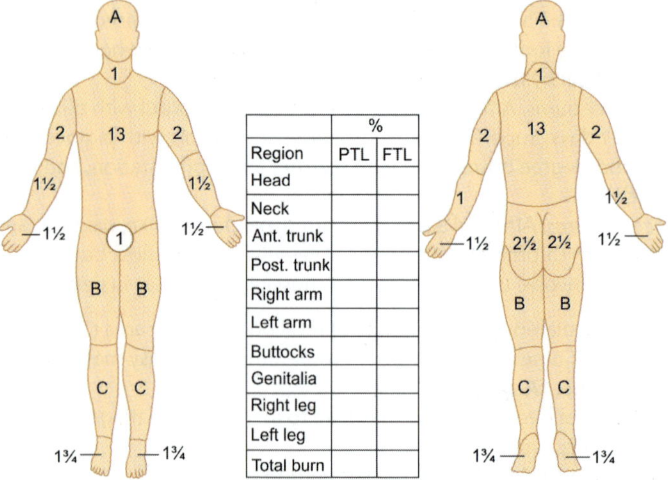

	%	
Region	PTL	FTL
Head		
Neck		
Ant. trunk		
Post. trunk		
Right arm		
Left arm		
Buttocks		
Genitalia		
Right leg		
Left leg		
Total burn		

Area	Age 0	1	5	10	15	Adult
A = 1/2 of head	9½	8½	6½	5½	4½	3½
B = 1/2 of one thigh	2¾	3¼	4	4½	4½	4¾
C = 1/2 of one lower leg	2½	2½	2¾	3	3¼	3½

Fig. 2: Lund and Browder chart for adult and child. (FTL: full thickness loss; PTL: partial thickness loss)

BOX 4: Primary assessment of burns.

- A—Airway maintenance—cervical spine protection, intubation, tracheostomy, assessment, and management of inhalational burns
- B—Breathing—to achieve adequate ventilation and rule out pneumothorax; concentric thoracic burns will need lateral escharotomy of thorax region
- C—Circulation—resuscitation of fluid as per total body surface area (TBSA) calculation with caution of overresuscitation and proper urine output (UO) monitoring. Evaluation of cardiac status
- D—Disability—carboxyhemoglobin, hydrogen cyanide, shock, trauma assessment
- E—Environment—moving the patient away from the source of burns to safety and prevention of additional injury

History is essential in understanding the nature and severity of burns, exact time of burn, and possibility of medicolegal case

Physical examination: Important factors include depth of burns, cause of burns, associated trauma, and premorbid disease

Criteria for burn injury requiring admission:
- Partial thickness burns >15% TBSA in adults and >10% TBSA in pediatric age group
- Third-degree burns >5% TBSA
- Burns which involve the face, hands, feet, genitalia, perineum, and joints
- Electrical burns (ECG to rule out arrhythmias)
- Chemical burns
- Inhalational burns
- Burns with associated comorbidity and additional risk factors
- Burns in extreme age (children have smaller body surface area and thin dermis)

Criteria for fluid resuscitation:
- For >20% TBSA burns in adult or >15% TBSA burn in children
- High voltage electric burns
- Burns in extreme age

BOX 5: Fluid resuscitation in burns.

Burns in excess of about 20% TBSA, more likely to cause shock, are manifested by decreased circulating blood volume, decreased cardiac output (CO), and inadequate end-organ perfusion. Fluid resuscitation to address burn shock is one of the key lifesaving interventions in the early care of burn patients. Inadequate or delayed fluid resuscitation causes organ failure and death

Note: Time since burn (not since presentation or admission) is taken into consideration while calculating fluid for resuscitation

Modified Parkland formula:
- Initial 24 hours—Ringers Lactate solution 4 mL/kg/% burn (half volume in first 8 hours, rest given in 16 hours)
- Next 24 hours—begin colloid infusion of 5% albumin 0.3–1 mL/kg/% burn/16 h

Modified Brookes formula:
- First 24 hours: Ringer lactate (RL): 4 mL/kg/% burns in 24 hours. Colloid not to be given in first 24 hours
- Second 24 hours: Crystalloids to maintain UO. Colloids: 0.3–0.5 mL/kg/% burns—24 hours

Pediatric age group fluid management—Pediatric age group modified Brooke formula: This formula estimates 3 mL/kg/TBSA of lactate ringer (LR). For the first 24 hours, with half given over the first 8 hours and the remaining 1/2 half LR is the titrated based on UO (target UO is 0.5–1.5 mL/kg/h). Children are also given 5% dextrose in one-half normal saline at a maintenance rate

BOX 6: Management of burns.

- Urinary catheterization monitor UO, 30–50 mL/h should be the output
- Tetanus toxoid injection
- Hourly pulse, BP, PO_2, electrolyte analysis, blood urea, and nasal oxygen
- Ryles tube insertion initially for aspiration, later for feeding
- Tissue culture of wound discharge, total white blood cell (WBC) count, platelet count at regular intervals to identify sepsis along with fever, tachycardia, and tachypnea
- Total parenteral nutrition for faster recovery via central venous pressure (CVP) line
- Tracheostomy/intubation tube may be required in impending respiratory failure
- Definitive management—admit the patient, maintain ABC emergency endotracheal intubation may be assess percentage, degree, and type of burn
- Isolation: Keep patient in a clean environment
- Sedation and proper analgesia
- Patient should be in burns unit [ideally air conditioned, high efficiency particulate air (HEPA) filter rooms] with barrier nursing, sterile clothes, sterile bed sheets, and all aseptic methods

Local wound management:
Wound cleaning: Wounds are cleaned thoroughly before application of suitable dressing using normal saline to remove any debris or contamination. Filtered tap water or antiseptic solution like chlorhexidine may also be used in acute setting (<48 hours of burns)

Chemical burns: Initial management of patient with chemical injury involves:
- Remove clothing to prevent further contact
- Remove chemical: For dry chemical: Brushing away (not wiping)
- For wet chemical: Copious flushing of areas with water
- Phenol the use of vegetable oil/or polyethylene glycol
- If suspected injury is with metallic sodium or potassium: Do not use water
- For hydrofluoric acid burn—treat the area with calcium and water lavage
- Drink water: If chemical is swallowed. Avoid attempting to vomit as it may cause more damage to esophagus
- Chemical injuries can cause erosions, perforations, strictures esophagus, pyloric stenosis, and mediastinal injury. Others: deep vein thrombosis (DVT), pulmonary embolism, urinary infection, bedsores, and severe malnutrition with catabolic status

Wound dressing: Dressing at regular intervals under general anesthesia using paraffin gauge, hydrocolloids, plastic films vaseline impregnated gauze, biological dressings like amniotic membrane or synthetic biobrane

Open method with application of silver sulfadiazine without any dressings used in burns of face, head, and neck

Tangential excision of burn wound with skin grafting can be done within 48 hours in patients with <25% burns. Usually done in deep dermal burn where dead dermis is removed layer by layer until fresh bleeding occurs. Later skin grafting is done

Once the area granulates well, in 3 weeks usually, split skin grafting is done

For wider area meshed split skin graft is used

Contd...

Contd...

Negative pressure wound therapy is widely used as coverage dressing over sheet grafts with good success

Various biological and synthetic skin substitutes are available, which plays an important role in wound coverage

Eschar: If there is an eschar, escharotomy is required to prevent compression of vessels

Burns over extremities and circumferential burns over torso are more prone for compartment syndrome and may warrant urgent decompression

For wounds over areas like face and ear, full-thickness graft (Wolfe graft) or flap may be required for coverage

Role of cadaver skin graft:
- Act as biological dressing
- Used as a stage between excision and autograft in critical areas
- Used in questionable wound bed to assess graft take
- Overlay dressing for wide meshed autograft
- Temporary coverage in massive area burns

Supportive therapy: Physiotherapy of joints for contracture prevention, compression dressing to prevent hypertrophy of scars, psychotherapy, and rehabilitation therapy with timely counseling

BOX 7: Complications of burn.

Early: Burn shock, renal failure, smoke inhalation syndrome, and septicemia

Late: Contractures, ectropion, microstoma, hypertrophic scar, and keloid formation

BOX 8: Airway management.

Airway management algorithm for patients at risk of inhalational injury:
- *Patient at risk of inhalational injury:*
  - Facial burn
  - Hoarseness
  - Evidence of smoke exposure
  - Other classic signs of thermal injury
- *Advanced trauma life support (ATLS) primary survey:*
  - If the patient shows significant respiratory distress or other indications of intubation (e.g., massive burns and apnea), proceed with intubation directly after the ATLS primary survey
  - If the patient shows mild respiratory distress but no other indications of intubation:
    - Perform a flow volume loop and/or fiberoptic bronchoscopy
  - If no flow loop evidence of obstruction and no concern findings on bronchoscopy:
    - Continue observation and repeat the study if clinical changes occur
  - If there are mild flow volume changes but no significant obstruction on bronchoscopy:
    - Conduct serial examinations
  - If there are glottic or subglottic changes with significant obstruction observed:
    - Intubate immediately

SUGGESTED READING

1. Austin RE, Schlagintweit S, Jeschke MG, MacDonald R, Ahghari M, Shahrokhi S. The cost of burn transfers: a retrospective review of 7 years of admissions to a regional burn center. J Burn Care Res. 2018;39:229-34.
2. Herndon DN (Ed). Total Burn Care. Elsevier; 2007.
3. Jackson D. The diagnosis of the depth of burning. Br J Surg. 1953;40:588-96.
4. Lagziel T, Asif M, Born L, Quiroga LH, Duraes E, Slavin B, et al. Evaluating the efficacy, safety, and tolerance of silver sulfadiazine dressings once daily versus twice daily in the treatment of burn wounds. J Burn Care Res. 2021;42:1136-9.
5. Lund CC, Browder NC. The estimation of areas of burns. Surg Gynecol Obstet. 1944;79:352-8.
6. Nielson CB, Duethman NC, Howard JM, Moncure M, Wood JG. Burns: pathophysiology of systemic complications and current management. J Burn Care Res. 2017;38:e469-e481.
7. Noone RB, Goldwyn RM, McGrath M, Spear S, Evans GRD. 50th anniversary Plastic Surgery Research Council panel on the future of academic plastic surgery. Plast Reconstr Surg. 2007;120:1709-21.
8. Padalko A, Cristall N, Gawaziuk JP, Logsetty S. Social complexity and risk for pediatric burn injury: a systematic review. J Burn Care Res. 2019;40:478-99.
9. Peck MD. Epidemiology of burns throughout the world. Part I: distribution and risk factors. Burns. 2011;37:1087-100.
10. Pham C, Collier Z, Gillenwater J. Changing the way we think about burn size estimation. J Burn Care Res. 2019;40:1-11.
11. Rae L, Fidler P, Gibran N. The physiologic basis of burn shock and the need for aggressive fluid resuscitation. Crit Care Clin. 2016;32:491-505.
12. Seidenari S, Giusti G, Bertoni L, Magnoni C, Pellacani G. Thickness and echogenicity of the skin in children as assessed by 20-MHz ultrasound. Dermatology. 2000;201:218-22.
13. Slavin B, Shoucair S, Klifto K, Grzelak M, Shetty P, Cox C, et al. Inappropriate transfer of burn patients: a 5-year retrospective at a single center. Ann Plast Surg. 2021;86:29-34.
14. Vrouwe SQ, Pham CH, Minasian RA, Yenikomshian HA, Garner WL, Gillenwater TJ. The state of burn care training during plastic surgery residency. Ann Plast Surg. 2020;85:122-6.
15. Wang C, Zhang F, Lineaweaver WC. Clinical applications of allograft skin in burn care. Ann Plast Surg. 2020;84(Suppl 2):S158-S160.
16. Whitaker IS, Prowse S, Potokar TS. A critical evaluation of the use of Biobrane as a biologic skin substitute: a versatile tool for the plastic and reconstructive surgeon. Ann Plast Surg. 2008;60:333-7

15.2.6 Electric Injuries

Pinank Pandya

BOX 1: Introduction.

- Electrical injuries can manifest with a variety of pathologies
- The direct impact of electrical current, conversion of electrical energy to thermal energy, and blunt mechanical trauma can lead to tissue damage and organ dysfunction
- Complications such as respiratory or cardiac issues, burns, and tissue injuries often necessitate multiple surgical interventions, including procedures like fasciotomy and skin grafting, along with extended periods of supportive and rehabilitative care
- While most electrical injuries arise from household appliances (100–240V), large scale industries might have people dealing with currents in excess of 600V, which can be fatal

BOX 2: Risk stratification of electrical injuries.

Factors that aid in predicting the severity of the injury include:

- Voltage
- Alternating current (AC) or direct current (DC)
- Duration of contact and
- Degree of wetness/humidity of the environment

Low voltage (<600V), such as household or office exposures are generally lower risk injuries

High voltage (>600V), such as industrial settings, subway rails, power lines are generally higher risk injuries

Alternating current causes prolonged muscle contraction due to its alternating nature, which prevents the victim from releasing the electrical source quickly, resulting in prolonged contact and more extensive tissue damage compared to DC

	Low voltage (<600V)	***High voltage (>600–1,000V)***	***Lightning***
Exposure	Household or office	Industrial	Environment
Voltage	Canada: 110–240 volts Europe: up to 400 volts	> 600–1,000 volts	Up to 1 billion volts
Contact	Prolonged	Brief	Very brief (ms)
Current	AC	AC or DC	DC
Injuries	Superficial burns, unlikely rhabdomyolysis, cardiac dysrhythmias [ventricular fibrillation (VF)] rare	Deep burns, tetany, rhabdomyolysis, cardiac dysrhythmias (VF/asystole)	Burns variable, rhabdomyolysis unlikely, cardiac dysrhythmias (asystole), respiratory arrest, autonomic dysfunction

Caveat: It is important to utilize *reverse triage* in mass casualty incidents, caused by lightning strikes. Patients who appear deceased may actually be more easily resuscitated with favorable survival rates, and therefore should be prioritized for immediate attention

BOX 3: Mechanism of injuries.

- Direct strike
- Contact strike
- Side flash or splash
- Ground strike

The following phenomena distinguish lightning strikes from other electrical injuries:

- *Flashover effect:* This effect in lightning strikes involves a high current rapidly passing over the skin, facilitated by reduced resistance from wet skin due to rain or sweat. This intense flow can effectively short-circuit and momentarily reset the central nervous system, leading to temporary shutdown of cardiac and respiratory centers and inducing a state akin to "suspended animation" at the cellular level. Unlike other electrical injuries, lightning strikes typically do not result in deep burns, because the current remains on the skin surface without penetrating deeply into tissues, ultimately dissipating into the ground
- *Keraunoparalysis*
- *Autonomic dysfunction*
- *Secondary trauma from shock wave* (Refer Chapter 15.2.7: Lightening Injuries)

BOX 4: Organ/systemic injuries.

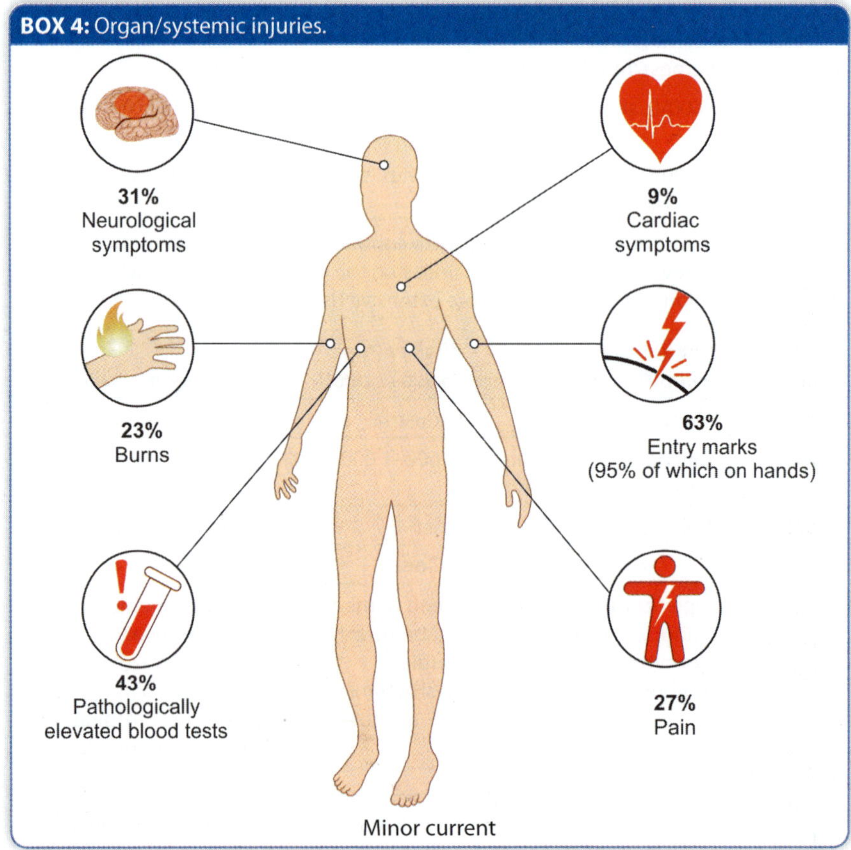

Contd...

Contd...

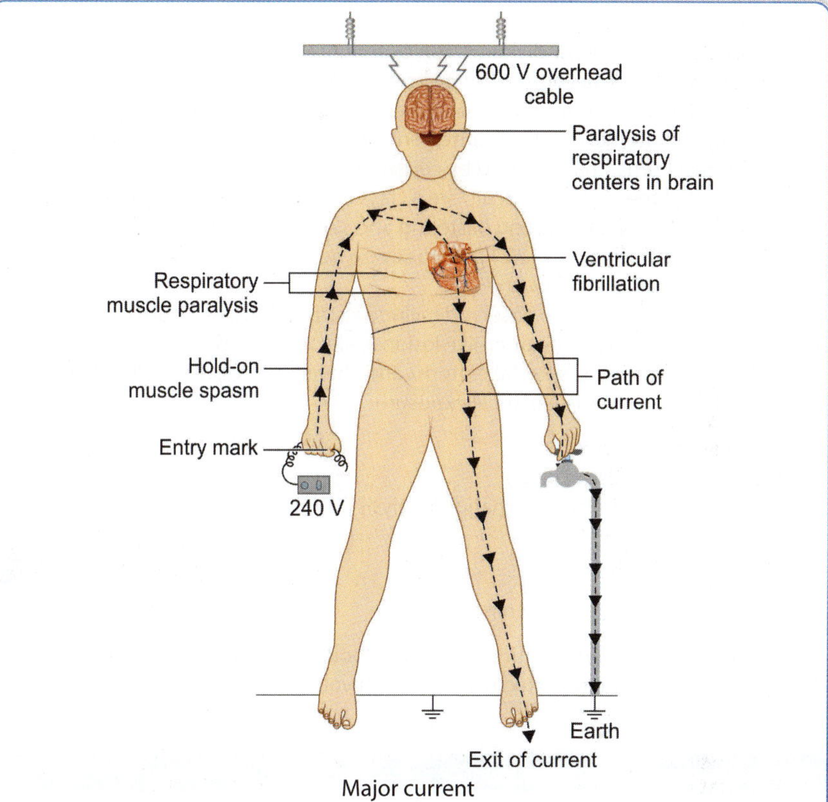

Major current

Cardiac:

- *Dysrhythmias:* Most are benign, but ventricular fibrillation is the most common fatal arrhythmia. Timing is important as they may occur from immediately to as later as 12 hours after high voltage current. Fatalities and malignant arrhythmias are very uncommon in low-voltage injuries. AC current is more dangerous than DC current in which dysrhythmias appear more common
- *Conduction disturbances:* Conduction disturbances in electrical injuries can lead to first- and second-degree atrioventricular (AV) blocks as well as bundle branch blocks. These disturbances typically resolve on their own without specific treatment but may persist in some cases
- *Myocardial damage:* Injury to myocardium, although rare, can result from electrothermal injury, electroporation, which means formation of cell membrane pores due to electrical current, myocardial contusion due to blast effect, or secondary blunt trauma

Neurological:

- Respiratory arrest
- Peripheral nerve injury
- Other common sequelae of electrical injuries include loss of consciousness, neuropsychological issues, and memory disturbances

Contd...

Contd...

Skin:

Following electrical injury, individuals can experience superficial, partial-thickness, and full-thickness thermal burns. The protective barrier of dry intact skin is compromised with wet skin, which has lower resistance, allowing more current to pass through to internal organs despite generating less heat for a given voltage. Electrothermal burns, characterized by contact point wounds where the body becomes part of the electrical circuit, are a classic injury pattern. These burns generate significant heat, causing blistering and swelling when skin temperature reaches approximately 50°C (122°F). More severe burns and charring can occur, raising skin temperature to around 90°C

Additional types of injuries observed include kissing burns, oral burns, flame burns, Lichtenberg figures (feather-like lesions), electric flash burns, and electric arc burns. Each type presents specific patterns and characteristics, depending on the nature and intensity of the electrical exposure

Musculoskeletal and renal:

- Bones and nearby tissue injury
- Compartment syndrome and rhabdomyolysis
- Acute Kidney injury
- Secondary trauma

Eye and ear: It is mainly in lightening injuries

Vascular and related injuries: Injuries to major blood vessels and organs like gastrointestinal tract have been reported mainly in high voltage or lightening injuries

BOX 5: Evaluation and management.

Physical examination	
Typical airway, breathing, and circulation (*ABC*) and *vital signs*	
Do a thorough *cardio/respiratory examination*	
Assess for signs of *trauma*	• Falls, fractures, lacerations, etc.
Perform a thorough *eye examination*	• Including visual acuity, inspecting the conjunctiva, and perhaps a slit lamp if warranted • *Rare* to have damage in *low* voltage
Do a thorough *neurologic* examination	• Motor, sensory, and reflexes
Look for *burns* everywhere	• Discoloration, blisters, charred skin, and other lesions • Look closely at skin creases and areas around joints • In a young *child*—closely examine the *mouth* • Remember surface burns may underestimate degree of injury
Inspect the *tympanic membranes* for rupture	• *Rare* in *low* voltage

Contd...

Contd...

Get blood tests such as creatine kinase (CK), troponins, and electrolytes for all and *most important—get ECG for all*

- Discoloration, blisters, charred skin, and other lesions
- Look closely at skin creases and areas around joints
- In a young child—closely examine the mouth
- Remember surface burns may underestimate degree of injury

Do the primary and secondary survey like the trauma protocol [advanced trauma life support (ATLS)] and get necessary X-rays and CT scans if needed according to the nature of the injury

High-voltage injuries usually have underlying blunt trauma, which may need imaging

Monitor for degree of burns and deep tissue injuries along with any possibility of compartment syndrome

Fluids: They are the cornerstone to management as the degree of burns may be underestimated in majority of cases. Can use *Parkland formula* and *balanced salt solutions* for resuscitation (refer to Chapter 15.2.5: Burns)

If rhabdomyolysis is suspected as is usually the case with high voltage injuries, resuscitate adequately to maintain urine output around 2 mL/kg/h (refer to Chapter 5.2: Rhabdomyolosis)

Get the initial bloodwork done along with the creatine phosphokinase (CPK) total levels

Tetanus shot is indicated if there is a visible wound, and sometimes along with tetanus globulin if the individual is not vaccinated and the degree of injury is significant (especially in lightning burns)

You can *discharge* the patient if:

- Low voltage (<600V)
- Asymptomatic—no chest pain, no current symptoms
- No reported loss of consciousness
- Normal physical examination
- Normal ECG
- *Note: No cardiac monitoring, no bloodwork/troponin needed*

Contd...

Contd...

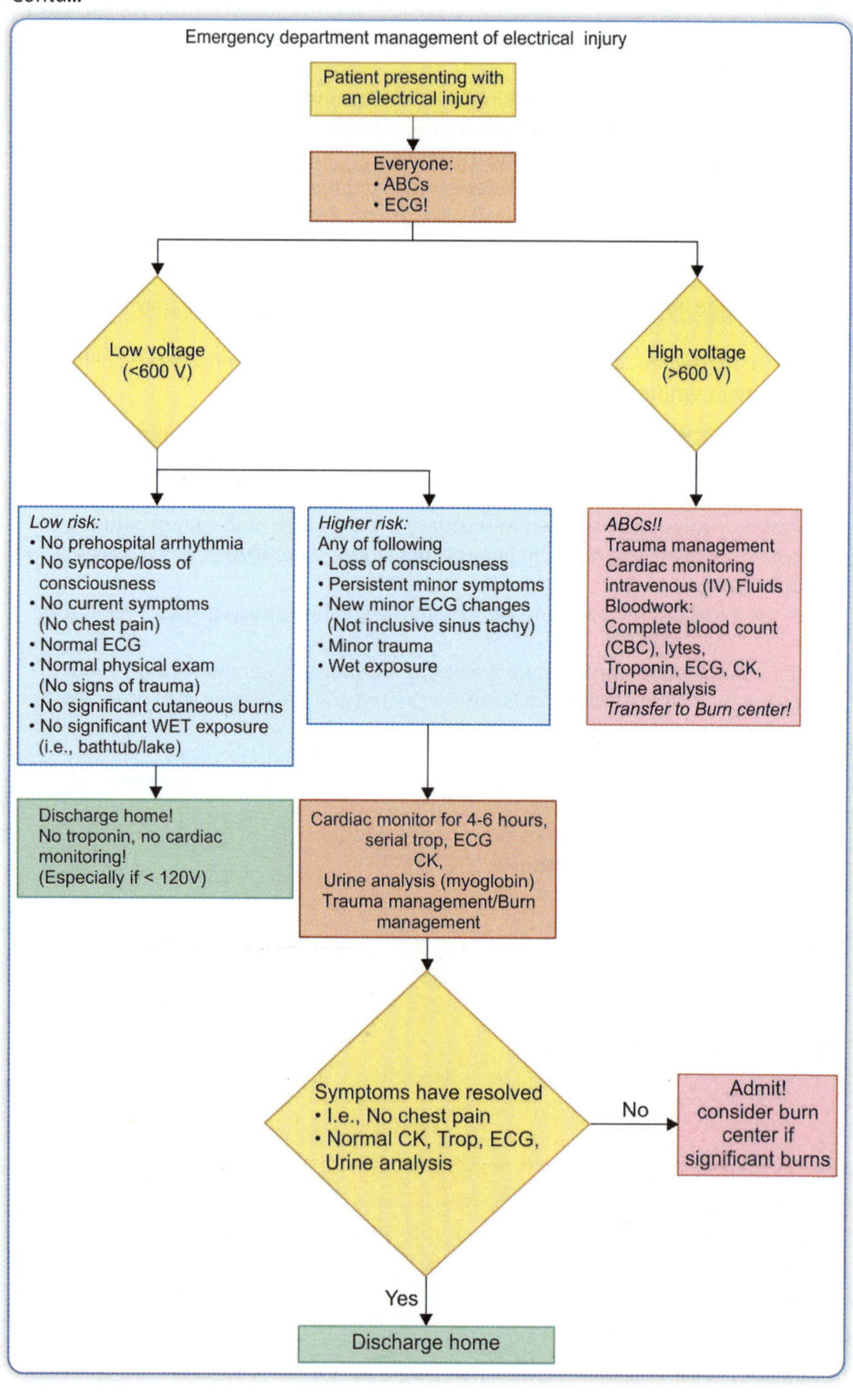
Emergency department management of electrical injury
Patient presenting with an electrical injury
Everyone:
• ABCs
• ECG!
Low voltage (<600 V)
High voltage (>600 V)
Low risk:
• No prehospital arrhythmia
• No syncope/loss of consciousness
• No current symptoms (No chest pain)
• Normal ECG
• Normal physical exam (No signs of trauma)
• No significant cutaneous burns
• No significant WET exposure (i.e., bathtub/lake)
Higher risk:
Any of following
• Loss of consciousness
• Persistent minor symptoms
• New minor ECG changes (Not inclusive sinus tachy)
• Minor trauma
• Wet exposure
ABCs!!
Trauma management
Cardiac monitoring
intravenous (IV) Fluids
Bloodwork:
Complete blood count (CBC), lytes,
Troponin, ECG, CK,
Urine analysis
Transfer to Burn center!
Discharge home!
No troponin, no cardiac monitoring!
(Especially if < 120V)
Cardiac monitor for 4-6 hours, serial trop, ECG
CK,
Urine analysis (myoglobin)
Trauma management/Burn management
Symptoms have resolved
• I.e., No chest pain
• Normal CK, Trop, ECG, Urine analysis
No
Admit! consider burn center if significant burns
Yes
Discharge home

BOX 6: *Observation* in emergency room (ER) with *cardiac monitoring* if:

- *Low-voltage exposure* (<600V) but *higher risk:*
  - Skin wet during injury
  - May have had tetany/significant muscle contractions
  - Symptomatic: Such as chest pain
  - High risk for cardiac complications: Significant cardiovascular history, etc.
  - Loss of consciousness
  - Mild cutaneous burns
  - Minor abnormalities on ECG
- *Note:* Can *discharge* these patients after 4–6 hours of cardiac monitoring if:
  - No more symptoms
  - Normal ECG:
    - (Or has normalized after monitoring)
  - Normal blood work—troponins, CK, and urine myoglobin
  - Normal cardiac monitoring

Admit the patient if:

High-voltage burns:

- *Deep skin and local soft tissue burn:*
  - *Rare*—but happens if patient was unable to "let go" of current
    - May have *deeper burns* than seen externally
  - *Transfer to burn* center for evaluation—may need more extensive repair
- *Major ECG* abnormalities
- *Failed* above *discharge* criteria

Any discharge instructions?

- Advise patients that:
  - Delayed neurologic symptoms may occur, even psychological—difficulty concentrating, etc.
  - They should return if signs of chest pain, palpitations, syncope, and compartment syndrome—increased pain/swelling in a particular limb

SUGGESTED READING

1. Gentges J, Schieche C. Electrical injuries in the emergency department: An evidence-based review. Emerg Med Pract. 2018;20(11):1-20.
2. Goffeng LO, Skare Ø, Brinchmann BC, Bjørnsen LP, Veiersted KB. Low-voltage electrical accidents, immediate reactions and acute health care associated with self-reported general health 4 years later. Burns. 2023;49(2):329-43.
3. Helman A. (2022). Electrical injuries. Emergency Medicine Cases.
4. O'Keefe KP. (2023). Electrical injuries and lightning strikes: Evaluation and management. [online] Available from https://www.uptodate.com/contents/electrical-injuries-and-lightning-strikes-evaluation-and-management [Last accessed September, 2024].
5. Zemaitis MR, Foris LA, Lopez RA, Huecker MR. Electrical injuries. U.S. National Library of Medicine. Treasure Island (FL): StatPearls Publishing; 2024.

15.2.7 Lightening Injuries

Altaf Patel, Hasnain Patel

BOX 1: Introduction.

- Lightning injuries differ from electrical shock injuries in several aspects
- The prevalence and severity of lightning injuries vary across developed and developing countries. In developed countries, lightning injuries are usually superficial and do not cause myoglobinuria
- They are also more preventable, as people have access to safe shelters such as habitable buildings or metal vehicles
- Most injuries occur outdoors, but indoor contact injuries with plumbing and wiring are also possible
- Using cell phones and other electronic devices may alter the pathway of lightning around a person, but they do not increase the risk of injury

BOX 2: Clinical presentation.

- The most common feature of lightning injuries is neurological impairment, as people who are struck by lightning and suffer cardiac arrest have a better survival rate than other causes of cardiac arrest
- Resuscitation should be initiated immediately
- Classification lightning injuries can be classified as mild, moderate, or severe
- Mild injuries may result in loss of consciousness, confusion, and other nonspecific symptoms
- Moderate injuries may cause seizures or cardiac arrest, which may resolve spontaneously
- Superficial burns are more common in this type of injury
- Severe injuries present with cardiopulmonary arrest, and unless cardiopulmonary resuscitation (CPR) is rapidly instituted, survival is rare

BOX 3: Diagnostic investigation in the emergency room.

Cardiac evaluation

- Obtain ECG and 2D echo in high-risk patients, including those who have a direct strike or complain of chest pain or dyspnea. In those patients who have a direct strike or abnormal screening ECG, obtain telemetry

CNS evaluation

- Check the central pulse before starting CPR, as keraunoparalysis may mimic a pulseless patient
- *Keraunoparalysis is paralysis, mottling, coldness, and lack of pulse, affecting the lower extremities and sometimes the upper extremities. It is caused by injury to the sympathetic nervous system. Such patients require admission, and it usually resolves within 7 hours*
- Occasionally, some degree of permanent paralysis may remain
- Diagnostic imaging should be done to rule out spinal cord injury. If there is loss of consciousness, a CT scan of the head is advisable
- It is possible to have neuropsychiatric dysfunction from lightning, and in such cases, a mental health expert should be consulted

Contd...

Contd...

Skin evaluation:

Transient feathering pattern on the skin, also known as Lichtenberg figure, is diagnostic of lightning strikes. It is not a burn and generally appears within 1 hour of lightning and resolves in <24 hours. It requires no treatment

Ophthalmic evaluation:

Assess if there is any vision loss, corneal burn, retinal detachment, or vitreous hemorrhage

ENT Evaluation

Evaluate the tympanic membrane in all lightning patients

BOX 4: Management.

- Resuscitation is the first step to management and should be started at the site of injury before the patient is brought to the ER
- In the ECG, look for atrial fibrillation, prolonged QT interval, and ST segment elevation or depression
- Look for hypotension, usually from vasomotor instability
- Look for fixed and dilated pupils, as they may indicate autonomic disturbances and may recover. This should not be used as an index to stop resuscitation
- There may be disorientation, respiratory paralysis, loss of consciousness, sudden death, or significant hypoxic brain injury. Cerebral edema should be managed in the usual way
- Therapy for burns should include cleaning of the wound and use of an antimicrobial cream
- Tetanus prophylaxis should be given
- Also, evaluate if the patient has had a fall and has received any blunt injuries, and in such cases, perform appropriate investigation

SUGGESTED READING

1. Johnson RM. Cardiovascular Implications of Lightning Injuries: A Review. Cardiology Clinics. 2021.
2. Smith AK. Lightning injuries: Mechanisms and management. Journal of Trauma and Acute Care Surgery. 2018.
3. Thompson LJ. Electromagnetic and neurological effects of lightning strikes. Neurology. 2020.

15.2.8 Diving Disorders

Sachna P Shetty

BOX 1: Diving disorders.

- Diving disorders can cause disorders related to drowning (discussed in individual chapter)
- Barotraumas
- Decompression illness
- Marine trauma in the form of bites and stings

BOX 2: Barotrauma clinical presentation and treatment.

Barotrauma of descent:

- **Middle ear barotraumas:** Pain, fullness, vertigo, conductive hearing loss from inability to equalize middle ear pressure—decongestants; consider antibiotics
- **Sinuses barotrauma:** It is commonly seen is pain over sinuses, epistaxis—decongestants; consider antibiotics
- **Inner ear barotraumas:** Nausea, ataxia, nystagmus sensorineural hearing loss, tinnitus, and severe vertigo (peripheral giddiness-like symptoms)
- **Head of bed up, no nose blowing, antivertigo medications and with early need of ENT specialist interventions**

Barotrauma of ascent:

- Lung barotraumas—in the form of pneumomediastinum (self-resolving)
- Pneumothorax (details in Chapter 37.2)
- **Arterial gas embolism (AGE)** is diagnosed when in presence of pulmonary barotrauma symptoms like sudden onset of neurological symptoms like headache, confusion, motor or sensory loss, and convulsions manifest
- Airway, breathing, circulation, oxygen, intravenous (IV) fluids, and immediate recompression **[hyperbaric oxygen (HBO)]**

BOX 3: Decompression sickness (DCS).

Type 1:
- It involves musculoskeletal, lymphatics, and skin
- Deep pain in joints and extremities
- Skin changes—mottling and color changes, and marbling
- Lymphatic obstruction causing extremity edema

Type 2:
- "Serious" involves any organ, but spinal manifestations predominate
- Lung/chest—cough, hemoptysis, shortness of breath, and substernal chest pain
- Hypotension
- Neurologic—ascending paralysis, usually rapid in onset
- Vestibular—vertigo, hearing loss, tinnitus, and imbalance
- Autonomic dysfunction may be seen

Type 3:
- Combination of DCS and arterial gas embolism
- *Caveat:* All the symptoms and signs can coexist

Diagnosis of mainly Arterial gas embolism (AGE) by San Diego
- Criteria >2 is an indicator
- Mainly is clinical, based on history and physical examination, with limited laboratory testing
- The San Diego Diving and Hyperbaric Organizations criteria uses a point system to identify dive injuries resulting in DCS
- **San Diego Diving and Hyperbaric Organizations Criteria for Arterial Gas Embolism Time Criteria Points**

Any of the following signs or symptoms within 5 minutes of surfacing:
- Disorientation, sudden loss of consciousness, aphasia, hemiplegia—three points
- Hemiparesis or monoparesis seizures (new onset) Cortical blindness—two points:
- With resurfacing or discovered during emergency room (ER) evaluation
  - A rapid uncontrolled ascent, or any ascent with panic and the onset of symptoms
  - Hemoptysis
    - Presence of barotrauma on chest radiograph (pneumomediastinum, pneumopericardium, or pneumothorax)
    - Creatine phosphokinase greater than two times normal in the absence of musculoskeletal trauma—1 point

Other tests: Complete blood count (CBC) (for hematocrit), creatinine kinase for musculoskeletal, cardiac enzymes, imaging for pulmonary and neurological involvement

Treatment:
- Manage ABCs; recompression is the main stay of the treatment administering 100% oxygen, IV fluids
- HBO is the main stay of treatment in arterial embolism
- Supine position over Trendelenburg is preferred

BOX 4: Caveat.

- Analgesics and sedatives can mask recompression responses
- After intubation inflate the endotracheal (ET) cuff with water instead of air as it will deflate the tube and cause dislodgement
- Aspirin can be prophylactically given to decrease capillary sludging, which accompanies severe DCS
- Hypothermia is common (Chapter 15.2.1)
- Steroids: No significant improvement in the outcome
- Anticoagulants should not be used for all patients with DCS or AGE, only as a prophylaxis for deep vein thrombosis (DVT) for the ones who have lower extremity weakness and are immobilized even after recompression therapy

BOX 5: Disposition.

- Flying time should be post 12 hours in a normal diver, 24 hours in multiple time diver, and 72 hours post recompression in DCS or AGE
- DCS type II symptoms or AGE should be discouraged from future diving again

SUGGESTED READING

1. Edmonds C, Bennett M, Lippmann J, Mitchell S. Diving and Subaquatic Medicine. 5th ed. CRC Press; 2015.
2. Hyperbaric oxygen therapy. In: UpToDate, Post TW, editor. Available from: https://www.uptodate.com/contents/hyperbaric-oxygen-therapy [accessed on November, 2024].
3. McFall GB, Heine JN, Bozanic JE. NOAA Diving Manual: Diving for Science and Technology. 6th ed. Best Publishing Company; 2017.
4. Undersea & Dive Medicine [Internet]. UC San Diego Health. Available from: https://health.ucsd.edu/care/undersea/

15.2.9 Drowning

Sachna P Shetty

BOX 1: Definition.

- The definition of drowning has been standardized by World Health Organization (WHO), recognizing it as "the process of experiencing respiratory impairment due to submersion/immersion in liquid"
- Fatal drowning refers to a drowning incident resulting in death
- Nonfatal drowning denotes a drowning event where respiratory impairment is interrupted before death, allowing the victim to survive
- *Further classification includes:*
  - Mild impairment: Alert but experiencing involuntary coughing
  - Moderate impairment: Difficulty breathing and/or disorientation while remaining conscious
  - Severe impairment: Unconsciousness accompanied by cessation of breathing

BOX 2: Risk factors.

- *Age:* Particularly the pediatric age group
- Influence of alcohol or other intoxicants
- Incidents of syncope, especially during diving
- Presence of seizures
- Cardiac conditions such as dysrhythmias (including prolonged QT syndromes, Brugada syndrome, and ischemic heart disease)
- Conditions like dementia
- Intentional incidents (suicide or homicide)

BOX 3: Clinical features.

- Pulmonary is the main component of drowning
  - Noncardiogenic pulmonary edema
  - Acute respiratory distress syndrome (ARDS) (Chapter 2.6) mainly secondary to aspiration
  - Increased respiratory rate and wheezing
  - CT chest localized, perihilar, or diffuse pulmonary edema
- *Cardiovascular:*
  - Dysrhythmia, ventricular fibrillation, or tachycardia might also be noted
  - Can have coronary artery spasm, takotsubo cardiomyopathy with ST-T changes
- *Neurological:*
  - Hypoxia-related ischemia to brain
  - Raised intracranial pressure (ICP) and cerebral edema
- Metabolic and/or respiratory acidosis
- Electrolyte imbalance
- Renal failure due to acute tubular necrosis (ATN) or rhabdomyolysis
- Hemolysis and coagulopathy
- Infected water can cause sepsis, hence multiple organ dysfunction syndrome (MODS)
- Hypothermia (Chapter 15.2.1)

Caveat: Salt water generally causes cardiac arrest and has worst prognosis

BOX 4: Management.

- *Prehospital care:*
  - Rapid, cautious rescue
  - Cervical spine stabilization
  - Cardiopulmonary resuscitation (CPR) if arrested
  - Transport (all patients)
  - Oxygen (all patients)
- *Emergency room care:*
  - The primary examination involves assessing airway, breathing, circulation, disability [including Glasgow Coma Scale (GCS) assessment], and exposure/environmental factors
  - Assess and manage any associated conditions postexposure, such as hypovolemia, hypothermia, seizures, myocardial infarction, alcoholic intoxication, and acute poisoning
  - **If GCS is >13**
    - Conduct both primary and secondary examinations to rule out spinal or head injuries. Observe the patient for 4–6 hours
  - If oxygen saturations and physical examination are normal, consider safe discharge home
  - If SaO_2 is <95% or abnormal physical findings are present, manage as if GCS is <13
  - **If GCS is <13:**
    - Manage airway with cervical spine stabilization, prioritize breathing and circulation
    - Administer supplemental oxygen to maintain SaO_2 ≥95%
    - Perform endotracheal intubation and provide positive-pressure ventilation as necessary [continuous positive airway pressure (CPAP) and positive end-expiratory pressure (PEEP)]
    - Conduct investigations including chest X-ray (CXR), complete blood count (CBC), electrolytes, glucose, troponin I, prothrombin time (PT)/partial thromboplastin time (PTT), urine analysis (U/A), creatine kinase (CK), urine myoglobin, urine drug screen, and arterial blood gases
    - Monitor body temperature, oxygen saturation, and urine output
    - Implement appropriate measures for ARDS and hypothermia as per respective protocols
    - Address bronchospasm and consider diuretics if edema develops
  - Steroids are of no role in routine use
  - Prophylactically administer antibiotics in cases of exposure to contaminated water
  - Ensure baroprotective measures are applied when using high PEEP to manage excess lung fluid
- Cardiac arrest in drowning to follow algorithm as per hypothermia-induced cardiac arrest (Chapter 15.2.1)

SUGGESTED READING

1. Idris H, Berg RA, Bierens J, Bossaert L, Branche C, Gabrielli A, et al. Drowning Definition and Epidemiology. Recommended guidelines for uniform reporting of data from drowning: the "Utstein style". Circulation. 2003;108(20):2565-74.
2. In: Tintinalli JE, Ma OJ, Yealy DM, Meckler GD, Stapczynski JS, Cline DM, et al. (Eds). Tintinalli's Emergency Medicine: A Comprehensive Study Guide, 9th edition. Mc Graw Hill Education; 2020.
3. Management of drowning. Long-term prognosis, incidence, and cost of drowning. In Bierens JJLM (Ed). Drowning: Prevention, Rescue, Treatment. Springer; 2014. pp. 299-306.
4. Szpilman D, Bierens JJLM, Handley AJ, Orlowski JP. Drowning. Drowning Risk Factors and Clinical Features. N Engl J Med. 2012;366(22):2102-10.
5. Walls RM, Hockberger RS, Gausche-Hill M (Eds). Rosen's Emergency Medicine: Concepts and Clinical Practice. 9th edition. Elsevier; 2018.

15.2.10 High Altitude Disorders

Manali Patel, Sachna P Shetty

BOX 1: Introduction.

- The most common syndromes are:
  - Acute hypoxia
  - Acute mountain sickness (AMS)
  - High altitude pulmonary edema (HAPE)
  - High altitude cerebral edema (HACE)
  - Others include: Retinopathy, altered sleep patterns, neurological symptoms, and peripheral edema
- Contributing factors are individual susceptibility, elevation reached, and the rate of ascent
- Treatment is mainly descent and supplemental oxygen

BOX 2: Acute mountain sickness.

- Acute mountain sickness is a syndrome characterized by headache along with combination of nausea or vomiting, dizziness, fatigue, or sleep disturbance similar to alcohol hangover
- A headache that occurs during ascent, along with any one of the associated symptoms, is sufficient for diagnosing altitude sickness
- The condition is further categorized into mild, moderate, and severe levels using tools like the Lake Louise AMS Self-Questionnaire, which assists in assessing the severity
- **Mild altitude sickness:** Symptoms typically appear within six hours of ascent and include headache, gastrointestinal discomfort, and irritability
- **Treatment:** The primary intervention involves descending to a lower altitude and administering oxygen. To accelerate acclimatization, acetazolamide can be prescribed at a dose of 125–250 mg orally twice a day, analgesics and antiemetics
- **In cases of moderate to severe altitude sickness**, there may be further neurological deterioration, with the risk of developing High Altitude Cerebral Edema (HACE) or High Altitude Pulmonary Edema (HAPE)
- **Immediate treatment:** An urgent descent is crucial to prevent complications
- *Medications:* Acetazolamide at 250 mg taken orally twice daily can aid in acclimatization. Additionally, dexamethasone, administered at 4 mg orally every six hours, may be used to reduce cerebral swelling
- *Additional Interventions:* Hyperbaric therapy can also be employed to simulate a lower altitude and alleviate symptoms
- **For HACE:**
  - *Administer dexamethasone:* Start with 8 mg orally, intramuscularly, or intravenously, followed by 4 mg every six hours
  - If descent is not feasible, hyperbaric therapy can be used to lower the effective altitude and alleviate symptoms
- **For HAPE:**
  - Provide supplemental oxygen as the primary treatment
  - Medications:
    - Nifedipine: 30 mg of extended release taken orally every 12 hours to reduce pulmonary artery pressure.
    - Alternatively, if oxygen or descent is unavailable, use tadalafil: 10 mg orally every 12 hours.
    - Hyperbaric therapy is also recommended if descent is not an option.
  - For Periodic Breathing or Insomnia:
    - Acetazolamide: Administer 62.5–125 mg at bedtime to manage symptoms.

BOX 3: Lake Louise AMS Self-Questionnaire.

Headache:
- No headache—0
- Mild headache—1
- Moderate headache—2
- Severe headache, incapacitating—3

Gastrointestinal (GI) symptoms:
- No symptoms—0
- Poor appetite or nausea—1
- Moderate nausea or vomiting—2
- Severe nausea and vomiting, incapacitating—3

Fatigue/weakness:
- Not tired or weak at all—0
- Mild fatigue or weakness—1
- Moderate fatigue or weakness—2
- Severe fatigue or weakness, incapacitating—3

Dizzy/lightheadedness:
- No dizziness/lightheadedness—0
- Mild dizziness/lightheadedness—1
- Moderate dizziness/lightheadedness—2
- Severely light-headed, fainting/passing out—3

Difficulty sleeping:
- Slept well—0
- Did not sleep as well as usual—1
- Woke many times, poor night's sleep—2
- Could not sleep at all—3

Total symptom score:
- Diagnosis of AMS requires headache plus 1 or more of the above symptoms
- Mild AMS: Score of 2–4
- Moderate AMS: Score of 5–9
- Severe AMS: 10–15

SUGGESTED READING

1. The Lake Louise consensus on the definition and quantification of altitude illness. In: Roach RC, Wagner PD, Hackett PH (Eds). Hypoxia and Mountain Medicine. 1993.
2. Tintinalli JE, Ma OJ, Yealy DM, Meckler GD, Stapczynski JS, Cline DM, et al (Eds). Tintinalli's Emergency Medicine: A Comprehensive Study Guide, 9th edition. Mc Graw Hill Education; 2020.
3. Walls RM, Hockberger RS, Gausche-Hill M (Eds). Rosen's Emergency Medicine: Concepts and Clinical Practice. 9th edition. Elsevier; 2018.

15.3 VACCINATION AND POSTEXPOSURE PROPHYLAXIS IN EMERGENCY ROOM

Sachna P Shetty

BOX 1: Introduction.

- Emergency room (ER) physicians must have a thorough understanding of the protocols for postexposure prophylaxis (PEP) for various vaccine-preventable diseases
- Proper management is critical, as failure to administer PEP appropriately can result in life-threatening outcomes
- This chapter outlines the indications and scheduling for PEP in conditions such as rabies, tetanus, occupational exposures, and certain respiratory illnesses

RABIES

BOX 2: Transmission of virus by animals and site.

Frequent	***Occasionally***	***Not reported***
Dogs	Cats, monkeys, cattle and buffaloes, mongoose, foxes/wolves, jackals, sheep, goats, bears, pigs, donkeys, horses, camels, spotted, and deer and squirrel	Bats, rodents, birds

Common	***Rare***
• Bites from infected animals • Licks on broken skin or mucous membrane • Scratches	• Inhalation • Organ transplantation (cornea) • Ingestion

- *Caveat:* However bats and rodents, if unusual circumstances, need rabies vaccination
- Incubation period 2–3 months but vary depending on the site and amount of inoculation

BOX 3: Rabid bite – grading and treatment.

- Category-based decision to treat
- The most crucial aspect of treatment is wound care, as improper management can lead to infections
- Suturing is covered in a different chapter
- Vaccination is essential, [as detailed in the accompanying box]

Category	***Type of exposure***	***Recommended PEP***
Category I	• Touching or feeding animals, licks on intact skin (i.e., no exposure) • Contact of intact skin with secretions, excretions from rabid animals/human cases	• None or proper washing of exposed areas

Contd...

Contd...

Category II	• Nibbling of uncovered skin, minor scratches or abrasions without bleeding	• Wound care • Rabies vaccination
Category III	• Single or multiple transdermal bites or scratches, contamination of mucous membrane with saliva from licks, licks on broken skin, and exposure to bats	• Wound care rabies vaccination active and passive with immunoglobulin [human rabies immunoglobulin (HRIG)/equine rabies immunoglobulin (ERIG)]

BOX 4: Dose of active and passive immunization.

Active Immunization				
Type of prophylaxis	***Route of administration***	***Dose of vaccine***	***Day of dose***	***Injection per visit***
PEP	Intradermal	0.1 mL/dose	Day 0, 3, 7, and 28	2
	Intramuscular (IM)	1 entire vaccine vial	Day 0, 3, 7, 14, and 28	1
Pre-exposure prophylaxis	Intradermal	0.1 mL/dose	Day 0, 7, 21, and 28	1
	IM	1 entire vaccine vial	Day 0, 7, 21, and 28	1
Re-exposure	Intradermal	0.1 mL	Day 0 and 3	1
	IM	1 vaccine vial	Day 0 and 3	1

- *Passive immunization:* Only one dose is administered because it provides immediate antibodies, and it should be given either immediately or within seven days of the bite.
  - *Nonvaccinated individual in grade 2/3 category bites:*
    - HRIG 20 international unit/kg body weight, on day 0 full dose to infiltrated locally around the wound, remaining dose IM on different site from vaccination
    - ERIG 3.33 IU/kg similar site and day as above
    - Types of vaccine: Human diploid cells, purified chick embryo, and vero cells
  - *Previously vaccinated individual:*
    - No immunoglobulin needs to be given

Caveat:
- **Immunocompromised might need to check antirabies titer to check the efficiency of vaccines**
- **Same dose to be given to pregnant women and children**
- **No disrupting the regimen if mild reaction develops to the vaccine**
- **Vaccination site adults—deltoid only**
- **3–18 years of age—deltoid or anterolateral thigh only if there is no alternative**
- **Less than 2 years anterolateral thigh if deltoid is not adequate**

Caveat:
Preexposure prophylaxis
- **High-risk groups should have their neutralizing antibody titers**
- **A booster would be recommended only if rabies virus-neutralizing antibody titers have dropped to <0.5 IU/mL**

BOX 5: Tetanus vaccination postexposure to injury or soiling.

- *Wound management and immunization:*
  - *Clean minor wounds:*
    - Unknown or less than three doses of tetanus toxoid: Tdap or Td IM and tetanus immunoglobulin (TIG) 250 units IM
    - Three or more doses of tetanus toxoid: No additional immunization required if the last dose was within 10 years
  - *All other wounds:*
    - Unknown or less than three doses of tetanus toxoid: Tdap or Td IM and TIG 250 units IM
    - Three or more doses of tetanus toxoid: Tdap or Td IM if the last dose was >10 years ago; TIG is not required
- *Additional recommendations:*
  - If age is 5–10 years and priming vaccination with booster taken no immunization required
  - If above 11 years and previous vaccination prior to 10 years, immunization is required
  - For children under 7 years, use DTaP or DT
  - For individuals 7 years or older, use Td, with a single booster dose of Tdap recommended for adolescents and adults
  - During pregnancy, Tdap should be administered during each pregnancy, preferably between 27 and 36 weeks gestation
  - Adverse reactions include erythema, induration, and pain at the injection site. Severe reactions may occur in adults with high serum tetanus antitoxin levels
- *Contraindications:*
  - History of serious allergic, neurological reactions, or severe illness attributable to the vaccine within 7 days
  - Consider passive immunization with TIG if tetanus toxoid is contraindicated

BOX 6: Definition.

Occupational hazards:

- The US Occupational Safety and Health Administration defines occupational exposure as a "reasonably anticipated skin, eye, mucous membrane, or parenteral contact with blood or other potentially infectious materials that may result from the performance of the employee's duties"
- Healthcare workers should treat all bodily secretions, fluids, and tissues as potentially infectious

BOX 7: Protocols for management of exposures to blood or body fluids.

- Do not squeeze or suck blood out if needle prick
- Irrigate and wash wounds with soap and water
- Medical evaluation in the emergency room (ER)
- Obtain history regarding type of exposure, source patient and vaccination, and history of exposed person **(Box 3)**
- Obtain blood samples for laboratory studies (using consents when required) from exposed person like hepatitis B/C, HIV for baseline
- If needle prick by a known source of human immunodeficiency virus (HIV)/ hepatitis B surface antigen (HBsAg)/hepatitis C virus (HCV), also send complete blood count (CBC), liver function tests, hepatitis B virus (HBV) DNA viral load, consider urine pregnancy test for women of childbearing potential
- Order laboratory studies from source patient if known, like HHH (using consents when required)
- Determine need for tetanus immunization **(Box 5)**
- Determine need for hepatitis B PEP **(Box 9)**
- Determine need for human immunodeficiency virus PEP and mechanism **(Box 9)** for dosing as rapidly as possible
- Counsel exposed person regarding risk of specific blood borne pathogens and discuss risks/benefits of available treatment options

BOX 8: Recommendations for needle stick injury/body fluid exposure report.

- Document the date and time of exposure
- Detail the procedure being performed and the device used
- Describe the type and amount of fluid or material, and the severity of the exposure
- Provide details about the exposure source and the exposed person

Caveat:

- For unknown source, consider exposure to high-risk source

BOX 9: Postexposure prophylaxis (PEP) for hepatitis B.

Vaccination/ antibody status of worker	***Source is HBsAg positive***	***Source is HBsAg negative***	***Source status unknown/ unavailable***
Unvaccinated/ nonimmune	Administer hepatitis B immunoglobulin (HBIG) once and start HB vaccine series	Start HB vaccine series	Start HB vaccine series
Previously vaccinated			
Known responder	No treatment required	No treatment required	No treatment required
Unknown antibody response	Test for anti-HBs	No treatment required if adequate; if inadequate, administer HBIG once and a vaccine booster	Test for anti-HBs; if adequate, no treatment; if inadequate, administer vaccine booster and recheck titer after 1–2 months

BOX 10: Need for HIV prophylaxis on basis of Risk Assessment Stratification Protocol (RASP) score.

When to use?

High- vs. low-risk exposure, helps determine whether or not to start PEP

- *Source population:*
  - Known HIV + acute AIDS +1
  - Known HIV + asymptomatic HIV +10
  - Unknown HIV status, high-risk situation +100
  - Unknown HIV status, low-risk situation +1,000
- *Inoculum type:*
  - Fresh blood +1
  - Other high-risk fluid (semen) +10
  - Dried old blood +100
  - Low-risk secretion (saliva, tears, urine) +1,000
- *Method of transmission:*
  - Intravenous +1
  - Deep IM +10
  - Deep transcutaneous with visible bleeding +100
  - Superficial transcutaneous without bleeding +200
  - Mucosal contact only +500
  - Intact skin +1,000
- *Volume of inoculum:*
  - Massive (transfusion) +100
  - Measurable >1 mL +10
  - Moderate; large bore, hollow needle >22 g +5
  - Small hollow needle <22 g +3
  - Trace surface only suture needle +1
  - Interpretation:
    - Basic risk = 1/(source population × inoculum type × method of transmission)
    - Total risk = Basic risk × volume of inoculum
    - 1/1,000—PEP definitely indicated
    - 1/1,000–1/10,000—recommended but optional
    - 1/10,001–1/100,000—optional
    - 1/100,000—not indicated

BOX 11: HIV PEP regimens.

Preferred HIV PEP regimen (tenofovir DF 300 mg + emtricitabine 200 mg once daily) *plus* raltegravir (400 mg twice daily) or dolutegravir (50 mg once daily)

Duration: 28 days
Alternative regimens: May combine one drug or drug pair from the left column with one drug or drug pair from the right column

Prescribers unfamiliar with these agents/regimens should consult with a physician familiar with these agents and their toxicities

• Raltegravir • Dolutegravir • Darunavir + Ritonavir • Etravirine • Rilpivirine • Atazanavir + Ritonavir • Lopinavir/ritonavir	• Tenofovir disoproxil fumarate + emtricitabine • Tenofovir disoproxil fumarate + lamivudine • Zidovudine + lamivudine • Zidovudine emtricitabine

Other alternative antiretroviral regimens should be used for PEP only with expert consultation

BOX 12: Prophylaxis for needle stick injury with HCV exposure.

Evaluation and testing:
- *Baseline testing:* Test the exposed individual for HCV antibodies (anti-HCV) and liver function tests
- *Source patient testing:* If the source is known, test them for HCV RNA and anti-HCV to determine if they are actively infected

Postexposure management:
- *No immediate prophylaxis:* Currently, there is no effective PEP for HCV
- *Monitoring:* Conduct follow-up testing for HCV RNA at 4–6 weeks postexposure to detect early infection. Test for anti-HCV at 4–6 months postexposure if earlier RNA testing is not performed
- *Consult specialist:* If the exposed person is found to be HCV RNA positive, refer them to a specialist for further evaluation and potential treatment

Counseling and support:
- *Inform exposed person:* Educate the exposed individual about the signs and symptoms of HCV infection, such as jaundice, fatigue, abdominal pain, loss of appetite, nausea, and vomiting
- *Supportive care:* Provide psychological support and counseling as needed

Conclusion: While there is no specific prophylactic treatment for HCV after a needle stick injury, immediate wound care, proper evaluation, and regular monitoring are crucial for early detection and management of potential HCV infection

BOX 13: Vaccination for high-risk infectious disease in health care providers.

- *Tuberculosis:* Airborne—no recommended vaccine
- *Measles:* Airborne—two doses of the vaccine are recommended for previously unvaccinated individuals (helpful if vaccine administered within 72 hours of exposure)
- *Varicella:* Respiratory and contact precautions—vaccination is recommended, works best if given within 4 days of exposure, and postexposure management includes quarantine for exposed employees
- *Influenza:* Respiratory and droplet—annual vaccination is recommended, with chemoprophylaxis for high-risk employees after exposure withy oseltamivir or zanamivir in higher-risk employees
- *Meningococcus:* Respiratory and droplet—chemoprophylaxis for those with high-risk exposure, such as mouth-to-mouth contact without a mask
- In the setting of confirmed meningococcus:
  - Rifampin 10 mg/kg (maximum 600 mg/dose) every 12 hours for 2 days
  - Ceftriaxone 250 mg in single dose
  - Ciprofloxacin 500 mg in single

Conclusion: Proper knowledge and implementation of PEP protocols for vaccine-preventable diseases are essential for ER physicians to protect patients and healthcare workers from potentially life-threatening infections

SUGGESTED READING

1. Advisory Committee on Immunization Practices. (2021). Immunization Recommendations for Healthcare Workers. [online] Available from https://www.cdc.gov/MMWR/preview/mmwrhtml/00050577.htm [Last accessed September, 2024].
2. American Association for the Study of Liver Diseases. (2020). HCV Guidelines: Recommendations for Testing, Managing, and Treating Hepatitis C. [online] Available from https://www.hcvguidelines.org/ [Last accessed September, 2024].
3. Centers for Disease Control and Prevention. (2021). Tetanus Vaccination Guidelines. [online] Available from https://www.cdc.gov/vaccines/vpd/tetanus/index.html [Last accessed September, 2024].
4. Centers for Disease Control and Prevention. (2021). Updated U.S. Public Health Service Guidelines for the Management of Occupational Exposures to HIV and Recommendations for Postexposure Prophylaxis. [online] Available from https://www.cdc.gov/mmwr/preview/mmwrhtml/rr5409a1.htm [Last accessed September, 2024].
5. Occupational Safety and Health Administration. (2020). Occupational Exposure to Blood-borne Pathogens: Final Rule. [online] Available from https://www.osha.gov/laws-regs/federalregister/1991-12-06 [Last accessed September, 2024].
6. World Health Organization. (2018). Rabies: Surveillance, prevention and control. [online] Available from https://www.who.int/rabies/resources/who_hse_see_2018.03/en/ [Last accessed September, 2024].

CHAPTER 16

Oncological Emergency

16.1 MEDICAL ONCOLOGICAL EMERGENCIES

Anjana Sainani

PARANEOPLASTIC SYNDROMES

BOX 1: Definition.

- Endocrine-mediated secretion of bioactive substances by the tumor

BOX 2: Syndrome of inappropriate antidiuretic hormone (SIADH).

Syndrome of inappropriate antidiuretic hormone (SIADH):

Underlying cancer	• Small cell lung cancer, aerodigestive tract tumors, nonsmall cell lung cancer, breast cancer, and lymphomas
Diagnostic criteria	• Euvolemic hypotonic hyponatremia: Urine osmolarity >100 mOsm with corresponding serum sodium levels: – Mild: 130–134 mEq/dL – Moderate: 125–129 mEq/dL – Severe: <125 mEq/dL
Symptoms	• Severe hyponatremia can lead to headaches, cognitive slowing, seizures, and even death
Differential diagnosis	• Hypovolemic hyponatremia due to excessive gastrointestinal losses where urine osmolarity >300 mOsm but urine sodium <20 mEq/L
Management	• Infuse intravenously 100 mL 3% NS bolus to acutely raise serum sodium by 2–3 mEq/L. Total increase of serum sodium by no >4–6 mEq/L in 24 hours to avoid central pontine myelinolysis • Free water restriction

BOX 3: Paraneoplastic hypercalcemia.

Paraneoplastic hypercalcemia:

Hypercalcemia in malignancy is due to either of the following:

- Tumor-based parathyroid hormone-related protein secretion

Underlying cancer	• Squamous cell cancers, renal cell cancer, gynecologic malignancies, breast cancer, and some lymphomas or • Secretion of ectopic vitamin D or parathyroid hormone • Osteolytic metastases in breast cancer and multiple myeloma
Diagnostic criteria	• Serum calcium levels: – Mild: 10.5–11.9 mg/dL – Moderate: 12.0–13.9 mg/dL – Severe: ≥14.0 mg/dL • In patients with hypoalbuminemia, observed serum calcium must be further increased by 0.8* (4.0 – serum albumin) mg/dL
Symptoms	• Altered mental status • Generalized muscle weakness • Constipation due to generalized slowing of central, peripheral, and autonomic nervous systems • Dehydration with ensuing acute kidney injury • Urolithiasis can be observed with subacute presentations
Management	• Immediate aggressive intravenous hydration with normal saline, 1–2 L in the first hour followed by 2 L at 200 mL/hour with close monitoring of volume status • Intravenous bisphosphonate administration (Zolendronic acid) • Calcitonin administered during the first 48 hours • Denosumab (monoclonal antibody inhibitor of osteoclast activity) in bisphosphonate-refractory cases • Loop diuretics avoidable as they can exacerbate hypercalcemia and kidney injury in inadequately hydrated patients

BOX 4: Ectopic adrenocorticotropic hormone syndrome.

Ectopic adrenocorticotropic hormone syndrome:

Underlying cancer	• Small cell lung cancer and bronchial carcinoid, tumors with neuroendocrine differentiation such as small cell prostate tumors, upper gastrointestinal neuroendocrine tumors
Symptoms	• Acute severe hypertension • Hypokalemia and associated muscle weakness • Generalized edema
Management	• Acute management of electrolyte disturbances and hypertensive crisis • Ketoconazole and metyrapone (inhibit steroid genesis)

BOX 5: Tumor lysis syndrome.

Tumor lysis syndrome:

Underlying cancers	• High-grade non-Hodgkin lymphoma (NHL), acute lymphoblastic leukemia, Burkitt lymphoma, leukemia, and chronic lymphocytic leukemia (CLL) and nonhematological malignancies with high tumor burden such as breast cancer, small cell carcinoma, neuroblastoma, germ-cell tumors, medulloblastoma, ovarian, and others
Diagnostic criteria	• Serum levels of uric acid >8 mg/dL • Potassium >6 mEq/L • Phosphorus >6.5 mg/dL in children and >4.5 mg/dL in adults • Calcium <7 mg/dL or, • A 25% change in these values or ≥2 abnormal values seen within 3 days before or 7 days after initiation of cytotoxic chemotherapy
Management	• Aggressive hydration with crystalloid improves renal perfusion and glomerular filtration as well as reduces uric acid or calcium phosphate crystallization and tubular deposition • Hyperkalemia destabilizes myocardial and other muscular conductivity and can trigger nausea, numbness, heart palpitations, arrhythmias, seizures, and possible sudden death • Continuous cardiac monitoring and re-evaluation of serum electrolytes, creatinine, and uric acid every 4 hours track the clinical course • Both uric acid and calcium phosphate can precipitate in the renal tubules to trigger an intrarenal acute kidney injury • In patients with urine output <2 mL/kg/hour, a loop diuretic may be considered • Flank pain raises concern for ureteral stones • Allopurinol reduces the formation of uric acid and is prophylactically administered to at-risk patients • Rasburicase metabolizes uric acid and is the preferred medication for extreme hyperuricemia; 0.2 mg/kg is initially administered with repeated dosing as necessary but should be avoided in patients with *G6PD* deficiency because it can lead to methemoglobinemia and hemolysis

BOX 6: Febrile neutropenia.

Febrile neutropenia:

Diagnostic criteria	• A single oral temperature measured at ≥38.3°C (101°F) or a temperature of ≥38.0°C (100.4°F) sustained over a 1-hour period combined with severe neutropenia, defined as an absolute neutrophil count (ANC) <500 cells/mm^3 or an ANC that is expected to decrease to <500 cells/mm^3 during the next 48 hours • Hypotension, dehydration, mucositis, recent history of cytotoxic chemotherapy, indwelling central venous catheter, breathlessness, and cough without expectoration
Management	• Initiate intravenous antibiotic therapy <1–3 hours after presenting at emergency room as there can be a fast progression to hypotensive shock • Immediately send blood cultures aerobic, anaerobic, and fungal (peripheral and from in-dwelling lines), a chest X-ray and a complete blood count and start IV antibiotics • Empiric monotherapy with an antipseudomonal β-lactam (piperacillin-tazobactum 4.5 g IV 6 hourly or cefepime 2 g IV 8 hourly) is recommended with the following exceptions: – Carbapenems (meropenem 1 g IV 8 hourly or imipenem-cilastin 500 mg IV 6 hourly for patients with a high risk of infection by an extended-spectrum β-lactamase-expressing organism) – Polymyxin-colistin in patients at high risk for a carbapenemase-producing *Klebsiella* – Aztreonam, fluoroquinolones, or aminoglycosides for patients with an anaphylactic β-lactam allergy – Vancomycin, linezolid, or daptomycin for methicillin-resistant *Staphylococcus aureus (MRSA)* or indwelling catheter infections are suspected and should be discontinued, if cultures are negative • Empiric antifungal coverage is not recommended at the time of presentation however to start upfront in patients with prolonged, profound neutropenia, invasive fungal disease markers positive • Empiric therapy begun after 4–7 days of persistent fevers and no apparent bacterial source with • Echinocandins being the preferred choice • The Multinational Association for Supportive Care in Cancer (MASCC) criteria defines patients with scores ≥21 as low-risk patients safe for emergency room (ER) discharge and outpatient management with appropriate regimens comprised of broad-spectrum β-lactams combined with a fluoroquinolone • Renal replacement therapy may be required for severe kidney injury or persistent electrolyte abnormalities

BOX 7: Hemorrhagic cystitis.

Hemorrhagic cystitis	• Bleeding into urinary bladder is primarily microscopic; however, persistent bleeding can precipitate intravascular blood clot formation with subsequent urinary tract obstruction
Management	• Blood transfusion to correct anemia • Continuous bladder irrigation using a large-bore, three-way catheter with saline infusion

SUGGESTED READING

1. Cairo MS, Bishop M. Tumour lysis syndrome: new therapeutic strategies and classification. Br J Haematol. 2004;127:3-11.
2. Daniels LM, Durani U, Barreto JN, O'Horo JC, Siddiqui MA, Park JG, et al. Impact of time to antibiotic on hospital stay, intensive care unit admission, and mortality in febrile neutropenia. Support Care Cancer. 2019;27:4171-7.
3. Gould Rothberg BE, Quest TE, Yeung SJ, Pelosof LC, Gerber DE, Seltzer JA, et al. Oncologic emergencies and urgencies: A comprehensive review. Ca Cancer J Clin. 2022;72:570-93.
4. Zimmer AJ, Freifeld AG. Optimal management of neutropenic fever in patients with cancer. J Oncol Pract. 2019;15:19-24.

16.2 SURGICAL ONCOLOGICAL EMERGENCIES

Mehul S Bhansali, Snehal A Bhange

BOX 1: Introduction.

- An oncologic emergency is defined as an acute, potentially life-threatening condition in a cancer patient that has developed as a result of the malignant disease or its treatment. Many oncologic emergencies are signs of advanced and end-stage malignant disease
- This write up is nowhere exhaustive, but it seeks to provide a basis for approach to any patient presenting with some emergency and how to manage that effectively

BOX 2: The most common presentation of surgical complications in gastrointestinal (GI) tract malignancy.

- The most common emergency that we see in our day-to-day practice is the *obstruction of the GI tract secondary to a malignancy*. The presentation may be in a patient who is a known case of malignancy undergoing neoadjuvant treatment, or it may be a de novo presentation with an obstructive malignancy. The obstruction may be at the gastric outlet level, small intestine or the large intestine
- The other mode of presentation we may encounter is an episode of severe *GI bleed*, either hematemesis (vomiting of fresh blood or coffee ground vomitus) or lower GI bleed (hematochezia/fresh per rectum (PR) bleed or black tarry stools/melena)
- A few patients may even present to us with severe *abdominal pain* of a few days duration. These patients may have an obstructing malignancy which was initially misdiagnosed or ignored, eventually leading to a perforation peritonitis
- It has been observed that such patients present to the emergency room with sepsis and acute renal failure; initially misdiagnosed in the peripheral hospitals and referred to us as a case of renal failure. A detail history and physical examination have revealed the true nature of the disease
- Patients presenting to the emergency room with complications of malignancy as a first presentation usually have a poorer prognosis than if they had presented earlier in the stage of disease (Vandyk AD, et al., 2012)
- Majority of these patients may also need intervention either surgical or radiological or ICU admission which adds to the morbidity and mortality
- A high index of suspicion should be entertained when any patient >50 years if age comes to the emergency room with gradually progressive abdominal pain associated with nausea, vomiting, symptoms of constipation or obstipation and/or recent onset of bleeding per rectum
- A detailed history should be taken of such patients. Patients presenting to the OPD with gradually progressive dysphagia may also then present to the emergency room with severe chest pain, respiratory distress, subcutaneous emphysema with or without sepsis, suggestive of a perforated esophageal malignancy
- A detailed history and physical examination, ably supported by laboratory investigations and appropriate imaging, can guide the diagnosis and management for such patients

BOX 3: Management.

- The primary management of these patients is emergency resuscitation, ventilatory support if needed, imaging studies and laboratory tests to arrive at a diagnosis. Depending on the patient's condition, intervention radiology, endoscopy services, or surgical intervention may then be required
- In cases of advanced malignancies, palliation may be the only way ahead and this should be discussed openly with the next of kin and immediate caregivers
- All treatment must be tailored based on patient's age, physiological reserve, nutritional status and performance score
- Patients with left-sided colonic malignancies presenting with obstruction may be offered self-expanding metal stent (SEMS) as the primary treatment with further staging after recovering from the acute episode
- Primary resectional surgery in the emergency setting has high chances of stoma formation which may or may be reversed in the future
- Stenting has been shown to reduce morbidity and no difference in stoma rates with future definitive surgery (CReST Collaborative Group, 2022)
- Right-sided colonic malignancies presenting with bleeding or obstruction may benefit with emergency surgery where resection with primary anastomosis is feasible. Small bowel obstruction necessarily needs resection in view of high possibility of perforation peritonitis
- Patients of gastric malignancies, presenting with gastrointestinal (GI) bleed may benefit from interventional radiology for bleeding source rather than surgery
- Patients presenting with gastric outlet obstruction may safely proceed to various types of gastrectomies based on tumor location and staging
- Patients with esophageal malignancies may present with obstruction, bleeding, perforation, some may even come to us with respiratory distress
- Most of the patients with obstruction may benefit from stenting which allows them to have liquids orally to maintain nutrition
- In highly constrictive tumors, feeding enterostomy may be considered with palliative radiotherapy
- Patients presenting with perforation and sepsis pose a diagnostic challenge
- Patients with duodenal or pancreatic malignancies may present with *cholangitis* and sepsis and palliation for the obstruction and jaundice both are emergency situations needing specialized interventional radiology and gastroenterology support

BOX 4: The most common presentation of complications secondary to aerodigestive tract and head and neck malignancies.

- Upper *aerodigestive tract and head neck malignancies* are quite common in India and we encounter many such patients in our practice
- Most of the head, neck, and oral malignancy patients present to OPD and are either undergoing chemoradiotherapy postsurgery or as primary treatment modality in view of inoperability
- A few present with recurrence and are undergoing palliative treatment for the same. These patients can present to the OPD with *acute airway obstruction, severe bleeding, or sepsis*

Management: First choice in case of airway obstruction is endotracheal intubation, which, if not possible then can consider for cricothyroidotomy or tracheostomy (Chapter 2). Patients may present with severe bleeding and need acute surgical or radiological intervention

BOX 5: The most common presentation of complication post lung cancer.

- Patients of lung cancer may present to us with acute severe *hemoptysis* or severe bleeding, airway obstruction, or massive pleural effusion (hemothorax) compromising ventilation (details in Chapter 2)
- Interventional bronchoscopy and radiology, if available in house, are the first-line management options and such patients may still be amenable to surgical resections after primary resuscitation and staging
- Even though there are no definite guidelines for oncosurgical emergencies, our treatment should be based on the patient's performance score
- In India, where the cost of cancer treatment is out of reach to a majority of population even today, sometimes palliation (Chapter 23) may be the best treatment we can offer

SUGGESTED READING

1. Astin M, Griffin T, Neal RD, Rose P, Hamilton W. The diagnostic value of symptoms for colorectal cancer in primary care: a systematic review. Br J Gen Pract. 2011;61(586):e231-43.
2. Biondo S, Martí-Ragué J, Kreisler E, Parés D, Martín A, Navarro M, et al. A prospective study of outcomes of emergency and elective surgeries for complicated colonic cancer. Am J Surg. 2005;189:377-83.
3. CReST Collaborative Group. Colorectal Endoscopic Stenting Trial (CReST) for obstructing left-sided colorectal cancer: randomized clinical trial. Br J Surg. 2022;109(11):1073-80.
4. Sheibani S, Kim JJ, Chen B, Park S, Saberi B, Keyashian K, et al. Natural history of acute upper GI bleeding due to tumours: short-term success and long-term recurrence with or without endoscopic therapy. Aliment Pharmacol Ther. 2013;38(2):144-50.
5. Tuca A, Codorniu N, Garzón, Serrano G. Malignant bowel obstruction due to advanced cancer in palliative care: Observational and descriptive study. Trodheim, Norway: 5th Research Forum of European Association for Palliative Care; 2008.
6. Vandyk AD, Harrison MB, Macartney G, Ross-White A, Stacey D. Emergency department visits for symptoms experienced by oncology patients: a systematic review. Support Care Cancer. 2012;20(8):1589-99.

CHAPTER 17

Eye Emergencies

Phiroze Patel, Janhvi Mehta

BOX 1: Red eye in emergency room.

At presentation note the following:

- Mild or severe congestion, pain present, discharge present, lid swelling
- Obvious white opacity in the cornea
- Loss of vision
- Injury to the eye or foreign body sensation

Management:

- Mild redness–viral–nonsteroidal anti-inflammatory drop (e.g., Nevanac eye drops)
- Redness with discharge—bacterial infection, advice antibiotic drops (e.g., Toba eye drops)
- Severe pain and lid swelling—could be iritis, acute glaucoma, or other conditions
- If below 7 years of age—preorbital cellulitis is a strong possibility and it is an emergency. Refer to ophthalmologists or immediately to the pediatrician as intravenous antibiotics will be required
- If associated with corneal involvement, the eye can be stained with fluorescein in dye to check if it stains green in color then it suggests active inflammation of the cornea, give antibiotic drops and refer to ophthalmologists
- If a foreign body is seen on the cornea, place a drop of local anesthetic and remove it with a cotton bud, if not possible refer to ophthalmologists
- Acid or alkali burns on presentation do copious saline irrigation, antibiotic eye drops and refer to ophthalmologists
- Subconjunctival hemorrhage—eye looks red, no congestion, no discharge, and no history of trauma then check blood pressure, ask for history of severe cough or constipation. They take 7–10 days to disappear
- Keep eye drops, fluorescein in staining strips, and cotton buds in the ophthalmologists
- Do remember it is safe to use anti-inflammatory or antibiotic eye drops but do not use steroid-based eye drops

BOX 2: Trauma to the eye.

Severe trauma to face and eye	• Ask for nature of the injury, carefully look at the eye • Do not apply pressure on the eye, to prevent prolapse of its content. The lids and surrounding to be examined and noted • Blunt, penetrating, perforating injuries, and foreign bodies, patch the eye and refer to ophthalmologists
Painless sudden loss of vision	• Take history of systemic illness • Note diabetes, hypertension and blood dyscrasias can cause retinal venous and arteriolar occlusions leading to loss of vision • Severe pain above the eyebrow, look for dilated blood vessels on skin, as giant cell arteritis could be the cause (age 60 years and above). High erythrocyte sedimentation rate (ESR) confirms the clinical suspicion • Complaints of flashes of light and black shadows. Retinal detachment is a possibility refers to ophthalmologists
Acute glaucoma	• Age group of 50 years and above, loss of vision with a very red painful eye and severe headache • Loss of vision • May occur in the evenings while watching television • Intraocular pressure will be very high (>50 mm Hg) • Diamox tablets two stat and even a mannitol drip started and a painkiller • Take advice from ophthalmologists
Uveitis	• Iritis is inflammation of the iris presenting as circumcorneal congestion with pain and reduced vision • Start painkiller, speak to the eye doctor before starting steroid eye drops

BOX 3: Most common used drugs.

Class	***Common drug***	***Indication***	***Dosage***
Mydriatic-cycloplegic	Tropicamide	• Short term for examination • Contraindicated in glaucoma	1–2 drops 20 minutes duration 6 hours action
Antihistamine	Olopatadine	Allergic conjunctivitis	1 drop twice daily
Mast cell stabilizer	Nedocromil sodium (Alocril)	Allergic conjunctivitis	1–2 drops twice daily
Anesthetic	Tetracaine/ proparacaine	For foreign body removal or procedure	1–2 drops 30 seconds to 1 minute onset
Antibiotic	• Ciprofloxacin • Moxifloxacin	Conjunctivitis and corneal abrasion	• 1–2 drops 4 hourly • 1–2 drops twice a day
Lubricant	Tear/refresh	Dryness	

SUGGESTED READING

1. Salmon JF. Kanski's Clinical Ophthalmology, 10th edition. Amsterdam: Elsevier; 2024.

CHAPTER 18

ENT Emergencies

Divya Prabhat

BOX 1: Wax.

- Complaints of earache, ear blockage, or reduced hearing **(Fig. 1)**
- Oral analgesics are enough
- Removal done by wax hook or any curved instrument
- Syringing the ear **(Fig. 2)** with 20cc syringe directed in the upward-backward direction
- Wax dissolving drops advised if incomplete removal of wax after the procedure. Analgesic and anti-inflammatory agents are given if pain persists

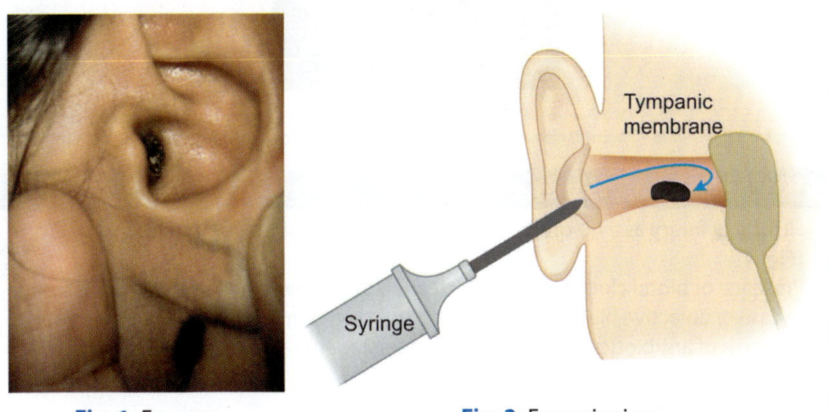

Fig. 1: Ear wax.

Fig. 2: Ear syringing.

BOX 2: Otitis externa.

- Earache which gets aggravated on pulling the pinna **(Fig. 3)**
- Ear canal is narrow and discharge is seen. Specifically enquire about diabetes as in these patients fungal infections are very common and of severe nature, therefore referred as malignant otitis externa
- Analgesics with local anesthetic drops advised. Antibiotic/antifungal drops advised depending on the clinical findings

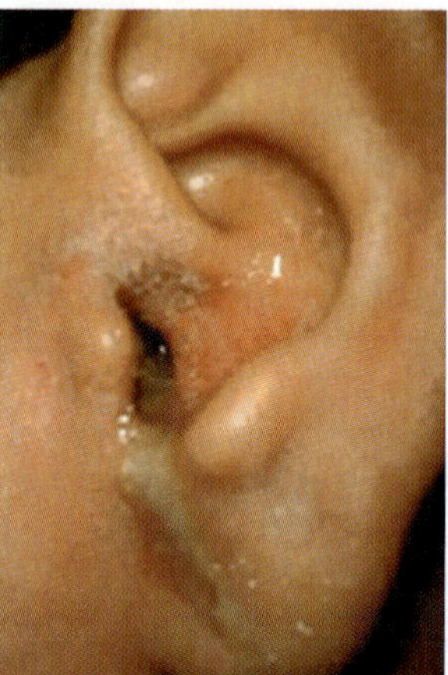

Fig. 3: Otitis externa.

BOX 3: Tympanic membrane rupture.

- History of injury as a hit on the ear, instrumentation of the ear, scuba diving, etc. **(Fig. 4)**
- Presence of blood clots needs to be cleaned to examine the tympanic membrane
- In case of an active bleed, just keep a cotton plug or gel-foam piece in the canal
- A course of antibiotics and anti-inflammatory agents are advised
- No ear drops to be given

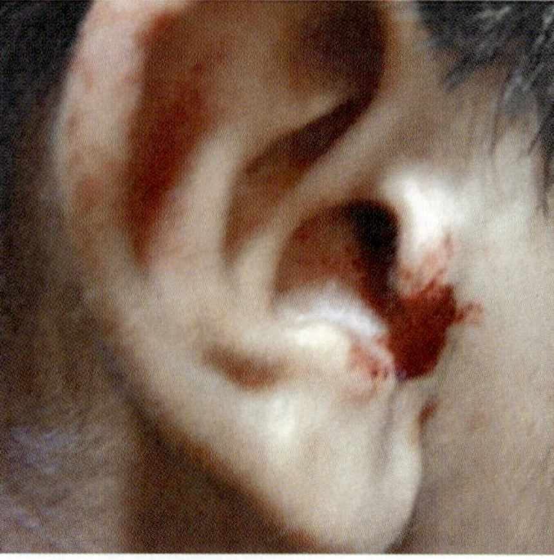

Fig. 4: Ear bleed.

BOX 4: Acute otitis media.

- Severe earache, which is unilateral with a preceding respiratory tract infection. It is the most common cause of a crying child coming to a hospital emergency **(Fig. 5)**
- Examine the respiratory tract for focus of infection viz. tonsils and for sinusitis
- Advise antibiotics, analgesics, nasal-decongestants, and local anesthetic ear drops
- Headache, vomiting, facial weakness, and dizziness may need a myringotomy

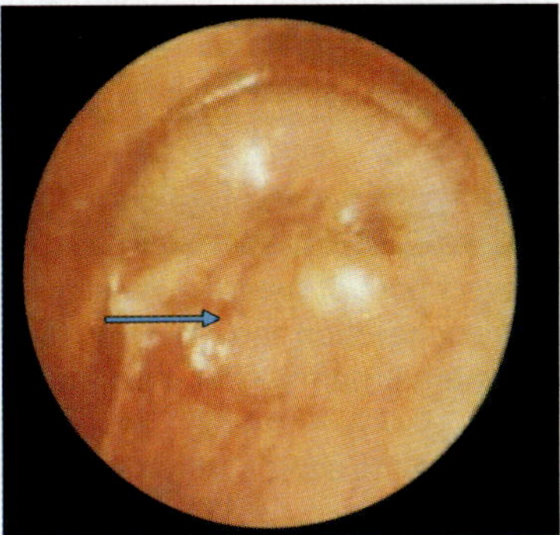

Fig. 5: Bulging tympanic membrane.

BOX 5: Epistaxis.

- Bleeding may be unilateral or bilateral and need to stop the active bleed.
- Lower part of the nose is pinched between two fingers for 5 minutes to stop the bleed. Ice compresses are applied on either sides of the nose, if not then pack the nose with gel-foam or then may need to do anterior nasal packing with Netcell/ Merocel. The throat is examined for any postnasal bleeding, which if present will require a postnasal pack (Foley's catheter) if history of hypertension. Monitoring the blood pressure is essential if history of hypertension. Renal or hepatic conditions are to be noted and accordingly managed
- Stopping any active bleeding is of prime concern. Intravenous (IV) fluids, tranexamic acid, antihypertensive agents, and sedatives.
- *Caveat:*
  - Avoid the usage of adrenaline soaked gauge pieces packed into the nose as the blood pressure (BP) will rise further
  - Pinch nostrils to stop nose bleed **(Fig. 6)**

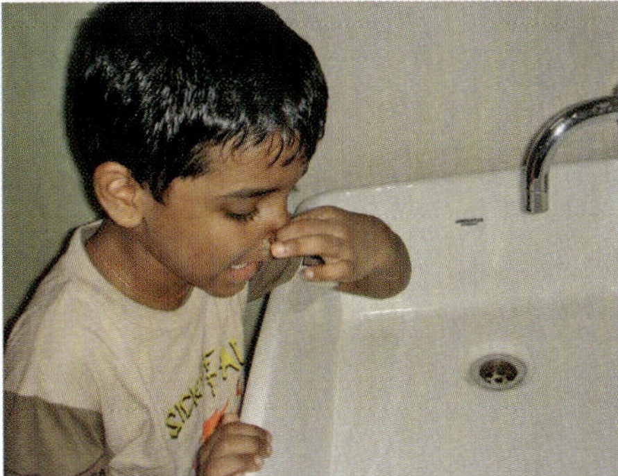

Fig. 6: Epistaxis.

BOX 6: Sinusitis.

- Patients come with headaches, fullness over the face, nasal blockage, nasal discharge, voice changes, fever, or cough which worsens on lying down
- On nasal examination see for nasal congestion, pus from the middle meatus and a postnasal drip; along with tenderness at the canine fossa over the maxillary sinus
- A CT scan of the paranasal sinuses (plain) is diagnostic
- Rule out migraine, dental neuralgia, temporomandibular neuralgia, etc.
- Manage with antibiotics, analgesics, antihistamines, and nasal decongestants
- An X-ray or CT scan of the paranasal sinuses will be diagnostic

BOX 7: Allergic rhinitis.

- Patients present with a severe bout of sneezing, nasal discharge, and nasal block
- May be associated with eye congestion and wheezing (asthma)
- Patient is given nasal drops, antihistamine's, and depending upon the severity a bolus of steroids
- Always one needs to auscultate the chest as this is one airway-one disease condition **(Fig. 7)**

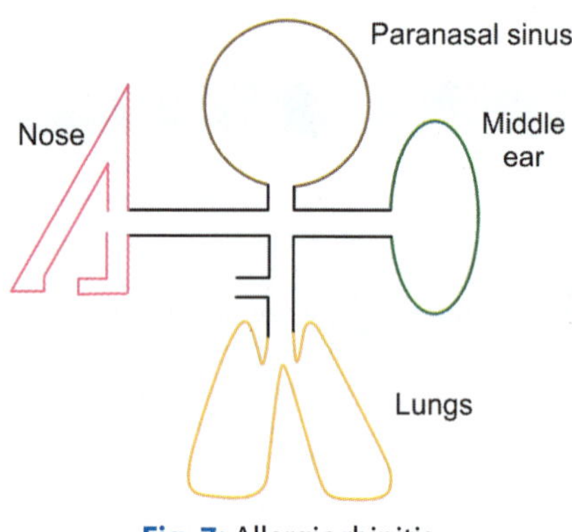

Fig. 7: Allergic rhinitis.

BOX 8: Septal hematoma.

- Complaints of complete nasal block, pain, headaches, and fever
- History of injury, surgery performed or nose picking
- On examination both the nostrils septum shows a bulge and anterior rhinoscopy is not possible
- The septal hematoma needs to be drained immediately as delay results in cartilage resorption and a permanent nasal deformity **(Fig. 8)**

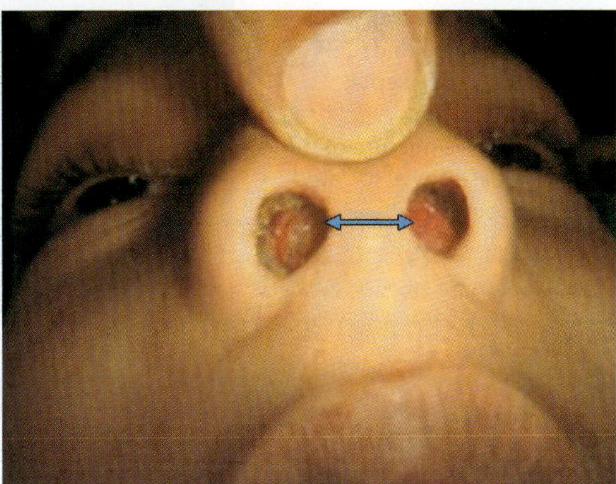

Fig. 8: Septal hematoma.

BOX 9: Unilateral facial swelling.

- The patients present as an acute presentation and a detailed history need to be taken
- Clinical examination an external injury or an insect bite, vesicles in the external auditory canal as herpes zoster oticus, infra-auricular swelling, i.e., parotid gland tenderness, furunculosis on the nasal vestibule, or any gingivitis or dental/gingival infections on the involved side
- For reducing the edema a bolus of steroids can be given, antibiotics, anti-inflammatory agents, and any pointing abscess can drained
- Associated facial palsy will require physiotherapy and care of the eye too

BOX 10: Fracture nasal bone.

- Always a history of fall or an injury is present
- Clinical signs of blood clots, swelling, and tenderness over the nose are noted
- Firstly, any active bleeding is stopped and vital parameters need to be checked
- Then examine for associated complications viz. active postnasal bleeding, eye movement is tested for orbital injury, nose is examined for cerebrospinal fluid (CSF) rhinorrhea and septum for any septal hematoma **(Fig. 9)**
- X-rays are done to confirm a fracture of the nasal bones and CT in case any associated complications are suspected

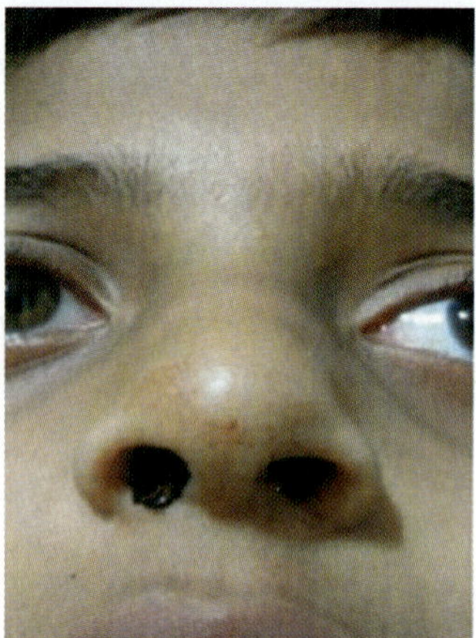

Fig. 9: Fracture nasal bone.

BOX 11: Foreign body.

- **Ear foreign bodies** are removed by syringing or using a hook-shaped instrument. Syringing the ear is done with patient in the sitting position (to avoid a vasovagal attack), water used is always at body temperature, and direction of fluid is upward and backward
- **Nose foreign bodies** are removed by passing a hockey shaped instrument, by carefully going beyond the object and gradually bringing it out. One needs to be very careful and prevent further slipping of the foreign body toward the nasopharynx. Impacted foreign bodies or rhinolith will require general anesthesia for removal **(Fig. 10)**

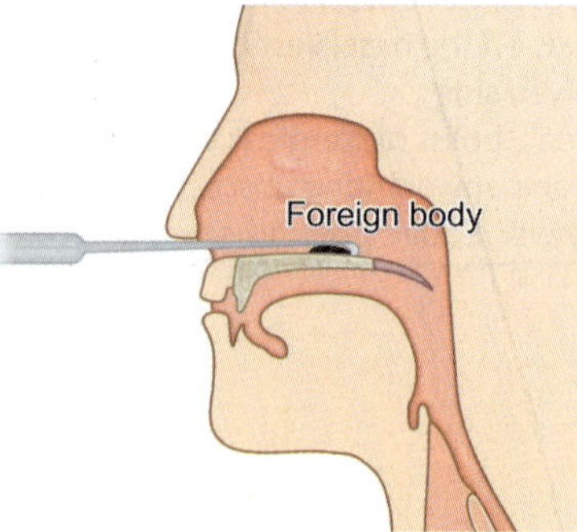

Fig. 10: Foreign body in nose.

BOX 12: Foreign body in left bronchus.

- Foreign bodies in the airway need urgent attention
- Clinical assessment along with oxygen saturations need to be monitored, nasal oxygen may be required, clinical signs for distress noted and the radiological assessment is done
- In worsening conditions an endotracheal intubation or SOS a tracheotomy could be required
- Various heroic procedures of removal of foreign bodies should be avoided in as can dislodge them from the bronchus to the subglottis or from the cricopharynx to the laryngeal inlet **(Figs. 11 and 12)**

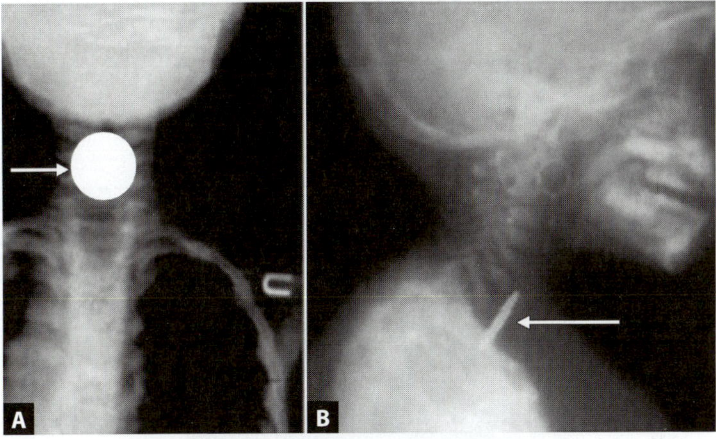

Figs. 11A and B: Esophageal foreign body.

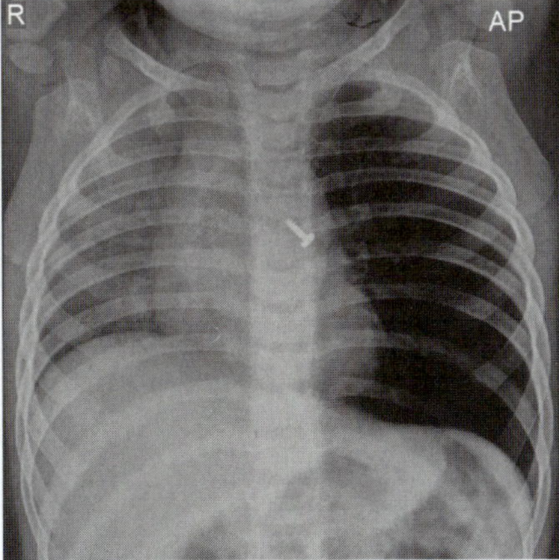

Fig. 12: Foreign body in left bronchus.

BOX 13: Deep neck infections.

- **Quinsy (peritonsillar abscess)** patients present with severe throat pain, trismus, fever, earache, and salivation. Treatment is by IV antibiotics, analgesics, and needle drainage of the abscess
- **Parapharyngeal abscess** may be consequence of a quinsy, dental infections, neck injuries, infections from parotid, or submandibular glands. Patients present with neck swellings, neck tenderness, high fever, and trismus. Managed by IV antibiotics, analgesics, anti-inflammatory, and later drainage
- **Acute retropharyngeal abscess** presents as croupy cough, difficulty in breathing, torticollis, neck swelling due to lymphadenitis, and pyrexia. An X-ray lateral neck is diagnostic and IV antibiotics and anti-inflammatory agents are given, later drainage is mandatory **(Figs. 13 and 14)**

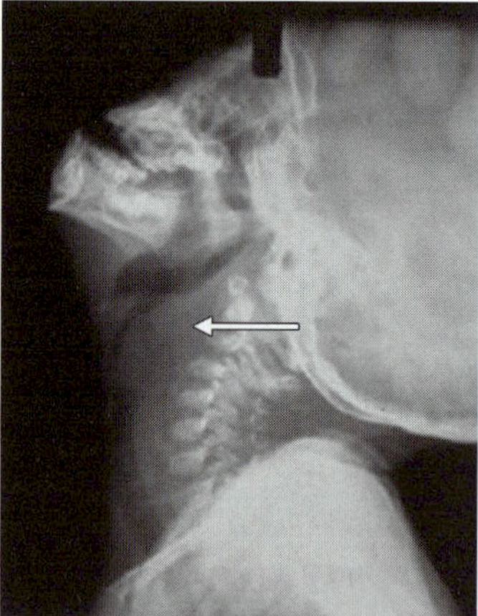

Fig. 13: Retropharyngeal abscess.

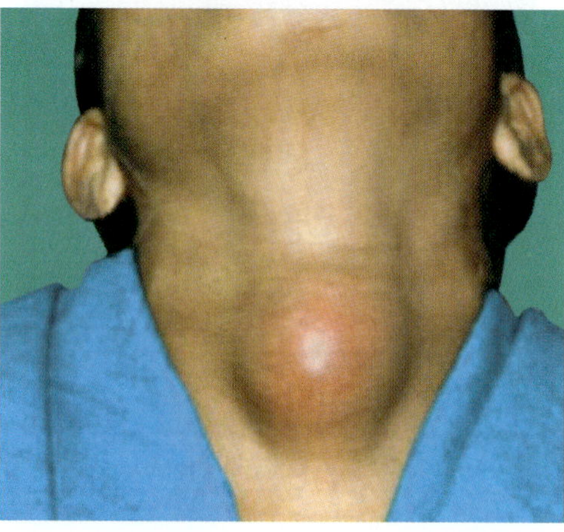

Fig. 14: Neck node (tubercular).

BOX 14: Stridor.

- The presentation is classical-noisy breathing
- A continuous stridor is an absolute emergency and constant monitoring of vital signs is mandatory
- Determine the site of obstruction as whether stridor occurring on inspiratory (laryngeal), expiratory (bronchial), or both (tracheal) phases of respiration **(Fig. 15)**
- The common causes are epiglottis, laryngitis, trachea-bronchitis; malignancies of base tongue, larynx or pyriform fossa; foreign body in the larynx or trachea, laryngeal papilloma, angioneurotic edema, vocal cord paralysis or even cardiac/hepatic or renal conditions
- Monitoring of vital signs is mandatory and rising pulse rate is a matter of concern
- Management includes oxygen and nebulization, steroids, bronchodilators, endotracheal intubation, or last resort is a tracheostomy

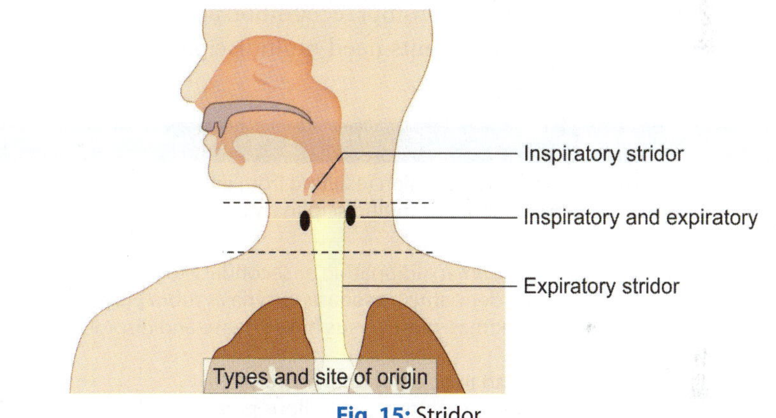

Fig. 15: Stridor.

SUGGESTED READING

1. Prabhat D. Practical ENT, 11th edition. New Delhi: CBS Publishers and Distributors; 2020.
2. Shah N. Clinical ENT, 3rd edition. New Delhi: CBS Publishers and Distributors; 2020.
3. Tysome J, Kanegaonkar R. ENT: An Introduction and Practical Guide, 2nd edition. United States: CRC Press; 2017.

CHAPTER 19

Dermatological Emergencies

Malavika Kohli, Sanyogita Warang

INTRODUCTION

Dermatological emergencies can have fatal consequences, if neglected. Manifestations may range from severe local reactions to multisystem failure depending on the causative agents. Prompt recognition and correct diagnosis is very important. Many times, patients need multidisciplinary approach in management.

BOX 1: Acute skin failure.

Acute skin failure is a state of total dysfunction resulting from different dermatological conditions. It is an emergency and needs multidisciplinary approach

Principal causes:

- Erythroderma which could be primary idiopathic or secondary to dermatitis (atopic, seborrheic, or contact dermatitis), psoriasis, pityriasis rubra pilaris, drug rashes, cutaneous T cell lymphomas, graft versus host disease and disorders of keratinization
- Stevens–Johnson syndrome and toxic epidermal necrolysis
- Immuno-bullous disorders like pemphigus and bullous pemphigoid
- Infections like staphylococcal-scalded skin syndrome and febrile viral exanthems

Complications:

- Infections leading to sepsis
- Deranged thermo and immune regulations
- Imbalance of electrolytes and fluids
- Endocrine deficiencies, e.g., vitamin D
- Renal failure, cardiac failure and gastrointestinal abnormalities like malabsorption
- Hypoproteinemia and loss of calories

Investigations: Routine investigations like complete blood count, liver, and renal function tests, C-reactive protein levels, serum protein levels, blood sugar levels, pus culture, and sensitivity from raw areas

Treatment:

- Sufficient oral intake has to be ensured, nasogastric tube feeding or IV supplements need to be given if necessary
- Vitals monitoring and correction of electrolytes
- IV fluid administration according to fluid loss given according to extent of skin involvement
- Temperature regulation, IV antibiotics if infection for suspected infection
- Causative disease or agents like drugs need to be investigated once the patient is stabilized
- If a drug is found to be responsible, it needs to be stopped immediately
- Barrier nursing has to be followed strictly
- Paraffin gauze bedding and dressing when necessary

BOX 2: Erythroderma (Refer figure in Chapter 7.5: Soft Tissue Infection in the Emergency Room).

Definition:
- Erythroderma is defined as skin inflammation involving around 80–90% of body surface area

Clinical features:
- Most cases present with erythema preceding the development of exfoliation by 2–6 days
- Larger and crusted scales are usually present in acute cases whereas in chronic phases tend to present with smaller and drier scales
- Pruritus is observed in almost all patients with a pink-red to deep-purple hue of underlying skin
- Nails may present with discoloration, brittleness, dullness, subungual hyperkeratosis, "shiny nails", Beau lines, paronychia, and splinter hemorrhages
- Staphylococcal infections are common and may lead to bacteremia
- Eyes may develop ectropion and purulent conjunctivitis, few may present with palmoplantar keratoderma
- Systemic involvement is suggested by tachycardia, edema, anemia, lymphadenopathy, hepatomegaly, hyperthermia, and high output cardiac failure

Causes:
- Idiopathic cause
- Chronic diseases like psoriasis and pityriasis rubra pilaris
- Various types of dermatitis, e.g., seborrheic, atopic, and allergic contact dermatitis
- Drug-induced erythroderma—phenytoin, carbamazepine, lithium, gold salts, etc.
- Immunobullous disease like pemphigus foliaceous
- Hereditary causes like ichthyosiform erythroderma
- Malignancies like lymphomas, leukemias, and Sezary syndrome
- Infections like dermatophytosis and Norwegian scabies

Complications:
- Hypoproteinemia
- Hypothermia
- Sepsis
- High output cardiac failure
- Death due to infections and heart failure
- Cutaneous sequelae include ectropion, nail dystrophy, diffuse hair loss, etc.

Investigation:
- Complete blood count, liver and renal function tests, C-reactive protein levels, serum protein levels, blood sugar levels, and serum electrolytes monitoring
- Sequential kin biopsies at different time intervals to find out the causative condition
- If malignancy is suspected, lymph node biopsy should be done

Treatment:
- Initial stabilization measures include nutritional assessment, correction of fluid and electrolyte imbalances, thermoregulation, and both prevention and treatment of secondary infections
- Severe pruritus may be dealt with by sedating oral antihistamines
- Systemic corticosteroids to be initiated at an initial prednisone dose of 1–2 mg/kg/day and a maintenance dose of 0.5 mg/kg/day or less, gives rapid improvement
- Topical therapy includes open wet dressings and bland emollients or low-potency corticosteroid ointments
- In neonates and children with erythroderma, management of fluid and electrolyte balance is critical in order to prevent hypernatremic dehydration
- Emollients, topical antibiotics and, depending upon the extent and severity of the secondary infections, systemic antibiotics are administered

BOX 3: Stevens–Johnson syndrome (SJS) and toxic epidermal necrosis (TEN) **(Fig. 1).**

- Stevens–Johnson syndrome (SJS) and toxic epidermal necrosis (TEN) are severe drug reactions characterized by extensive mucocutaneous erythema, blistering, and necrosis followed by extensive skin loss with an unpredictable course
- Stevens–Johnson syndrome and TEN represent different spectrums of the same entity depending on body surface involvement and mortality. TEN has higher mortality

Causes:

- Strong genetic susceptibility is known
- Most common drugs: Sulfa drugs, tetracyclines, nonsteroidal anti-inflammatory drugs (NSAIDs), and allopurinol
- Anticonvulsants include carbamazepine, lamotrigine, phenobarbital, and phenytoin
- Antiretroviral drugs like nevirapine, etc.
- *Mycoplasma pneumonia* has also been implicated apart from drugs, especially in children

Clinical features:

Latency period is usually 7–10 days, but may vary

- Initial symptoms may begin with malaise, fever, prostration, stinging of eyes, difficulty in swallowing, and symptoms associated with upper respiratory tract
- Rash begins with trunk and rapidly spreads to face, and extremities including palms and soles
- Lesions may begin as dusky macules or targetoid lesions with irregular size evolving into flaccid blisters
- Lesions may be painful and rapidly coalesce and progress forming sheets of erythema resembling wet "cigarette paper"
- Positive Nikolsky's sign (Gentle lateral pressure on lesional intact epidermis leads to separation from dermis indicating epidermal necrosis)
- Mucosal involvement of eyes, mouth, nose, and genitalia usually starts early and leads to painful erosive and hemorrhagic mucositis

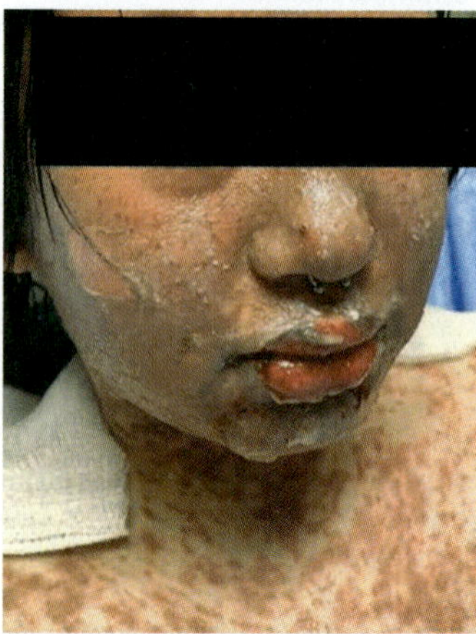

Fig. 1: Steven–Johnson syndrome.

Contd...

Contd...

- Fever, lymphadenopathy, hepatitis, cytopenia, and cholestasis due to vanishing bile duct
- Based on body surface area (BSA) involvement disease can be classified as:
  - *Stevens–Johnson syndrome:* Body surface area <10%
  - *Stevens–Johnson syndrome and TEN overlap syndrome:* Body surface area 10–30%
  - *Toxic epidermal necrosis:* Body surface area >30%
- Increasing age, comorbid conditions, and higher surface area involvement are poor prognostic factors

Differential diagnosis:
- Erythema multiforme major
- Immuno-bullous diseases such as pemphigus vulgaris, paraneoplastic pemphigus, and bullous pemphigoid
- *Lupus erythematosus:* Bullous varient
- Generalized fixed drug eruption (FDE)
- Acute graft-versus-host disease
- Staphylococcal-scalded skin syndrome (SSSS)

Complications:
- Secondary infections and septicemia
- Acute skin failure
- Hematological abnormalities—anemia and leukopenia
- Hepatitis
- Epithelial necrolysis resulting into bronchial erosions and airway obstruction
- *Sequalae:* Corneal damage, Sicca syndrome, oral adhesions, gastrointestinal adhesions, vaginal and urethral adhesions

Treatment:
Promptly discontinue any, and all, possible offending drugs
- Admit to skilled nursing care unit, e.g., ICU or burn unit, nutritional supplementation
- Correct fluid and electrolyte imbalances, caloric replacement, gastric care—antacids, and removal of oral and nasal debris
- Protect from secondary infections with topical antibiotic ointments
- Ophthalmology consultation and good eye care
- Periodic cultures of mouth, eyes, skin, sputum, and oral hygiene
- Physiotherapy to prevent contractures
- If extensive denuded areas, use biological dressings or skin equivalents
- Skin care includes gentle bathing; normal saline soaks, vaseline gauze dressing, and bullae aspiration
- Prompt intubation and ventilatory support at the earliest sign of acute respiratory distress
- Prevention of deep venous thrombosis, patient may require low molecular weight heparin
- Acute phase management: Consider one of the following—
  - Intravenous immunoglobulin (IVIg) (0.5–1 g/kg daily for 3–4 consecutive days)
  - Systemic corticosteroid (e.g., prednisolone 0.5–1 mg/kg daily for 10 days, and tapered)
  - IV methylprednisolone 500 mg on 3 consecutive days
  - Ciclosporin (3 or 5 mg/kg/day in divided doses for 10 days, and tapered)

BOX 4: Urticaria **(Fig. 2)**.

Definition:
- Urticaria refers to recurrent pruritic healing of the skin, with or without angioedema
- Wheals are pruritic, pink or pale, of variable number and sizes, swellings of the upper dermis; and have an initial erythematous flare around them, which typically resolving within 24 hours
- Angioedema has deeper dermis and subcutaneous tissue involvement, forming painful rather than pruritic areas with normal or erythematous overlying skin, lasting for 2–3 days

Clinical features:
- Multiple itchy wheals of different sizes erupt anywhere on the body and usually disappear within 2–24 hours without bruising
- Angioedema may last up to 72 hours when severe
- Wheals may occur at any time, but tend to be nocturnal in nature, patients tend to rub rather than scratch
- Symptoms tend to be more severe at night; may disturb sleep
- The differential diagnosis of urticaria includes insect bite reactions, prebullous phase of pemphigoid, acute eyelid contact dermatitis, urticarial drug reactions, and urticaria pigmentosa

Diagnosis:
- A comprehensive history and physical examination are important to confirm the diagnosis
- A detailed questionnaire includes duration and frequency of the attacks, associated illness, known adverse drug reactions, past and family history, occupation, and an assessment of the impact of the disease on the patient's quality of life
- A complete blood count and erythrocyte sedimentation rate (ESR) are important part of initial evaluation
- Investigation should be targeted at specific features identified in the clinical assessment, may include blood tests, skin biopsy (obtained in all patients with lesions lasting >24 hours), challenges for physical urticarias, food additives and drugs, and, infrequently as an extended investigation, skin tests for allergy

Treatment:
- Antipruritic lotions and avoidance of precipitating factors, including medicines like NSAIDs
- H1-antihistamines are the mainstay of the treatment for most patients with urticaria, includes cetirizine, levocetirizine, chlorpheniramine, and desloratadine
- Although systemic corticosteroids completely eliminate lesions, recurrences often occur with tapering of the dosage, and long-term use is unacceptable. In addition, combination of therapies can nearly always control symptoms and significantly improve quality of life

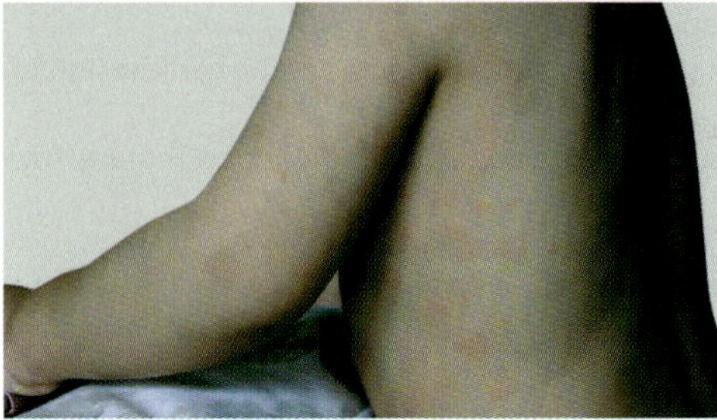

Fig. 2: Urticaria with hives.

BOX 5: Drug reaction with eosinophilia and systemic symptoms (DRESS) (Refer figure in Chapter 7.5: Soft Tissue Infection in the Emergency Room).

Drug reaction with eosinophilia and systemic symptoms is an idiosyncratic, life-threatening drug hypersensitivity reaction characterized by skin rash, eosinophilia, and internal organ involvement; most commonly liver

Causes:

Drug reaction with eosinophilia and systemic symptoms is known to have genetic predisposition and probable viral reactivation [human herpesviruses (HHV)-6 and 7]

- *Causative medications:*
  - Antiepileptics like phenytoin, carbamazepine, etc.
  - Antibiotics include amoxicillin, vancomycin, piperacillin-tazobactam, minocycline, etc.
- *Diuretics:* Furosemide
- Allopurinol
- Ibuprofen
- Dapsone

Clinical features:

- Symptoms develop 2–6 weeks after drug initiation, initially involving the face and gradually spreading to the trunk
- Cutaneous involvement usually begins as a morbilliform, maculopapular, purpuric, or papulopustular eruption, which later becomes edematous, often with a follicular accentuation
- Associated symptoms may include fever, systemic symptoms, and lymphadenopathy
- Mucosal involvement includes cheilitis, oral mucosal, and ophthalmic involvement
- Systemic features include fever, eosinophilia, hepatitis, renal involvement, pericarditis, myocarditis, and any thyroid dysfunction

Complications:

- Acute fulminant hepatic failure
- Nephritis
- Erythroderma
- Autoimmune phenomenon like lupus erythematosus and thyroiditis

Differential diagnosis:

- Stevens–Johnson syndrome (SJS) and TEN syndrome
- Erythema multiforme

The differential diagnosis includes other cutaneous drug eruptions, acute viral infections, hypereosinophilic syndrome, lymphoma, and pseudolymphoma

Investigation:

- Routine blood tests like complete blood count, liver and kidney function tests, erythrocyte sedimentation rate, peripheral smear for atypical lymphocytes, viral serology, electrocardiogram, chest X-ray, and thyroid function tests

Management:

- Withdrawal of the causative drug, patient's counseling, and education
- Daily oral prednisolone 1 mg/kg or intravenous methylprednisolone pulse therapy 1 g for 3 consecutive days
- Other options include IVIg, ciclosporin, cyclophosphamide, rituximab, ganciclovir, and N-acetylcysteine for severe hepatitis

BOX 6: Immuno-bullous disorders.

Pemphigus vulgaris:

- Immunobullous disorders represent group of chronic mucocutaneous blistering skin diseases antibody-mediated blistering disorders which can have fatal consequences if not managed effectively. Most common and severe among them is *"Pemphigus vulgaris (PV)"*
- Pemphigus vulgaris can be associated with other autoimmune diseases like autoimmune thyroiditis and rheumatoid arthritis
- Mortality can be high if not treated adequately. Morbidity is mainly due to chronic nature of the disease and side effects of medicines
- Major types are *Pemphigus vulgaris, Pemphigus foliaceus* (show only cutaneous lesions), and "paraneoplastic pemphigus" (associated with malignancies)

Clinical features:

- Pemphigus vulgaris usually presents after 4th and 5th decade of life
- Patients may present as two subgroups: (1) the mucosal-dominant type with mucosal erosions but minimal skin involvement; and (2) the mucocutaneous type with extensive skin blisters and erosions in addition to mucosal involvement
- Mucous membrane lesions usually present as painful erosions of variable sizes, irregular borders commonly involving the buccal and palatine mucosa with supra-added candidiasis
- Skin lesions present on head, chest, and back as flaccid, thin-walled vesicles that easily rupture forming painful erosions with expansive nature that ooze and bleed easily, show positive Nikolsky sign, healing without scarring

Complications:

- Secondary infections and sepsis
- Acute skin failure
- Drug-related side effects

BOX 7: Bullous pemphigoid.

Bullous pemphigoid (BP) is the most common autoimmune subepidermal bullous disease presenting in older age group with substantial morbidity

Clinical features:
- *Nonbullous phase:* In the prodromal phase, symptoms begin with mild to severe pruritus that may be associated with excoriated, papular, eczematous, urticarial lesions. This phase may last several weeks to months

Bullous phase:
- This stage is marked by development of clear fluid containing vesicles and tense bullae of varying size
- Vesicles and bullae may appear on normal or urticarial skin, together with urticarial and infiltrated papules and plaques
- Lesions mostly involve flexural aspects of the extremities and the lower trunk, including the abdomen with a symmetrical distribution
- Intertriginous areas may show vegetative plaques
- Lesions resolve with hypopigmentation or hyperpigmentation, milia, and scarring is rare
- Only 10–30% patients develop mucosal lesions, 50% patients show blood eosinophilia

Diagnosis:
- Classic clinical presentation, histopathology of lesion skin, and positive direct immunofluorescence (DIF) microscopy studies confirm the diagnosis
- Detection of specific circulating immunoglobulin G (IgG) autoantibodies (anti-BP180 and anti-BP230) via either indirect immunofluorescence (IIF) microscopy or enzyme-linked immunosorbent assay (ELISA) provides a supporting evidence for diagnosis

Differential diagnosis:
- Adverse drug reactions, arthropod reactions, allergic contact dermatitis, urticarial dermatoses, prurigo (simplex and nodularis), and infestations like scabies
- Bullous arthropod bite reactions, porphyrias, allergic contact dermatitis, dyshidrotic eczemas, Stevens–Johnson syndrome, etc.
- In pediatric age group, bullous impetigo, inherited epidermolysis bullosa, and bullous mastocytosis are possible differential diagnoses

Treatment of chronic bullous disorders:
- Local care including saline, potassium permanganate dressings, bland emollients, and paraffin gauze dressings help to alleviate discomfort
- Potent topical corticosteroids, e.g., clobetasol propionate 0.05% cream, can control the disease as efficiently as oral corticosteroids with fewer side effects
- The steroid sparing agents commonly used include azathioprine, mycophenolate mofetil (1.5–3 g/day), methotrexate (7.5–15 mg/week), and cyclophosphamide (1–3 mg/kg/day)
- The choice of a particular immunosuppressive drug depends on its side-effect profile, the patient's overall condition, and the experience of the physician
- Longstanding, recalcitrant, and extensive bullous disorder may develop sepsis and hemodynamic compromise and must be approach like acute skin failure

BOX 8: Post burn blisters (Refer figure in Chapter 15.2.5: Acute Burns).

Delayed blisters have been observed weeks to months after the initial healing of second-degree thermal burns, donor sites of split-thickness skin grafts, and recipient sites of split-thickness skin grafts

Clinical features:
- Tense vesicles or blisters develop after the injured skin (burned, donor site, and recipient site) has completely healed
- Lesions are not present on the uninvolved areas
- The blisters tend to resolve spontaneously; however, they show a tendency of recurrence

Differential diagnosis:
- Herpes zoster infection
- Immunobullous disease
- Diabetic bullae
- Irritant contact dermatitis

Treatment:
- These blisters heal spontaneously with simple care, topical antibiotics, wound dressings, and local compression

BOX 9: Infections (Refer figure in Chapter 7.5: Soft Tissue Infection in the Emergency Room).

Staphylococcal-scalded skin syndrome:
Staphylococcal-scalded skin syndrome (SSSS) is a toxin-mediated blistering syndrome caused by *Staphylococcus aureus* exfoliative toxins. Toxin-mediated separation of epidermis at granular layer

Etiology:
- *Staphylococcus aureus* phage group II toxins like exfoliative toxin A and B
- Minor infections like staphylococcal impetigo or throat infections can precipitate SSSS
- Toxin destroys desmoglein 1 which functions as skin adhesion molecule
- Risk factors—children <6 years of age, kidney diseases, immune-suppression

Clinical features:
- Staphylococcal-scalded skin syndrome begins with malaise, fever, irritability, and tender erythematous skin, initially involving the face and intertriginous areas, and gradually becoming generalized within 2 days
- This is followed by formation of flaccid, sterile bullae within the superficial epidermis with positive Nikolsky sign
- Initially, the flexures exfoliate leaving behind superficial erosion with periorificial crusting and radial fissuring
- Scaling and desquamation continue for the next few days, followed by re-epithelialization without scarring over weeks
- If treated promptly, SSSS resolves within few weeks without any sequelae

Diagnosis:
- Staphylococcal-scalded skin syndrome is a clinical diagnosis
- Cultures taken from skin lesions are usually negative but *S. aureus* may be cultured from the conjunctiva, nasopharynx, perianal area, or pyogenic foci on the skin

Contd...

Contd...

- Leukocytosis is a common finding; histopathology helps in confirming the level of split
- Enzyme-linked immunosorbent assay (ELISA), double immunodiffusion and slide latex agglutination can identify the toxins responsible for SSSS

Differential diagnosis:
- Stevens–Johnson syndrome and toxic epidermal necrolysis
- Epidermolysis bullosa and pemphigus foliaceus
- Erythema multiforme, Graft versus host reaction
- Drug reactions and sunburn
- Kawasaki disease

Investigation:
- Diagnosis of SSSS is mostly clinical, however, certain investigations are required during management
- Swabs from raw areas and suspected areas and blood cultures
- Tzanck smears from fresh erosions to check for acantholytic cells
- Complete blood test, liver and renal function tests, and electrolyte monitoring

Treatment:
- Most patients with SSSS require hospitalization and parenteral antibiotics
- Beta-lactamase-resistant antibiotic (e.g., dicloxacillin and cephalexin) for a minimum of 1 week should be administered
- Clindamycin administration is also effective but up to 50% of strains may be resistant, so monotherapy is not recommended
- It is crucial to identify possible carriers of staphylococcus among the handlers

BOX 10: Impetigo (Refer figure in Chapter 7.5: Soft Tissue Infection in the Emergency Room).

- Impetigo is a common, contagious, and superficial bacterial skin infection which presents as nonbullous and bullous forms
- *Staphylococcus aureus* is most common pathogen in both nonbullous and bullous forms. Group A β-hemolytic *Streptococcus (Streptococcus pyogenes)* is another important cause of nonbullous impetigo
- The infection is transmitted via direct contact or through fomites, and is common in children <6 years of age
- Risk factors include a warm temperature, high humidity, poor hygiene, atopic dermatitis, skin trauma, and contact during sports

Clinical features:
- *Nonbullous impetigo:* Single erythematous maculae rapidly develops into transient vesicles gradually leading to formation of superficial erosions typically showing "honey-colored" crusts
- May be associated with lymphadenopathy, is benign and self-limiting, and resolves over 2 weeks without any scarring
- Bullous variant is seen less commonly, beginning with small vesicles enlarging to superficial flaccid bullae that rupture forming colarette scales with minimal erythema
- Commonly seen on face, trunk, perineum, axillae, and extremities, resolves in 3–6 weeks with no scarring

Contd...

Contd...

Diagnosis:

Diagnosis is usually clinical; however, exudate can be sent for culture to confirm the diagnosis and determine antibiotics sensitivity

- Leukocytosis and regional lymphadenopathy are common findings

Differential diagnosis:

- *Bullous impetigo:* Bullous insect bite reactions, herpes simplex infection, and burn injury
- *Nonbullous impetigo:* Herpes simplex infection, eczema, candidiasis, and insect bite reaction

Treatment:

- Topical mupirocin, retapamulin, or fusidic acid are often equally effective as oral antibiotics
- Cleansing affected area and removing crusts are important part of management

BOX 11: Herpes simplex infection.

Herpes simplex virus (HSV)-1 and HSV-2 primarily cause orolabial and genital infections. It is one of the most common sexually transmitted infections

Clinical features:

- Painful and grouped vesicles appear on normal or an erythematous base, sometimes progressing to pustules and eventually to erosions and ulcerations with a characteristic border **(Fig. 3)**
- Crusting and resolution of symptoms usually take 2–6 weeks
- A prodrome of tender lymphadenopathy, malaise, anorexia, and fever may occur before the onset of mucocutaneous lesions
- Orolabial infections may present as gingivostomatitis, pharyngitis, and an infectious mononucleosis-like syndrome
- Recurrent lesions usually minimally painful and most often present on the vermilion border of the lips but can also present as an excruciatingly painful, erosive balanitis, vulvitis, or vaginitis

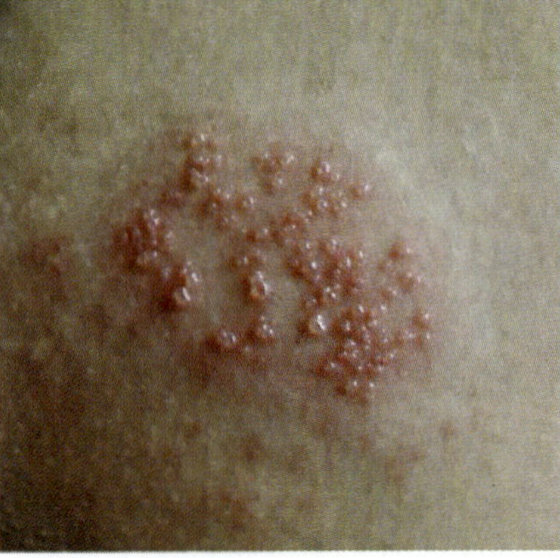

Fig. 3: Herpes.

Contd...

Contd...

- In women, it may involve cervix, buttocks, and perineum. It is also associated with inguinal adenopathy and dysuria
- Genital lesions in men occur on the glans, prepuce, or shaft of the penis
- Extragenital lesions, urinary retention, and aseptic meningitis may be late sequelae

Diagnosis:

- Clinical
- Laboratory tests include viral culture, direct fluorescent antibody assays, Tzank smear, molecular techniques, and serology

Differential diagnosis:

- *Orolabial herpes:* Aphthous stomatitis, erythema multiforme, Stevens–Johnson syndrome, Coxsackievirus infections, oral candidiasis, Behçet disease, and chemotherapy-induced mucositis
- *Genital herpes:* Trauma, syphilitic chancres, chancroid, Epstein-Barr virus (EBV)-related ulcers, and lymphogranuloma venereum

Treatment:

Acyclovir:

- *Primary herpes genitalis:* 3 × 400 mg tablets PO daily for 7–10 days
- *Severe primary herpes genitalis:* 3 × 5 mg/kg IV daily for 5–7 days
- *Recurrent herpes genitalis (<5–6 episodes/year):* 2 × 800 mg PO daily for 5 days
- *Prophylaxis:* 2 × 400 mg PO daily for 6 months

Valacyclovir:

- *Primary herpes genitalis:* 2 × 500 mg tablets PO daily for 7–10 days
- *Recurrent herpes genitalis (<5–6 episodes/year):* 2 × 500 mg PO daily for 3 days or 1 × 1,000 mg tablet daily for 5 days
- *Prophylaxis:* 1 × 500 mg PO daily for 6 months

BOX 12: Varicella **(Fig. 4)**.

- Varicella zoster virus (VZV) is the etiology of varicella (chickenpox) and herpes zoster (shingles)
- Herpes zoster represents reactivation of latent VZV infection with significant morbidity and develops in ~20% of healthy adults and 50% of immunocompromised persons

Clinical features:
- A prodrome of mild fever, malaise, and myalgia may occur, especially in adults
- This is succeeded by erythematous maculopapular pruritic eruption of pruritic, starting on head and enact and gradually involving the body
- Lesions rapidly evolve over ~12 hours into 1–3 mm several clear vesicles surrounded by narrow red halos ("dew drops on a rose petal")
- Distal extremities may be spared, and oral mucosa may be involved
- Older vesicles evolve to form pustules and crusts, may be hemorrhagic or umbilicated, with individual lesions healing within 7–10 days
- The presence of lesions in all stages of development is a hallmark of varicella
- The disease course is usually self-limited and benign in healthy children

Complications:
Secondary bacterial infection, scarring, less commonly encephalitis, acute cerebella's ataxia, Reye syndrome, keratitis, arthritis, hepatitis, glomerulonephritis, pancreatits, hepatitis, and myocarditis

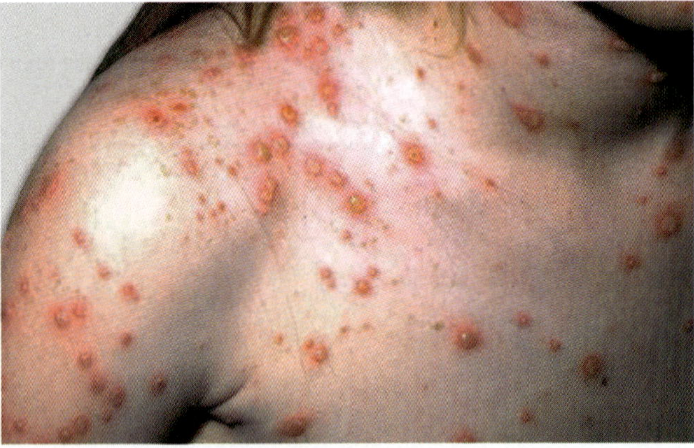

Fig. 4: Varicella.

BOX 13: Herpes zoster.

Clinical features: Begins with a prodrome of pruritus, tingling, tenderness, hyperesthesia, and/or intense pain, with or without skin lesions

- Most patients develop a painful eruption of grouped vesicles on an erythematous base in a dermatomal distribution which may be preceded by edematous plaques more commonly seen on the trunk and face
- Herpes zoster usually resolves without sequelae in immunocompetent children and young adults with most common sequalae being posthermetic neuralgia
- Other complications can include secondary bacterial infection, scarring, meningoencephalitis, pneumonitis, and hepatitis

Diagnosis:

- A clinical diagnosis is made based upon the history, including previous varicella or vaccine administration and physical examination
- A Tzanck smear, polymerase chain reaction (PCR), or direct fluorescent-antibody testing (DFA) can assist in quickly confirming the diagnosis
- Immunohistochemical staining can distinguish between the two viruses
- Serologic assays are diagnostic of VZV if the convalescent serum has at least a fourfold increase in the VZV titer relative to the acute serum

Differential diagnosis:

The differential diagnosis of varicella may include vesicular viral exanthems, disseminated herpes simplex virus (HSV) infection, pityriasis lichenoides et varioliformis acuta (PLEVA), rickettsial pox, drug eruptions, bullous insect bite reactions, and scabies

Treatment:

- *Acyclovir:* 800 mg PO five times daily for 7–10 days
- *Famciclovir:* 500 mg PO three times daily for 7 days
- *Valacyclovir:* 1 g PO three times a day for 7 days
- Immunocompromised persons requiring hospitalization or severe neurologic

Complications:

- Acyclovir (intravenous) 10 mg/kg IV 8 hourly

BOX 14: Approach to fever with rash **(Fig. 5)**.

Several febrile illnesses can present with skin eruptions
These eruptions may present as macules, papules, wheal, or even purpuric patches

Etiology in brief:
Bacterial causes: Staphylococcal infections [Impetigo, SSSS, toxic shock syndrome, septicemia (*Streptococcus, Staphylococcus, Pneumococcus,* etc.), *Vibrio vulnificus, Mycoplasma,* meningococcemia, and disseminated gonococcal infection

Viral causes: Measles, rubella, erythema infectiosum, exanthem subitum, eczema vaccinatum, enterovirus, infectious mononucleosis, Gianotti–Crosti syndrome, leptospirosis, hand foot mouth disease, HIV, and herpes simplex infection

Rickettsial diseases: Rickettsia africae, Q fever, scrub typhus, and murine typhus autoimmune diseases—systemic lupus erythematosus (SLE), acute rheumatic fever, and hypersensitive vasculitis

Others: Erythematous multiforme, hematologic malignancy, pityriasis rosea, drug eruption, plant dermatitis, toxic erythematous neonatorum, and idiopathic
- A complete history must be taken, including underlying diseases, recent travel, medications, and exposure to flora and fauna and other natural environments
- The onset of symptoms and the characteristics of the rash itself (morphology, location, and distribution) could be helpful in the clinical diagnosis
- Immediate treatment includes supportive management and hydration
- The patient should be thoroughly investigated and treated accordingly after establishing appropriate diagnosis

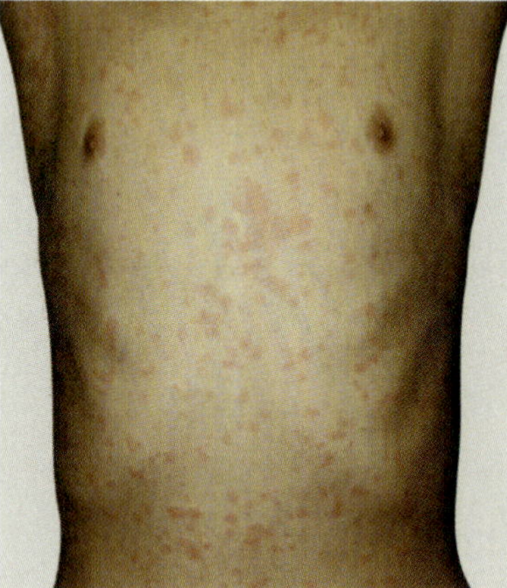

Fig. 5: Viral exanthems.

BOX 15: Insect bite reaction.

- Hypersensitivity to mosquito bites with bullous and necrotic skin lesions may occur in few individuals
- Lesions begin with burning sensation with erythematous papules which may be accompanied by edema that resolves spontaneously but can be persistent in a few
- Exaggerated insect bite reactions (e.g., papulovesicular and nodular) can represent a manifestation of chronic lymphocytic leukemia and less often other hematologic malignancies

Differential diagnosis:

- Arthropod reactions account for many "cryptic" chronic skin eruptions. Features that should suggest an arthropod reaction include grouping of papules, patterns of eruption that correlate with exposure, and the histologic features noted above. When an arthropod reaction is suspected, a detailed history of outdoor exposures, pets, work, and hobbies may prove helpful

Treatment:

- Zinc oxide, camphor, and menthol lotion and gel formulations may be useful in the control of pruritus
- For more persistent bite reactions and topical corticosteroids are often required
- In young children, mid-strength corticosteroid preparations may suffice, while in older children and adults, class 1 or 2 corticosteroids are preferable
- These agents can be applied under occlusion to enhance efficacy, but for a predetermined time period to avoid potential side effects of cutaneous atrophy and striae

BOX 16: Dermatophytosis **(Figs. 6A to F).**

Superficial fungal infection is defined as a dermatophyte infection of keratinized tissues including skin, hair, and nails. It is also known as Ring worm in common language

Dermatophyte species are divided into three genera (*Epidermophyton, Microsporum*, and *Trichophyton*). Their ability to attach to, invade, and use keratin as a source of nutrition underlies the pathogenesis of superficial fungal infection of skin, hair, and nails, and is termed *"dermatophytosis"*

Clinical features:
- Pruritic, erythematous, and raised brown red ring like plaques with sharply defined borders are seen on body. Vesicles may form along the edge of the rash
- Depending on involvement of body area, dermatophytosis can be classified as "Tinea corporis, Tinea cruris, Tinea barbae, Tinea capitis, Tinea pedis, Tinea mannum," etc.

Diagnosis:
- Clinical
- Skin scraping potassium hydroxide (KOH) wet mount for fungal hyphae
- Skin scraping for culture

Treatment:

Oral antifungals:
- Griseofulvin, 20–25 mg/kg/day × 6–8 weeks
- Terbinafine, 250 mg/day × 2–8 weeks
- Itraconazole, 5 mg/kg/day × 2–4 weeks
- Fluconazole, 6 mg/kg/day × 3–6 weeks

Topical antifungals:

Miconazole, luliconazole, eberconazole, sertaconazole, and ketoconazole creams to be applied once or twice daily

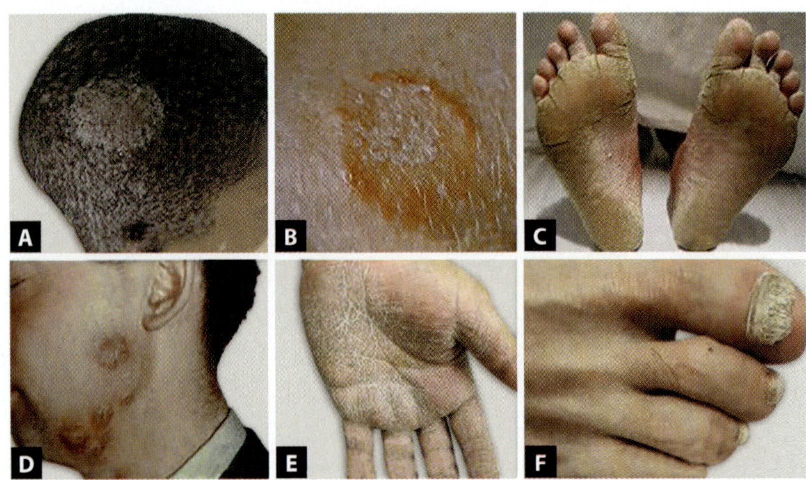

Figs. 6A to F: Dermatophytosis. (A) Tinea captits; (B) Tinea corporis; (C) Tinea pedis; (D) Tinea barbae; (E) Tinea manuum; (F) Tinea unguium.

BOX 17: Scabies **(Fig. 7)**.

Human infestation caused by the *Sarcoptes scabiei* var. hominis mite which completes his entire lifecycle within human epidermis

Clinical features:

- Scabies presents with intense pruritus associated with a characteristic flexural distribution of lesions and history. Onset is usually insidious with intense nocturnal pruritus. Symptoms appear 4–6 weeks after initial infestation
- Excoriations and eczematous dermatitis at interdigital webs, sides of fingers, volar aspects of the wrists and lateral palms, elbows, axillae, scrotum, penis, labia, and areolae in women. The head and neck are usually spared in adults, but may be involved in infants
  Indurated and crusted nodules may be present in severe cases called "Nodular scsbies"
- The pathognomonic lesion of scabies is a burrow, which is a thin, thread-like, linear, or often J-shaped structure and measures 1–10 mm in length

Diagnosis:

- Clinical
- Microscopic examination of skin scrapings for mites, eggs, or fecal pellets (scybala)

Treatment:

- Permethrin 5% cream to be applied on entire body (neck down) for 8–14 hours then wash, repeat after 7 days; if crusted scabies use daily for 7 days, then twice weekly until cured
- Oral ivermectin 200 ug/kg single dose for patients above 6 years of age

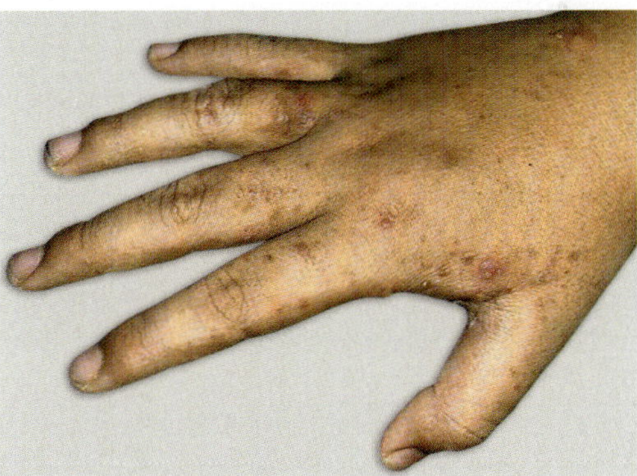

Fig. 7: Scabies.

SUGGESTED READING

1. Bolognia JL, Schaffer JV, Cerroni L. Dermatology, 4th edition. Amsterdam, The Netherlands: Elsevier; 2017.
2. Griffiths CEM, Barker J, Bleiker TO, Chalmers R, Creamer D. Rooks textbook of Dermatology, 9th edition. United States: Wiley-Blackwell; 2016. p. 4992.
3. Inamadar AC, Palit A. Acute skin failure: concept, causes, consequences and care. Indian J Dermatol Venereol Leprol. 2005;71:379-85.

4. Inamadar AC, Palit A. Critical care in Dermatology. New Delhi: Jaypee Brothers Medical Publishers (P) Ltd.; 2013.
5. Kang JH. Febrile Illness with Skin Rashes. Infect Chemother. 2015;47(3):155-66.
6. Kang S, Amagai M, Bruckner A, Enk AH, McMichael A, Orringer JS, et al. Fitzpatrick's Dermatology, 9th edition. United States: McGraw-Hill Education; 2019. p. 1866.
7. Mallory S, Bree AF, Chern P. Illustrated manual of Pediatric Dermatology: Diagnosis and management. London: CRC press; 2005. p. 432.
8. McLendon K, Sternard BT. Anaphylaxis. [Updated 2023 Jan 26]. In: StatPearls [Internet]. Treasure Island (FL): StatPearls Publishing; 2024.
9. Usatine RP, Sandy N. Dermatologic emergencies. Am Fam Phys. 2010; 82(7):773-80.

CHAPTER 20

Pediatric Emergencies

Fazal Nabi, Varshil Shah

FEVER AND SEVERE BACTERIAL INFECTION

BOX 1: Definition.

- Fever is a common presenting symptom in pediatric patients and can indicate a wide range of conditions
- It is crucial to assess the child's overall appearance, vital signs, and clinical history to determine the appropriate management

BOX 2: History.

- Inquire about the duration of fever, associated symptoms (e.g., cough and vomiting), recent travel or exposures, and immunization status
- Also, ask about any recent antibiotic use, as this can affect the presentation of bacterial infections

BOX 3: Physical examination.

- Look for signs of serious illness, such as lethargy, poor perfusion, abnormal breathing, or a nonblanching rash
- Assess the child's hydration status and perform a thorough examination of the respiratory, cardiovascular, and gastrointestinal systems

BOX 4: Investigations.

- Consider performing blood tests (complete blood count, inflammatory markers such as C-reactive protein or procalcitonin) and cultures (blood and urine) based on the clinical suspicion
- Imaging studies, such as chest X-ray or ultrasound, may also be indicated in certain cases

BOX 5: Treatment.

- Administer antibiotics promptly if a severe bacterial infection is suspected. Choose antibiotics based on the likely pathogens and local resistance patterns. Ensure appropriate dosing based on the child's weight and age
- Monitor the child closely for any signs of deterioration and adjust treatment as needed
- Manage fever with antipyretics such as acetaminophen or ibuprofen
- Ensure adequate hydration, especially if the child has signs of dehydration

BOX 6: Complications.

- *Septic shock:* In severe cases, bacterial infections can lead to septic shock, characterized by hypotension, tachycardia, and altered mental status. Prompt recognition and management with fluid resuscitation and vasopressors are essential to prevent morbidity and mortality
- *Meningitis:* Bacterial meningitis can occur as a complication of severe bacterial infections. It presents with fever, headache, neck stiffness, and altered mental status. Lumbar puncture with cerebrospinal fluid analysis is required for diagnosis, and treatment with appropriate antibiotics is essential

SUGGESTED READING

1. Edwards MS, Baker CJ. Sepsis in the Neonate and Child. In: Feigin RD, Cherry JD, editors. Feigin and Cherry's Textbook of Pediatric Infectious Diseases. 8th ed. Philadelphia: Elsevier; 2020. pp. 1279-1312.
2. Mackowiak PA. Fever: Basic Mechanisms and Management. 1st ed. Philadelphia: Lippincott Williams & Wilkins; 2005.
3. Wright SW, Lovelace-Macon L. Recognition and Management of Febrile Children. Emerg Med Clin North Am. 2018;36(2):275-92.

VOMITING, DIARRHEA, AND DEHYDRATION

BOX 1: Definition.

- Vomiting and diarrhea are common in pediatric patients and can lead to dehydration, especially in young children
- Prompt recognition and management are essential to prevent complications

BOX 2: History.

- Inquire about the frequency and duration of vomiting and diarrhea, associated symptoms (e.g., fever and abdominal pain), recent dietary changes, and urine output
- Ask about recent travel or exposure to sick contacts, as this can help to determine the etiology

BOX 3: Physical examination.

- Assess the child's hydration status, including skin turgor, mucous membranes, and capillary refill time
- Look for signs of dehydration, such as sunken eyes, decreased skin turgor, and dry mucous membranes
- Assess for signs of systemic illness, such as fever or abdominal tenderness

BOX 4: Management.

- *Rehydration:* Offer oral rehydration solutions (ORS) for mild-to-moderate dehydration. Encourage frequent and small sips to prevent vomiting. For severe dehydration or inability to tolerate oral fluids, intravenous fluids may be necessary
- *Nutrition:* Continue breastfeeding or formula feeding if the child is tolerating it. Avoid solid foods initially, as they can worsen vomiting and diarrhea. Gradually, reintroduce a normal diet as tolerated

BOX 5: Complications.

- *Electrolyte imbalance:* Prolonged vomiting and diarrhea can lead to electrolyte imbalances, such as hyponatremia or hypernatremia. Monitor electrolyte levels and correct imbalances as needed
- *Acidosis:* Severe dehydration can lead to metabolic acidosis. Monitor for signs of acidosis, such as Kussmaul breathing or altered mental status, and manage accordingly
- *Shock:* In severe cases, dehydration can lead to hypovolemic shock. Monitor for signs of shock, such as tachycardia, hypotension, and altered mental status, and provide fluid resuscitation as needed

SUGGESTED READING

1. Bhutta ZA, et al. Acute Gastroenteritis in Children. Pediatrics in Review. 2018;39(10):500-511.
2. Guarino A, et al. Management of Acute Diarrhoea in Children: An Update. Lancet Infect Dis. 2021;21(6):e250-e265.
3. Walker CLF, et al. Diarrhoea in Children: Epidemiology, Prevention, and Treatment. Lancet. 2013;381(9875):51-59.

ABDOMINAL PAIN

BOX 1: Definition.

Abdominal pain in children can be challenging to diagnose due to the wide range of possible causes, including gastrointestinal, genitourinary, and gynecological issues

BOX 2: History.

- Obtain a detailed history, including the location, onset, duration, and character of the pain
- Inquire about associated symptoms such as vomiting, diarrhea, fever, and urinary symptoms
- Also, ask about dietary habits, recent travel, and any family history of gastrointestinal or inflammatory conditions

BOX 3: Physical examination.

- Perform a thorough abdominal examination, including inspection, auscultation, percussion, and palpation
- Look for signs of peritonitis (e.g., guarding and rebound tenderness), organomegaly, or masses
- Assess for signs of systemic illness, such as fever or tachycardia

BOX 4: Investigations.

- Consider imaging studies (ultrasound and CT scan) and laboratory tests (complete blood count, electrolytes, and amylase/lipase) based on the clinical suspicion
- Stool studies may be indicated if infectious etiologies are suspected
- Consider consulting pediatric surgical or gastroenterology services for further evaluation and management

BOX 5: Treatment.

- Manage pain with analgesics as needed
- Treat the underlying cause, such as antibiotics for infections (e.g., appendicitis and urinary tract infection) or surgical intervention for conditions like appendicitis or intussusception

BOX 6: Complications.

- *Perforation:* In cases of severe abdominal pain, consider the possibility of perforated viscus, especially in conditions like appendicitis. Monitor for signs of peritonitis and shock, and expedite surgical consultation, if suspected
- *Intestinal obstruction:* Abdominal pain accompanied by vomiting and constipation may indicate intestinal obstruction. Consider imaging studies and surgical consultation for further evaluation and management
- *Inflammatory bowel disease (IBD):* Chronic or recurrent abdominal pain with associated symptoms such as diarrhea or weight loss may indicate IBD. Refer to pediatric gastroenterology for further evaluation and management

SUGGESTED READING

1. Stringer MD, Pablot SM. Diagnostic Approaches to Pediatric Abdominal Pain. Clin Gastroenterol Hepatol. 2018;16(1):e1-e10.
2. van den Bosch GE, et al. Chronic Abdominal Pain in Childhood: New Insights in Pathophysiology and Management. Nat Rev Gastroenterol Hepatol. 2021;18(9):528-544.
3. Sultan M, et al. Surgical Emergencies in Pediatric Patients Presenting with Acute Abdominal Pain. J Pediatr Surg. 2020;55(1):42-48.

RASHES

BOX 1: Definition.

Rashes are common in pediatric patients and can be caused by a variety of factors, including infections, allergies, and inflammatory conditions

BOX 2: History.

- Obtain a detailed history, including the onset, duration, and progression of the rash
- Inquire about associated symptoms such as fever, itching, and exposure to potential triggers (e.g., new medications and foods)

BOX 3: Physical examination.

- Perform a thorough skin examination, noting the distribution, morphology, and color of the rash
- Look for signs of systemic illness, such as mucous membrane involvement or lymphadenopathy
- Consider performing a full-body skin examination to identify any other lesions

BOX 4: Identification of underlying cause.

- Consider infectious causes (viral, bacterial, and fungal), allergic reactions (medications, foods, and insect bites), and inflammatory conditions (eczema and psoriasis)
- Perform appropriate investigations, such as skin scrapings, cultures, or serologic tests, based on the clinical suspicion

BOX 5: Treatment.

- Treat the underlying cause if identified. Provide symptomatic relief, such as antihistamines for itching or topical steroids for inflammation
- Educate the family on proper skin care and hygiene practices

BOX 6: Complications.

- *Secondary infection:* Scratching or irritation of the rash can lead to secondary bacterial or fungal infections. Educate the family on proper wound care and hygiene practices to prevent infections
- *Systemic illness:* In some cases, rashes may be a manifestation of a systemic illness, such as Kawasaki disease or meningococcemia. Monitor for signs of systemic illness and manage accordingly

SUGGESTED READING

1. Cohen BA. Pediatric Dermatology: A Quick Reference Guide. American Academy of Pediatrics, 2021.
2. Hay RJ, et al. Skin Disorders in Children: Diagnosis and Treatment. Lancet Child Adolesc Health. 2019;3(5):338-349.
3. Hurwitz S. Clinical Pediatric Dermatology: A Textbook of Skin Disorders of Childhood and Adolescence. Saunders, 2020.

NEONATAL EMERGENCIES AND COMMON ISSUES

BOX 1: Definition.

Neonatal emergencies require prompt recognition and management to prevent adverse outcomes. Common issues in the neonatal period include respiratory distress, sepsis, and congenital anomalies

BOX 2: History.

- Obtain a detailed prenatal, perinatal, and postnatal history, including maternal health, gestational age, birth weight, and any complications during delivery
- Inquire about the infant's feeding and voiding patterns, as well as any concerns raised by the parents

BOX 3: Physical examination.

- Perform a thorough physical examination, focusing on vital signs, respiratory status, heart sounds, and presence of any anomalies
- Assess the infant's color, tone, and activity level

BOX 4: Management.

- *Respiratory support:* Provide oxygen therapy and respiratory support as needed, including mechanical ventilation or continuous positive airway pressure (CPAP). Monitor oxygen saturation and respiratory effort closely
- *Infection control:* Administer antibiotics promptly if sepsis is suspected, based on clinical and laboratory findings. Perform appropriate cultures (blood, urine, and cerebrospinal fluid) and imaging studies as indicated
- *Nutrition:* Ensure adequate nutrition, either through breastfeeding or formula feeding. Monitor weight gain and feeding tolerance closely
- *Temperature regulation:* Maintain a neutral thermal environment to prevent hypothermia or hyperthermia. Use incubators or radiant warmers as needed

BOX 5: Complications.

- *Respiratory distress syndrome (RDS):* Premature infants are at risk for RDS due to surfactant deficiency. Manage with surfactant replacement therapy and respiratory support
- *Neonatal sepsis:* Infants are at risk for sepsis due to immature immune systems. Monitor for signs of sepsis, such as fever, lethargy, or poor feeding, and treat promptly with antibiotics
- *Neonatal jaundice:* Physiological jaundice is common in newborns but can progress to severe hyperbilirubinemia. Monitor bilirubin levels and treat with phototherapy or exchange transfusion as needed

BOX 6: Pharmacopoeia.

1. **Antibiotics**
    - **Antimicrobial dosage in normal renal function**
        - Ampicillin* 25–50 mg/kg/dose IV every 6 hours (every 8 hours for neonates <7 days old)
        - Gentamicin 2.5 mg/kg/dose IV given every 8 hours or 7.5 mg/kg/dose IV every 24 hours
        - Ceftriaxone 50–75 mg/kg/dose IV every 24 hours, contraindicated in neonates
        - Cefotaxime 50 mg/kg/dose IV every 8 hours
        - Ceftazidime 50–75 mg/kg/dose IV every 8 hours
        - Cefepime 50 mg/kg/dose IV every 12 hours to a maximum of 1 g per dose
        - Oral antibiotics
    - **Antimicrobial oral dosage in normal renal function:**
        - Oral antibiotics not recommended for neonates and infants <2 months of age
        - Cephalexin 25 mg/kg/dose PO every 8 hours, maximum 500 mg/dose
        - Cefdinir 14 mg/kg/dose PO every 24 hours
        - Cefixime 16 mg/kg/dose PO on day 1 followed by 8 mg/kg every 24 hours
        - Cefpodoxime 5 mg/kg/dose PO every 12 hours
        - Ceftibuten 9 mg/kg/dose PO every 24 hours
        - Amoxicillin-clavulanate 25 mg/kg/dose PO every 8 hours
        - Trimethoprim/Sulfamethoxazole 6 mg/kg PO every 12 hours

Contd...

Contd...

2. **Antipyretic dose/pain management:**
    - Ibuprofen (10 mg/kg PO every 6 hours PRN)
    - Acetaminophen (15 mg/kg/PR every 4 hours PRN)
3. **Fluid choice oral rehydration with standard ORS is preferred in mild-to-moderate dehydration**

    Give 50–100 mL of oral rehydration solution per kilogram of body weight, plus additional oral rehydration solution to compensate for ongoing losses (approximately 10 mL/kg/stool and 2 mL/kg/emesis)

    If intravenous degree of dehydration to be assessed:

    Severe with uncompensated shock:
    - 20 mL/kg 0.9% saline bolus over 5 minutes, repeated until hemodynamically stable
    - 5–10 mL/kg 0.9% saline or 5% dextrose in 0.9% saline for each watery diarrheal stool
    - And, 2 mL/kg 0.9% saline or 5% dextrose in 0.9% saline for each emesis

    Moderate-to-severe without signs of shock:
    - 20 mL/kg 0.9% saline bolus over 1 hour followed by 5% dextrose in 0.9% saline at 1–2 × maintenance rate for 1 hour

    Antiemetic dose—ondansetron is the most common 0.15 mg/kg/dose which can be given in neonates: 5–10% dextrose is the fluid of choice

SUGGESTED READING

1. Cloherty JP, Stark AR, editors. Manual of Neonatal Care. 8th ed. Philadelphia: Lippincott Williams & Wilkins; 2020.
2. Gomella TL, Cunningham MD, Eyal FG, et al., editors. Neonatology: Management, Procedures, OnCall Problems, Diseases, and Drugs. 8th ed. New York: McGraw-Hill Education; 2020.
3. Wyckoff MH, Aziz K, Escobedo MB, et al. Neonatal Resuscitation Program (NRP) Guidelines. Elk Grove Village, IL: American Academy of Pediatrics; 2021.

CHAPTER 21

Psychiatric Emergencies

Nirmee N Shah

INTRODUCTION

The emergency room is the portal of entry for the most acute patients that need treatment.

Many patients who may have psychiatric problems, may also present to the "emergency room" seeking treatment.

BOX 1: Definition of agitation.

- Agitation is a broad term used for behaviors marked by excessive motor or verbal activity
- Patients may present as irritable in mood or may not be cooperative. They may display psychomotor restlessness and agitation, aggression or even violent behavior

BOX 2: Clinical presentation of agitation.

- Inability to stay calm
- Display excessive purposeless motor and/or verbal activity
- Repetitive and restless behavior
- Irritable or hostile mood, emotional lability
- Paranoia
- Escalating tone of voice
- Intense eye contact
- Confusion, disorientation, and delirium
- Fluctuating awareness and attention
- Intoxication
- Inability to communicate
- Muscle tension and pacing
- Suicidal ideation

BOX 3: Etiology of acute agitation.

Medical:

- *Neurological:* Traumatic brain injury, intracranial hemorrhage, seizures, and cardiovascular event
- *Infectious:* Encephalitis, sepsis, and meningitis
- *Metabolic:* Electrolyte disturbance, hypoglycemeia, diabetic ketoacidosis
- *Respiratory:* Pneumonia, hypoxia, and pulmonary embolism
- *Cardiac:* Arrhythmia, myocardial infarction, and heart failure
- *Others:* Neuroleptic malignant syndrome, serotonin syndrome, medication reactions, and pain
- *Delirium:* New onset agitation in someone who is older than 45 years with no previous psychiatric history is suggestive of medical etiology

Substance related:

- Substance misuse and dependence can occur either in isolation or comorbid with other psychiatric illness
- *Common substances:* Alcohol, opioids, stimulants, and hallucinogens
- Newer substances such as bath salts, street drugs like spice or K2
- It may not be possible to detect the newer drugs in available toxicology screens
- Misuse as well as withdrawal from alcohol or substances can contribute to agitation. Withdrawal from alcohol or benzodiazepines can be life-threatening, making early diagnosis vital to management

Psychiatric illness:

- Severe depression particularly of the agitated type
- Bipolar disorder
- Schizophrenia
- Personality disorders

Modifiable risk factors:

- Acute clinical presentation
- Physical illness
- Substance misuse
- Psychiatric illness

Nonmodifiable risk factors:

- Previous history of agitation or violence
- Previous psychiatric hospitalization
- Traumatic brain injury
- Cognitive decline
- Borderline or antisocial personality disorder
- History of sexual or physical abuse
- Interpersonal violence

BOX 4: Assessment.

- Patients who display agitated and disturbed behavior must be assessed in thoughtfully designed environments keeping in mind the safety of both patients and staff
- Designated space for crisis assessments should be available in the emergency room
- Observe the patient in the waiting room to assess their mental status
- Based on agitation level, prepare interview approach
- Work together as a team to manage agitated patients
- Goal is to achieve calmness using minimal restraint
- Triage of the agitated patient in the emergency room must include vital signs, oxygenation level, and blood glucose level
- Laboratory testing must target suspected etiology
- Urine drug screen is recommended
- Gather collateral information from available family/friends. This information may help to gather vital information suggesting possible etiology
- Risk assessment and suicide risk assessment is an integral part of every psychiatric assessment, even more in the emergency room

BOX 5: Assessment of suicide risk.

- *History of suicidal thoughts:* Enquire about active or passive thoughts of death, intent, prior suicidal ideation, any plans made, and previous suicidal attempts
- Enquire about access to means of suicide
- Also screen for associated symptoms of anxiety, mood changes, hopelessness, and impulsivity
- Check for use of alcohol and substances
- Enquire about psychosocial stressors
- Also discuss protective factors which must be discussed and documented when present or absent
- Documentation of risk must be made clearly
- Psychiatrists may be best suited to assess risk

BOX 6: Management of acute agitation.

The goal is to calm the patient. Ideally, the least invasive way possible is recommended. Oversedation should be avoided

Nonpharmacological interventions
Verbal de-escalation:
- Key is early recognition of agitation or aggression
- Try understanding the likely cause of agitation or aggression
- One designated individual should engage the patient
- Respect personal space—at least two arms' length allowing space for both you and the patient to exit
- Response to anger and agitation must be measured and reasonable
- Use simple clear instructions
- Validate the patients' emotions
- Focus on what can be done to help the patient
- Provocation must be avoided at all times
- Use distraction and calming techniques, encourage relaxation

Environment change:
- Environment can impact agitation. Crowding, bright lights, and longer waiting times can contribute to agitation
- Moving the patient to a low stimulation environment can aid in de-escalation

Contd...

Contd...

Physical restraint:
- Staff should be aware of restraint policy at the institute
- Restraint should only be used in exceptional circumstances

Pharmacological management
Medication management:
- Broadly, two classes of medication are used in treating acute agitation—Benzodiazepines and antipsychotics (first and second generation antipsychotics)
- Interventions target modifiable risk factors, treat underlying illness and address substance use
- At all times possible, oral medication should be preferred over parenteral route of administration when patient is cooperative
- In more agitated patients, parenteral route of administration may be required for quicker onset

Antipsychotic medication:
- These are used in treating agitation as they are sedating and are useful in treating underlying psychiatric illness
- First generation antipsychotics such as haloperidol and second generation drugs such as olanzapine, risperidone, and qutipin are used

First-generation drugs:
- *Haloperidol:* Usually between 2–10 mg dose is used with a maximum dose of 20 mg/24 hours. Can be used orally or parenteral administration
- *Per oral (PO)/IM:* Effect expected within 15–30 minutes
- Intravenous (IV): Expect quicker onset of action. If used intravenous, cardiac monitoring is recommended

Second-generation antipsychotics:
- *Olanzapine:* 5–10 mg oral administration
- Risperidone can be used orally. Liquid formulations are also available. Recommended dose 0.5–2 mg

Benzodiazepines:
- These are sedating and calming
- Lorazepam and midazolam are most commonly used drugs in this category
- *Midazolam:* 2–5 mg IM/IV is used. Average time to sedation is 13–18 minutes if used IM and 1–5 minutes, if used IV
- *Lorazepam:* 0.5–2 mg IM/IV. Longer acting compared to midazolam

Rapid tranquillization:
- This means the use of parenteral route of administration (IM/IV)
- Used when oral medication is not possible or not appropriate
- Can be used for quicker sedation
- *Preferred choice:* Intramuscular lorazepam on its own or a combination of intramuscular haloperidol with intramuscular promethazine
- If the patient is antipsychotic naïve, intramuscular lorazepam is the preferred option
- In case of partial response to IM lorazepam, consider further dose
- If no response, IM haloperidol + IM promethazine
- In case of partial response to this combination, repeat dose
- Monitor pulse, blood pressure, respiratory rate, level of hydration, and level of consciousness every hour till there is no further concern
- The former practice of rapid tranquillization wherein large cumulative doses of medication was used in a short span of time to induce sedation is no longer preferred

BOX 7: Special considerations.

- In *elderly population*, there is higher risk of medication interactions. Start at half the adult dose. Consider risk of QTc prolongation and monitor ECG. In this population, benzodiazepines are associated with poorer outcomes and antipsychotics are preferred as first choice
- In *alcohol intoxication*, haloperidol is preferred choice. Alternatively, olanzapine or risperidone can also be used. Benzodiazepines should be avoided

In *stimulant intoxication or alcohol withdrawal or benzodiazepine withdrawal*

- *Lorazepam:* 1–2 mg PO/IM
- *Diazepam:* 5–10 mg PO
- If psychotic symptoms are prominent, add antipsychotics
- *Pregnancy:* Medication should be avoided where possible. Risperidone is recommended as first line as no teratogenic effects
- With haloperidol, there is increased risk of fetal limb defects but this risk is considered to be small and typically seen with long-term use of the drug
- Benzodiazepines should be avoided due to the risk of malformations and cleft lip, particularly after prolonged use especially in the first trimester

SUGGESTED READING

1. Lofchy J, Boyles P, Delwo J. Emergency psychiatry: clinical and training approaches. Can J Psychiatry. 2015;60(6):1-7.
2. National Institute for Health and Care Excellence. Overview | Violence and aggression: short-term management in mental health, health and community settings | Guidance | NICE [Internet]. NICE; 2015. Available from: https://www.nice.org.uk/guidance/ng10

CHAPTER 22

Pain Management

Preeti P Doshi

BOX 1: Introduction.

Pain management is an integral part of patient care in "Emergency Room (ER)" as pain accounts for 78% visits to "Emergency Room" and it can be attributable to variety of etiological causes. The management of pain still remains suboptimal in most EDs, in view of the fact that it is invisible and other symptoms often get preferential attention.

Providing appropriate analgesia is important, since undertreated acute pain is associated with significant negative consequences, including the risk of pain chronification, delayed recovery, impaired sleep, reduced mobility, and poorer quality of life.

Studies have shown that patients whose primary pain is well managed and treated in the ER have a higher overall satisfaction with hospital services.

Given the diversity of healthcare setups across India, including the use and availability of medications, it is clear that any protocol developed needs to be adapted to suit the needs of individual institutions and units.

The ER physicians needs to be conversant with:

- Pain assessment and updated protocols for safe, effective, and timely analgesic administration
- Identifying any serious life-threatening pathology such as myocardial infarction or cerebral hemorrhage requiring urgent attention
- Individualized approach depending on the likely pain generator and patient's condition and profile
- Opioid risk tool to identify patients who are at high risk of abusive drug behaviors

BOX 2: There are a multitude of causes for pain in patient presenting to emergency room (ER).

System	***Example***
Musculoskeletal	Fracture, sprain, dislocation, and severe back and neck pain
Cardiac	Myocardial infarction, aortic dissection or rupture
Neurological	Headache, intracranial hemorrhage—aneurysm, arteriovenous malformation (AVM), hypertension
Gastrointestinal	GI perforation, intestinal obstruction, and appendicitis
Urogenital	Renal colic
Obstetric	Ruptured ectopic pregnancy
Gynecological	Twisted ovarian cyst
Dermatological	Cellulitis and abscess
Chest pain	Noncardiac
Hematological	Vaso-occlusive sickle cell crisis

Pain management forms an important component of patient care in ER after a primary assessment of airway, breathing, and circulation (ABC), and triage tools, such as the Manchester Triage scale.

Depending on the clinical symptoms, an appropriate referral to a relevant specialist is made for further management. This article provides broad outline about the possible options to manage pain until a specialist care is initiated.

BOX 3: Assessment of acute pain in the emergency room.

A numeric rating score (NRS) is a simple quick method to assess pain for majority of patients presenting to ER. FLACC or Wong-Baker facial scales may need to be used for patients with cognitive impairment or pediatric patients. It may, however, not accurately reflect the multidimensional nature of pain.

It is important to attend to severe pain within 15 minutes of arrival in the ER, preferably with intravenous medication. Try to re-assess the pain control within 15–30 minutes in severe and moderate pain.

	No pain	***Mild***	***Moderate***	***Severe***
	0	***1–3***	***4–6***	***7–10***
Initial assessment (NRS)	Within 15 minutes of arrival	Within 15 minutes of arrival	Within 15 minutes of arrival	Within 15 minutes of arrival
Re-evaluation	Within 60 minutes of initial assessment	Within 60 minutes of analgesia	Within 30 minutes of analgesia	Within 15 minutes of analgesia

In patients who have instituted RICE at home, it can be continued while analgesics are administered.

Following reassessment, if analgesia is still found to be inadequate, stronger or increased dose of analgesics should be used along with the use of nonpharmacological measures.

- Assess pain severity
- Use sling, splint, and dressing
- Find any other source of distress
- Consider regional blocks if possible

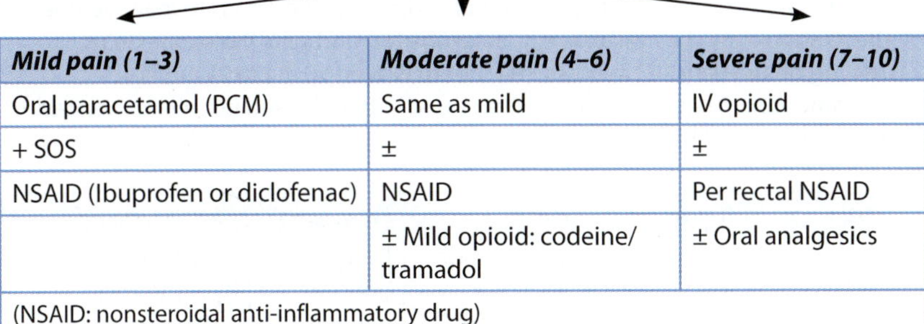

Mild pain (1–3)	***Moderate pain (4–6)***	***Severe pain (7–10)***
Oral paracetamol (PCM)	Same as mild	IV opioid
+ SOS	±	±
NSAID (Ibuprofen or diclofenac)	NSAID	Per rectal NSAID
	± Mild opioid: codeine/ tramadol	± Oral analgesics
(NSAID: nonsteroidal anti-inflammatory drug)		

BOX 4: Pharmacological management.

After a quick assessment, multimodal pharmacological management generally forms the mainstay of treatment. Rapid pain relief is a fundamental element of the treatment of trauma patients in the ER.

Three categories:

1. *Nonopioid drugs:* Nonsteroidal anti-inflammatory drugs (NSAIDs)/Muscle relaxants/antineuropathic drugs: Paracetamol and/or NSAIDs are often used as first-line therapy for mild-to-moderate pain; the route of administration is usually oral or intravenous (IV), depending on the patient's condition and needs. Analgesic dose is titrated by factors such as the age, weight, comorbidities, or special requirements (pregnancy) of the patient.

   Common simple analgesics/NSAID drugs and doses:

Drug	Route	Dose	Frequency SOS	Adverse effects
Paracetamol	Oral/IV	500 mg/650 mg/1 g	Every 6 hours	Liver toxicity
Diclofenac	Oral/IV	50 mg/75 mg/100 mg	Every 12 hours	Gastritis/Ulcer/ Renal toxicity
Ibuprofen	Oral/IV	400 mg	Every 8 hours	Gastritis/Ulcer/ Renal toxicity
Naproxen	Oral	250–500 mg	Every 8 hours	Gastritis/Ulcer/ Renal toxicity
Ketorolac	IV	30 mg	Every 6 hours	Gastritis/Ulcer/ Renal toxicity

2. *Opioid drugs:* Availability of opioids may be challenging in the ER of many hospitals in India. One should be aware about the contraindications and potential side-effects and abuse potential of opioids before administering. Drugs to manage side effects should also be available, e.g., naloxone for morphine [Naloxone bolus 0.04 mg bolus every 2–3 minutes PRN; not to exceed 10 mg (0.01 mg/kg)]

   Intramuscular/transdermal routes have poor titrability and not recommended unless IV access is impossible

Drug	Route	Dose	Frequency	Risks vs. benefit
Morphine	Intravenous (IV)	0.1–0.2 mg/ kg IV is a typical adult dose, or 2–3 mg bolus every 5 minutes	Every 6 hours as needed	Sedation, nausea, hypothermia, and respiratory depression

Contd...

Contd...

Drug	***Route***	***Dose***	***Frequency***	***Risks vs. benefit***
Fentanyl	Intravenous	0.1–0.15 µg/kg Repeat after 10 minutes 0.075 µg/kg	Every 10 minutes with monitoring vital signs/ SpO_2	Rapid onset watch for respiratory depression, hypotension, nausea, vomiting pruritus, and chest wall rigidity
Fentanyl	Nebulization	Nebulization of 4 µg/kg		Pediatric patients found analgesic efficacy equivalent IV morphine (0.1 mg/kg)
Codeine	Oral	30 mg	8 hourly	Nausea/vomiting
Tramadol	Oral/IV	50–100 mg	4–6 hourly	Nausea/vomiting
Tapentadol	Nasal spray	22.5 mg/spray	6 hourly	Nausea/vomiting

3. *Other drugs for analgesia:*

Ketamine	IV	0.1–0.3 mg/kg over 15 minutes	Equal pain relief at 60 minutes (Like morphine)	Nausea, vomiting, dizziness, diplopia (double vision), drowsiness, and dysphoria
Lignocaine	IV	1–1.5 mg/kg dose over 10 to 15 minutes	NP-PHN; lipopolysaccharide binding protein (LBP); renal colic	Use on case-to-case basis—not regularly

(NP-PHN: neuropathic pain e.g., postherpetic neuralgia)

Other routes:

Inhalation: Entonox®, a 50% mixture of nitrous oxide and oxygen, is very useful for short term and rapid relief of severe pain—Caution in head or chest injury, pregnancy, middle ear disease, etc.

Regional blocks:

- Point-of-care ultrasound (POCUS) is a rapidly accepted concept in the care of patients in EMS
- Ultrasound-guided "Regional Anesthesia" can be a useful tool to provide significant pain reduction, alleviates the need for rescue opioid analgesia, and decreases the length of stay in the ER (Details are mentioned in a separate chapter)

BOX 5: Nonpharmacological methods.

Cryotherapy/Heat therapy/Manipulation/Splints/Acupuncture/Acupressure

BOX 6: Keypoints to keep in mind while treating pain in emergency room (ER).

1. Identify the underlying medical or surgical cause for pain
2. Pain cannot be treated if it cannot be assessed
3. Pain should be addressed within a reasonable amount of time
4. Pain relief has medical benefits
5. Consider targeted analgesia
6. When pain is severe, intravenous (IV) analgesia is usually preferable
7. Pain care is an ongoing process in the ER
8. Pain care is an ongoing process after ER discharge
9. Keep it simple

Transition care/Discharge care:

If the patient is advised hospital admission or discharge, a full report on treatment received including details of administration of drug (dose, frequency, response, and side effects) should be provided to the receiving medical team or caregiver, respectively.

BOX 7: Conclusion.

Education and training of ER staff to assess and manage pain in a timely, safe, and effective manner as per individual patient needs can help to improve outcomes and patient's satisfaction. Nonopioids analgesics such as NSAIDs and acetaminophen are commonly used in the treatment of acute pain. However, the relief of acute moderate to severe pain usually requires opioid agents. Opioid medications do not come without risk, patients should be evaluated frequently for drug interactions and adverse events. Discharge planning requires a collaborative effort to ensure patient safety.

SUGGESTED READING

1. Cordell WH, Keene KK, Giles BK, Jones JB, Jones JH, Brizendine EJ. The high prevalence of pain in emergency medical care. Am J Emerg Med. 2002;20:165-9.
2. Emergency Triage: Manchester Triage Group, 3rd Edition. New Jersey: Wiley Blackwell; 2013.
3. Motov SM, Vlasica K, Middlebrook I, LaPietra A. Pain management in the emergency department: a clinical review. Clin Exp Emerg Med. 2021;8(4):268-78.
4. Thomas SH. Management of Pain in the Emergency Department. ISRN Emerg Med. 2013.
5. Todd KH, Ducharme J, Choiniere M, Crandall CS, Fosnocht DE, Homel P, et al. Pain in the emergency department: results of the pain and emergency medicine initiative (PEMI) multicenter study. J Pain. 2007;8(6):460-6.

CHAPTER 23

Comprehending Palliative Care in Emergency Medicine

Manali Patel

BOX 1: Concept and benefits.

- Palliative care is comfort-oriented care without hastening process of dying. Life-prolonging interventions can delay dying and add days of suffering end of life phase. Decisions about life-sustaining interventions like invasive mechanical ventilation, cardiopulmonary resuscitation (CPR) are made rapidly in emergency room (ER), thus, every ER physician should be aware of basic concept of palliative care
- Many acute deterioration lead to repeated admission in the background of chronic, life limiting, and advanced illness. These episodes increase toward end of life. Early integration of palliative care can reduce these repeated visits by better understanding these diseases and connecting patients to home-based care services, which will reduce cost, burden of ER visit, and hospitalization
- Comfort care options should be discussed with families of these patients with deteriorating quality of life. It has significant impact on improving quality of life as well as quality of death. It should include acute condition without significant chronic illnesses like prolonged CPR (Null-Please Score or CREST score >5 high mortality risk)

BOX 2: Palliative care common terminology.

- World Health Organization (WHO) defines palliative care as an approach that improves the quality of life of patients—adults and children—and their families who are facing problems associated with life-threatening illness. It prevents and relieves suffering through the early identification, impeccable assessment and treatment of pain and other problems, whether physical, psychosocial, or spiritual. Thus, whether the cause of suffering is cardiovascular disease, cancer, major organ failure, drug-resistant tuberculosis, severe burns, end-stage chronic illness, acute trauma, extreme birth prematurity or extreme frailty of old age, and palliative care may be needed and has to be available at all levels of care
- *Hospice:* Hospice is a place to provide palliative care at the end of life with intention to comfort care only and not to hospitalize
- *End-of-life care:* Palliative care does not mean end of life. End-of-life care is part of palliative care when treatment options are exhausted. It improves quality of death by measures to reduce symptoms burden

Contd...

Contd...

- *Advanced directive:* Advance directives are the documents the person fills out while still having the capacity to make decisions concerning their healthcare in a situation in which they become incompetent of performing so. These are legal papers that appoint surrogate decision-makers and/or offer guidance for choices regarding treatment
- *Living will:* Living will is a written statement of a person's wishes for their medical treatment in the future. A living will usually covers resuscitation and life support; however, it can also cover preferences for hospitalization, pain management, and other possible treatments (e.g., chemotherapy for cancer, ventilatory support for respiratory disease, or inserted defibrillators for heart failure, or feedings through tubes for dementia). Importantly, a living will cannot be made by a surrogate on the patient's behalf
- *Surrogate:* Persons who represent patients when they lose their capability to make decision for themselves
- *Decision-making capacity versus competence:* Decision-making capacity is ability to understand information about illness and treatment options to choose as per his preference which is decided by clinician. Competence is decided by legal judgment if patient has legal right to decide for oneself. Consultation of psychiatry may be necessary, if decisional capacity is difficult to assess
- *Withholding versus withdrawing of nonbeneficial life sustain interventions:* Preventing medical therapy before it begins is referred to as withholding care. The term "withdrawal of care" describes the end of a medical intervention that has already been started, such as ventilator support. The emotional burden of terminating a treatment is more for some doctors and family members than it is for withholding it, even when there is no morally significant distinction among the two
- *Comfort measures only:* Treatment which improves comfort irrespective of disease

BOX 3: Eastern Cooperative Oncology Group (ECOG).

Performance status	*Definition*
0	Fully active; no performance restrictions
1	Strenuous physical activity restricted; fully ambulatory and able to carry out light work
2	Capable of all self-care but not able to carry out any work activities. Able to be up and about for about >50% of waking hours
3	Capable of only limited self-care; confined to a bed or chair >50% of waking hours
4	Completely disabled; not able to carry out any self-care; totally confined to a bed or chair

Source: Table adapted and modified from Oken MM, Creech RH, Tormey DC, Horton J, Davis TE, McFadden ET, et al. Toxicity and response criteria of the Eastern Cooperative Oncology Group. Am J Clin Oncol. 1982;5(6):649-55.

BOX 4: Indication of emergency room (ER) visit patients with advanced diseases.

- New acute event [acute coronary syndrome (ACS), cerebrovascular accident (CVA), trauma, bleeding, acute abdomen, urine retention, spinal cord compression, etc.]
- Exacerbation of progressive disease
- Increase intensity of previous chronic symptom, e.g., pain, dyspnea, constipation, nausea and vomiting, and weakness
- Malfunction/malposition/accidental extubation of feeding tube, tracheostomy tube, and urinary catheter
- Reduced performance status, worsened frailty
- Altered sensorium (e.g., delirium)
- Psychological distress
- Social problems (e.g., lack of home-based palliative care availability or awareness, a caregiver burnout, and poor coordination of care)
- Logistic issues (lack of space in house and caregiver support)
- Inability to witness suffering of patient
- Conflicts about prognosis and treatment options

BOX 5: Expected palliative care skills of emergency room (ER) physician.

- Recognition and screening of palliative care need
- Assessment and treatment of basic distressing symptoms and their objective in context of situation
- Communication about prognosis, goals of care, recommendation about only comfort care, futility of interventions [ventilator, cardiopulmonary resuscitation (CPR), vasopressor, and ICU admission], and death disclosure
- Providing suggestions regarding the code status
- Clearly identifying primary treatment group
- Seeking agreement from treating medical practitioners and the patient's relatives
- Identifying end of life issues and imminently dying patient
- Further coordinating expert care-disposition
- Monitoring the shift to hospice care/home as per patient's wishes
- Connect to home care services team for support at home
- Monitoring discharges from the hospital

BOX 6: How to proceed?

- In an already overwhelmed emergency room (ER), considering palliative care can seem daunting, let alone implementing it. The ER is frequently inundated with acute cases, and patients who have no other place to go after outpatient hours often end up there. The focus of the ER team should not be on providing palliative care directly. Instead, they should identify candidates for palliative care and assign a team to discuss alternative options with the patient and their relatives
- When making assessments quickly on life-saving procedures (such as intubation for respiratory failure), it is important to first establish the primary goals of care
- Find the legal decision-maker and check if any advance directives have been completed
- Finish the quick goals-of-care evaluation
- Make a plan recommendation ("Based on the goals you describe, I would recommend doing...")
- In the event that the patient is in the process of dying
- Determine the patient's or family's desired location for the dying process (e.g., return home with home-based medical support; private hospital room; and private place in the ER); consider the patient's cultural and spiritual needs; ensure privacy
- Diagnostic assessment
- Testing should wait, whenever possible, until after discussing with the hospice care team. The goals of care as expressed by the patient should guide testing
- Low-burden, noninvasive procedures that might reveal reversible pathology or provide explanation on the prognosis should be carried out first, if testing is needed
- Palliative-care screening tools such as "Palliative Care and Rapid Emergency Screening (P-CaRES) and Screen for Palliative and End-of-life care needs in the ER (SPEED)" can be utilized

BOX 7: Symptom management.

- *Dyspnea:*
  - Assessment reversible cause like congestive cardiac failure, pulmonary edema, airway obstruction, reversible airway obstruction, pleural effusion, arrhythmia, angioedema, pericardial effusion, pneumothorax, acute coronary syndrome, gross ascites, and psychosocial factor
  - *Treatment:* Opioids are drug of choice
  - *Morphine opioid naïve:* Tablet morphine IR 5–10 mg can be repeated after 60 minutes/Injection 2–5 mg IV
- For acute dyspnea treatment intravenous 2 mg every 5–10 minutes until symptoms improve
- Patients taking morphine for pain 10% of daily dose—increase regular morphine dose by 25%
- Watch for sedation, respiratory depression, and confusion
- If morphine allergy (nausea/hypotension)—oxycodone or hydromorphone to consider
- Oxycodone 5 mg orally can repeat after 1 hour
- Hydromorphone 0.2 mg subcutaneously (SC) every 5–10 minutes as needed

BOX 8: Other interventions.

- Treat psychosocial factors—relaxation techniques, distraction, activity and behavioral modification, cognitive therapy, and antidepressant for depression component
- Pulmonary rehabilitation benzodiazepines for anxiety-related dyspnea, secretion management, fan, oxygen, and noninvasive ventilation (NIV) are other options, nutrition, and energy conservative activity planning

Following issues are covered in other chapters:

- Delirium
- Pruritus
- Swelling
- Nausea vomiting
- Cough hemoptysis
- Malignant bowel obstruction
- Chronic wounds including malodorous or bleeding malignancy-related wound
- Acute urinary retention
- *Pain*—causes of pain in chronic illness (Chapter 22: Pain Management)
- Constipation (Chapter 4.8)

BOX 9: End-of-life symptom management.

- Delirium, nausea/vomiting—haloperidol 1–2 mg 2nd hourly till it settles then 6–8 hourly
- Agitation/delirium midazolam 1–5 mg every 5–15 minutes or infusion 1 mg/hour IV/SC titrate
- Death rattle—noisy breathing C = due to secretions in throat
- Keep throat dry
- Glycopyrrolate 0.2 mg SC 4 hourly or 0.1 mg SL orally
- Scopolamine patch 1.5 mg apply behind ear every 72 hourly or 20 mg SC 4–6 hourly

SUGGESTED READING

1. Givens J. (2024). What's new in palliative care? UpToDate. [online] Available from https://sso.uptodate.com/contents/palliative-care-for-adults-in-the-ed-goals-of-care-communication-consultation-and-patient-death [Last accessed September, 2024].
2. Indian Association of Palliative Care. IAPC Textbook for certificate course in essentials of palliative care. New Delhi: Indian Association of Palliative Care; 2012.
3. Tan AJ, Swartz J, Wilkins C, Grudzen C. Leveraging Emergency Department Information Systems to Address Palliative Care Needs of ED Patients During the COVID Pandemic. Am J Hosp Palliat Care. 2022;39(5):581.

CHAPTER 24

Anaphylaxis

Indraneel P Raut

BOX 1: Introduction.

- Anaphylaxis is a rapid and widespread allergic reaction triggered by exposure to a foreign substance
- It can involve mechanisms such as immunoglobulin E (IgE)-mediated reactions, complement-mediated responses, or mechanisms that are not fully understood
- Common triggers include drugs, insect stings/bites, food, and latex

BOX 2: Clinical manifestations of anaphylaxis.

Eye:
- Conjunctivitis
- Itching
- Increased lacrimation

ENT (Ear, Nose, Throat):
- Throat fullness
- Tongue swelling
- Uvular edema

Skin:
- Urticaria and/or angioedema
- Flushing
- Pruritus

Respiratory:
- Shortness of breath and/or wheezing
- Pharyngeal or laryngeal edema
- Stridor (rare)
- Rhinitis

Cardiovascular:
- Hypotension
- Chest pain

Gastrointestinal (GI):
- Nausea, emesis, cramps, or diarrhea

Contd...

Contd...

Neurological:
- Headache
- Seizure
- Sense of impending doom
- Confusion

Hematologic:
- Disseminated intravascular coagulation
- Abnormal bleeding and bruising
- Mucous membrane bleeding
- Increased uterine tone
- Vaginal bleeding

Genitourinary:
- Pelvic pain
- Urinary incontinence

Caveat: Any system can be involved but history of foreign exposure needs to be there

BOX 3: Diagnosis of anaphylaxis on basis of clinical criteria.

Anaphylaxis is probable if exposure to a known allergen is associated with involvement of multiple organs as below:

- Sudden onset of illness with skin or mucosal involvement, plus:
  - Respiratory system involvement in the form of fall in saturation, increased respiratory rate or wheeze
  - Reduced blood pressure or symptoms of end-organ dysfunction

Or

- Rapid onset of two or more symptoms after exposure to a likely allergen:
  - Skin or mucosal tissue involvement
  - Respiratory system involvement in the form of fall in saturation, increased respiratory rate or wheeze
  - Reduced blood pressure or symptoms of end-organ dysfunction
  - Gastrointestinal symptoms

Or

- A significant drop in blood pressure following exposure to a recognized allergen can be observed as follows:
  - *Infants and children:* A notably low systolic blood pressure or a decrease of >30% in systolic blood pressure
  - *Adults:* A systolic blood pressure below 90 mm Hg or a reduction of >30% from the baseline level

BOX 4: Differential diagnosis of anaphylaxis.

Caveat: It can be a wide range of differentials, hence, history of exposure to allergens is important

- Acute generalized urticaria
- Asthma exacerbation
- Myocardial infarction
- Pulmonary embolism
- Syncope
- Adverse cutaneous drug reactions
- Anxiety/panic attacks

Flush syndrome
Conditions causing flushing:

- Food-related reactions
- Alcohol
- Scombroidosis
- Carcinoid tumors
- Perimenopause
- Thyrotoxicosis

Shock syndromes:

- Septic
- Hypovolemic
- Cardiogenic
- Distributive

Miscellaneous:

- Hypoglycemia
- Red man syndrome (Vancomycin)
- Central nervous system disorders (seizure and stroke)
- Dysfunctioning vocal cord

BOX 5: Diagnosis.

Diagnosis of anaphylaxis is primarily clinical, based on symptoms and presentation. (As serum histamine and tryptase levels may be elevated but are not typically used in acute settings).

BOX 6: Management.

Emergency measures (simultaneously):
- Remove the triggering agent
- Assess and stabilize airway, breathing, and circulation
- Initiate rapid infusion of isotonic crystalloid (normal saline)
- Anaphylaxis treatment medications

First-line agent

Epinephrine is the primary medication for anaphylaxis:
- *Adults:* 0.3–0.5 mg IM (1:1,000 concentration) injected into the anterolateral thigh every 5–10 minutes as needed
- *Pediatrics:* 0.01 mg/kg IM (1:1,000 concentration) injected into the anterolateral thigh every 5–10 minutes as needed

Alternatively, you can use an EpiPen (0.3 mL) or EpiPen Jr (0.15 mL) for administration in the anterolateral thigh

Second-line agents

After administering epinephrine:
- Antihistamines (e.g., diphenhydramine)
- H_2-receptor antagonists (e.g., ranitidine)
- Aerosolized β-agonists (for bronchospasm)

Glucocorticoids

Though not effective for immediate management, glucocorticoids may be utilized:
- *Methylprednisolone:* Adults—125–250 mg IV; Pediatrics—12 mg/kg IV
- *Prednisone/Prednisolone:* Adults—40–60 mg orally; Pediatrics—12 mg/kg orally

Refractory hypotension

For persistent hypotension, consider a continuous IV epinephrine infusion [dilute 1 mg (1 mL of 1:1,000) in 1,000 mL of normal saline or D5W to achieve a concentration of 1 μg/mL):
- *Adults:* 1–10 μg/min IV
- *Pediatrics:* 0.1–1.5 μg/kg/min IV

Other vasopressors

In cases where epinephrine is insufficient:
- Dopamine, norepinephrine, phenylephrine, or vasopressin can be considered

Beta-blockade

For patients on β-blockers:
- *Administer glucagon:* 1–5 mg IV over 5 minutes, followed by a continuous IV infusion of 5–15 μg/min

BOX 7: Important notes.

- Epinephrine remains underutilized despite being the preferred treatment for anaphylaxis
- Injections in the thigh are more effective than those in the deltoid
- In suspected anaphylactic respiratory arrest, administer epinephrine/adrenaline before attempting intubation
- If the symptoms of anaphylaxis post sc adrenaline subsides, patient can be discharged after 2 hours of observation as very unlikely for a patient to have delayed peak response of anaphylaxis, and if any the patient should be trained to self-administer adrenaline via injector pens

SUGGESTED READING

1. Kemp SF, Lockey RF. Anaphylaxis: A review of causes and mechanisms. J Allergy Clin Immunol. 2002;110(3):341-8.
2. Lieberman P, Nicklas RA, Oppenheimer J, Kemp SF, Lang DM, Bernstein DI, et al. The diagnosis and management of anaphylaxis practice parameter: 2010 update. J Allergy Clin Immunol. 2010;126(3):477-80.e1-42.
3. Muraro A, Roberts G, Worm M, Bilò MB, Brockow K, Fernández Rivas M, et al. Anaphylaxis: Guidelines from the European Academy of Allergy and Clinical Immunology. Allergy. 2014;69(8):1026-45.
4. Sampson HA, Muñoz-Furlong A, Campbell RL, Adkinson NF Jr, Bock SA, Branum A, et al. Second symposium on the definition and management of anaphylaxis: Summary report—Second National Institute of Allergy and Infectious Disease/ Food Allergy and Anaphylaxis Network symposium. J Allergy Clin Immunol. 2006;117(2):391-7.
5. Simons FE, Ardusso LR, Bilò MB, El-Gamal YM, Ledford DK, Ring J, et al. (2011). World Allergy Organization anaphylaxis guidelines: Summary. J Allergy Clin Immunol. 2011;127(3):587-93.e1-22.
6. Tintinalli JE, Ma OJ, Yealy DM, Meckler GD, Stapczynski JS, Cline DM, et al. Tintinalli's Emergency Medicine: A Comprehensive Study Guide, 9th edition. New York, NY: McGraw-Hill Education; 2020.
7. Walls RM, Hockberger RS, Gausche-Hill M (Eds). Rosen's Emergency Medicine: Concepts and Clinical Practice, 9th edition. Amsterdam, Netherlands: Elsevier; 2018.

CHAPTER 25

Wound Management

Snehal A Bhange

Wound—Any breach in the natural continuity of any tissues of the living body.

Types of wounds commonly encountered in EMS are mentioned in **Box 1**:

Evaluation: Primary survey and resuscitation is the main stay in all ER patients.

BOX 1: Types of wounds encountered in the emergency medical services (EMS).

- *Contusion:* Hemorrhage in the dermis, subcutaneous tissues, deep soft tissues or internal organs as a result of blunt force trauma
- *Abrasion:* Superficial denudation of the epithelium due to scraping or pressure They have high chances of being contaminated and getting infected if not primarily treated
- Lacerations are *a pattern of injury in which skin and underlying tissues are cut or torn exposing the underlying tissue*. They can be clean incised wounds, e.g., from sharp instruments or with contused jagged edges due to direct forceful trauma that splits open the skin. Most of the wounds encountered in trauma patients have a high chance of being contaminated and infection
- Diabetic foot wounds
- Venous or arterial ulcers and nonhealing wounds ± Gangrene
- *Stab wounds:* Wound by a sharp penetrating object where the depth of the wound is more than the visible length
- Animal bites [punctures and clean lacerated wound (CLW)]
- Gunshot wound (GSW)
- Crush injuries seen due to excessive compressive forces on the body in between two hard surfaces
- Burns
- Pressure sores

BOX 2: Management.

Mainstay in wound management:
- *Proper history taking:* Mode of injury/onset of symptoms and duration of the wound
- Associated complaints such as fever, pain, and discharge
- Comorbidities and list of medications being taken (performance status is important to guide treatment modalities)

General physical examination:
- *Pyrexia:* Points to presence of infection
- *Pulse:* Guide to sepsis and/or degree of hemorrhage
- Hypotension in major trauma will guide resuscitation and promptness of intervention
- *High BP:* In case of lower limb ulcers will point to atherosclerotic changes and possible arterial ulcers
- *Respiratory rate:* Guide to sepsis and ongoing hemorrhagic shock

Laboratory investigations:
- White blood cell (WBC) count
- Anemia
- Blood urea nitrogen (BUN)/Creatinine
- Glycated hemoglobin (HbA1c)
- Blood gas analysis in severe sepsis

In case of a trauma patient, the wound assessment is a part of the primary and secondary survey and management is basis advanced trauma life support (ATLS) guidelines, 10th edition.

For all other wounds secondary to systemic illness, following is important:

BOX 3: Wound assessment.

- Location of wound
- Dimensions
- *Joint involvement and patient mobility:* Proximity to any joint which can restrict movement
- Vascularity distal to the wound area
- Assess for signs and symptoms of infection, which include the following:
    - Redness
    - Warmth of surrounding tissue
    - Swelling
    - Tenderness or pain
    - Type of drainage
    - Fever and increased white blood cell count
    - Drainage, if any, can point toward the nature of illness and the degree of infection and may also guide to modality of intervention
        - *Sanguineous:* Fresh bleeding (sometimes seen in varicose ulcers)
        - *Serous:* Clear, thin, and watery plasma seen during inflammatory phase. In small amounts this is normal
        - *Serosanguinous:* Serous drainage with small amounts of blood
        - *Purulent:* Thick sticky exudate. It can be tan, yellow, green, or brown in color depending on causative organism. Its presence is never normal

BOX 4: Classifications of wounds.

Sometimes we may encounter patients with surgical site infections or dehiscence of surgical wounds, in such circumstances it is beneficial to know the classification of surgical wounds as per the Centers for Disease Control and Prevention

- *Class 1 wounds:* Clean wounds. Neither infected nor have any signs of inflammation. They are closed primarily. They do not involve the respiratory, alimentary, genital, or urinary tracts, e.g., open inguinal hernia repair, thyroidectomy, and mastectomy
- *Class 2 wounds:* Clean-contaminated. Low level of contamination which is controlled with no spillage. These involve entry into the respiratory, alimentary, genital, or urinary tracts, e.g., laparoscopic cholecystectomy and laparoscopic hernia repairs
- *Class 3 wounds:* Contaminated. They result from a breach in sterile techniques or leakage from the gastrointestinal tract, e.g., major bowel resections with controlled spillage. Incisions resulting from acute or nonpurulent inflammation are also considered
- *Class 4 wounds:* Dirty or infected. These injuries usually occur from inadequate treatment of traumatic wounds, gross purulence, and evident infections, e.g., crush injury, perianal or any other abscess

BOX 5: Management of traumatic wounds.

- *Contused abrasions:*
  - Simple cleansing with antiseptics and disinfectants (betadine and alcohol-based disinfectants, e.g., AHD)
  - Analgesics and anti-inflammatories help
- Minor CLW which are present on limbs, scalp, trunk, and face in adults can be very well managed in the EMS by primary suturing under local anesthesia after a thorough debridement if needed
- Some wounds which are contaminated or have ragged devitalized edges may need minor debridement. This can be achieved with hydrogen peroxide along with mechanical sharp debridement before considering primary closure

BOX 6: Suturing: Why?

- Closing dead space to prevent collections and delayed healing
- Approximating skin edges for a cosmetic and functional result
- Minimizing the risks of bleeding and secondary infection
- Supporting tissues till such time as natural healing returns the tensile strength

BOX 7: Suture technique.

The choice of suture technique depends on the following:

- Type and anatomic location of the wound
- Thickness of the skin/depth of wound
- Degree of tension/degree of gaping of edges
- Desired cosmetic result
- Proximity to major joints
- Whether closure needs to be done in separate layers or en masse

BOX 8: Which suture to use where?

- Use the smallest suture that adequately holds the healing wound edges. The tensile strength of the suture should be equal or less than the tensile strength of the tissue
- Nonabsorbable suture should be considered in skin, fascia, and tendons (slowly healing tissues) (prefer 3-0/4-0 ethilon for skin and 4-0/3-0 prolene for fascia and tendons), whereas mucosal wounds (rapidly healing tissues) may be closed with absorbable sutures (3-0/4-0 polyglactin/vicryl)
- Areas such as the eyelid, periorbital area, nose, pinna, lip, vermillion, etc. where the tensile strength requirements tend to be less, smaller suture sizes are preferred (4-0/5-0 prolene or ethilon)
- No standardized sizing system is available for needles. The main concern should be minimal trauma. A taper-point needle is sufficient for tissues that are easy to penetrate (in essence, all tissues except skin). Cutting needles are typically reserved for tough tissues like skin and fascia. The length, diameter, and curvature of the needle will depend on the thickness and depth of wound and layers involved

BOX 9: Suturing techniques.

Suturing technique: The most versatile suture in cutaneous surgery is the simple interrupted suture

Few other suturing techniques are:
- Simple running suture (for areas like scalp or extremity wounds which bleed from skin edges)
- Running locked suture (for areas like scalp or extremity wounds which bleed from skin edges)
- Vertical mattress suture (for CLW which are relatively deeper till muscle and need closure in single layers, where skin loss is more for a simple approximation, and we expect delay in healing)
- Horizontal mattress suture (same as above)
- Running subcuticular sutures (for clean incised wounds, for better cosmetic results)

BOX 10: Alternative methods of wound closure.

- *Wound closure tapes (e.g., Steri-Strips):* Reinforced microporous surgical adhesive tape. They provide extra support to a suture line, either when running subcuticular sutures are used or after sutures are removed
- Stainless steel staples are used to approximate wound edges in wounds under high tension, e.g., scalp or the trunk
- *Tissue adhesive:* Cyanoacrylate glues may be applied to superficial wounds to block pinpoint skin hemorrhages and to precisely coapt wound edges **(Figs. 1 to 3)**

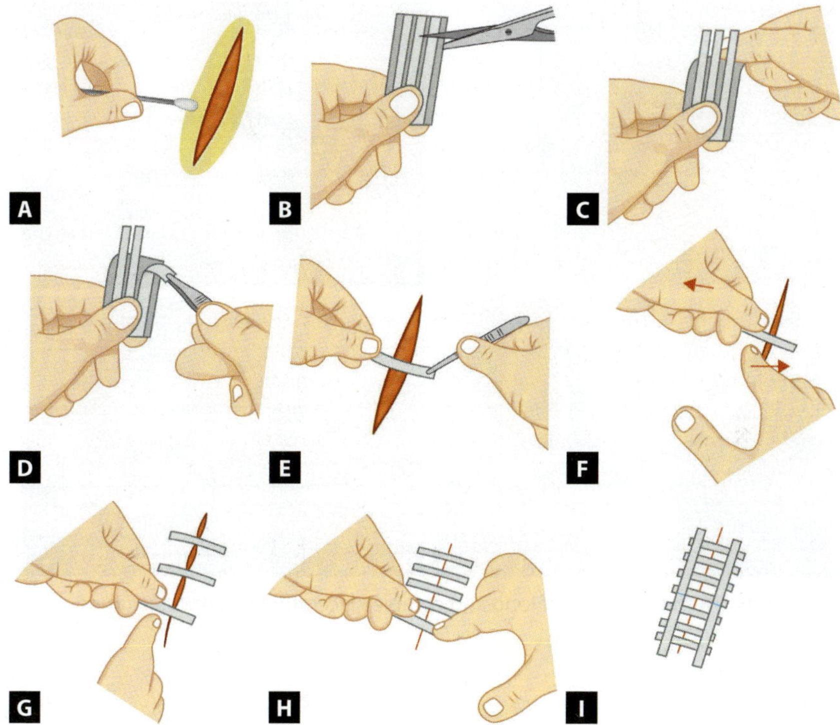

Figs. 1A to I: Laceration repair with adhesive tapes.

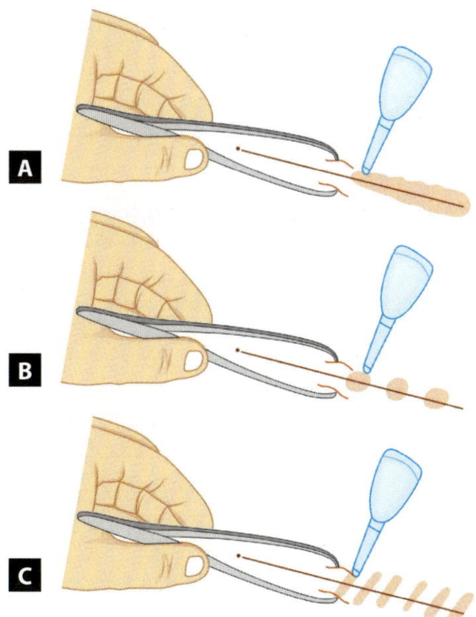

Figs. 2A to C: Laceration repair with tissue adhesives.

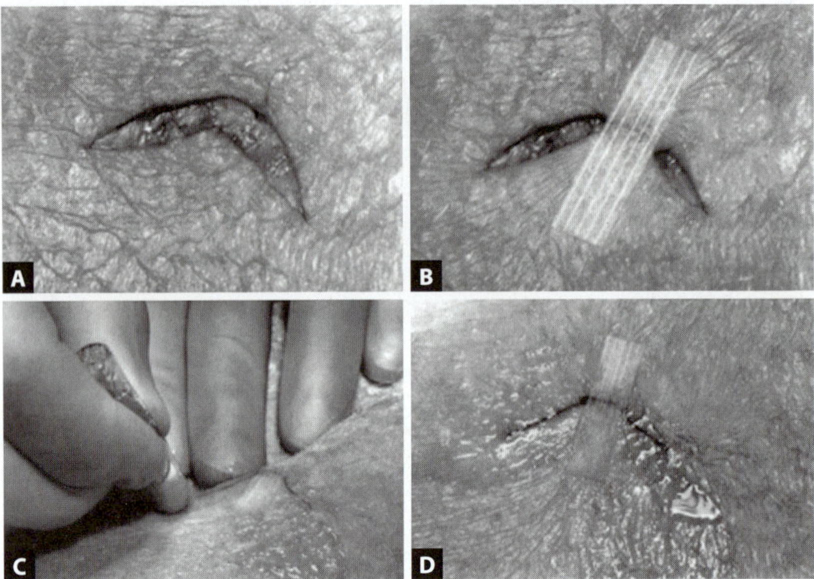

Figs. 3A to D: Closure of long and complex laceration by adhesive tapes.

BOX 11: Management of diabetic foot wounds.

- Patients with uncontrolled diabetes present with infected wounds mostly over their feet secondary to minor trauma which goes unnoticed, the extent may be involvement of few toes to the entire foot being involved in the disease process and cellulitis extending to the leg too. These patients are mostly septic, and need inpatient multidisciplinary care. Wound management is important to get the sepsis under control and majority of the times such patients need debridement under anesthesia
- The following classification systems will help to decide which patient needs admission:
  A. *The Wagner–Meggitt classification* is based mainly on wound depth and consists of 6 wound grades:
    1. Grade 0 (intact skin)
    2. Grade 1 (superficial ulcer)
    3. Grade 2 (deep ulcer to tendon, bone, or joint)
    4. Grade 3 (deep ulcer with abscess or osteomyelitis)
    5. Grade 4 (forefoot gangrene)
    6. Grade 5 (whole foot gangrene)

  B. *University of texas classification:*

	Grade 0	*Grade 1*	*Grade 2*	*Grade 3*
Stage 1	Preulcerative or postulcerative lesions completely epithelialized	Superficial wound not involving tendon, capsule or bone	Wound penetrating tendon or capsule	Wound penetrating to bone or joint
Stage 2	Infection	Infection	Infection	Infection
Stage 3	Ischemia	Ischemia	Ischemia	Ischemia
Stage 4	Infection and ischemia	Infection and ischemia	Infection and ischemia	Infection and ischemia

It is advisable to send cultures from the EMS before starting empiric antibiotics

- Many diabetic patients present to us with stage 2 and above wounds which need surgical debridement and admission for sugar and sepsis control
- Sharp extensive mechanical debridement under all aseptic precautions preferably under anesthesia is the best way forward
- Many patients also have concomitant atherosclerotic disease and may benefit from revascularization procedures (peripheral angioplasty) before major surgery like amputations

BOX 12: Management of venous ulcers.

Some patients may present with varicose ulcers, usually seen on the medial malleolus area (gaiter area)

Signs and symptoms of venous ulcers include:
- Shallow sore with a red base, sometimes covered by yellow tissue
- Unevenly shaped borders
- Surrounding skin may be shiny, tight, warm or hot, and discolored
- Leg pain more by the end of the day, in calf area
- If the sore becomes infected, it may have a bad odor, and pus may drain from the wound

Rarely, these patients may present as an emergency with severe bleeding from the ulcer base. This can be treated easily with compression and limb elevation

These wounds need simple dressings with normal saline and antiseptic solutions. The main treatment of varicose ulcers is *graduated pressure dressings.* Different class of compression dressings are readily available

The pressure dressings need to achieve a higher pressure at the calf area than the ankle area, hence known as graduated compression dressings. The various compression grades are:
- Class 1: <20 mm Hg
- Class 2: 20–30 mm Hg
- Class 3: >30 mm Hg

Usually, we prefer class 2 compression stockinette over simple sterile dressings

BOX 13: Management of arterial ulcers.

Distinguishing features of arterial ulcers include:
- Located on the lower legs and tops of the feet or toes, especially on weight bearing areas
- Rest pain
- Punched-out appearance
- Minimal bleeding
- Cool, pale, or bluish surrounding skin that appears shiny, with loss of hair and brittle nails and thinning of affected extremity
- Faint or absent ankle pulses
- These patients do not usually present with sepsis but mostly nonhealing chronic ulcers. These need proper angiographic evaluation and consideration for revascularization,
- Simple wound dressings SOS small debridement can be offered in EMS

Note: Be careful not to use local anesthetic with adrenaline during debridement

BOX 14: Wound dressings.

Wound dressings: An ideal dressing not only protects a wound and maintains wound humidity but is also biocompatible, biodegradable, nontoxic, and nonallergenic while promoting gas exchange, granulation, and re-epithelialization

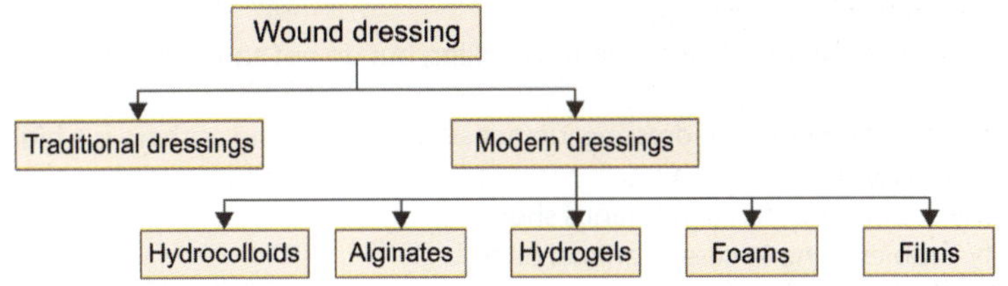

The newer dressing materials help by reducing frequency of change of dressings by being more absorptive and less painful

BOX 15: Management of other high velocity wounds.

Stab injuries/gunshot wound (GSW): [Manage as per advanced trauma life support (ATLS) guidelines]
- Often present in a state of hemodynamic instability depending on the site of the stab wounds (limb, trunk, face, neck, etc.) and the number of wounds
- Initial resuscitation is very important and permissive hypotension may be advisable in stab wounds with arterial injuries
- Application of tourniquet to limbs may be weighed cautiously against options of pressure dressings and immediate surgical exploration in theater
- Preoperative imaging is desirable if hemodynamic stability can be maintained
- Immediate transfer to theater in case of hemodynamic instability

The most common organs injured are the small bowel (50%), large bowel (40%), liver (30%), and intraabdominal vascular (25%)

Puncture wounds:
- Wash with lots of flowing water and soap
- Do not squeeze out the blood
- Bits of clothing or debris might be present in the wound so thorough washing is important
- Usually do not bleed but risk of infection depending on mode of injury (rusty nail, thorn, needle, etc.)
- Can apply pressure to stop bleeding
- Apply antibiotic ointment and dress it with bandage
- Do not leave open, reduce chances of secondary infection
- Serial monitoring to look for signs of infection
- Tetanus shot, if not received one within last 5 years

Contd...

Contd...

Bite wounds: Can be both from animals or humans. Both have a lot of bacteria in their mouths, which can cause an infection if a bite breaks the skin

- Clean the wound immediately by running warm tap water over it for a couple of minutes even if skin intact
- Remove any debris, if present
- Allow to bleed slightly, helps to remove toxins, but do not squeeze out surrounding area
- Proper debridement then dressing, do not suture the wound as there is a higher risk of infection
- Prophylactic antibiotics and tetanus shot
- Verify if rabies or no in case of animal bites
- Prophylactic antirabies vaccine to be given

Foreign body in wounds:

- Proper evaluation of all contaminated CLW
- Thorough cleaning with antiseptics
- *Exploration under local anesthesia:* Explore layer wise and try to mechanically remove all particles
- Through antiseptic cleansing is required afterward with sterile dressings
- Regular site checks and dressing to detect early infection

Postsurgical wounds: Depending on the grade of the surgery whether clean, contaminated or dirty the risk of wound infection differs. Contaminated and dirty cases have higher chances of wound infection

- History of systemic symptoms of fever with chills
- History of discharge from the wound, color, and smell
- Carefully examine and see if any signs of burst abdomen (copious salmon-colored discharge, defect seen in rectus sheath, underlying bowel visible or protruding out from wound)
- Involve the operating surgeon

SUGGESTED READING

1. American Burn Association White Paper. (2009). Surgical management of the burn wound and use of skin substitutes. [online] Available from www.ameriburn.or [Last accessed September, 2024].
2. Everett E, Mathioudakis N. Update on management of diabetic foot ulcers. Ann N Y Acad Sci. 2018;1411(1):153-65.
3. Forsch RT, Little SH, Williams C. Laceration repair: A practical approach. Am fam phys. 2017;95(10):628-36.
4. Monteiro-Soares M, Boyko EJ, Jeffcoate W, Mills JL, Russell D, Morbach S, et al. Diabetic foot ulcer classifications: A critical review. Diabetes Metab Res Rev. 2020;36(S1):e3272.
5. Onyekwelu I, Yakkanti R, Protzer L, Pinkston CM, Tucker C, Seligson D. Surgical wound classification and surgical site infections in the orthopaedic patient. JAAOS Glob Res Rev. 2017;1(3):e022.

Part 3

Resuscitation in Emergency Room

CHAPTER 26

Cardio-respiratory Resuscitation

Sachna P Shetty, Sunil B Jain

BOX 1: Introduction.

Effective cardiopulmonary resuscitation (CPR) depends on several key factors:
- A fully equipped emergency room (ER)
- A skilled and trained resuscitation team
- A capable and efficient team leader
- A reliable system for data monitoring, post-CPR feedback, and quality control
- Most importantly, high-quality basic life support (BLS), including effective CPR **(Box 3)** and early defibrillation **(Box 4)**. for shockable rhythms, is crucial for successful outcomes.

BOX 2: Steps.

As soon as the patient is unconscious and cardiac arrest is identified, activate the emergency response system and follow these steps:

Step 1:
- Connect the monitor, identify the rhythm, and follow the Advanced Cardiac Life Support (ACLS) algorithm for cardiac arrest
- Remember the "C-A-B" mantra: Circulation, Airway, and Breathing

Step 2:
- Begin uninterrupted high-quality CPR, then open the airway and provide rescue breathing

Step 3:
- Analyze and assess the cardiac rhythm. Cardiac rhythms are categorized as below:
  - Shockable rhythm
    - Pulseless ventricular tachycardia (monomorphic/polymorphic)
    - Ventricular fibrillation (coarse/fine)
  - Nonshockable rhythm
    - Asystole (flat line)
    - Pulseless electric activity (PEA) (any rhythm without a pulse)

Step 4:
  - If there is ventricular fibrillation (VF)/ventricular tachycardia (VT) (refer figure in Chapter 3.2: Cardiac Rhythm Disorders), attempt defibrillation as early as possible and continue CPR for 2 minutes
  - If asystole/PEA, continue CPR for 2 minutes

Step 5:
- Administer epinephrine every 3–5 minutes
- After three shocks, administer amiodarone/lidocaine

Step 6:
- Focus on advanced primary assessment and treatments for shockable rhythms

Contd...

Contd...

- ***Airway:* Place airway device as soon as possible**
  - **Only advanced trained person should attempt intubation and CPR should not be stopped for more than 10 seconds**
  - **Airway devices with bag-mask ventilation (BMV) (Chapter 30) are sufficient to maintain patency and ventilation (Box 18)**
  - **Extraglottic devices are also sufficient**
  - **If the patient is not intubated and using a bag-mask valve (BMV), the recommended compression-to-ventilation ratio is 30:2**
  - **For intubated patients, deliver 10–12 unsynchronized ventilations per minute to ensure the administration of 100% oxygen**
  - **Cricoid pressure should not be applied during intubation**
- ***Breathing:* Confirm airway device placement, oxygenation, and ventilation**
- **Assess end-tidal carbon dioxide ($EtCO_2$) to check CPR quality, correct placement of tracheal tube, and to check if there is a return of spontaneous circulation (ROSC)**
- **Access intravenous or intraosseous line, endotracheal (ET) route may be used for administration of drugs**
- **Do a secondary survey**
- **Remember 5H/5T for reversible cause during primary and secondary survey**
- **Role of arterial line as a quality indicator of CPR and monitoring in ACLS 2020 is highlighted**

Caveat:

- Overzealous ventilation elevates intrathoracic pressure thereby decreasing venous return, ventricular filling, and stroke volume with compression, hence causing inadequate cerebral perfusion
- Also, it causes inadequate gastric inflation, thus leading to regurgitation and aspiration
- Standard BMV has volume of 1,000–1,500 mL and even if some air is lost to environment, full squeeze is not necessary to deliver 600 mL volume
- Remember the drugs given in cardiac arrest **(Box 5)**
- Drugs can also be given via ET tube if there is no intravenous (IV) access **(Box 5)**

BOX 3: Excellent cardiopulmonary resuscitation (CPR).

- *No interruption:* Ensure there is no interruption in CPR, not even for airway management or while defibrillator is being charged
- *Proper timing:* 100–120 compressions per minute
- 5–6 cm [2–2.5 inch] depth
- Allow complete recoil of chest
- Prioritize over ventilation

BOX 4: Excellent defibrillation.

- Attach and charge defibrillator while continuing excellent chest compressions
- Stop compression and assess rhythm (no more than 5 seconds)
- If VT/VF, deliver shock
- Resume CPR immediately after shock is delivered
- Pad placement for defibrillator is shown in **Figure 1**
- It may be unsuccessful when insufficient energy transits the fibrillating ventricle
- Biphasic defibrillator is recommended—lower energy levels are required (200 J)
- One should resume CPR after delivering shock
- Only check rhythm after 2 minutes of complete CPR post defibrillator

Caveat:

- Minimize interruption, do not stop compression while defibrillator is being charged
- Remember to focus on excellent quality compression and early defibrillation for shockable rhythm
- Keep the defibrillator pads attached tightly to the chest/back for few seconds approx 5 seconds after delivering shock
- According to some studies, changing location of the defibrillator from lateral to anterior post maybe required if refractory arrhythmia, for the defibrillator to detect ventricles
- Certain trials for dual sequential defibrillator are being conducted and vector change are being conducted, some studies support benefits, especially in refractory arrhythmia
- Currently, newest studies suggest using a 270 J biphasic defibrillator [Modern defibrillator machines are equipped with a maximum output of 270 joules.]
- Agonal breathing or transient convulsive activity may accompany dysrhythmia, therefore do not delay CPR
- Extracorporeal membrane oxygenation (ECMO) during CPR is widely studied and practiced (Chapter 34)

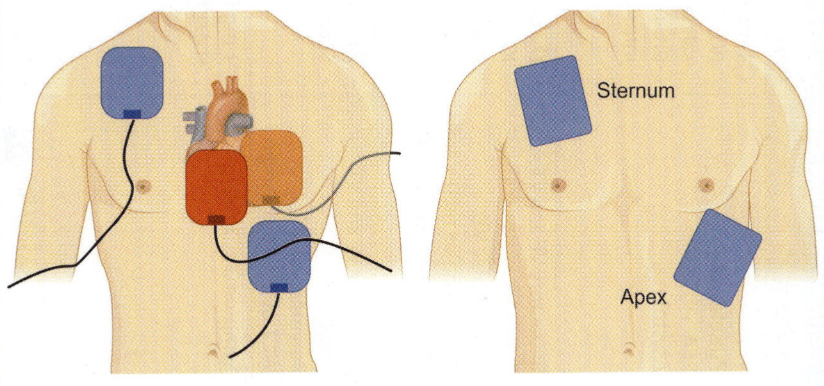

Fig. 1: Pad placement for defibrillator.

BOX 5: Overview of drugs used in cardiac arrest.

Drugs	***Indications***	***Dosage***	***Pediatric dose***
Adrenaline	• VF • Pulseless VT • PEA • Asystole	• 1 mg (1:1,000) IV/ intraosseous (IO) diluted in 10 mL normal saline (NS) every 3–5 minutes • 0.1–0.5 µg/kg/min continuous infusion	• Bradycardia: – *IV/IO:* 0.01 mg/kg (0.1 mL/kg of 1:10,000) – *Endotracheal:* 0.1 mg/kg (0.1 mL/kg of 1:1000) • *Pulseless arrest* – *IV/IO:* 0.01 mg/kg (0.1 mL/kg of 1:10,000) – *Endotracheal:* 0.1 mg/kg (0.1 mL/kg of 1:1000) – *Maximum dose:* 1 mg IV/IO; 2.5 mg ET tube
Amiodarone	• Refractory VF and VT • Stable VT • Polymorphic VT • Wide complex tachycardia (WCT) of unknown origin	• *During cardiac arrest:* 300 mg IV/IO first dose. If VT persists, 150 mg IV/IO push second dose • *In case of arrhythmias:* 150 mg over 10 minutes followed by 1 mg/min infusion for 6 hours	• *IV/IO:* 5 mg/kg over 20–60 minutes; then 5–15 µg/kg/min infusion • Maximum bolus repetition to 15 mg/kg/day
Lignocaine/ Lidocaine	• Refractory VF and VT • Stable VT • Polymorphic VT • WCT of unknown origin	• *First dose:* 1–1.5 mg/kg • Second dose: 0.5–0.75 mg/kg	• *IV/IO:* 1.0 mg/kg bolus • *Endotracheal:* Double IV dose and dilute with NS to 3–5 mL
Atropine	• Symptomatic bradycardia	• 1 mg IV every 3–5 minutes, maximum dose: 3 mg	• *IV/IO:* 0.02 mg/kg, repeat in 5 min (minimum single dose is 0.1 milligram) • *Endotracheal:* 0.04–0.06 mg/kg diluted with NS to 3–5 mL • *Maximum single dose:* 0.5 milligram (child) and 1.0 milligram (adolescent) • *Maximum cumulative dose:* 1.0 mg (child) and 2.0 mg (adolescent)
Magnesium sulphate	• Torsades de pointes	• 1–2 g diluted in 5% dextrose over 20 minutes	

BOX 6: Reversible causes of cardiac arrest.

5H	*5T*
• Hypoxia • Hypovolemia/hemorrhage • Hyper/Hypokalemia • Hypothermia • Hydrogen ion (acidosis)	• Tablet/Toxin • Trauma • Tamponade (Cardiac) • Tension pneumothorax • Thrombosis (Coronary) • Thrombosis (Pulmonary)
Caveat: PEA evaluation	
• **Narow complex PEA** • Mechanical cause • Tamponade, pulmonary embolism (PE), high hypovolemia, bleeding, tension pneumothorax • Acute myocardial infarction (MI) (bedside. ultrasound (US)—hyperdynamic left ventricle (LV)	• **Wide complex PEA** • Consider metabolic course • Hyperkalemia • Sodium channel blocker overdose • Severe acidosis, agonal rhythm, and acute MI with pump failure • *Bedside:* Hyperkinetic and akinetic LV

BOX 7: Algorithm for pulseless arrest.

Flowchart 1: Pulseless arrest.

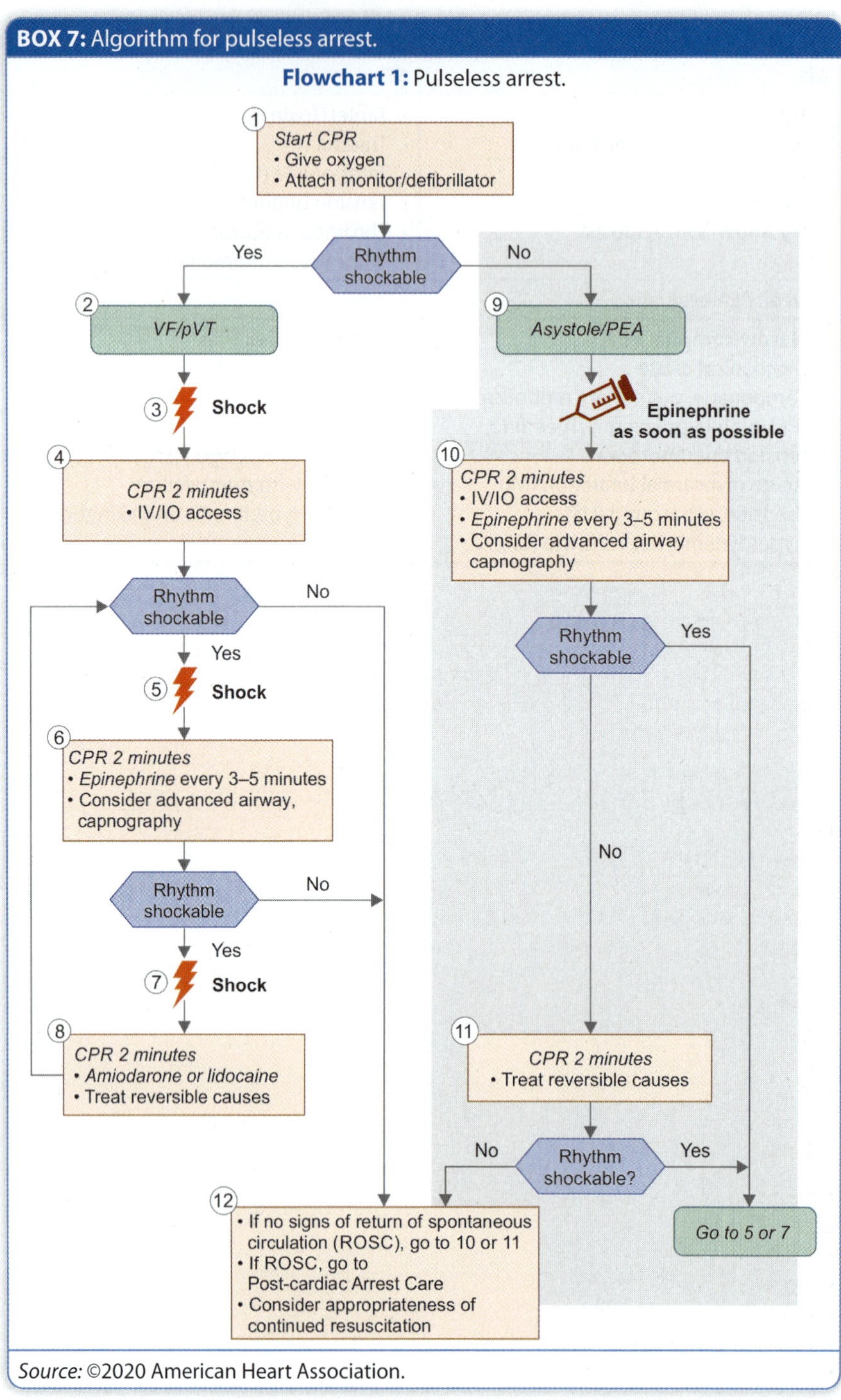

Source: ©2020 American Heart Association.

BOX 8: Intra-arrest monitoring target.

- $EtCO_2$ >10 mm Hg
- Arterial diastolic >20 mm Hg
- Point-of-care (POC) ultrasonography (USG)

BOX 9: Special scenario in cardiopulmonary resuscitation (CPR).

- Hypothermia/drowning (Chapter 15.2)
- Trauma (Chapter 10)
- Pregnancy **(Flowchart 2)**
- Pediatric **(Box 18)**
- Neonatal **(Box 19)**

BOX 10: Practical advice for resuscitation scenarios.

- Identify patient wishes (advance directive and prior communications)
- Communicate with family and loved ones during and following resuscitative efforts
- Allow family to be present during resuscitative efforts, if appropriate
- Assess prognosis, based on scientific evidence
- Enroll patient in research trials, with surrogate consent, or using the United States Food and Drug Administration waiver of consent rule, as appropriate
- Provide spiritual, psychosocial, and educational support to family and loved ones throughout and after termination of resuscitative efforts

BOX 11: Outcomes.

Poor:

- Asystole
- PEA, if out of hospital
- Absence of vital signs on arrival
- Sepsis
- Severe cerebrovascular accident (CVA)
- Cancer/Alzheimer's disease
- More than two chronic diseases
- Cardiac disease
- Prolonged CPR
- Prolonged VF
- Delayed time to resuscitate

If the patient survives until reaching the hospital, factors that may contribute to a poor outcome include:

- Persistent coma
- Hypotension, pneumonia, or renal failure after CPR
- Need for intubation or pressor
- Heart failure
- Older age

Contd...

Contd...

Better:
- If converted to shockable rhythm, in witnessed arrest
- Younger patient age
- Shorter time to arrival, no need for atropine postrevival
- VT arrhythmia (MI commonest cause for VT)
- *Noncardiac causes:* Better if reversible cause is known (in-house factors)
- Pulse regained in first 10 minutes
- Arrest during on duty hours
- Early warning sign identification
- Dedicated resuscitation team
- Bystander CPR better prognosis as compared to delay
- Chest compression only, no difference
- *Automated CPR:* Unclear
- Early defibrillator is better

BOX 12: ROSC scores to predict outcome.

NULL-PLEASE score:
- Nonshockable rhythm
- Unwitnessed arrest
- Long no time flow period >30 minutes before ROSC
- Ph <7.2
- Lactate >7
- End-stage renal disease (ESRD) on hemodialysis (HD)
- Age >85 years
- Ongoing CPR on arrival
- Extracardiac disease

>5 score poor outcome

CREST scores:
- Coronary artery disease (CAD)
- Nonshockable rhythm
- Ejection fraction (EF) <30
- Shock at presentation
- Time for ROSC >25 minutes

BOX 13: Good Outcomes Following Attempted Resuscitation (GO-FAR).

Mentioned in Chapter 44 – Scoring in ER.

BOX 14: Termination.

- National Association of Emergency Medical Services (EMS) Physicians Standards for Termination of Resuscitation in Nontraumatic Cardiopulmonary Arrest
- Termination of resuscitation may be considered when, at the time of decision of termination, all of the following conditions have been met:
  - The arrest was not witnessed by an EMS provider
  - There is no shockable rhythm identified by an automated external defibrillator (AED) or other electronic monitor
  - There is no ROSC prior to EMS transport

BOX 15: Pregnant resuscitation.

- Potential cause of sudden cardiac arrest could be obstetric or nonobstetric:
  - **A:** Anesthetic complication/accident/trauma
  - **B:** Bleeding
  - **C:** Cardiac
  - **D:** Drugs
  - **E:** Embolic causes
  - **F:** Fever
  - **G:** General including hypoxia, and electrolyte disturbances
  - **H:** Hypertension
- Main priority of resuscitation remains the mother
- Estimate gestational age to determine viability of fetus, if nonviable focus singly on mother
- Assemble the maternal resuscitation team, adult resuscitation, obstetrician gynecologist (OB-GYN), and neonatologist
- Use standard ACLS algorithm with a few modifications
- IV access must be secured above diaphragm, for drug delivery to not be altered by gravid uterus compressing inferior vena cava (IVC)
- **During CPR, tilt the patient to left 15°–30° (Fig. 2)**
- Defibrillator position remains same
- In pregnant airway, oxygenation should be prioritized as it can be prone to failure
- No fetal monitoring during arrest
- In maternal mortality, perform perimortem cesarean (CS) delivery within 5 minutes of no ROSC
- If attains ROSC and signs of fetal distress persist, perform perimortem CS within 5 minutes (Chapter 27)

Flowchart 2: Cardiac arrest in pregnancy.

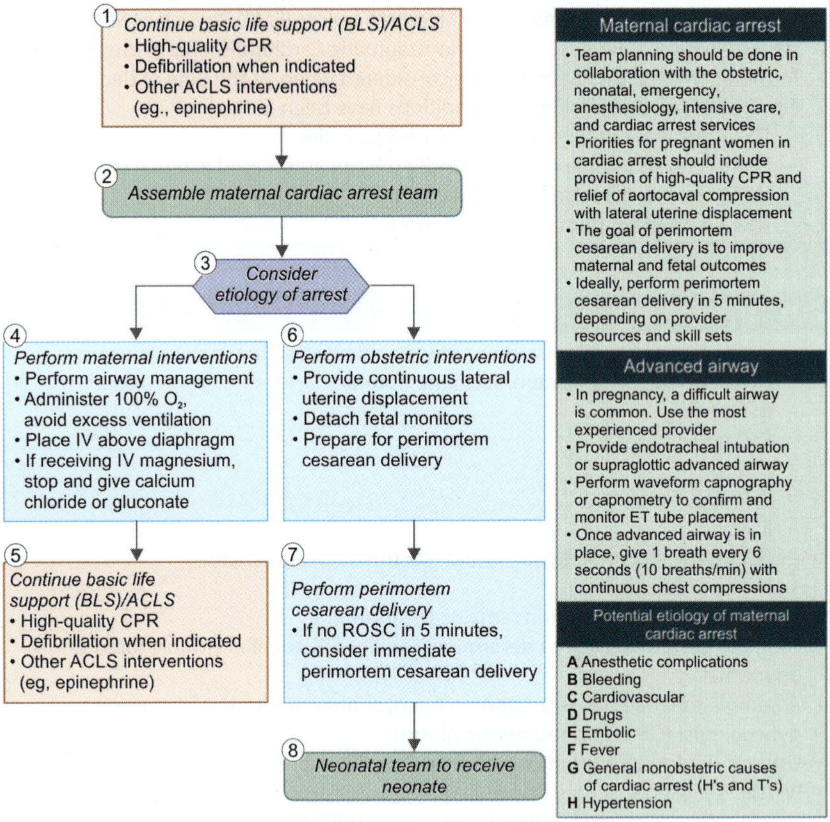

① *Continue basic life support (BLS)/ACLS*
- High-quality CPR
- Defibrillation when indicated
- Other ACLS interventions (eg., epinephrine)

↓

② *Assemble maternal cardiac arrest team*

↓

③ *Consider etiology of arrest*

④ *Perform maternal interventions*
- Perform airway management
- Administer 100% O_2, avoid excess ventilation
- Place IV above diaphragm
- If receiving IV magnesium, stop and give calcium chloride or gluconate

↓

⑤ *Continue basic life support (BLS)/ACLS*
- High-quality CPR
- Defibrillation when indicated
- Other ACLS interventions (eg, epinephrine)

⑥ *Perform obstetric interventions*
- Provide continuous lateral uterine displacement
- Detach fetal monitors
- Prepare for perimortem cesarean delivery

↓

⑦ *Perform perimortem cesarean delivery*
- If no ROSC in 5 minutes, consider immediate perimortem cesarean delivery

↓

⑧ *Neonatal team to receive neonate*

Maternal cardiac arrest
- Team planning should be done in collaboration with the obstetric, neonatal, emergency, anesthesiology, intensive care, and cardiac arrest services
- Priorities for pregnant women in cardiac arrest should include provision of high-quality CPR and relief of aortocaval compression with lateral uterine displacement
- The goal of perimortem cesarean delivery is to improve maternal and fetal outcomes
- Ideally, perform perimortem cesarean delivery in 5 minutes, depending on provider resources and skill sets

Advanced airway
- In pregnancy, a difficult airway is common. Use the most experienced provider
- Provide endotracheal intubation or supraglottic advanced airway
- Perform waveform capnography or capnometry to confirm and monitor ET tube placement
- Once advanced airway is in place, give 1 breath every 6 seconds (10 breaths/min) with continuous chest compressions

Potential etiology of maternal cardiac arrest

A Anesthetic complications
B Bleeding
C Cardiovascular
D Drugs
E Embolic
F Fever
G General nonobstetric causes of cardiac arrest (H's and T's)
H Hypertension

Source: ©2020 American Heart Association.

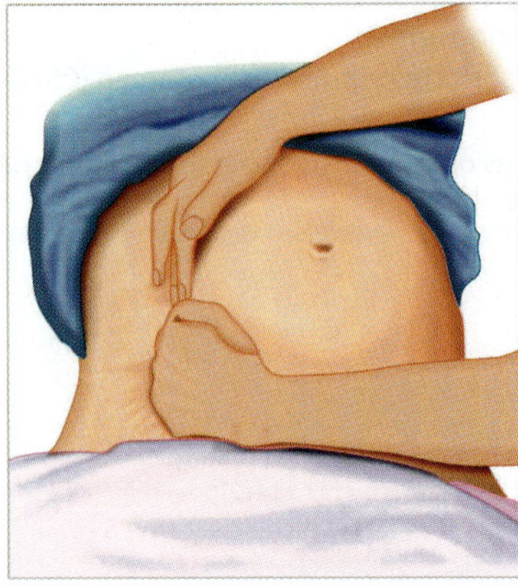

Fig. 2: Manual left uterine displacement performed with the two-handed technique.

BOX 16: Pediatric.

- Arrest secondary from respiratory failure, hence oxygenation and ventilation are a high-priority
- At least 3 cm gap between paddles of defibrillator
- For >1 year, large adult paddles
- For <1 year, small infant paddles

BOX 17: Guidelines to pediatric cardiac arrest support.

Maneuver	***Newborn***	***Infant <1 years***	***Child = 1 year to puberty***	***Onset of puberty to adult***
Airway	Head tilt/chin lift	Head tilt/chin lift	Head tilt/chin lift	Head tilt/chin lift
If trauma	Jaw thrust	Jaw thrust	Jaw thrust	Jaw thrust
If foreign body—conscious	Suction	Back blows and chest thrusts	Abdominal thrusts	Abdominal thrusts
If foreign body—unconscious	Suction	Chest compressions	Abdominal thrusts	Abdominal thrusts
Breathing rate	30–60 breaths/minute (every 1–2s)	12–20 breaths/minute (every 3s)	12–20 breaths/minute (every 3s)	10–12 breaths/minute (every 5s)
Circulation pulse check	Umbilical	Brachial	Carotid or femoral	Carotid or femoral
Compression				
Location	One finger below intermammary line	One finger below intermammary line or lower half of sternum	Lower half of sternum	Lower half of sternum
Method	Two fingers or two thumbs	Two fingers or two thumbs	Heel of one hand or two hands	Two hands
Depth	One-third of chest	One-third to one-half of chest	One-third to one-half of chest	One-third of chest
Rate	120/min	100/min	100/min	100/min
Compression-to-ventilation ratio	3:1	15:2 (single rescuer—30:2)	15:2 (single rescuer—30:2)	30:2

Source: Adapted from Tintinalli JE, Ma OJ, Yealy DM, Meckler GD, Stapczynski JS, Cline DM, et al. Tintinalli's Emergency Medicine: A Comprehensive Study Guide, 9th edition. New York, NY: McGraw- Hill Education; 2019.

BOX 18: Pediatric pulseless arrest decision tree.

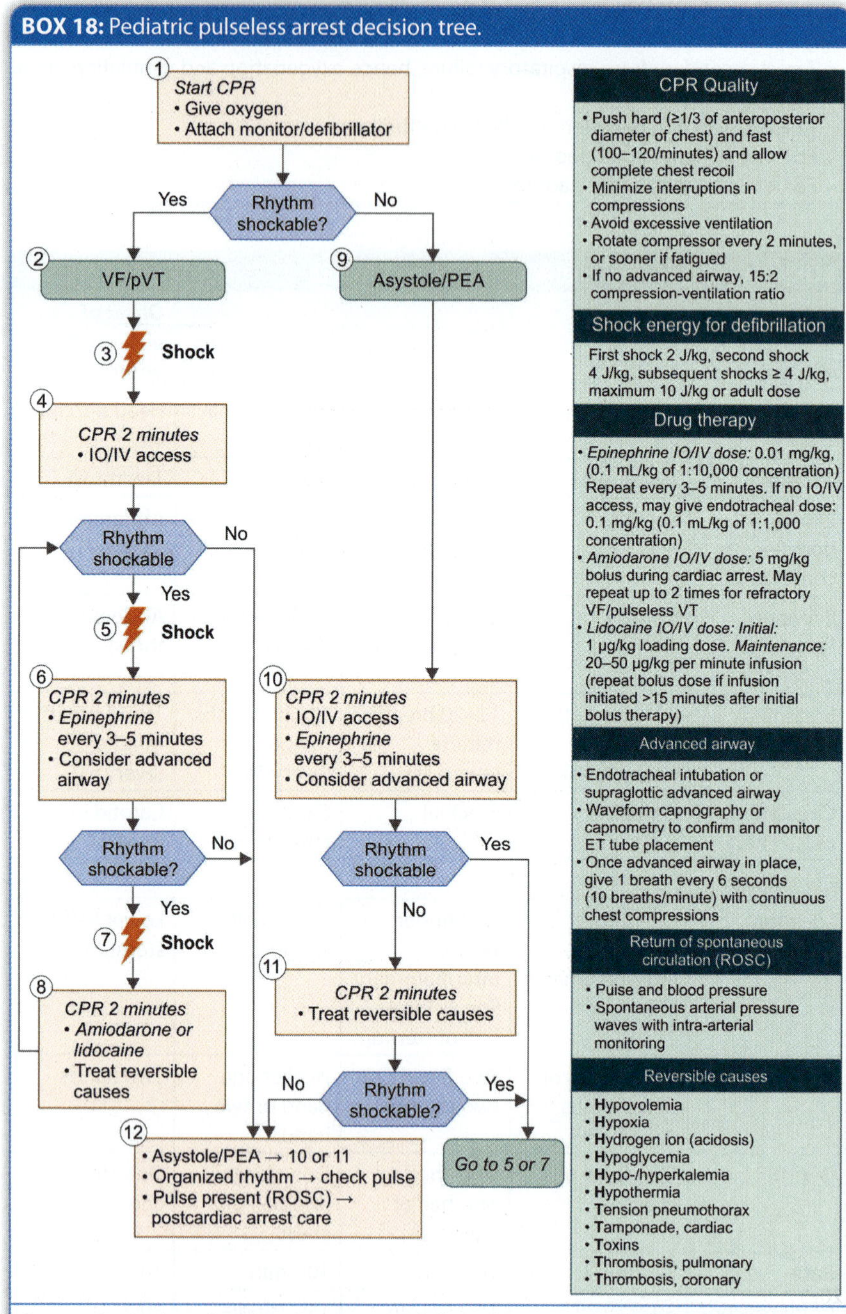

Source: Reproduced with permission: Web-based integrated 2010 & 2015 American Heart Association Guidelines for CPR and ECC Part 12: Pediatric Advanced Life support © 2015 American Heart Association, Inc.

BOX 19: Neonatal resuscitation.

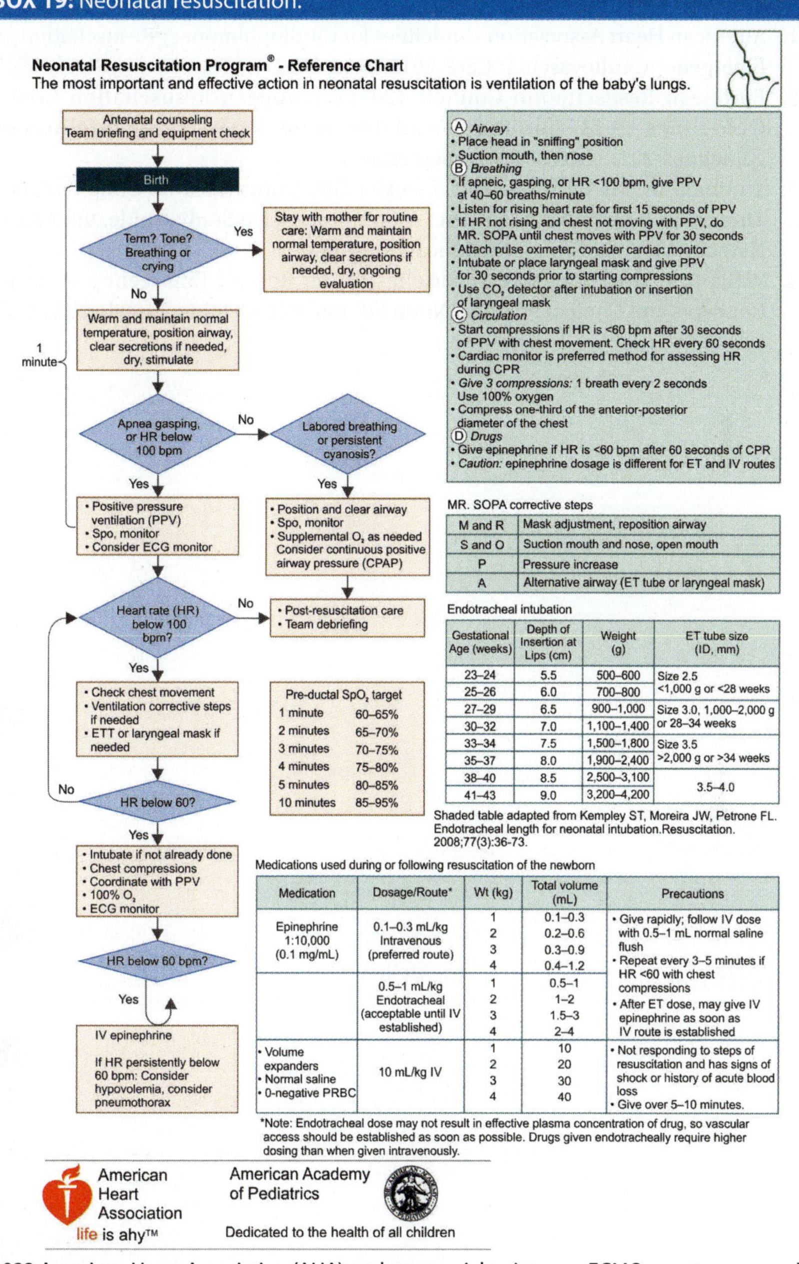

Neonatal Resuscitation Program® - Reference Chart

The most important and effective action in neonatal resuscitation is ventilation of the baby's lungs.

Pre-ductal SpO_2 target	
1 minute	60–65%
2 minutes	65–70%
3 minutes	70–75%
4 minutes	75–80%
5 minutes	80–85%
10 minutes	85–95%

Ⓐ *Airway*
- Place head in "sniffing" position
- Suction mouth, then nose

Ⓑ *Breathing*
- If apneic, gasping, or HR <100 bpm, give PPV at 40–60 breaths/minute
- Listen for rising heart rate for first 15 seconds of PPV
- If HR not rising and chest not moving with PPV, do MR. SOPA until chest moves with PPV for 30 seconds
- Attach pulse oximeter; consider cardiac monitor
- Intubate or place laryngeal mask and give PPV for 30 seconds prior to starting compressions
- Use CO_2 detector after intubation or insertion of laryngeal mask

Ⓒ *Circulation*
- Start compressions if HR is <60 bpm after 30 seconds of PPV with chest movement. Check HR every 60 seconds
- Cardiac monitor is preferred method for assessing HR during CPR
- *Give 3 compressions:* 1 breath every 2 seconds Use 100% oxygen
- Compress one-third of the anterior-posterior diameter of the chest

Ⓓ *Drugs*
- Give epinephrine if HR is <60 bpm after 60 seconds of CPR
- *Caution:* epinephrine dosage is different for ET and IV routes

MR. SOPA corrective steps

M and R	Mask adjustment, reposition airway
S and O	Suction mouth and nose, open mouth
P	Pressure increase
A	Alternative airway (ET tube or laryngeal mask)

Endotracheal intubation

Gestational Age (weeks)	Depth of Insertion at Lips (cm)	Weight (g)	ET tube size (ID, mm)
23–24	5.5	500–600	Size 2.5 <1,000 g or <28 weeks
25–26	6.0	700–800	
27–29	6.5	900–1,000	Size 3.0, 1,000–2,000 g or 28–34 weeks
30–32	7.0	1,100–1,400	
33–34	7.5	1,500–1,800	Size 3.5 >2,000 g or >34 weeks
35–37	8.0	1,900–2,400	
38–40	8.5	2,500–3,100	3.5–4.0
41–43	9.0	3,200–4,200	

Shaded table adapted from Kempley ST, Moreira JW, Petrone FL. Endotracheal length for neonatal intubation.Resuscitation. 2008;77(3):36-73.

Medications used during or following resuscitation of the newborn

Medication	Dosage/Route*	Wt (kg)	Total volume (mL)	Precautions
Epinephrine 1:10,000 (0.1 mg/mL)	0.1–0.3 mL/kg Intravenous (preferred route)	1 2 3 4	0.1–0.3 0.2–0.6 0.3–0.9 0.4–1.2	• Give rapidly; follow IV dose with 0.5–1 mL normal saline flush • Repeat every 3–5 minutes if HR <60 with chest compressions • After ET dose, may give IV epinephrine as soon as IV route is established
	0.5–1 mL/kg Endotracheal (acceptable until IV established)	1 2 3 4	0.5–1 1–2 1.5–3 2–4	
• Volume expanders • Normal saline • 0-negative PRBC	10 mL/kg IV	1 2 3 4	10 20 30 40	• Not responding to steps of resuscitation and has signs of shock or history of acute blood loss • Give over 5–10 minutes.

*Note: Endotracheal dose may not result in effective plasma concentration of drug, so vascular access should be established as soon as possible. Drugs given endotracheally require higher dosing than when given intravenously.

American Heart Association life is ahy™ | American Academy of Pediatrics Dedicated to the health of all children

2023 American Heart Association (AHA) updates crucial points are: ECMO or extracorporeal management in cardiac arrest is helpful in only certain situations like hypothermia, toxicology, some cases of pulmonary embolism, younger group and most importantly with immediate cannulation, possible with a multidisciplinary committee agreement.

Cardiac intervention in patients is might be of some value only if there is a strong suspicion of cardiac arrest secondary to thrombosis and an ST elevation post ROSC or before cardiac arrest

SUGGESTED READING

1. American Heart Association Guidelines for Cardiopulmonary Resuscitation and Emergency Cardiovascular Care. 2015, 2020, 2023.
2. European Resuscitation Council. (2021). European Resuscitation Council Guidelines 2021. [online] Available from https://cprguidelines.eu/guidelines-2021 [Last accessed September, 2024].
3. Tintinalli JE, Ma OJ, Yealy DM, Meckler GD, Stapczynski JS, Cline DM, et al. Tintinalli's Emergency Medicine: A Comprehensive Study Guide, 9th edition. New York, NY: McGraw- Hill Education; 2019.
4. Walls RM, Hockberger RS, Gausche-Hill M. Rosen's Emergency Medicine: Concepts and Clinical Practice, Ninth Edition. Philadelphia: Elsevier; 2018.

Postcardiac Arrest Care (PCAC) after Return of Spontaneous Circulation (ROSC)

Jamshed D Sunavala

BOX 1: Definition.

- Return of spontaneous circulation (ROSC) is defined as return to normal or near normal pulse and rhythm following cardiac resuscitation
- Postcardiac arrest care (PCAC) is the resuscitation that will need to continue following ROSC with the goal to initiate and maintain hemodynamic and respiratory stabilization

BOX 2: Checklist.

Check list is a rapid checklist to identify correctable causes and comorbidities, which need to be immediately recognized after ROSC in order to avoid recurrence of arrests, serious arrhythmias, and hemodynamic instability **(Box 3)**

BOX 3: Clinical, laboratory, and bedside tests to identify correctable causes and comorbidities, which could result in recurrence of cardiac arrest, and also help to stabilize the patient.

P: Rule out tension Pneumothorax (postresuscitation complication)	Can be immediately diagnosed on clinical examination
O: Oxygen-persistent hypoxia (requiring immediate intubation and mechanical ventilation)	
S: Stroke/decreased sensorium (requiring further respiratory support)	
T: HypoTension (requiring volume or vasopressors)	
A: Acidosis [arterial blood gas (ABG)]	Tests for confirmation at bedside
T: Coronary *T*hrombosis [electrocardiography (ECG)]	
T: Pericardial *T*amponade (2D Echocardiography)	
A: Aortic Tear (X-ray chest and 2D Echocardiography)	
C: Congestive cardiac failure (X-ray chest)	
K: Hypo*K*alemia (Serum electrolytes)	

BOX 4: Essential interventions and therapies to be considered after cardiac arrest.

During cardiopulmonary resuscitation (CPR):

- Uninterrupted good quality cardiac compression [As per American Heart Association (AHA) guidelines for CPR]
- *Defibrillation* for ventricular fibrillation (VF)/ventricular tachycardia (VT)
- *For pulseless electrical activity (PEA):* Intravenous (IV) epinephrine and continue CPR. If shockable rhythms appears, defibrillate
- *Oxygen (O_2) delivery and ventilation:* Studies have shown that maintaining higher O_2 levels during prolonged CPR, improved neurological outcomes

After ROSC:

- Checklist **(Box 3)**
- Stabilization **(Box 5)**
- Therapeutic hypothermia **(Box 6)**
- Predicting neurological recovery **(Box 7)**
- Triage for percutaneous coronary intervention **(Box 8)**

BOX 5: Stabilization after ROSC—Outcome associated with O_2, CO_2 and blood pressure (BP) optimization.

Oxygenation:

- *Recommended:* Lowest fraction of inspired oxygen (FiO_2) to maintain partial pressure of oxygen (PaO_2) of 94% in order to avoid hyperoxia
- Emerging evidence suggests that very high PaO_2 values in the first 24 hours may be detrimental

Carbon dioxide:

- It is recommended to maintain $PaCO_2$ between 35 mm Hg and 40 mm Hg
- Hypocarbia due to hyperventilation has shown poor neurological outcomes

Mean arterial pressure (MAP):

- Maintaining higher MAP of 90–100 mm Hg has shown better neurological outcomes than maintaining MAP of 60–70 mm Hg

BOX 6: Therapeutic hypothermia—management.

Indications:
Patients with decreased sensorium who cannot be aroused

Contraindications:
Serious bleeding, preexisting temperature below 34°C, and cryoglobulinemia

Aim:
- To begin immediately after ROSC
- To induce hypothermia to 34°C
- To maintain hypothermia between 34°C and 36°C

(Latest studies have shown no difference in outcomes on maintaining temperature between 34°C and 36°C)

Method:
- *Induction:* Ice cold (4°C) infusion of normal saline to a core body temperature of 34°C
- *Maintenance:* To maintain core temperature preferably to 34°C, however up to 36°C is acceptable
- *Cooling:* By using endovascular cooling or surface cooling or using both simultaneously

Monitoring:
Intracerebral temperatures are best measured by pulmonary artery catheter or tympanic thermometer. However, in practice, core (rectal or lower esophageal) temperatures are measured

Complications:
Shivering, bleeding, bradycardia, hypotension, hypokalemia, and infection

BOX 7: Predicting neurological outcomes at discharge.

Cerebral performance capacity (CPC) Scale:
1. Conscious and alert
2. Conscious and alert but with moderate disability
3. Conscious with severe disability
4. Comatose or persistent vegetative state
5. Brain dead

Modified Rankin Scale (mRS):

0. No symptoms
1. Some symptoms with usual activities possible
2. *Slight disability:* Unable to do all previous activities, but independent
3. *Moderate disability:* Requiring some help but able to walk without help
4. *Severe disability:* Bedridden and incontinent
5. Dead

Patients at discharge having a mRS score of 0–3 or CPC scale score of 1–2 generally have a good neurological outcomes.

BOX 8: Triage for percutaneous coronary intervention (PCI).

- Majority of patients after cardiac arrest particularly those occurring out of hospital (OHCA) would have succumbed to acute coronary syndrome if no other oblivious cause was ascertained
- These group of patients may benefit from PCI
- Survivors from cardiac arrest with post recovery ECG showing ST-segment elevation myocardial infarction (STEMI) have a particularly good prognosis from neurological point of view. Hence, these patients should be triaged for PCI
- PCI is contraindicated in patients with major complication such as bleeding. However, clinician's judgment is required for patients with advanced age or doubtful neurological recovery. In case of the later, a CPC scale score of 1–2 or mRS score of 0–3 is generally acceptable as a good neurological outcome **(Box 7)**

SUGGESTED READING

1. Drebek T, Patrick K. Is there a role of therapeutic hypothermia in critical care? In: Deutschmann CS, Neligon PJ (Eds). Evidence-based Practice of Critical Care, 3rd edition. Amsterdam, Netherlands: Elsevier; 2020.
2. Holzer M. Targeted temperature management for comatose survivors of cardiac arrest. N Engl J Med. 2010;363(10):1256-64.
3. Merchant RM, Topjian AA, Panchal AR, Cheng A, Aziz K, Berg KM, et al. Part 1: Executive Summary: 2020 American Heart Association Guidelines for Cardiopulmonary Resuscitation and Emergency Cardiovascular Care. Circulation. 2020;142:S337-57.

CHAPTER 28

Choking

Janhavi Gholap

BOX 1: Introduction.

Choking is a sudden airway obstruction experienced while a person is eating due to food getting lodged in the upper respiratory tract

The universal sign of choking for an individual is to grab his or her neck with both hands, in between the meals

BOX 2: Types of airway obstruction.

- In cases of partial airway obstruction with sufficient air exchange, the individual may still be able to talk and breathe, though they will likely experience persistent coughing
- If partial obstruction worsens and signs of respiratory distress such as stridor, difficulty speaking, or cyanosis develop, it indicates that the airway is becoming more severely blocked. This progression can lead to unconsciousness due to insufficient oxygen supply
- With a complete airway obstruction, the individual will show diminished respiratory effort, little to no chest movement, and inadequate ventilation, eventually resulting in loss of consciousness

BOX 3: Management depending on severity of airway obstruction.

In partial airway obstruction with adequate air exchange, the person should be encouraged to cough, and no attempt should be made to blindly do a finger sweep

Check for any signs of deterioration or recovery.

If choking not relieved or signs of deterioration develop but the patient is conscious, Heimlich maneuver (subdiaphragmatic abdominal thrusts) and chest thrusts to be performed.

If the patient loses consciousness, initiate cardiopulmonary resuscitation (CPR) following the Advanced Cardiac Life Support (ACLS) protocol. While performing CPR, position the patient lying down and continue with the Heimlich maneuver (up to five attempts). If the obstruction is still not cleared, perform a finger sweep—but only if the foreign body is visible—and then begin ventilation.

Heimlich maneuver:

- A method of forceful expiration by elevating the diaphragm to remove obstruction, can be performed while standing, sitting, or lying down
- For a conscious person, the aid should stand behind the patient, place the thumb side of a fist above the navel and below the xiphoid process, grasp the fist with the other hand, and push forcefully upward **(Fig. 1)**

Contd...

Contd...

- For self-administration, the individual can lean against a firm surface to apply more pressure during the maneuver
- For an unconscious person, perform the maneuver with the individual lying supine on a solid surface. Place the heel of your dominant hand just above the navel, with the other hand placed on top. **Deliver upward thrusts (Fig. 2)**
- Possible complications may include injury to abdominal or thoracic organs and the risk of regurgitation

Chest thrusts:

- It is recommended for obese individuals or pregnant women
- Stand behind the person, make a fist and place the thumb side against the sternum, avoiding the costal margins and xiphoid process. Grasp the fist with the other hand and deliver quick **backward thrusts (Fig. 3)**
- If the patient becomes unconscious, place them supine and perform chest thrusts similar to CPR
- If the patient becomes unconscious:
  - Begin CPR according to ACLS protocol
  - Perform lying-down Heimlich maneuvers up to 5 times, if not successful, then perform a finger sweep if the foreign body is visible and start ventilation. Repeat until successful

Finger sweep maneuver:

- This is used only in unconscious patients
- Grasp the patient's tongue and mandible with one hand, lift them, and insert the index finger into the throat with the other hand to hook and remove the visible foreign body. Do not perform blind sweeps as they can push the object deeper **(Fig. 4)**

Caveats:

For infants, back blows and chest thrusts are recommended to clear the airway. The Heimlich maneuver should not be used on children under 1 year as per American Heart Association (AHA) guidelines

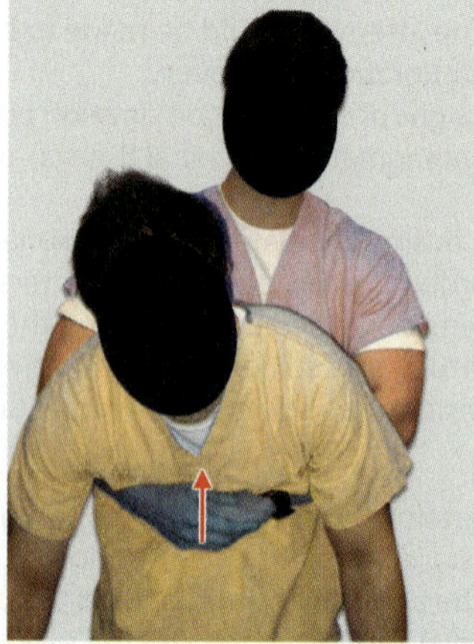

Fig. 1: Heimlich maneuver, if patient is sitting or standing.

Contd...

Contd...

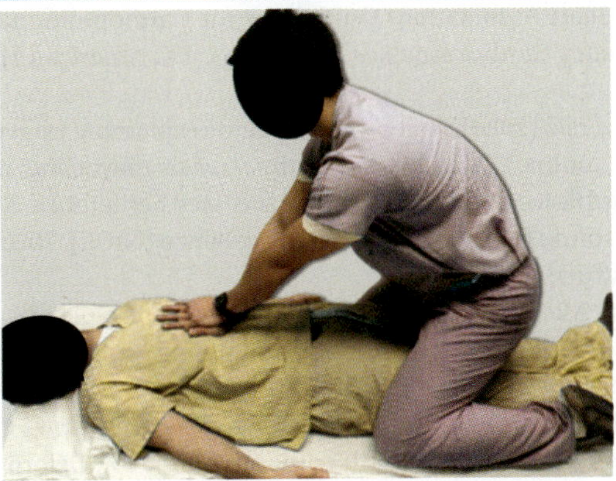

Fig. 2: Heimlich maneuver if patient is unconscious.

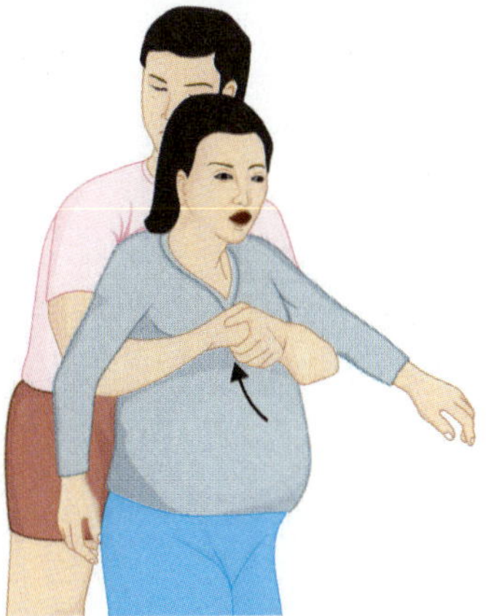

Fig. 3: Chest thrust.

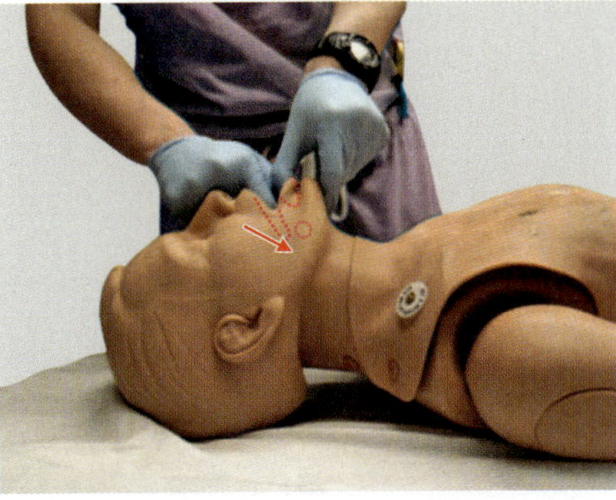

Fig. 4: Finger sweep maneuver.

SUGGESTED READING

1. American Heart Association. Guidelines for Cardiopulmonary Resuscitation and Emergency Cardiovascular Care. Dallas, TX: American Heart Association; 2021.
2. Mayo Clinic Staff. (2024). A step-by-step guide explaining what to do in a choking emergency. [online] Available from https://www.mayoclinic.org/first-aid/first-aid-choking/basics/art-20056637 [Last accessed September, 2024].
3. National Institute for Health and Care Excellence (NICE), 2020. Management of Airway Obstruction.
4. Tintinalli JE, Ma OJ, Yealy DM, Meckler GD, Stapczynski JS, Cline DM, et al. Tintinalli's Emergency Medicine: A Comprehensive Study Guide, 9th edition. New York, NY: McGraw-Hill Education; 2020.
5. Wyatt JP, Illingworth RN, Graham CA, Hogg K, Robertson C, Clancy M. Oxford Manual Emergency Medicine, 4th edition. Oxford, UK: Oxford University Press; 2012

CHAPTER 29

Approach to Hypotension in Emergency Room

Varun Deshmukh

BOX 1: Introduction.

Hypotension: Systolic blood pressure (BP) <90 mm Hg or mean BP <65 mm Hg or drop in systolic BP by over 40 mm Hg is defined as hypotension.

Shock: It is a life-threatening condition of circulatory failure that most commonly presents with hypotension.

It is a state of cellular and tissue hypoxia due to imbalance in oxygen demand and supply. This could be because of reduced oxygen delivery or increased oxygen consumption or inability to utilize oxygen at tissue level.

Suspect shock when patient has altered mentation, hypotension, tachycardia/bradycardia, tachypnea, cold-clammy peripheries, poor capillary refill, lactic acidosis, and oliguria.

In a hypotensive patient, actively look for signs of shock.

BOX 2: What will you do if your patient is hypotensive?

- Recheck BP
- Look at trend of BP
- Ask for history of diabetes mellitus (DM)/peripheral vascular disease (PVD) to suspect autonomic dysfunction
- Recent administration of medications (antihypertensives, heart failure medications, anxiolytics, antidepressants, and diuretics)
- Ask for symptoms after postural change
- Rule out food/drug allergy
- Look for external or internal bleeding
- History of loss of volume (Gastrointestinal losses, diuresis, and excessive perspiration)
- History of chest pain/breathlessness, which points towards cardiopulmonary causes
- History of fever points towards sepsis
- In case of post operative hypotension, whether any analgesics were given

BOX 3: Next steps of management.

- Secure airway, breathing, circulation, disability, and exposure (ABCDE)
- Airway protection may be needed for patients with low Glasgow Coma Scale (GCS) score (<8)
- Septic patients and those with severe shock may need intubation and ventilation to prevent them from getting into fatigue and respiratory arrest
- Choose your sedatives wisely in a hypotensive patient. Prefer ketamine, etomidate, or fentanyl over propofol or midazolam
- Once sedated and started on positive pressure ventilation, patients may soon have further drop in BP. So, start fluid challenge while preparing for intubation and keep vasopressors ready

Act in seconds in case of the following:
- Arrhythmias
- Tension pneumothorax
- Cardiac tamponade
- Anaphylaxis

Act in minutes in case of the following:
- Pulmonary embolism (PE)
- Myocardial infarction (MI)
- Bleeding patient
- Ruptured aortic aneurysm/aortic dissection
- Sepsis
- Adrenergic crisis

BOX 4: Investigate further to narrow down the etiology.

- Electrocardiography (ECG)
- Arterial blood gas (ABG) with lactate
- Complete blood count (CBC) and metabolic profile
- Coagulation profile
- Troponin/N-terminal pro-brain natriuretic peptide (NT ProBNP)
- C/S and Procalcitonin

BOX 5: Imaging.

- Point-of-care ultrasound (POCUS)
- Echocardiography (ECHO)
- Chest X-ray
- Computed tomography (CT)

BOX 6: Monitoring of hypotensive patients.

- *Cycling of BP:* Decide interval of BP monitoring
- ECG monitoring
- Arterial for patients who are unstable clinically and likely to have more fluctuations in BP
- *Central venous pressure (CVP):* Rather than just single CVP value, monitor the trend. In a hypovolemic patient, CVP may remain unchanged after fluid challenge. However, in a volume overloaded patient, CVP may start rising with fluid challenge; this can be used as a rough guide to decide if more fluids are needed or not. CVP is also going to help as access for administrating vasopressors/inotropes
- Stroke volume variation (SVV)/pulse pressure variation (PPV): Pulse index continuous cardiac output (PICCO), lithium dilution cardiac output measurement (LIDCO) (discussed in Hemodynamics)
- *POCUS:* Monitor inferior vena cava (IVC) collapsibility, systolic function of left and right ventricles, acute valvular lesions. Rule out cardiac tamponade, pneumothorax, and pulmonary embolism (discussed in USG in ER)
- *Pulmonary artery catheter:* It is rarely used in ER. But this is a very helpful tool in undifferentiated shock. (discussed in Hemodynamics)

BOX 7: Treatment.

- Fluid challenge for all patients; even cardiogenic shock patients may be fluid depleted
- Identify cause of hypotension
- Vasopressor and inotropes
- Treat primary cause of shock
- *Mechanical devices for refractory shock:* Intra-aortic balloon pump (IABP)/Extra corporeal membrane oxygenation (ECMO)/Ventricular assist devices

SUGGESTED READING

1. Rodgers KG. Cardiovascular shock. Emerg Med Clin North Am. 1995;13(4): 793-810.
2. Seymour CW, Liu VX, Iwashyna TJ, Brunkhorst FM, Rea TD, Scherag A, et al. Assessment of Clinical Criteria for Sepsis: For the Third International Consensus Definitions for Sepsis and Septic Shock (Sepsis-3). JAMA. 2016;315(8):762-74.
3. Vincent JL, De Backer D. Circulatory shock. N Engl J Med. 2013;369(18):1726-34.

Part 4

Emergency Support

CHAPTER 30

Airway Management and Support

Jamshed D Sunavala

BOX 1: Stepwise management of airways in an emergency to provide patent and secure airways for adequate ventilation and oxygenation.

- Clear the upper airways by simple maneuvers
- Correct hypoxia by delivering oxygen
  - Use appropriate delivery systems
  - For patent airways, use nasal cannula or simple oxygen mask
  - For delivery of high fraction of inspired oxygen (FiO_2), use partial rebreathing or nonrebreathing mask
  - If airways are not patent, obtain clear ventilation by using oro/nasopharyngeal airways
- Secure airways for short-term or long-term use
  - Endotracheal (ET) intubation
  - *Difficult intubation:* Attempt needle cricothyrotomy or surgical cricothyrotomy (Seldinger technique using min-trach kit)
- *Securing airways for long term:* Surgical tracheostomy
- *For artificial ventilation:* Noninvasive mechanical ventilation (NIV) or invasive mechanical ventilation (MV)

BOX 2: Simple maneuvers to clear airways.

- Clearing airways of extraneous material, food, saliva, denture, etc. can be done by suctioning or cleaning with the finger wrapped in gauze
- Triple airways maneuver involves "head-tilt" to extend the neck, "jaw-thrust" by pulling the mandible forward and mouth opening. This maneuver is often beneficial in obtunded patients. However, it is contraindicated in patients with trauma and spine instability. Here, immobilizing the spine is mandatory before performing the maneuver

BOX 3: Noninvasive oxygen delivery systems.

- *Nasal prong:* The main disadvantage is that it cannot deliver >30% oxygen
- Masks
  - *Simple mask:* It cannot give higher than 50% oxygen even at very high flow rates
  - Partial rebreathing or nonrebreathing mask with reservoir bag attached can give oxygen concentration up to 60–80%
  - *Venture mask:* Delivers an exact concentration of inspired oxygen ranging from 25–35%

BOX 4: Obtain clear ventilation.

- Oropharyngeal airways (OPA)/nasopharyngeal airways (NPA) is introduced between the tongue and posterior pharyngeal wall and used as a temporary measure to keep the airways patient
- Laryngeal mask airways (LMA) **(Fig. 1)** are used as a bridge before introducing ET in patients with difficult intubation. This is a mask mounted on a tube, which is placed blindly in the lower pharynx overlying the glottis with an inflatable cuff sealing the inlet allowing direct manual ventilation via an ambu bag. They come in various sizes usually 3 for females and 4 for males

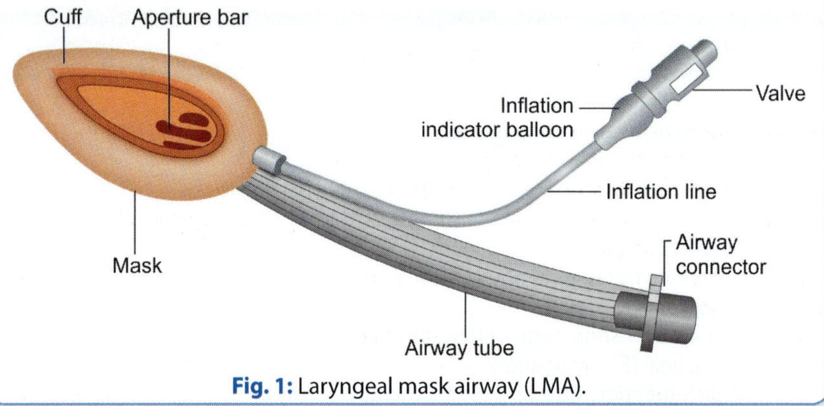

Fig. 1: Laryngeal mask airway (LMA).

BOX 5: Indications for ET intubation.

- Poor respiratory effort requires intubation and mechanical ventilator
- *Poor gag reflex:* Check for protective reflexes
- All patients with NIV contraindications

BOX 6: Rapid sequence intubation technique.

- Prepare and position the patient. Set the instrument tray with laryngoscope and different-sized blades. Check the light on laryngoscope
- Preoxygenate the patient
- Apply carotid pressure
- Administer induction agent rapidly
- Direct laryngoscopic-guided intubation
- Verify correct tube placement

BOX 7: Conditions associated with difficult intubation.

- Mouth bleeding
- Foreign body
- Small mouth
- Large tongue
- Acromegaly
- Facial muscle spasm
- Facial burns
- Tetanus
- Cervical spine trauma or surgery
- Short neck
- Neck stiffness
- Obesity
- Inability to reach base of epiglottis with laryngoscope blade

BOX 8: Protocol for cannot intubate–cannot ventilate.

- Call for appropriate help
- Do not keep struggling to force the ET
- Intubate with LMA as a bridge
- Continue with 100% oxygen by Ambu bag with mask or LMA
- Avoid giving further sedation or muscle relaxants instead wait for help from an anesthetist or a more experienced intensivist
- Needle cricothyrotomy in an absolute emergency is useful to maintain oxygenation for a short while
- Surgical cricothyrotomy is a more permanent procedure (see **Box 10** for procedure)
- Tracheostomy is indicated in case where more permanent airways patency is required **(Box 11)**

BOX 9: Procedure for needle cricothyrotomy **(Fig. 2)**.

- Done as an absolute emergency to maintain oxygenation for short periods
- It is not a stable airway
- Inadequate for carbon dioxide (CO_2) to escape through the needle-sized cannula

Procedure:

- 14-gauge intravenous (IV) cannula over a needle is attached to a syringe
- It is pierced through the cricothyroid membrane with the syringe
- Continuous negative pressure is applied while piercing through the cricothyroid membrane until there is a gap and air enters the syringe
- At this point, slide the cannula off the needle into the trachea

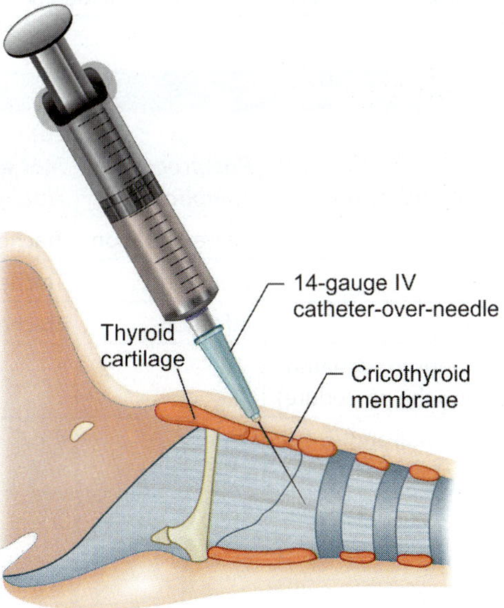

Fig. 2: Procedure for needle cricothyrotomy.

BOX 10: Procedure for surgical cricothyrotomy.

- Surgical cricothyrotomy is more permanent and a stable procedure with minimal risk of bleeding or surgical emphysema
- After injecting, a local anesthetic makes an incision of 1–1.5 cm over the cricothyroid membrane incising the superficial facial and subcutaneous fat
- Next, proceed to divide the membrane with blunt forceps or the handle of the scalpel, through which cuffed tracheostomy tube is inserted between the thyroid and cricoid cartilage
- Commercial prepacked "mini-trach" kits are available, enabling a small-sized cannula to be inserted through the cricothyroid membrane
- Here Seldinger technique is used, which accurately and safely guides the cannula into the trachea

BOX 11: Surgical tracheostomy.

- Surgical tracheostomy is indicated where a patent airway is required for long-term period
- It provides a better access for suctioning and maintaining a good tracheobronchial toilet
- It should be avoided or deferred if there is local inflammation over the operating area and also in patients with coagulation abnormalities
- Timing of tracheostomy is left to the judgment of the physician and often, it is deferred till the patient is transferred to the intensive care unit (ICU) where better bedside facilities are available
- Tracheostomy has its own inherent complications **(Box 11)**, which the treating physician should be alert to detect and mange immediately

BOX 12: Complications of tracheostomy.

During procedure complications	***Postprocedure complications***	***Late complications [not seen in the short emergency room (ER) stay]***
Bleeding	Self-extubation	Tracheal stenosis
Creating a false tract	Bleeding	Tracheoesophageal fistula
Pneumomediastinum	Infection	Tracheomalacia
Hypoxia (if patient is not oxygenated through the ET during the procedure)		
Injury to the posterior wall and oropharynx		

SUGGESTED READING

1. Andriolo BN, Andriolo RB, Saconato H, Atallah ÁN, Valente O. Early versus late tracheostomy for critically ill patients. Cochrane Database Syst Rev. 2015;1(1):CD007271.
2. Apfelbaum JL, HagbergCa, Caplan RA, Blitt CD, Connis RT, Nickinovich DG, et al. Practice guidelines for management of the difficult airway: An updated report by the American Society of Anesthesiologists Task Force on Management of the Difficult Airway. Anesthesiology. 2013;118(2):251-70.
3. Engels PT, Bagshaw SM, Meier M, Brindley PG. Tracheostomy: From insertion to decannulation. Can J Surg. 2009;52(5):427-33.
4. Frerk C, Mitchell VS, McNarry AF, Mendonca C, Bhagrath R, Patel A, et al. Difficult Airway Society 2015 guidelines for management of unanticipated difficult intubation in adults. Br J Anaesth. 2015;115(6):827-48.
5. Gurjar M. Manual of ICU Procedures. New Delhi: Jaypee Brothers Medical publisher; 2015.
6. Maxwell BG, Ganaway T, Lighthall GK. Percutaneous tracheostomy at the bedside: 13 tips for improving safety and success. J Intensive Care Med. 2014;29(2):110-5.

CHAPTER 31

Mechanical Ventilation

Jamshed D Sunavala

TABLE 1: Indications for mechanical ventilation.

Absolute indications	***Clinical judgment/ assessment***	***Supporting parameters***
Cardiorespiratory arrest	–	–
Severe shock	Severe hypotension, respiratory distress, and sensorium	Elevated serum lactate and venous oxygen saturation (SvO_2) <60% in cardiogenic shock
Type I acute respiratory failure (ARF)	–	• Partial pressure of oxygen (PaO_2) <60 mm Hg or • Arterial oxygen saturation (SaO_2) <90% despite supplemental O_2
Type II ARF	Declining mental status	Partial pressure of carbon dioxide ($PaCO_2$) ≥50 mm Hg or acute increase from baseline in $PaCO_2$ and pH <7.25
Potential indications	***Clinical judgment/ assessment***	***Supporting parameters***
Hypoventilation with inadequate lung expansion	Shallow and rapid breathing	Tidal volume (V_T) ≤5 mL/kg, volume controlled (VC) <15 mL/kg, respiratory rate (RR) ≥35
Respiratory weakness	Underlying clinical problem causing hypoventilation	VC <20 mL/kg
Acute decompensated heart failure	Signs of heart failure	Clinical judgment
Increased work on breathing	Respiratory distress, use of accessory muscles, and paradoxical respiration **(Box 1)**	Minute ventilation >15 L/min and dead space >50%

Contd...

Contd...

Absolute indications	***Clinical judgment/ assessment***	***Supporting parameters***
Postoperative pulmonary complications [noninvasive ventilation (NIV)/ invasive mechanical ventilation (IMV)]	Mainly, post-upper abdominal and cardiac surgery	Abnormal blood gas values
Acute exacerbation of chronic obstructive pulmonary disease (COPD) (NIV/IMV)	Progressively decreasing sensorium, degree of respiratory distress, and air hunger	Acute increase from baseline $PaCO_2$ pH <7.25
Contraindications to NIV	Impaired sensorium, poor respiratory drive, risk of aspiration, excessive secretions, head–neck and facial injuries, flail chest, upper airways obstruction, and severe acute respiratory distress syndrome (ARDS) PaO_2/ fraction of inspired oxygen (FIO_2) <150	

Source: Sunavala JD. Essentials of Critical Care Medicine for the Physician New Delhi: Jaypee Brothers Medical Publishers; 2022.

BOX 1: Physical signs of acute respiratory distress.

Hypoxemic respiratory failure:
- Tachypnea, hypertension, and at times hypotension
- *Use of accessory muscles for respiration:* Intercostals, abdominal muscles, and sternomastoid
- Tracheal tug
- Exaggerated retraction of the intercostals space
- *Facial signs:* Nasal flaring, open mouth breathing, and pursed lips with labored breathing, as in COPD
- Moaning and grunting during exhalation
- Profuse sweating
- Diminished mentation or vacant gaze

Hypercapnic respiratory failure:
- Mostly similar to hypoxemic respiratory failure
- Greater neurological manifestations
- Tremors of outstretched hands and asterixis
- Myoclonic jerks, irritability, behavioral changes, decreased sensorium, and seizures

BOX 2: Basics of mechanical ventilation (MV).

Volume-controlled ventilation (VCV) versus pressure-controlled ventilation (PCV) ***(Fig. 1)***
The VCV delivers a preset V_T and the ventilation automatically adjusts the inflation pressure, whereas in PCV, the pressure is preset to deliver the desired volume. Thus, in VCV, the V_T is always constant despite the changing compliance of the lung whereas in PCV mode, there is a little risk of barotrauma as the airway pressure remains within the fixed set limits though the V_T may vary

*Compliance (C_L)***(Fig. 2)***:* C_L is change in V_T per change in unit pressure (i.e., $C_L = \Delta V/\Delta P$)
A poorly compliant lung (stiff lung) will need increasing positive pressure to inflate it

Peak airway pressure (P-peak) is the pressure generated by the ventilator to overcome both the resistance to the flow of air, provided by the airway pressure and elastic forces of the lung and chest wall. (i.e., P-peak = Preset + P_{CL}). **Figure 2** gives an idea of the stiffness of the lung (a rise in plateau pressure) as in ARDS and airway obstruction reflected by the difference between the peak and plateau pressure

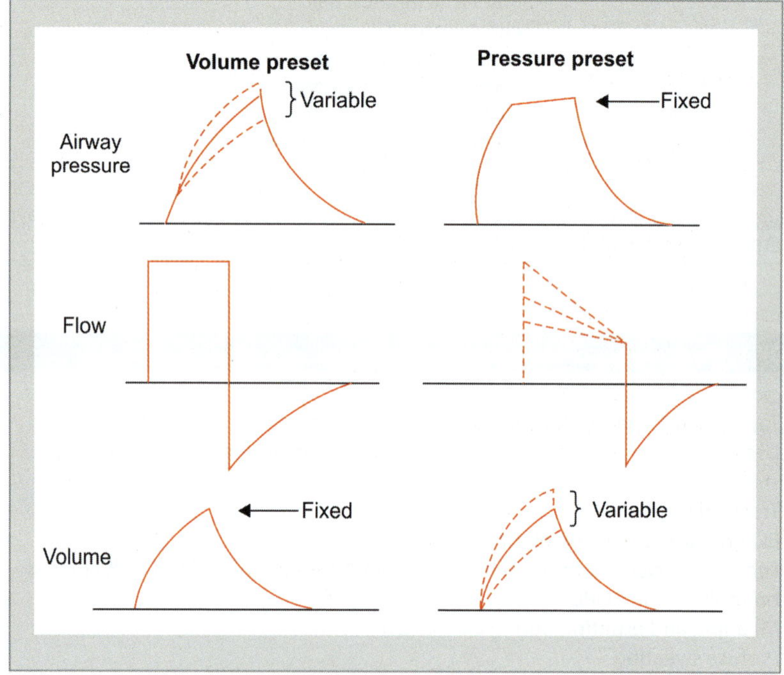

Fig. 1: Volume preset versus pressure preset ventilation.
Source: Sunavala JD. Essentials of Critical Care Medicine for the Physician. New Delhi: Jaypee Brothers Medical Publishers; 2022.

Contd...

Contd...

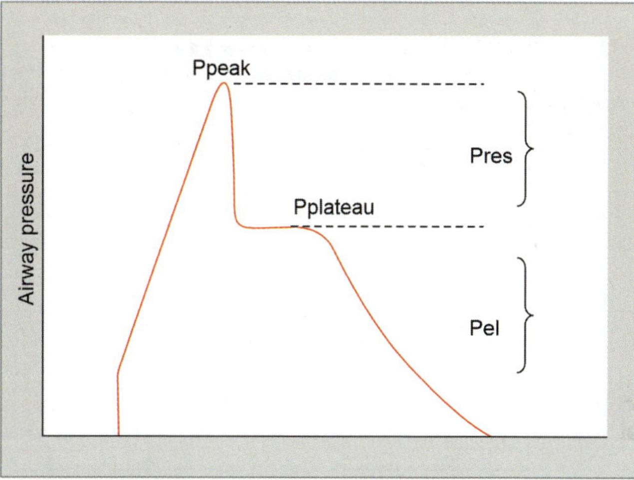

Fig. 2: Graph of a mechanically ventilated pressure curve of VC breath showing peak airway pressure (Ppeak) and plateau pressure (Pplateau).
Note: Pres is the pressure needed to overcome airway resistance and Pel is the pressure required to overcome the forces of elastic recoil.
Source: Sunavala JD. Essentials of Critical Care Medicine for the Physician. New Delhi: Jaypee Brothers Medical Publishers; 2022.

Positive end-expiratory pressure (PEEP) is the positive pressure in the alveoli during end-expiration. Normally, during spontaneous ventilation or on normal ventilator settings, the baseline of the pressure waveform is at zero. However, a positive pressure can be applied by selecting a ventilatory mode called PEEP. High level of PEEP prevents alveolar collapse during expiration and hence, decreases atelectasis and improves ventilation/perfusion (V/Q) mismatch in patient with hypoxic respiratory failure. More details on PEEP are given in chapter on ARDS. The normal physiological PEEP of 0–5 cmH_2O is used in normal ventilation as in the immediate post-op period

Auto PEEP or intrinsic PEEP ***(Fig. 3)****:* In asthmatic and COPD patients, PEEP can occur without applying the PEEP mode. This happens because the lungs are not capable of emptying air completely during expiration as a result of airflow limitation during a prolonged expiration and this process is commonly called "air-trapping"

Contd...

Contd...

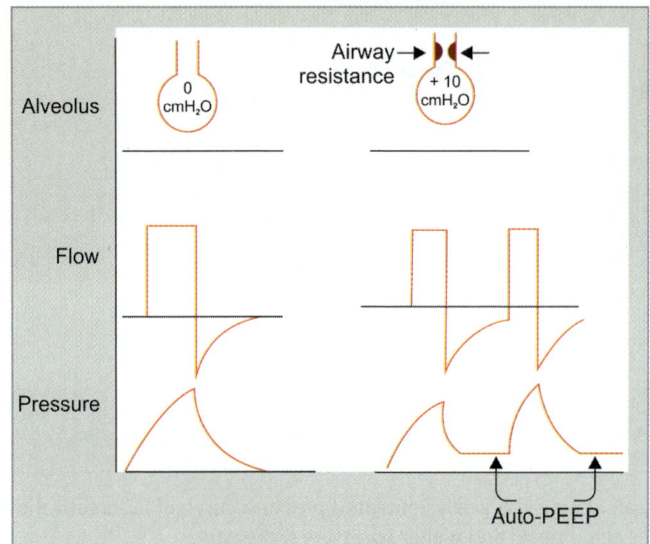

Fig. 3: Auto-positive end-expiratory pressure (Auto-PEEP).
Source: Sunavala JD. Essentials of Critical Care Medicine for the Physician New Delhi: Jaypee Brothers Medical Publishers; 2022.

BOX 3: General classification of ventilation modes.

Basic modes as per breath pattern:
- Breath pattern within the breaths:
  - VCV
  - PCV
- Breath sequence between breaths:
  - Continuous mandatory ventilation (CMV)
  - Intermittent mandatory ventilation (IMV)
  - Continuous spontaneous ventilation (CSV)

Strategic modes:
- Mainly for lung recruitment:
  - PEEP
  - Inverse ratio ventilation (IRV)
  - High-frequency oscillation ventilation (HFOV)
  - Pressure release volume control (PRVC)
  - Prone position ventilation
- Facilitate difficult weaning:
  - Pressure support ventilation (PSV)
- Lung protection ventilation (LPV):
  - Low-tidal-volume ventilation (LTV)
  - Permissive hypercapnia
- Noninvasive ventilation (NIV)

BOX 4: Basic modes of ventilation.

Assist control ventilation (ACV): Common ventilation mode to initiate ventilator support in most patients

Intermittent mandatory ventilation: Here the patient can spontaneously trigger a breath and breathe on his own but will take over at fixed intervals or earlier if required like a demand pacemaker. The ventilator breaths can be either VC or pressure-controlled (PC) and when the mandatory breaths are delivered in synchrony with the patient's breath, it is termed as synchronized intermittent mandatory ventilation (SIMV)

BOX 5: Advanced modes of mechanical ventilator.

- The *conventional modes* have fixed parameters as per the setting without the ability to adapt to the patient's changing lung parameters, hence these modes are not suitable for all patients. In patients where lung dynamics vary, there is a need for different modes and ventilation strategies such as PRVC, airway pressure release ventilation (APRV), proportional assist ventilation (PAV), and adaptive support ventilation (ASV)
- *PRVC:* This mode is mainly chosen in patients with varying lung compliance where the traditional PC mode does not deliver the required minute ventilation due to changing compliance and effort
  - Useful in patients with ARDS who need a constant V_T
  - It is a combination of VC and PC modes
  - Here, the initial breath is VC where Pplateau is assessed and the subsequent ones are PC with the previous Pplateau as the maximum pressure
  - This mode works well in delivering a fixed V_T at the lowest peak airway pressure enabling a low work of breathing
- *APRV or bilevel ventilation **(Fig. 4)**:*
  - This is a bilevel mode of open-lung ventilation used in patients with ARDS and refractory hypoxia with atelectasis. It is time-cycled and pressure-limited
  - It works at two levels (P-high and P-low). The former level (P-high) is maintained continuously at higher level of PEEP for a longer period whilst the later (P-low) is maintained for a short duration in expiration (IRV)
  - The longer P-high prevents alveolar collapse and improves recruitment while the P-low, following the release pressure, facilitates CO_2 removal
  - Here, the V_T is the difference in the driving pressure P-high and P-low
  - In this mode, spontaneous breathing is possible during any phase of the cycle, and hence, the need for sedation and paralysis is low and is better tolerated than the usual PC-IRV
  - It is contraindicated in COPD patients as there is a tendency for dynamic hyperinflation during the prolong inspiratory time
- *PSV **(Fig. 5)**:*
  - This is similar to bilevel positive airway pressure (BiPAP) as in the NIV but used in intubated patients with spontaneous breathing
  - Here, the pressure support (PS) is mechanical support given by the machine above the constant level of set PEEP in order to ease the effort of spontaneous breathing
  - To enable adequate spontaneous respiration, patient should be awake and alert
  - It is useful in spontaneously breathing patients and during weaning trials

Contd...

Contd...

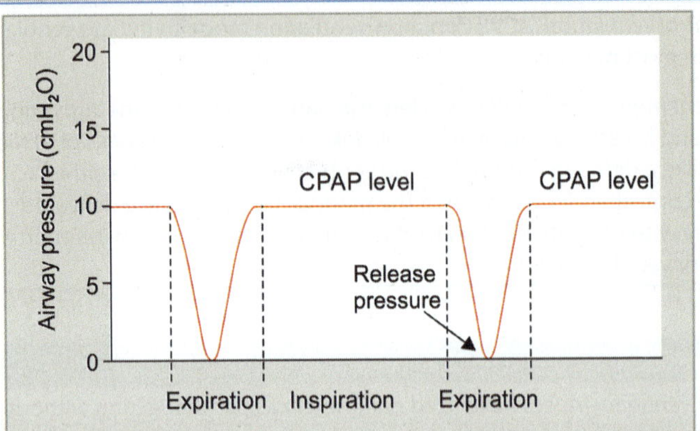

Fig. 4: Airway pressure release ventilation. (CPAP: continuous positive airway pressure)
Source: Sunavala JD. Essentials of Critical Care Medicine for the Physician. New Delhi: Jaypee Brothers Medical Publishers; 2022.

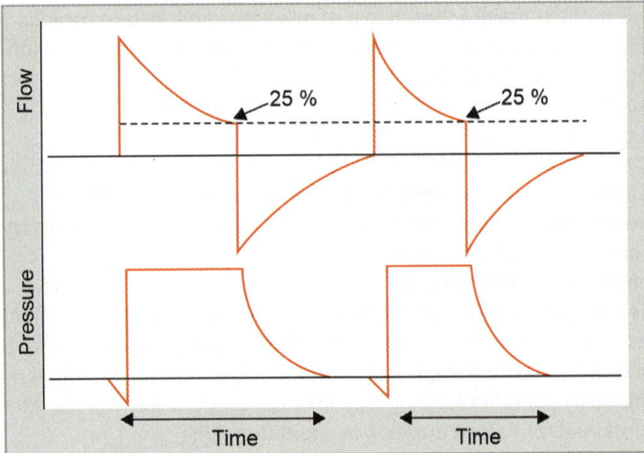

Fig. 5: Pressure and flow waveforms of PSV. Pressure support remains constant as long as the inspiratory flow continues and ends when the inspiratory flow reachs 25% of the peak inspiratory flow. Inspiratory flow and time are dependent on the patients' spontaneous breathing.
Source: Sunavala JD. Essentials of Critical Care Medicine for the Physician. New Delhi: Jaypee Brothers Medical Publishers; 2022.

BOX 6: Weaning from ventilator support.

- In the emergency room (ER), most patients are observed for a limited period and transferred to the intensive care unit (ICU) on MV
- Short duration (24–48 hours) of ventilation support can be weaned abruptly without weaning trial
- However, if longer duration of ventilation support is required, it is important to be aware of the possibilities of difficult weaning
- However, one should not attempt weaning in the ER in patients with severe lung pathology, hemodynamic instability, or worsening respiratory blood gases parameters. This is best done in the ICU
- Weaning failure may manifest as sudden rise or fall in blood pressure (BP), heart rate (HR), rising $PaCO_2$ or O_2 desaturation

BOX 7: Checklist for weaning failure.

- Increased airflow resistance due to blockage of endotracheal (ET) tube or reappearance of bronchospasm
- *Increased metabolic demands:* Occur when underlying disease is unresolved or partially resolved
- Decreased C_L as in unresolved ARDS, which increases the work of breathing
- Decreased respiratory drive due to lingering effect of sedatives or chest wall pain

SUGGESTED READING

1. Tobin MJ. Principles and Practice of Mechanical Ventilation, 3rd edition. New York: McGraw Hill Publication; 2014.

CHAPTER 32

Hemodynamic Monitoring

Jamshed D Sunavala

BOX 1: Main aims of hemodynamic monitoring.

Assessing and monitoring the determinants of:

- Cardiac performance **(Flowchart 1, Box 2, Tables 1 and 2)**
- Tissue oxygenation **(Boxes 8 and 9)**
- Fluid responsiveness **(Boxes 10 and 11)**

Flowchart 1: Determinants of cardiac performance.

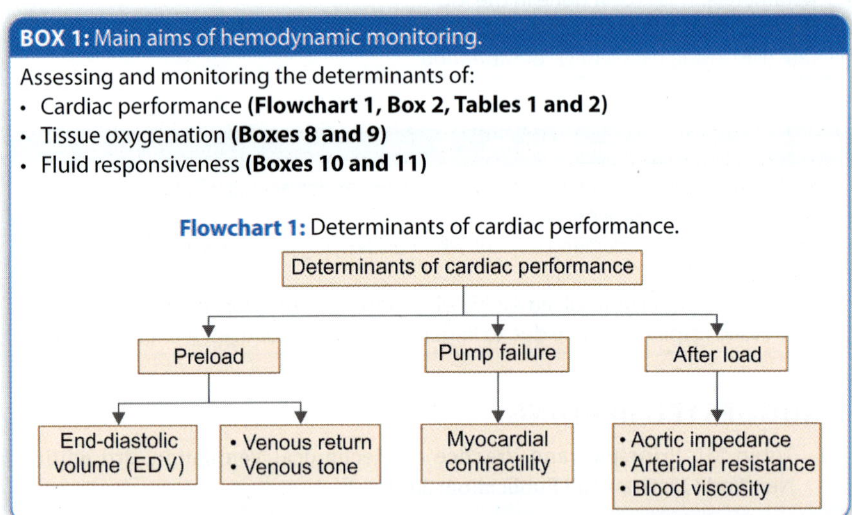

BOX 2: Determinants of cardiac performance.

- **Preload** is the force acting to stretch the left ventricular (LV) muscle fibers at end-diastole, which increases the strength of muscle contraction and this is one of the main determinants of cardiac performance. The force here is the returning venous blood that fills the ventricle in end-diastole, hence preload is end-diastolic volume (EDV)
- **Contractility** is defined as the inherent capacity of the myocardium to contract independently of the alteration in pre and afterload
- **Afterload** is defined as the impedance to blood flow from the ventricle as a result of systemic vascular resistance (SVR)

BOX 3: Measuring preload.

Central venous pressure (CVP) is equivalent to right atrial pressure (RAP) and in the absence of tricuspid valve dysfunction, RAP reflect**s** the right ventricular end-diastolic pressure (RVEDP). In a normal heart, the RVEDP/CVP correlates well with left ventricular end-diastolic pressure (LVEDP) in the absence of mitral valve dysfunction, provided the LV compliance is normal. Hence, CVP monitoring is practical at the bedside and can be used to guide fluid resuscitation for severe diarrhea and blood loss in young individuals without underlying heart problem. Normal CVP is 0–6 mm Hg (using transducer monitoring system) and 3–8 cmH_2O (using a simple water manometer)

Pulmonary capillary wedge pressure (PCWP) directly measures the left atrial pressure (LAP) and in the presence of a normal "mitral outflow tract", it is equivalent to LVEDP. However, LVEDP being a surrogate for left ventricular end-diastolic volume (LVEDV) is not entirely correct, but despite the limitations, the filling pressures are still important and practical bedside guiding to assist decision-making in patients with heart failure or volume overload. PCWP is measured by use of pulmonary artery catheter (PAC) also called Swan–Ganz catheter **(Fig. 1)** and for technique of insertion using pressure waveform as guide see **Figure 2**

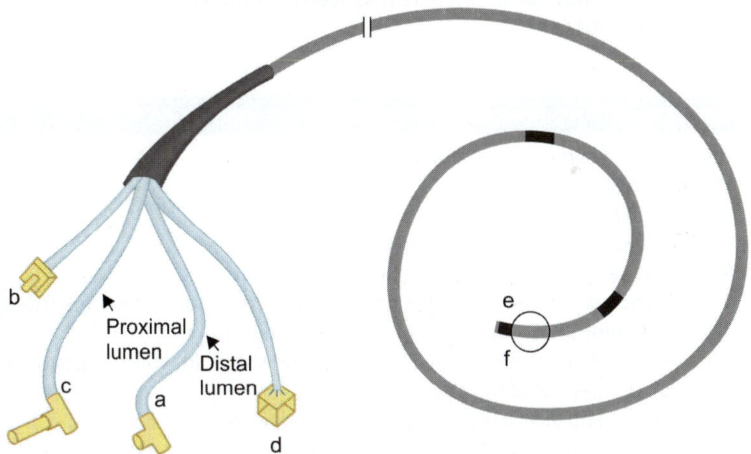

Fig. 1: Triple-lumen pulmonary catheter. a = distal pulmonary artery (PA) port, b = balloon inflation port, c = proximal right atrium (RA) port, d = thermistor hub, e = balloon, f = thermistor.
Source: Sunavala. (2014).

Contd...

Contd...

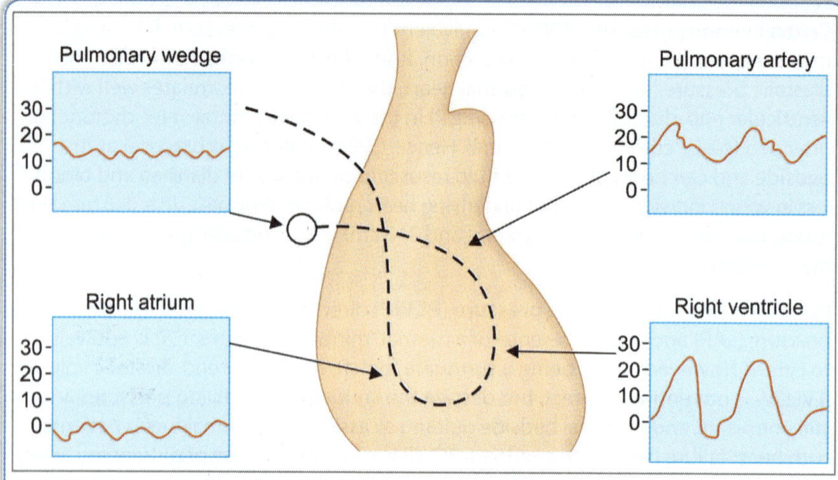

Fig. 2: Pressure waveform configuration as seen during the passage of the pulmonary artery catheter through the various chambers of the heart and in wedge position. The position of the catheter shown here is as seen in fluoroscopy.
Source: Sunavala. (2014).

BOX 4: Indications for pulmonary artery (PA) pressure monitoring.

- *In critically ill and hemodynamically unstable patients:*
  - Shock (of any etiology)
- *In cases, where the diagnosis is uncertain:*
  - Cardiogenic versus noncardiogenic pulmonary edema
  - Acute respiratory failure with uncertain cardiac status
  - Acute myocardial infarction with a new loud murmur indicating acute rupture of the interventricular septum or of a papillary muscle
  - In patients with acute myocardial infarction and shock, in whom hypovolemia has to be differentiated from pump failure
- *As a therapeutic guideline, under the following conditions:*
  - Massive fluid replacement in patients with severe fluid loss, especially in elderly patients or in those with a history of ischemic heart disease
  - Fluid management in patients with noncardiogenic pulmonary edema [acute respiratory distress syndrome (ARDS)]
  - In acute hemorrhage, necessitating massive transfusions, particularly in patients with associated cardiac or renal problems
  - Management of patients with shock or other critically ill patients on inotropic and/or vasodilator drugs
  - In patients with pump failure who respond unsatisfactorily to initial therapy
- *Patients at risk of hemodynamic decompensation:*
  - Preoperative monitoring in all seriously ill patients (cardiac or noncardiac surgery)
  - Patients with underlying cardiac disease on mechanical ventilator

Note: All the above are only a broad list of guidelines to be used with judgment so that the information available will alter treatment plan toward clinical benefit.
Source: Sunavala. (2014).

BOX 5: Complications directly attributable to PAC.

Complications	*Action/prevention*
Arrhythmias	• Decrease insertion time • Use fluoroscopic guidance in high-risk groups so that less maneuvering of catheter is necessary • Promptly remove catheter if arrhythmias persist
Infection	• Meticulous, sterile technique with all aseptic precautions during insertion and aftercare • Avoid repeated manipulations • Catheter is to be removed at the earliest
Balloon rupture	Inflation of balloon is typically associated with a feeling of resistance, the absence of resistance and failure to wedge suggest balloon rupture
Knotting	• Knots may be resolved by insertion of suitable guidewires and manipulation under fluoroscopy • If knot does not include any intracardiac structure, apply gentle traction to tighten the knot and then, withdraw slowly • Only in worst cases, a thoracotomy and cardiotomy may be required
Clotting and thromboembolic complications in RA or systemic veins	• Intermittent flushing of catheters with heparinized saline • Avoid long-standing catheter placements • Heparin-coated catheters may reduce catheter thrombogenicity
Pulmonary infarction and PA rupture	• Avoid prolonged or overinflation of the balloon in the wedge position • Avoid repeated inflation of balloon for PCWP measurements; instead use PADP for continuous monitoring, as pulmonary artery diastolic pressure (PADP) equals PCWP • Avoid inserting the catheter too far peripherally into a branch of PA. If catheter is seen beyond the hilum, there is an increased chance of infarction or rupture

Source: Sunavala. (2014).

BOX 6: Measuring contractility.

There is no bedside method of monitoring contractility alone; however, if two of the fundamental determinants of stroke volume (SV) (pre and afterload) can be kept constant, then obviously the changes in stroke work performed by the ventricle becomes the determinant ventricular function solely affected by the inotropic state of the heart

Stroke work for the two ventricles is calculated as follows:
- LVSWI = SI × (MAP – PCWP) × 0.0136 g/min/m^2
- RVSWI = SI × (MPAP – CVP) × 0.0136 g/min/m^2

Where LVSWI is the LV stroke work index, RVSWI is RV stroke work index, MAP is the mean arterial pressure, MPAP is mean pulmonary artery pressure and SI is the stroke index

2D Echocardiography measure of ejection fraction (EF) is frequently used a measure of ventricular contractility despite its limitations

BOX 7: Measuring afterload.

Resistance to the two ventricles [indexed to the body surface area (BSA)] is derived by the following equations:

- Systemic vascular resistance index (SVRI)

$$= \frac{\text{Mean arterial blood pressure} - \text{CVP}}{\text{Cardiac index}} \times 80$$

- Pulmonary vascular resistance index (PVRI)

$$= \frac{\text{Mean pulmonary artery pressure} - \text{PCWP}}{\text{Cardiac index}} \times 80$$

BOX 8: Determining tissue oxygenation **(Box 9)**.

- **Mixed venous oxygen saturation (SvO_2):** Tissue oxygenation depends on two important determinants, oxygen delivery (DO_2) and oxygen uptake (VO_2) by the tissues. This fractional uptake of O_2 into the tissue determines the oxygen extraction ratio (O_2ER); the normal O_2ER is 25% of DO_2 (i.e., $O_2ER = 0.250$). A reasonably good bedside marker of tissue oxygenation is the *SvO_2*, which varies inversely with the changes in oxygen extraction. Hence, in low cardiac output (CO) states where O_2ER is increased, the SvO_2 will fall below the normal of 75%, to improve tissue oxygenation. However, in a state of severe sepsis and shock, one may find the SvO_2 to be normal or even slightly higher. This is because of the tissues' inability to extract O_2 from the capillaries as a result of the severe mitochondrial damage at the cellular level
- **Serum lactate** measured from venous or arterial blood is a good marker of tissue oxygenation. The normal blood lactate level is <2 mmol/L is also a good prognostic marker. Early recovery of serum lactate levels within 24 hours of cardiorespiratory resuscitation has shown a good outcome

BOX 9: Determinants of tissue perfusion (oxygenation).

- **Mean arterial pressure (MAP)** = CO × SVR
- Arterial O_2 content (CaO_2) = [1.34 × hemoglobin (Hb) × arterial oxygen saturation (SaO_2)] + 0.0031 × partial pressure of oxygen (PaO_2)
- $DO_2 = CO \times CaO_2$ (*N* = 1,000 mL/min)
- $VO_2 = CO \times [CaO_2$ – central venous oxygen saturation (CvO_2)] (*N* = 250 mL/min)
- $O_2ER = VO_2/DO_2 = CaO_2 - CvO_2/CaO_2$ (N = 0.025)

TABLE 1: Normal hemodynamic values.

Variables	*Abbreviations*	*Units*	*Normal range*
Right atrial pressure	RAP	mm Hg	2–6
Mean pulmonary artery pressure	MPAP	mm Hg	11–15
Pulmonary capillary wedge pressure	PCWP	mm Hg	3–15
Cardiac index	CL	L/min-m^2	2.8–3.6
Left ventricular stroke work index	LVSWI	gm-m/m^2	44–68
Right ventricular stroke work index	RVSWI	gm-m/m^2	4–8
Systemic vascular resistance index	SVRI	dynes-sec/cm^5-m^2	1,700–2,600
Pulmonary vascular resistance index	PVRI	dynes-sec/cm^5-m^2	100–225
Oxygen delivery index	DO_2 I	mL/min-m^2	500–650
Oxygen consumption index	VO_2I	mL/min-m^2	110–150

TABLE 2: Hemodynamic changes caused by some commonly used IV drugs.

Drug	*Heart rate (HR)*	*MAP*	*PCWP*	*CO*	*SVR*
Nitroprusside	↑	↓	NC or ↓	↑	↓
Nitroglycerin	↑	↓	↓	↑	↓
Norepinephrine	NC or ↑	↑	↑↓	↑, NC	↑
Dopamine	NC or ↑	NC or ↑	NC or ↑	↑	↑
Dobutamine	NC or ↑	NC or ↑	NC	↑	NC
Amrinone	NC	↓	↓	↑	↓

Key: NC = No change; ↑ = increased; ↓ = decreased.

BOX 10: Means of predicting fluid responsiveness.

Modes and underlying principles	*Methodology*	*Comments*
• *Stroke volume variation (SVV) or pulse pressure variation (PPV)* • Cyclical changes in intrathoracic pressure with mechanical ventilator alter RV and LV pre and afterload	• PPV requires arterial line • SVV = CO monitoring device or esophageal Doppler or echocardiogram • Patient needs to be sedated and on mechanical ventilation (MV)	• False positive in presence of cardiac arrhythmias, spontaneous breathing, and RV dysfunction

Contd...

Contd...

Modes and underlying principles	***Methodology***	***Comments***
• Assess SVV as reflected by arterial PPV or by direct estimation of stroke volume by CO monitoring or esophageal echo	• Need to be in sinus rhythm • Should always start from semirecumbent position (45%) and not supine	• False negative in presence of low tidal volume of <8 mL/kg as it creates insufficient change in cardiac preload
• *Passive leg raising (PLR)* – Cardiac preload is transiently increased by recruiting about 200–300 mL of blood from the legs to the central circulation	• Leg raising is done along with lowering the trunk flat on bed, simultaneously elevating the legs to 30–45° • Assess passive leg raising (PLR) preferably by directly measuring CO and not BP • Baseline CO should be done in original recumbent position • Increase in CO by 10–15% predicts reliable assessment of fluid responsiveness	• Applicable to both patients with arrhythmias and patients on MV or spontaneously breathing • It is quite useful test at bedside because it is less complex and easily applicable • To be avoided in patients with intracranial hypertension and critically ill patients, where this maneuver best avoided
• *M-mode echocardiography* – Measures inferior vena cava (IVC) collapsibility with respiratory variation • Best used in patients on MV but also on patients with spontaneous breathing and good respiratory excursions	• Respiratory variations on IVC diameter using transthoracic echo • The difference in diameters in expiration and inspiration is expressed as collapsibility index or in percentage • >50% collapsibility is normal • <30% collapsibility is a warning against aggressive fluid challenge	This method is best applicable to patients with good imaging window

Source: Adapted with modification from Anstey JR, Deane AM, Bellomo R. Fluid in sepsis. In: Wiersinga WJ, Seymour CW (Eds). Handbook of Sepsis. Cham, Switzerland: Springer; 2018

BOX 11: Determinants of fluid responsiveness.

Methodology	***Equation***	***Suggestive of fluid responsiveness***
IVC: Distensibility index (dIVC) by echocardiogram	$dIVC = \frac{ID - ED}{ID}$	>18%
PPV	$PPV\% = 100 \times \frac{(PPVmax - PPVmin)}{PPVmax + PPVmin/2}$	>13%*
SVV	SVV over respiratory cycle on mechanical ventilation	>10%#

*Implies 85% probability of benefit from fluid challenge.
#Predicts increase in CO of ≥15% for bolus of 500 mL of fluid.
ID/ED = Inspiratory/expiratory diameter

BOX 12: Fluid challenge.

- *Fluid bolus:* Here, one administers fluid without any prior predictive test of responsiveness. It is based on clinical evidence of hypoperfusion (hypotension with MAP <60 mm Hg and or oliguria). Here, measuring MAP may be surrogate for CO. Surviving sepsis campaign guidelines (2016) recommend that in initial resuscitation of sepsis, induced hypotension at least 30 mL/kg of IV crystalloid fluid be given over 3 hours
- *Mini fluid challenge:* This is similar to "fluid bolus" but smaller amount of fluid (e.g., 250 mL over 10 minutes) is given and change in CO or MAP or repeated IVC collapsibility by ultrasound or echo is measured before the next challenge. Here, the end point is clinical improvement in perfusion. Mini fluid challenge is an alternative to fluid bolus in aged patients or in those suspected to have cardiac dysfunction
- *Fluid responsiveness:* As previously mentioned, static filling pressures measured by CVP and PCWP cannot predict preload (fluid) responsiveness; hence, dynamic parameters other than CVP/PCWP, such as SVV and PPV, are highly predictive of preload responsiveness. SVV and PPV measure dynamic changes in CO based on increase and decrease in intrathoracic pressure during respiratory cycle. Common measures of predicting responsiveness and their calculations are given in **Box 11**

BOX 13: Parameters used to guide end points of fluid resuscitation in septic shock.

- *Clinical*
  - HR/MAP
  - Cognition
  - Urine output
  - Capillary refill time
  - Skin temperature
  - Lung auscultation for moist sounds
- *Non-invasive*
  - IVC collapsibility index by ultrasonography (USG) or echocardiography
  - PPV using pulse index continuous cardiac output (PiCCO)
  - PLR
  - SpO_2
- *Invasive*
  - CVP
  - Central venous oxygen saturation ($ScVO_2$) response
  - PCWP

BOX 14: Use of echocardiography in hemodynamic instability.

Focused echocardiography: It accurately expedites identification and/or exclusion of potential causes of hemodynamic deterioration as follows:

- *Hypovolemic shock:* (a) A small LV cavity with hyperdynamic LV function, (b) an increase in SV with PLR, and (c) a collapsed IVC
- Obstructive shock as in (a) cardiac tamponade, (b) massive pulmonary embolism (PE) with acute RV failure/dysfunction, and (c) left ventricular outflow tract (LVOT) obstruction
- Cardiogenic shock due to (a) cardiomyopathy, (b) valvular disease, (c) ischemic heart disease, (d) papillary muscle rupture, and (e) acute ventricular septal defect (VSD)
- Septic shock needs fluid resuscitation by (a) providing assessment of volume status (IVC collapsibility) and (b) in detection of sepsis-induced myocardial dysfunction

Advanced echocardiography: Advanced echocardiography gives additional information in defining the etiology of undifferentiable shock and obtains quick and noninvasive hemodynamic data, and monitors hemodynamic changes in response to therapy as follows:

- It helps in obtaining *real-time monitoring of CO* by esophageal echocardiography or Doppler during dynamic measurement to predict fluid responsiveness. Also, in evaluating changes in IVC diameter to measure IVC collapsibility index and real-time monitoring of CO during PLR
- For measurement of *diastolic dysfunction* as there is some evidence to show that significant diastolic dysfunction in sepsis is associated with increased mortality
- Echocardiographic evaluation of pulmonary artery pressure (PAP) may be useful in assessing successful weaning from MV. Increased PAP during spontaneous breathing predicts weaning failure as a result of load-related heart failure

SUGGESTED READING

1. Carsetti A, Cecconi M, Rhodes A. Fluid bolus therapy: Monitoring and predicting fluid responsiveness. Curr Opin Crit Care. 2015;21(5):388-94.
2. Monnet X, Marik P, Teboul JL. Prediction of fluid responsiveness: An update. Ann Intensive Care. 2016;6(1):111.
3. Parienti J, Mongardon N, Mégarbane B, Mira JP, Kalfon P, Gros A, et al. Intravascular complications of central venous catheterization by insertion site. N Engl J Med. 2015;373(13):1220-9.
4. Pinsky MR. Hemodynamic evaluation and monitoring in the ICU. Chest. 2007;132(6):2020-9.
5. Sunavala JD. Procedures in the Intensive Care Unit. In: Udwadia FE (Ed). Principles of Critical Care, 3rd edition. New Delhi: Jaypeee Brothers Medical Publishers (P) Ltd.; 2014.

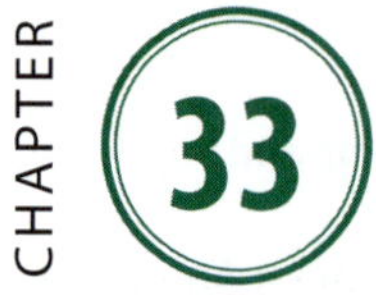

Emergency Support: Point-of-Care Ultrasound in Cardiac Arrest

Varun Deshmukh

BOX 1: Introduction.

Cardiac arrest or peri-arrest situations in emergency room (ER) need rapid and accurate management to achieve good outcomes. When we think about using point-of-care ultrasound (POCUS) in these circumstances, it is essential to have good command over basic critical care ultrasound skills and familiarity with the machine being used at your place.

We also need to make sure that performing POCUS with ongoing cardiopulmonary resuscitation (CPR) should not interfere with the quality of CPR.

The assigned roles for the team members should be clear. Also, there should be clear planning regarding where to keep the ultrasonography (USG) machine and who will perform scan.

Ideally, the machine should be as compact as possible with quick boot-up time and battery backup. We should try and minimize probe changes to optimize the use. It is imperative to save the images because this will help you to review them later and justify your decisions during management.

Also, we must continue to monitor clinical signs as per standard advanced cardiovascular life support (ACLS) guidelines.

BOX 2: POCUS in cardiac arrest management.

There are potentially five situations where POCUS can help in management

- **To confirm cardiac arrest:** Use phased array probe in subcostal view. A cardiac standstill can confirm arrest. You can also see pseudo-pulseless electrical activity (PEA) (cardiac activity with no palpable pulse). You can rule out cardiac tamponade (swinging heart, more details later) and pleural effusion in this view
- **Assess effective chest compressions:** Use phased array probe in subcostal view while CPR is going on. We can evaluate the effectiveness of chest compressions by real-time observation of compression/relaxation of the cardiac chambers during cardiac massage. We can adjust position of hands to perform more effective CPR
- **Aid interventions:** Linear probe can be used for intravenous (IV) access, intra-aortic balloon pump (IABP) insertion, draining pleural effusions/hemothoraces, and confirming position of endotracheal (ET) tube (rule out endobronchial and esophageal intubation). Phased array probe can be used to aid needle insertion for pericardiocentesis
- **Diagnose and treat reversible causes:** Looking at the 5Hs and 5Ts of reversible causes for cardiac arrest, we can diagnose pneumothorax, pulmonary embolism (PE), cardiac tamponade, hypovolemia, and myocardial infarction (MI) with help of POCUS
- **Immediate postreturn of spontaneous circulation (ROSC) care:** Immediately post-ROSC, we can use POCUS to: (a) Secure IV access and arterial lines, (b) rule out any complication of CPR like pneumothorax, pleural, or pericardial effusion, (c) hemodynamic monitoring [velocity–time integral (VTI) and complication of MI], (d) intubation and tracheostomy, and (e) neurological complications—optic nerve sheath diameter and transcranial Doppler

BOX 3: Diagnosis of reversible causes during CPR.

- **Tension pneumothorax:** While CPR is on hold for 10 seconds and breaths are being given, we can assess the lung sliding on both sides in 3rd intercostal spaces. Absent lung sliding with A profile and Barcode sign on M mode is highly suggestive of pneumothorax. We must clinically corelate to confirm reduced air entry and tympanic note on that side to aid to the diagnosis. We should understand that based on just the clinical signs which are vague, we cannot confirm our diagnosis. So, performing POCUS followed by clinical confirmation makes sense before we drain the pneumothorax
- **Pulmonary embolism (PE):** If we can demonstrate pleural sliding and A profile, the next step would be to scan both groins for presence of any thrombi in the femoral veins. PE is very likely in presence of thrombi with A-profile lungs and these patients should be considered for thrombolysis while ongoing CPR
- **Cardiac tamponade:** Use phased array probe in subcostal view when the CPR is on hold. If we can see large pericardial effusion with cardiac standstill, the cause of cardiac arrest is likely to be tamponade. If the heart is beating and swinging with systolic collapse of free wall of right atrium or diastolic collapse of free wall of left ventricle (LV), it is diagnostic of tamponade. These patients should be considered for pericardiocentesis with help of USG visualization. In these circumstances, 200–500 mL fluid drainage is also sufficient to reverse cardiac arrest and improve hemodynamics
- **Hypovolemia:** When we see A profile in lungs and rule out deep vein thrombosis (DVT)/PE, we should scan the abdomen for ascites/free fluid and both costophrenic angles for large effusions/hemothorax. If hypovolemia is the cause of arrest, we will also see small sized inferior vena cava (IVC) (<2 cm and small sized left ventricular cavity). If the patient is peri-arrest, we can see small ventricles with kissing LV walls and more than 50% collapsing IVC. In these patients pumping more fluids will be helpful
- **Myocardial infarction (MI):** We will see B profile on lungs with dilated IVC (>2 cm). We can also see LV free-wall rupture. If it is peri-arrest situation, we can see regional wall motion abnormality in blocked coronary artery territory. Once you have clear idea about all parameters, we can assess using POCUS during CPR and peri-arrest situations, you need to follow a systematic/protocolized assessment system to perform POCUS. There are various protocols published in last few years. One of the most prominent protocols is SESAME protocol **(Box 4)**, which you can read through to get more information

BOX 4: SESAME protocol.

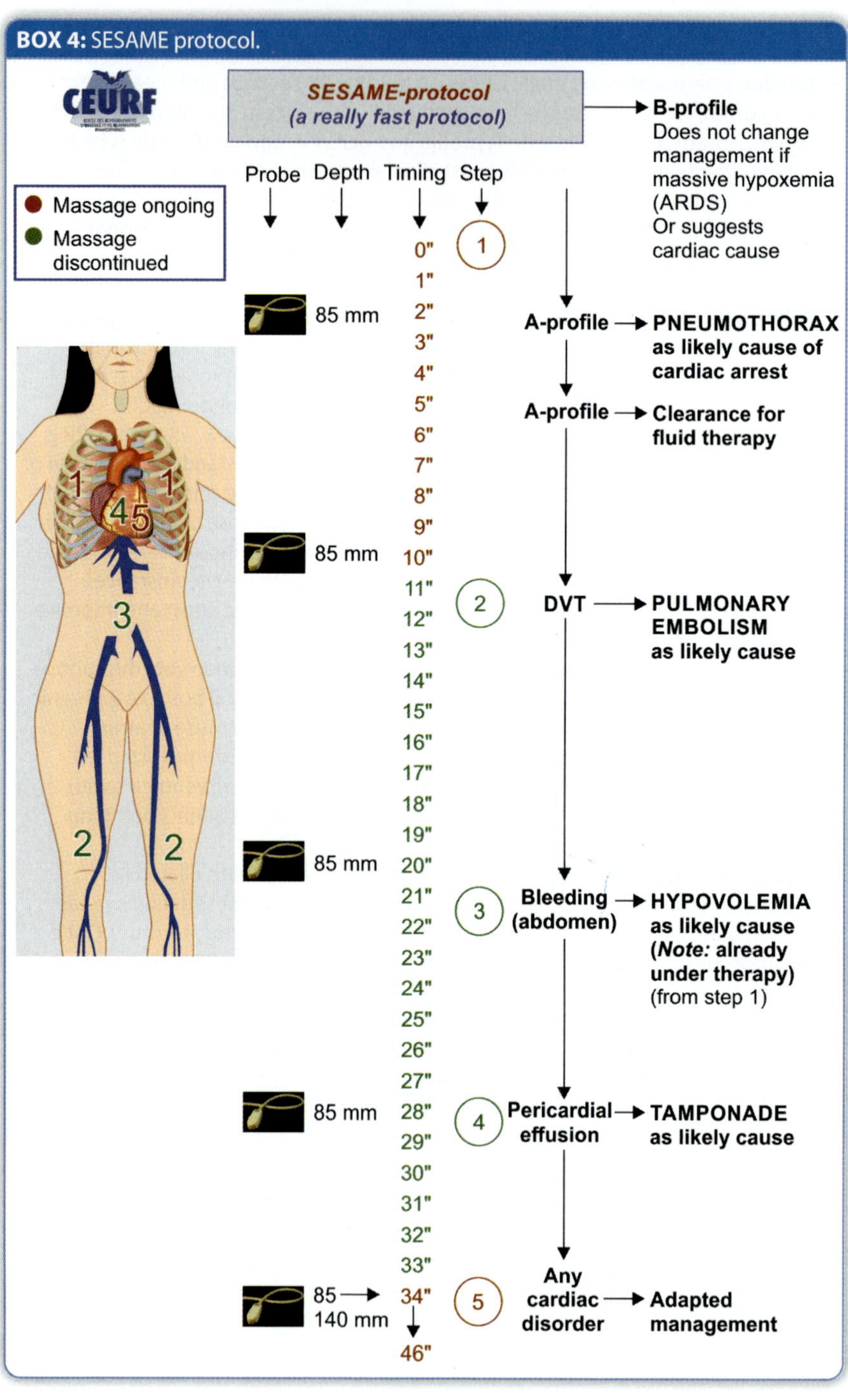

SUGGESTED READING

1. Lichtenstein D, Malbrain ML. Critical care ultrasound in cardiac arrest. Technological requirements for performing the SESAME-protocol—a holistic approach. Anaesthesiol Intensive Ther. 2015;47(5):471-81.
2. Wong A, Vignon P, Robba C. How I use ultrasound in cardiac arrest. Intensive Care Med. 2023;49(12):1531-4.
3. Zafiropoulos A, Asrress K, Redwood S, Gillon S, Walker D. Critical care echo rounds: Echo in cardiac arrest. Echo Res Pract. 2014;1(2):D15-21.

CHAPTER 34

Cardiac/Circulatory Support

34.1 EXTRACORPOREAL MEMBRANE OXYGENATION

Upendra D Bhalerao

BOX 1: Introduction.

Extracorporeal membrane oxygenation (ECMO) is an extracorporeal life support system in which a pump draws venous blood from the patient to an oxygenator where oxygen is replenished, and carbon dioxide is extracted. Oxygenated blood is then pumped back into the arterial system with the help of the centrifugal pump in patient's circulation. ECMO provides temporal organ support as life-saving procedure. ECMO may support the body for a long period of time (days to weeks) to allow heart and/or lungs time to rest and recover. ECMO is supportive therapy and not a disease-modifying treatment. The challenge remains to provide timely initiation of this technology in the appropriate critically ill patients.

BOX 2: Indications.

- *Cardiac:* ECMO provides time interval for recovery of the heart function or can act as intervening bridge to another treatment (heart transplant and ventricular assist device)
- *Respiratory:* The aim of ECMO therapy is to provide rest to the damaged lungs and allow them to recover while performing the function of gas exchange

Venovenous (V-V) ECMO is modality of ECMO therapy chosen in isolated respiratory dysfunction [acute respiratory distress syndrome (ARDS)] and venoarterial (V-A) ECMO is preferred in cardiac and combined cardiorespiratory dysfunction.

Extracorporeal cardiopulmonary resuscitation (ECPR) is defined as V-A ECMO cannulation during refractory cardiac arrest. Refractory cardiac arrest is considered as the absence of return of spontaneous circulation (ROSC) despite provision of appropriate cardiopulmonary resuscitation (CPR) for 15–30 minutes. Moreover, ECPR includes patients with on/off CPR and those without stable ROSC.

TABLE 1: Respiratory and cardiac conditions for ECMO.

Respiratory conditions for V-V ECMO	***Cardiac conditions for V-A ECMO***
Severe pneumonia	*Severe cardiogenic shock:* Myocardial infarction and consequent complications, not responding to conventional treatment such as inotropes, intra-aortic balloon pump (IABP), etc.
ARDS	*Postcardiac surgery:* Unable to wean safely from cardiopulmonary bypass using conventional supports
Supportive therapy prior to lung transplant	Pulmonary embolism
Pulmonary contusion	Myocarditis
Smoke inhalation	Primary graft dysfunction following heart transplant
Acute lung (graft) failure following transplant	• Acute anaphylaxis • Bridge to transplant • ECPR • Sepsis with profound cardiac depression

BOX 3: Contraindication to ECMO.

- Age >75 years, indicating significant frailty
- Nonrecoverable cardiac, respiratory, and neurological disease
- Preexisting cancers/conditions limiting the survival
- Advanced liver disease
- Unwitnessed cardiac arrest or CPR >60 minutes

BOX 4: Cannulation strategy for ECMO.

VV ECMO	***VA ECMO***
Peripheral cannulation: Drainage cannula is put in the femoral vein and positioned in the inferior vena cava (IVC) and returning cannula is put in the jugular vein	*Peripheral cannulation:* • Drainage cannula is put in the femoral vein and positioned in the IVC • Returning cannula is put in the femoral artery • Need distal perfusion cannula to supply the distal limb
• It needs intravenous (IV) heparin before cannulation • Percutaneous technique to put cannula is preferred • Transesophageal echocardiography (echo) guidance helps with the suitable placement of cannula in IVC	• Needs IV heparin before cannulation • Open/semiopen cannulation practiced to prevent arterial trauma • Transesophageal echo guidance helps for suitable placement of cannula in IVC

Contd...

Contd...

VV ECMO	*VA ECMO*
• Supports lung function • Blood is drained and put back in venous system • Low pressure in the venous system helps ECMO circuit to last longer • Lesser hemodynamic fluctuations • Target blood partial pressure of oxygen (pO_2) 60–90 mm Hg • Adjust the ECMO flow depending on the pO_2 levels • Changes in the sweep gas flow are done as per the blood partial pressure of carbon dioxide (pCO_2)	• Provides rest to the heart and lungs • Blood is drained from venous side and then put back in the arterial system • Improves function of both the ventricles • Helps to maintain the organ perfusion till suitable heart is available for transplantation in end-stage cardiac failure • ECMO flow equivalent to cardiac output • Changing flow rates affect cardiac output
Flow rate: 2/3 of parts cardiac output are enough to achieve adequate oxygenation	*Flow rate:* Flow rate equals to the cardiac output
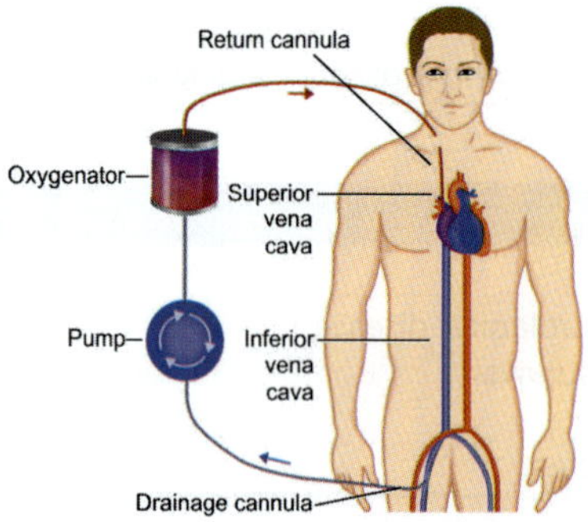 Return cannula; Oxygenator; Superior vena cava; Pump; Inferior vena cava; Drainage cannula	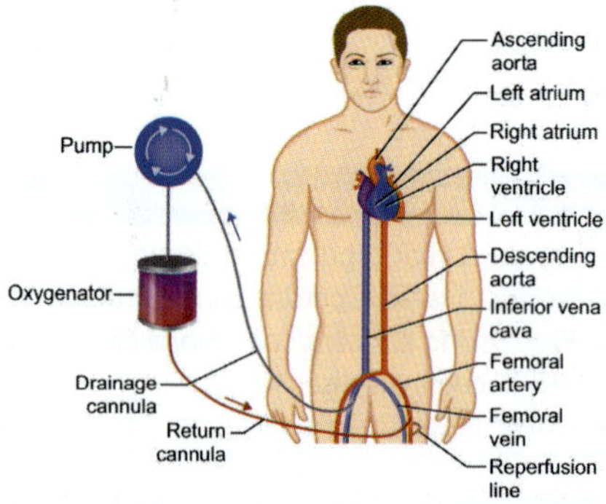 Ascending aorta; Left atrium; Right atrium; Right ventricle; Left ventricle; Pump; Descending aorta; Oxygenator; Inferior vena cava; Femoral artery; Drainage cannula; Return cannula; Femoral vein; Reperfusion line

BOX 5: Murray score.

Murray score stratifies severity of acute lung injury and is also used for ECMO patient selection

Parameter/score	*0*	*1*	*2*	*3*	*4*
Partial pressure of oxygen (PaO_2)/fraction of inspired oxygen (FiO_2) (mm Hg)	≥300	225–299	175–224	100–174	<100
Chest X-ray (quadrants infiltrated)	Normal	1	2	3	4
Positive end-expiratory pressure (PEEP) (cmH_2O)	≤5	6–8	9–11	12–14	≥15
Compliance (mL/cmH_2O)	≥80	60–79	40–59	20–39	≤19

Contd...

Contd...

Score >2.5 indicates severe lung injury and these patients are candidates for VV ECMO and therapy in the setting of ARDS/acute lung injury

Hemodynamic effects of ECMO

	ECMO
Cardiac flow	3–7 L/min
After load	↑↑↑
MAP	↑↑
LVSV	↓
Cardiac flow	↑↑
Cardiac power	↑↑
LVEDP	—
PCWP	—
LV preload	↓
Coronary perfusion	—
Myocardium O_2 consumption	—
Peripheral tissue perfusion	↑↑↑

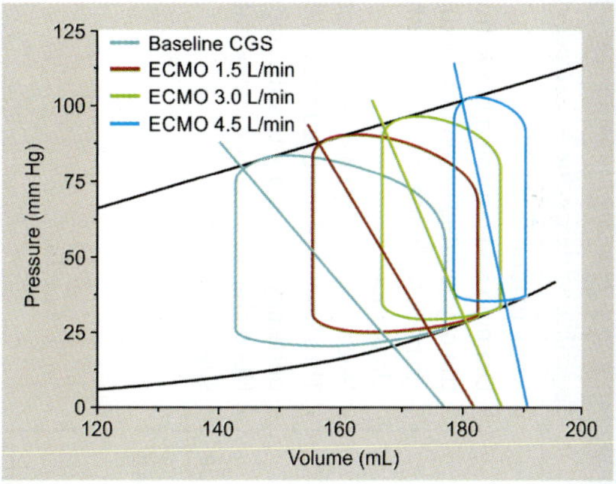

(LVSV: left ventricular stroke volume; LVEDP: left ventricular end-diastolic pressure; PCWP: pulmonary capillary wedge pressure, LV: left ventricle)

BOX 6: ECMO monitoring.

The outcome of ECMO therapy in a given patient depends on careful monitoring of patient and circuit

Parameter	***Determinant***
Hemodynamic variables	Heart rate and rhythm, respiratory rate, and temperature Pulsations in the limbs distal to cannula site, consciousness, and renal function
Blood gas	Arterial and venous saturation (paO_2, pCO_2, and mixed venous saturation)
Echocardiography	Assess cannula positions, right atrium (RA) and right ventricle (RV) decompression, tricuspid annular plane systolic excursion (TAPSE), status of LV and cardiac recovery
Coagulation parameters	• Systemic heparinization should be monitored by activated clotting time (ACT) every 4–6 hourly • VV ECMO ACT should be in range of 160–180 seconds • VA ECMO ACT should be in range of 200–240 seconds • Daily APTT monitored with target of 60–70 seconds

BOX 7: Complications of ECMO therapy.

During cannulation	***Patient-related***	***Specific problems due to extracorporeal life support (ECLS)***
• Bleeding during the cannula insertion or during ECMO flow (1–4%) • Injury to the vessel requiring surgical suturing	• Hemorrhage, gastrointestinal (GI) bleed, and intracerebral bleeds • Hematologic, thrombocytopenia, fibrinolysis, and disseminated intravascular coagulation (DIC) • Neurological embolic stroke, intracranial (IC) bleed, and hypoxic brain damage • Acute renal failure • Infection, bloodstream infections due to catheters and lines • Ventilator-associated pneumonia and Gram-negative sepsis • ECMO dependency, failure to wean off ECMO, needing heart transplant/durable ventricular assist device (VAD)	• Recirculation in VV ECMO • Draining and returning blood from two different veins and the oxygenated blood from returning cannula can directly go back to draining cannula without going into systemic circulation • Need to keep optimal cannula position to prevent this • Thrombosis of the circuit and failure of oxygenator, generally secondary to suboptimal anticoagulation • Need change of circuit/oxygenator to keep the ECMO support viable
• LV distension and hemorrhagic pulmonary edema – Reversal of blood flow toward the LV results in increase in left ventricular afterload, causing ventricle to dilate resulting in congestion and pulmonary edema	• Ischemia of the limb distal to the site of arterial cannula – *Lower extremity ischemia:* 16.9% – *Fasciotomy or compartment syndrome:* 10.3% – *Lower extremity amputation:* 4.2–8.3%	• *Differential hypoxemia upper body hypoxemia, Harlequin syndrome:* This occurs in femoral arterial cannulation with improved heart function but poor lung function • Poorly oxygenated blood from patient's native circulation gets mixed with blood supplied from femoral cannula in the aortic arch. This causes poor saturation/hypoxia in upper limbs and brain • This can be solved by placing additional venous return catheter in the internal jugular vein (IJV) to allow oxygenated blood from arterial pump to flow through it [veno-arteriovenous (VAV) ECMO]

BOX 8: Weaning from ECMO.

- **In the case of VV ECMO**, assessment of native respiratory function is performed by altering the gas flow through the ECMO circuit 5–65%. Usually, recovery of lungs takes around 1–3 weeks
- Signs of recovery can be a progressive increase in arterial oxygen saturation (SaO_2) greater than venous oxygen saturation (SvO_2); improvement in SaO_2 for a given circuit flow or requirement of a reduced circuit flow to achieve the target SaO_2; and improvement in chest X-ray or improving lung compliance
- Weaning is considered when the gas exchange can be maintained with low FiO_2 (<30%); <2 L/min fresh gas flow rates into the circuit at the respiratory rate of <25 breaths/minute; and <15 cmH_2O of PEEP
- **In the case of VA ECMO**, once the etiology of cardiogenic shock is addressed and native cardiac function is returned, weaning of ECMO can be planned
- Cardiac assessment is performed by reducing flows in the ECMO circuit
- To assess cardiac function and response to reduced flow rates, a transesophageal echocardiogram (TEE) is used
- Inotropic weaning is usually started several hours before the weaning
- Reduction in circuit flow should be 1–2 L/min. Weaning of VA ECMO is achieved with a gradual reduction in blood flow until the flow of 0.5–1.0 L/min is met. Close hemodynamic and serial echocardiographic monitoring is required. After 1–2 hours of minimal support or without any support, if the patient is stable, they can be decannulated in a surgical setting

BOX 9: Survival.

Benefits of ECMO are dependent on the underlying pathology and organ recovery. As per 2023 Extracorporeal Life Support Organization (ELSO) database, survival-to-discharge rate for VA ECMO used for cardiac indications is 48%. The survival-to-discharge rate when ECMO is used for pulmonary indication is 58%. The survival-to-discharge rate of ECPR is 30–35% in largest series

SUGGESTED READING

1. Delnoij TS, Driessen R, Sharma AS, Bouman EA, Strauch U, Roekaerts PM. Venovenous extracorporeal membrane oxygenation in intractable pulmonary insufficiency: Practical issues and future directions. Biomed Res Int. 2016;2016:9367464.
2. Extracorporeal Life Support Organization (ELSO). (2024). ECLS Registry Report and International Summary of Statistics. [online]. Available from https://www.elso.org/registry/internationalsummaryandreports.aspx [Last accessed September, 2024].
3. Lo Coco V, Lorusso R, Raffa GM, Malvindi PG, Pilato M, Martucci G, et al. Clinical complications during veno-arterial extracorporeal membrane oxygenation in post-cardiotomy and non post-cardiotomy shock: Still the achilles heel. J Thorac Dis. 2018;10(12):6993-7004.
4. Marasco SF, Lukas G, McDonald M, McMillan J, Ihle B. Review of ECMO (extra corporeal membrane oxygenation) support in critically ill adult patients. Heart Lung Circ. 2008;17(Suppl 4):S41-7.
5. Ortuno S, Delmas C, Diehl JL, Bailleul C, Lancelot A, Naili M, et al. Weaning from veno-arterial extra-corporeal membrane oxygenation: Which strategy to use? Ann Cardiothorac Surg. 2019;8(1):E1-8.
6. Wrisinger WC, Thompson SL. Basics of extracorporeal membrane oxygenation. Surg Clin North Am. 2022;102(1):23-35.

34.2 INOTROPES

Jamshed D Sunavala

BOX 1: Inotropes used in intensive care unit.

Agent	***Standard infusion***
Noradrenaline	4 or 8 mg/50 mL (mL/hour μg/min or μg/kg/min) *Dose:* 0.01–1 μg/kg/min
Adrenaline	3 or 4 mg/50 mL (mL/hour μg/min or μg/kg/min) *Dose:* 0.01–0.5 μg/kg/min
Dobutamine	500 mg/50 mL (mL/hour μg/kg/min) *Dose:* 2–10 μg/kg/min
Dopamine	200 or 400 mg/50 mL (mL/hour μg/kg/min) *Dose:* 2–20 μg/kg/min
Isoprenaline	4 mg/50 mL (mL/hour μg/min) *Dose:* 0.01–1 μg/kg/min
Levosimendan	12.5 mg/250 mL 5% dextrose *Loading dose:* 6–12 μg/kg over 10 minutes followed by infusion *Infusion:* 0.05–0.2 pg/kg/min for 24 hours only *NB:* Loading dose may cause marked hypotension, therefore may be omitted or reduced
Milrinone	10 mg/50 mL *Loading dose:* 50 pg/kg/20 minutes *Infusion:* 0.375–0.75 pg/kg/min
Vasopressin	40 units/40 mL (mL/hour = units/minute) *Dose:* 0.01–0.04 units/minute
Phenylephrine	10 mg/50 mL (mL/hour = pg/min or pg/kg/min) *Dose:* 10–100 pg/min 0.1–1 pg/kg/min

Notes:
- All inotropes are to be administered in a syringe pump via a central venous catheter.
- All dilutions are up to 50 mL. The amount of diluent will vary depending on the amount of drug. For example, 3 mg adrenaline = 3 mL of drug.
- Add 47 mL of 5% dextrose to make a total of 50 mL.
- All dilutions are preferred to be in 5% dextrose (isotonic), but 0.9% normal saline may also be used.
- May vary as per individualized institutional protocols.

SUGGESTED READING

1. Sunavala J. Essentials of Critical Care Medicine for the Physician, 1st edition. New Delhi: Jaypee Brothers Medical Publishers (P) Ltd; 2022.

34.3 TRANSVENOUS PACING

Jamshed D Sunavala

BOX 1: Indications.

- *Therapeutic:*
  - Life-threatening bradyarrhythmias
    - Sick sinus syndrome
    - Second-/third-degree heart block
    - High-degree atrioventricular (AV) block
    - Slow junctional
    - Idioventricular
  - Symptomatic bradycardia
    - Symptomatic conduction defects in patients presenting with recurrent STOKES ADAMS attacks
    - Syncope
    - Near syncope due to blocks
  - In selected patients with tachyarrhythmias, where overdrive temporary pacing is used to terminate or prevent tachycardia [temporary measure to buy time for stabilization with medical therapy]
- *Prophylactic in acute myocardial infarction with:*
  - Inferior myocardial infarction with Wenckebach phenomenon or second-degree heart block progressing to complete heart block
  - Anterior wall infarction with recent bifascicular blocks (especially right bundle block associated with a block in left posterior inferior division or new bundle branch block with transient complete heart block)

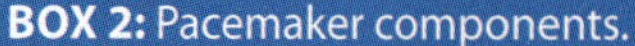

BOX 2: Pacemaker components.

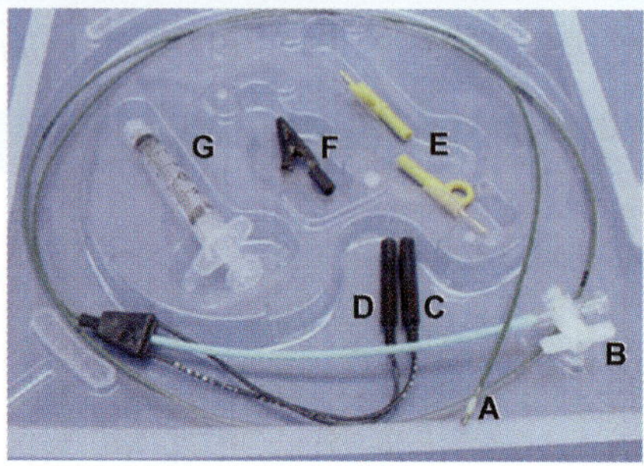

Transvenous pacemaker catheter; (A) Catheter tip with balloon; (B) Balloon inflation port; (C) Negative electrode; (D) Positive electrode; (E) Adapters to attach electrodes to external pacing generator; (F) Alligator clip to attach negative electrode to ECG V lead; (G) Syringe for balloon inflation.

A

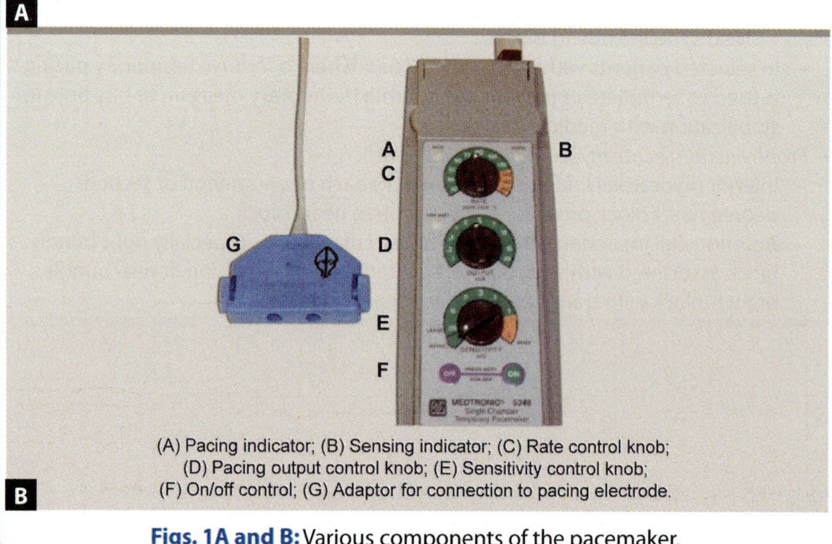

(A) Pacing indicator; (B) Sensing indicator; (C) Rate control knob; (D) Pacing output control knob; (E) Sensitivity control knob; (F) On/off control; (G) Adaptor for connection to pacing electrode.

B

Figs. 1A and B: Various components of the pacemaker.

BOX 3: Procedure.

- External pulse generator is used, which is ventricular inhibited (demand) units permitting the rate between 50 and 150 beats/min, with a sensing facility that allows use in full demand or in asynchronous mode.
- Both unipolar/bipolar of 5–7 French are available, but commonly used is bipolar lead.

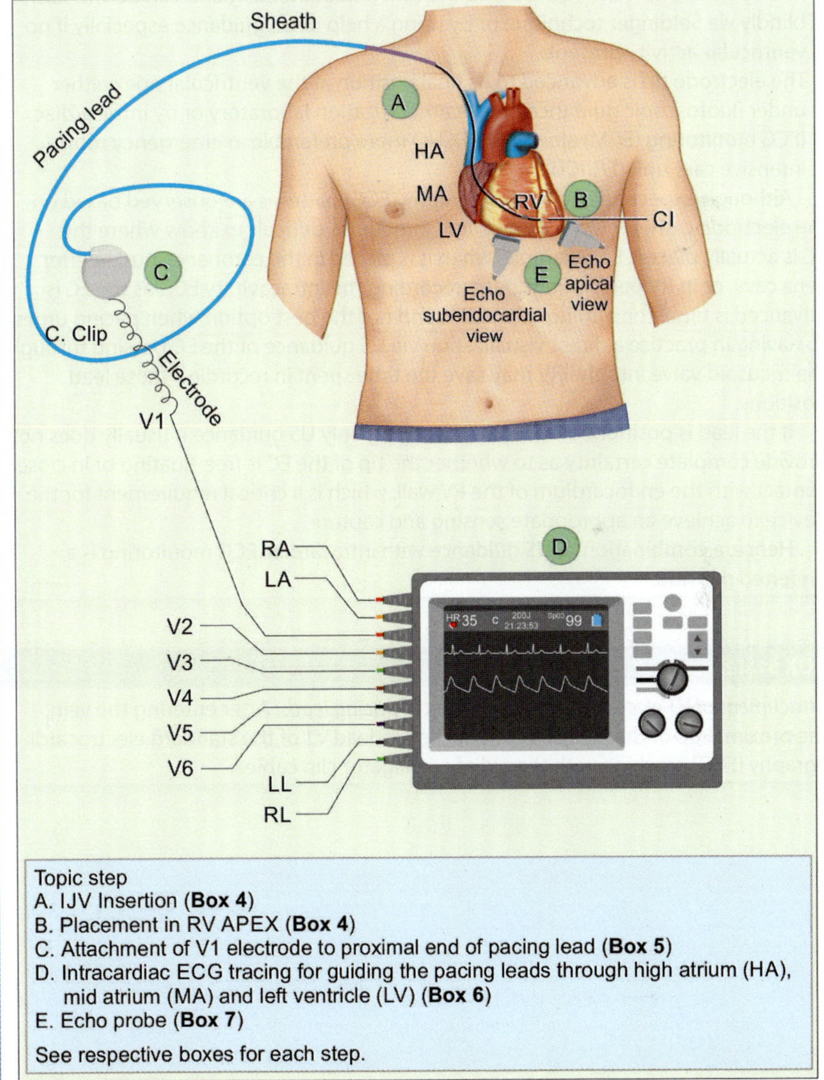

Topic step
A. IJV Insertion (**Box 4**)
B. Placement in RV APEX (**Box 4**)
C. Attachment of V1 electrode to proximal end of pacing lead (**Box 5**)
D. Intracardiac ECG tracing for guiding the pacing leads through high atrium (HA), mid atrium (MA) and left ventricle (LV) (**Box 6**)
E. Echo probe (**Box 7**)

See respective boxes for each step.

Fig. 2: Bedside intracardial pacing characteristics of intracardiac electrocardiograms. (CI: current of injury)

BOX 4: Steps A and B.

Commonly used veins are subclavian, internal jugular, and femoral, choice depends on accessibility and doctor's expertise.

Insertion and placement in right ventricular (RV) apex:

- Ultrasound (US) guidance for insertion of sheath into selected vein (mostly internal jugular vein) or alternatively, the subclavian/femoral vein
- Pacing electrode is introduced into the vein percutaneously and can do the same blindly via Seldinger technique or by using a help of US guidance especially if no ventricular activity present.
- The electrode tip is advanced to its final position at the ventricular apex either under fluoroscopic guidance in the catheterization laboratory or by intracardiac (ECG monitoring (ECM) along with ECHO more preferable in emergency room/ intensive care unit (ER/ICU) setting).

Although expected electrocardiography (ECG) patterns are observed based on the electrode catheter (EC) position, it is sometimes difficult to know where the EC is actually placed. For example, when it is placed in the coronary sinus, inferior vena cava, or in RV perforations. Also, recording the intracavitary ECG as the EC is advanced is time-consuming in practice and not the best option when pacing urges, so having in practice a direct visualization via US guidance of the EC passing through the tricuspid valve into the RV may save the time spent in recording these lead positions.

If the lead is positioned into the RV by using only US guidance it usually does not provide complete certainty as to whether the tip of the EC is free-floating or in close contact with the endocardium of the RV wall, which is a critical requirement for the device to achieve an appropriate sensing and capture.

Hence, a combination of US guidance with intracardiac ECG monitoring is a preferred method.

BOX 5: Step C.

Attachment of V1 electrode to proximal end of pacing leads: After entering the vein, the proximal tip of the electrode is attached to lead V1 of the standard electrocardiography (ECG) machine with the aid of an alligator clip cable.

BOX 6: Step D

Intracardiac ECG tracing for guiding the pacing lead through high atrium (HA), mid atrium (MA), and RV ***(as shown in Fig. 3)****:*

- Lead V1 shows a prominent *p* wave as the pacing electrode advances toward the heart, being inverted in the HA and biphasic in the MA.
- As electrode tip crosses the tricuspid valve and enters the right ventricular cavity, the intracardiac ECG changes markedly.
- A rS ventricular pattern with very deep S and T waves appears, this may necessitate decreasing the standardization by half.
- When the catheter tip abuts on the endocardial surface of the right ventricular wall an elevated ST segment is observed due to current of injury (CI).
- Ventricular ectopic beats are commonly observed when the catheter tip traverses the tricuspid orifice rarely ventricular fibrillation might occur necessitating withdrawal of the pacing catheter tip and prompt defib if necessary.
- The whole procedure of lead placing is made easy with the availability of the ballon tip floating electrodes.

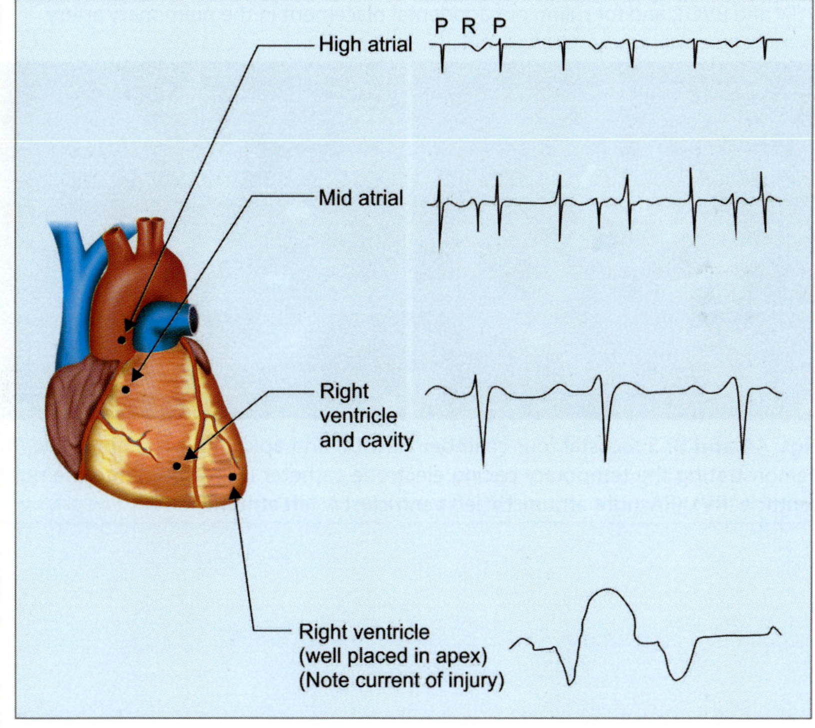

Fig. 3: Bedside intracardial pacing characteristics of intracardiac electrocardiograms.

BOX 7: Step E

ECHO probe placement:

- Key echocardiographic views for monitoring the electrode catheter include the subcostal four-chamber and the apical four-chamber views. These views are crucial for tracking the catheter as it moves through the right atrium (RA) and progresses through the tricuspid valve (TV) to its final position in the right ventricle (RV) apex. Alternative, albeit less stable, catheter positions may include the interventricular septum, RV free wall, or RV outflow tract (RVOT)
- Once the sheath is in place, a 5–7-F bipolar electrode catheter (preferably balloon-tipped) is advanced by one operator, while a second operator performs an echocardiogram. The electrode catheter appears as a bright, linear hyperechoic structure on the ultrasound
- If the catheter does not seem to advance into the RV, checking the inferior vena cava (IVC) view is recommended. Due to the anatomical continuity between the superior vena cava and IVC, the catheter may inadvertently enter the IVC, which is a common incorrect placement. Short-axis views (subcostal or parasternal) at the level of the great vessels are useful for detecting the catheter passing through the TV and RVOT, and for ruling out accidental placement in the pulmonary artery

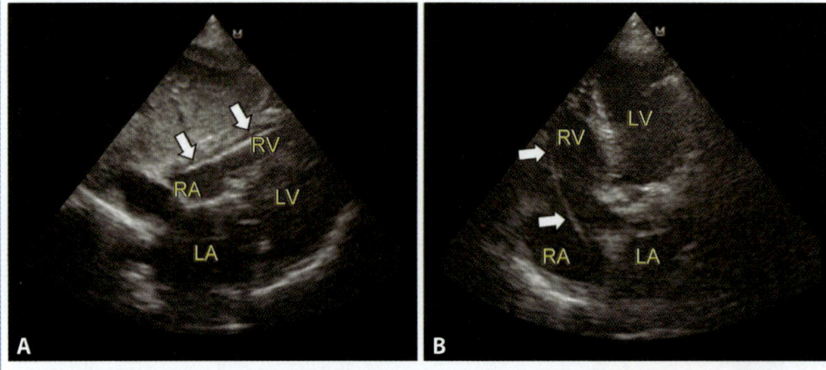

Figs. 4A and B: Subcostal four-chamber view (A) and apical four-chamber view (B) demonstrating the temporary pacing electrode catheter (EC, arrows) into the right ventricle (RV). (RA: right atrium; LV: left ventricle; LA: left atrium)

BOX 8: Step C (Contd...)

- Once electrodes correctly positioned at the apex of the right ventricle, the lead is connected to the battery operated pacemaker box
- It is now necessary to test the electric threshold of stimulation and if the pacemaker is set for demand mode the ability of the electrode tip to sense the R waves
- The electrical threshold is tested by slowly reducing the amperage of the pacemaker till the past QRS complexes disappear and only the pacemaker spikes and the patient's own spontaneous beats are present. Amperage is now slowly increased till pacing is reestablished this being the electrical threshold. If pacing does not occur at an electrical threshold of <2 mA it may be best to reposition the electrode
- Most temporary pacemakers have a low pacing threshold of 1 mA or less and should be capable of sensing spontaneous ventricular activities of 5 mV signals or larger. The pacemaker rate depends on the clinical needs of the patient and is generally kept between 70 and 80 beats/min
- To test the sensing function in the demand mode, the sensing dial is turned clockwise (in most pulse generates) to full demand mode and then gradually turn toward the asynchronous mode till sensing is just lost. In this way we can measure R wave amplitude to ensure adequate sensing of cardiac activity
- Unfortunately, most temporary pulse generators do not write the exact values over the dial but the full demand mode would usually indicate 1 mV and the opposite asynchronous mode about 20 mV Ideally the R wave < 6 mV should be sensed if this is not occur indicating that the sensing threshold for the R wave exceeds 6 mV then the lead should be repositioned

Caveat: Next is to check the surface ECG, which should show pacemaker spikes paired with broad QRS complexes consistent with left bundle branch block (LBBB) morphology. Sensing should be optimal at low thresholds, although a "benign" right bundle branch block (RBBB) pattern, though rare, can also be seen in some patients. If RBBB is observed, especially in left-sided catheter placements or coronary sinus insertions, ultrasound confirmation of the EC in the RV provides reassurance.

BOX 9: Rule out complication.

Immediate	• Screen for postprocedure complications using ultrasound • Issues such as septal perforations (interatrial and interventricular) • Right ventricular (RV) free wall perforation • Pericardial effusion, and possible cardiac tamponade can be detected • Misplacement of the catheter into the pulmonary artery or inferior vena cava (IVC) can also be identified by transthoracic echocardiography (TTE), allowing for repositioning • Additionally, a catheter mistakenly placed in the coronary sinus (CS) can occur, particularly if the CS is dilated or if a left-sided insertion (left internal jugular or subclavian vein) is used and a persistent left superior vena cava is present • Lung ultrasound should also be performed to rule out pneumothorax
Delayed	• Infection at a local site • Phlebitis • Thrombosis of peripheral veins • Systemic infection lead perforation through the ventricular wall diaphragmatic pacing and pacemaker-induced arrhythmias

SUGGESTED READING

1. Barold SS, Camm AJ. Recognition of pacemaker-associated ECG patterns. Heart Rhythm. 2018;15(2):232-8. (This review article focuses on ECG patterns associated with pacemakers and their recognition).
2. Elliott P, Nair M. Managing complications in temporary pacing. J Cardiovasc Electrophysiol. 2023;34(8):1235-44.
3. Fleming H, Ray R. Modern pacemakers: Components and functionality. J Cardiac Electrophysiol. 2021;32(4):1136-44. (This article explains the components and operational details of modern pacemakers).
4. Kotecha D, Pillai A. Temporary cardiac pacing: Indications, techniques, and complications. Euro Heart J. 2020;41(29):2744-56.
5. Liu L, Zha Y. Echocardiographic guidance in temporary pacemaker lead placement. J Am Soc Echocardiogr. 2022;35(6):621-30. (This article covers the use of echocardiographic guidance in the placement of temporary pacemaker leads).
6. Miller J, Wells C. Techniques in temporary pacing: A guide for the cardiologist. Heart Rhythm J. 2019;16(3):469-78. (This guide provides step-by-step techniques for temporary pacing, including lead insertion and positioning).
7. Tisdale JE, Reynolds T. (2020). Electrocardiographic monitoring for pacemaker placement. Am J Cardiol. 2020;125(12):1887-94. (This paper discusses the use of ECG for monitoring pacemaker lead placement and verification).
8. Udwadia FE. Principles of Critical Care, third edition. New Delhi: Jaypee Brothers Medical Publishers (Pvt Ltd.); 2014.

34.4 PERICARDIOCENTESIS

Rahul Chhabria, Kunal Dinesh Kale

BOX 1: Approaches.

- Fluoroscopy-guided fashion
- Computed tomography-guided fashion
- Echocardiography-guided technique

BOX 2: Equipment required to perform echocardiography-guided pericardiocentesis **(Fig. 1)**.

Echocardiography machine with probe, sterile probe cover, 16–18 gauge teflon sheathed needle, 6–8 Fr dilator and introducer sheath, j tipped guidewire, pigtail angiocatheter, and 18-gauge needle.

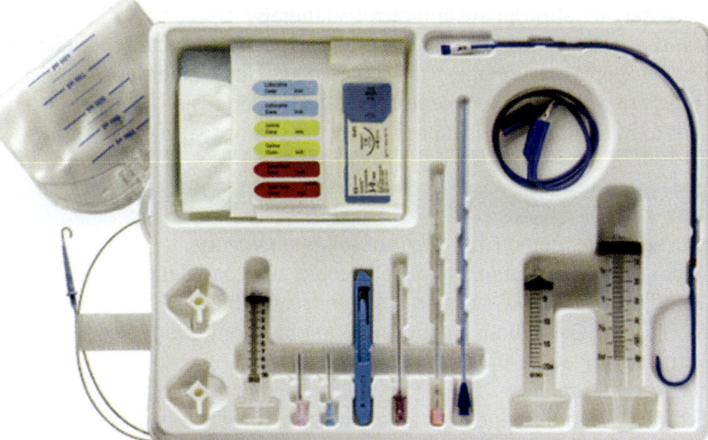

Fig. 1: Pericardiocentesis kit.

Pericardiocentesis kit contents. 1. Access needle; 2. Chiba access needle 18G; 3. Dilator 6 Fr; 4. 6 F Straight catheter; 5. J tipped guidewire; 6. Pigtail angiocatheter; 7. Medication needle; 8. Syringe with Luer Lock; 9. Disposal bag with drainage spout; 10. Suture material; 11. Double end clip cable.

BOX 3: Indications for emergency pericardiocentesis.

Emergency pericardiocentesis is indicated when there is a need to rapidly remove fluid from the pericardial sac to relieve cardiac tamponade, which is a life-threatening condition. The primary indications include:

- Cardiac tamponade
- *Diagnostic indications:*
  - Unexplained pericardial effusion: To determine the etiology of the effusion, such as infection, malignancy, or autoimmune conditions
  - Traumatic hemopericardium: Following chest trauma, where blood accumulates in the pericardial sac
- *Therapeutic indications:*
  - Acute hemodynamic compromise: When immediate relief of pressure on the heart is necessary to restore hemodynamic stability
  - Recurrent pericardial effusion: In cases, where there is a recurrent buildup of fluid causing symptoms
  - Infectious Pericarditis: When an infectious cause is suspected, fluid analysis is necessary for appropriate antimicrobial therapy

Contraindications: Relative contraindications include uncorrected coagulopathy or thrombocytopenia, though these may be managed in an emergency

In emergency settings, the procedure should be performed by experienced clinicians to minimize complications and ensure prompt relief of symptoms

BOX 4: Procedure.

- *Preprocedure preparation (can skip in absolute emergency):*
  - Laboratory tests ensure that platelet count and coagulation profile are checked
  - Blood products have packed red cell units available
  - Monitoring: Continuous electrocardiographic monitoring is required along with appropriate resuscitation equipment
- *Central venous catheter:*
  - Essential for monitoring right atrial pressure
  - Allows rapid infusion of fluids and medications if necessary
- Continuous arterial pressure monitoring is recommended to detect pulsus paradoxus and quickly address hemodynamic instability
- *Echocardiographic evaluation:*
  - Perform an initial echocardiographic evaluation with multiple views to assess the size and distribution of the effusion
  - Helps in selecting the optimal entry point and monitoring the procedure
- *Patient positioning:* Position the patient in a semireclining position at a 30° angle with slight left rotation to facilitate fluid collection in the inferior-anterior part of chest
- *Operative field preparation:*
  - Thoroughly disinfect the operative field
  - Administer a local anesthetic at the puncture site
- *Needle insertion:*
  - Define the needle path by the angle between the probe and the chest wall
  - Visualize the optimal needle path
  - Use a 16–18G Teflon-coated needle with an attached saline-filled syringe
  - Advance the needle toward the fluid-filled space, aspirate fluid, then advance the needle approximately 2 mm further

Contd...

Contd...

- *Sheath and guidewire insertion:*
  - Advance the sheath over the needle and withdraw the steel core, leaving the sheath in the pericardial space
  - Insert a guidewire through the sheath, the guidewire can be removed later
- *Fluid aspiration:*
  - Confirm the extracardiac position of the needle tip by injecting 5 mL of agitated saline and visualizing bubbles via echocardiography in the pericardial space
  - Make a small incision at the entry point
  - Insert a sheathed dilator (6–8 Fr) over the guidewire
  - Remove the dilator and fit a pigtail catheter into the sheath
  - Aspirate the pericardial effusion using syringe suction, then close the catheter after flushing with 5 mL of heparinized saline
  - Repeat aspiration every 4–6 hours until drainage decreases to <25–30 mL in 24 hours
- *Catheter care:*
  - Similar to central venous catheter care
  - Perform chest radiography postprocedure to rule out pneumothorax

BOX 5: Efficacy and safety.

- Echocardiography guidance significantly enhances the safety and efficacy of pericardiocentesis
- When performed by experienced practitioners using a careful approach, procedural outcomes are excellent with very low complication rates

BOX 6: Complications.

Possible complications include:
- Death
- Cardiac chamber injury (e.g., ventricular wall perforation)
- Coronary artery laceration
- Intercostal vessel damage
- Pneumothorax
- Pneumopericardium
- Ventricular arrhythmias
- Reaccumulation of pericardial effusion in pericardial recompression
- Myocardial and coronary perforations may initially be silent and present later with delayed hemopericardium or intrapericardial thrombus

SUGGESTED READING

1. Freeman LE, Hamid JL, Pael SD. Mayo Clinic Proceedings. 2017
2. Kim ST, Park JH. Journal of Cardiovascular Ultrasound. 2022.
3. Meyer CL, Goodman DL, Sanchez RJ. Circulation. 2018.
4. Shah MM, Nair SS, Zobhbi MA. Journal of the American College of Cardiology. 2016
5. Thompson RH, Williams JM. American Journal of Cardiology. 2019.

Part 5

Procedures Done in the Emergency Room

CHAPTER 35

Vascular Procedures

Prerna Gomes, Savi J Kapila

BOX 1: Central line insertion.

Indications:
- Central venous pressure (CPV) monitoring
- Pulmonary artery catheterization and monitoring
- Temporary hemodialysis
- Transvenous cardiac pacing
- *Drug administration:* Use of inotropic drugs, concentrated electrolytes such as potassium, and parenteral nutrition, in cancer patients a central port insertion is done for administration of chemotherapy drugs
- Infections requiring antibiotics for prolonged duration
- Surgeries with major fluid shifts, blood loss
- Aspiration of air in a case of air embolism
- Difficult intravenous access
- Patients requiring repeated investigations

BOX 2: Contraindications to central line insertion.

- Local site infection or burns
- Anatomic abnormalities
- Coagulopathy (ultrasound guidance will help)

BOX 3: Sites for central venous cannulation **(Fig. 1)**.

- Internal jugular vein (IJV)
- External jugular vein
- Subclavian vein
- Femoral vein
- Antecubital vein

Maxillary vein
Superficial temporal vein
Facial vein
Submental vein
Common facial vein
External jugular vein
Internal jugular vein
Anterior jugular vein
Common carotid artery
Sternocleidomastoid
Communicating vein
Trapezius
Retromandibular vein
Posterior auricular vein
Occipital vein
Sternocleidomastoid (cut)
Communicating vein
External jugular vein
Internal jugular vein
Left subclavian artery
Left subclavian vein
Sternocleidomastoid (cut)

Fig. 1: Veins for cannulation in the neck.

BOX 4: Precautions for central line insertion.

- Central venous line is inserted under all aseptic precautions
- Follow the hand wash steps after wearing cap, mask, and sterile gown
- Painting is done usually with betadine or 2% chlorhexidine in a circular manner from center to periphery so to cover adequate area and then sterile drapes are placed

BOX 5: Central line set **(Fig. 2)**.

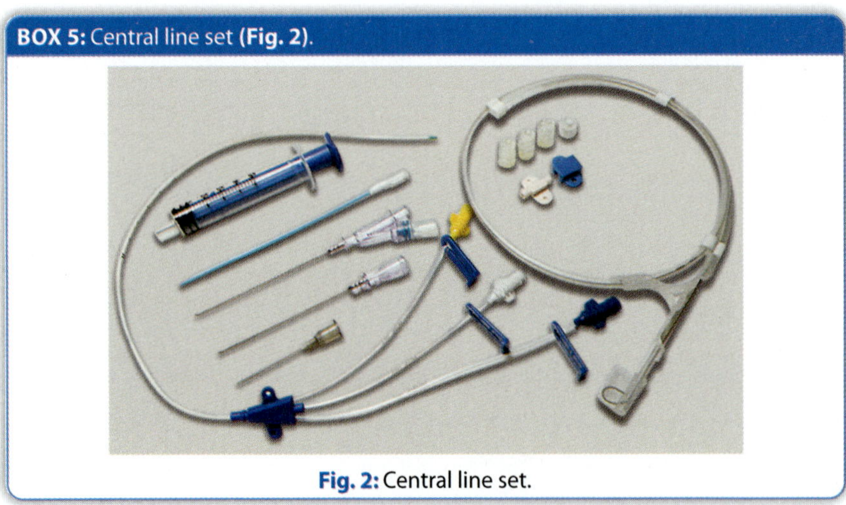

Fig. 2: Central line set.

BOX 6: Ultrasound techniques for central venous catheter (CVC) placement.

- "Static" US helps in the identification of the site of the central vein, its dimensions and depth before placement hence it is called US-assisted CVC placement
- In contrast, "real-time" US as the name suggests is placement of central line under ultrasound guidance

Short-axis/long-axis and out-of-plane/in-plane views: The in-plane and out of plane technique have been shown in the diagram below.

BOX 7: Ultrasound probe orientation and needle view **(Figs. 3A and B)**.

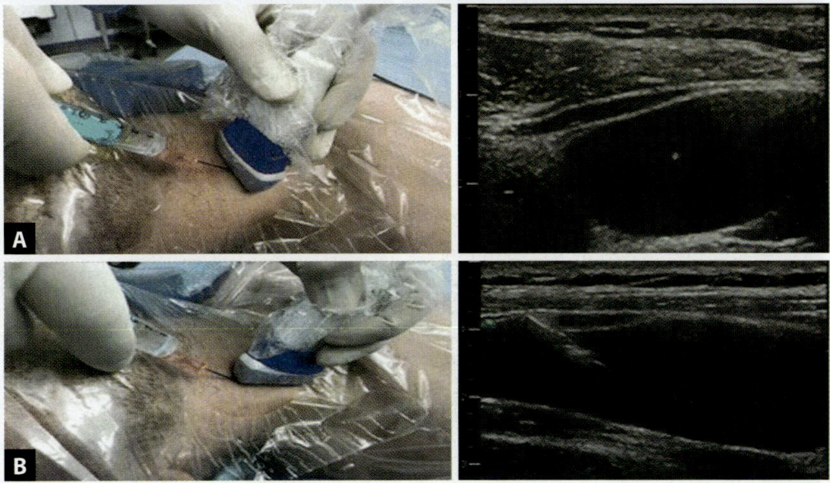

Figs. 3A and B: Ultrasound guidance during needle advancement can be performed using a (A) short-axis probe orientation and an out-of-plane view technique or a (B) long-axis probe orientation and an in-plane view of the needle.

BOX 8: Ultrasound-guided IJV catheterization **(Figs. 4 and 5)**.

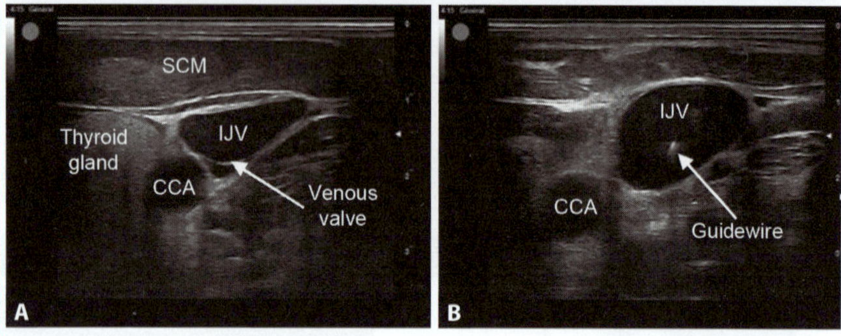

Figs. 4A and B: Ultrasound-guided IJV catheterization using the short-axis view of the vein in combination with out of plane needle approach. (A) Ultrasound visualization of IJV and common carotid artery (CCA). (B) Ultrasound visualization of the guidewire in the IJV.

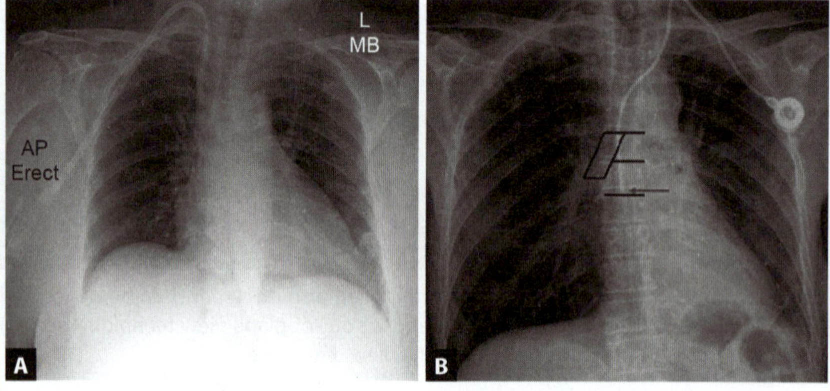

Figs. 5A and B: Showing the X-ray image of central line placement in right (A) and (B) left IJVs, respectively.

BOX 9: Subclavian vein cannulation position.

Subclavian vein cannulation is done in Trendelenburg position with or without using a shoulder with the patient's head turned in the opposite direction

- The puncture is done 2–3 cm caudal to the midpoint of clavicle facing the suprasternal notch, the needle when advanced further abuts the clavicle and is further advanced inferiorly till the vein is punctured

Care should be taken to avoid any injury to the pleura

- The central line is inserted using the Seldinger technique shown in **Figures 6A to E**

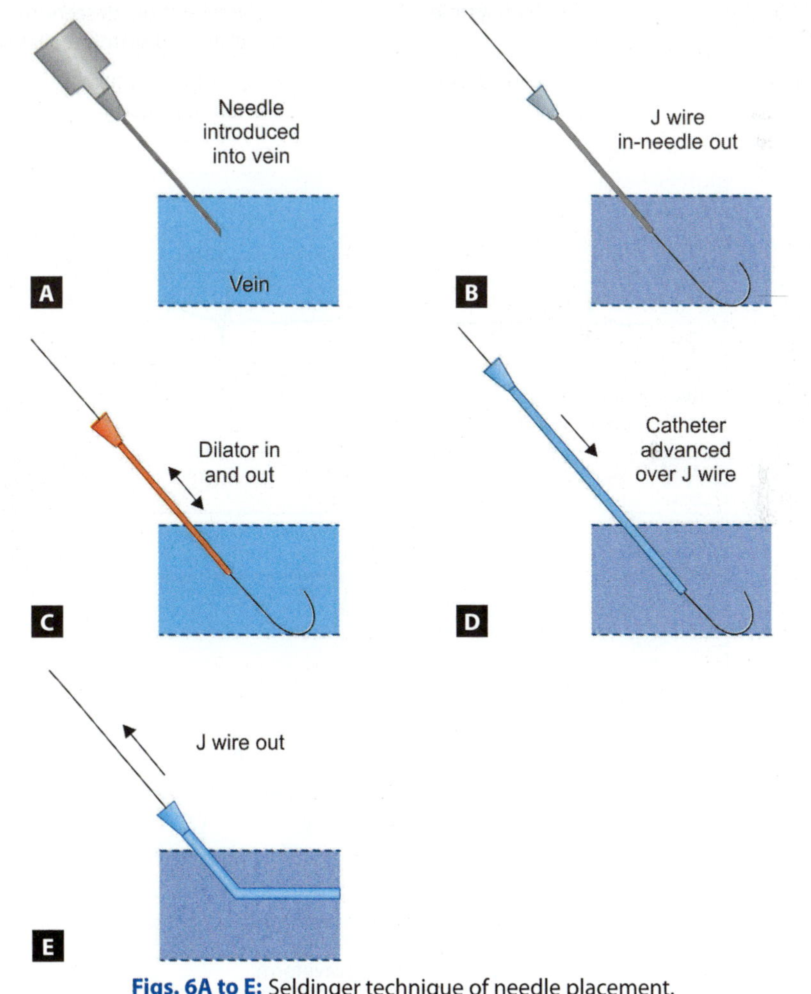

Figs. 6A to E: Seldinger technique of needle placement.

BOX 10: Central lines waveform **(Fig. 7)**.

Waveform component	*Phase of cardiac cycle*	*Mechanical event*
A wave	End-diastole	Contraction of atria
C wave	Early systole	Isovolumic ventricular contraction, tricuspid motion toward right atrium
V wave	Late systole	Systolic filling of atrium
H wave	Mid- to late diastole	Diastolic plateau
X descent	Mid-systole	Atrial relaxation, descent of the base, and systolic collapse
Y descent	Early diastole	Early ventricular filling, diastolic collapse

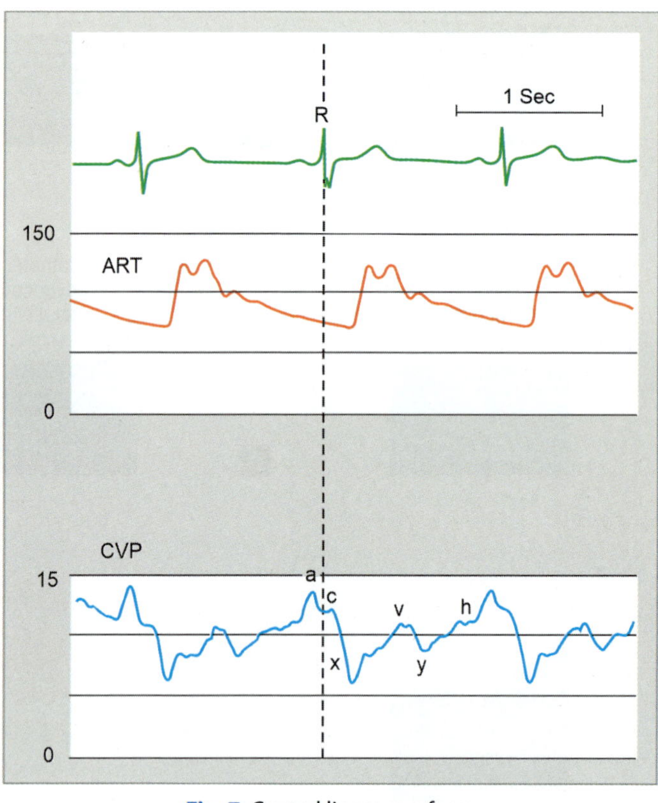

Fig. 7: Central lines waveform.

BOX 11: Complications of central line insertion.

Complications of CPV monitoring: Injury to adjacent vessels:
- Cardiac tamponade
- Thoracic duct injury
- Pneumothorax
- Arrhythmias
- Thromboembolic complications
- Infection
- Embolism of guidewire

BOX 12: Indications for arterial line cannulation.

- Continuous, real-time blood pressure monitoring
- Mechanical error like in obese patients or in surgeries with major fluid shifts, blood loss
- Patient needing frequent investigations or arterial blood gas monitoring
- Pulse pressure variation is a value that is derived from the arterial waveform and it has proved to be very useful in determining the fluid status of the patients, it has proven more useful than CVP for deciding on fluid status of patients

BOX 13: Contraindications for arterial line cannulation.

- Inadequate circulation to the involved extremity
- Uncontrolled bleeding
- Burns
- Skin infection
- Raynaud's phenomenon
- Thromboangiitis obliterans
- Locations near arteriovenous fistulas

BOX 14: Arterial line cannulation.

Arteries cannulated for invasive blood pressure monitoring: The radial artery is the most common site for invasive blood pressure monitoring because it is easy to cannulate with rare complications
- *Modified Allen's test:*
  - This test is done as a safety test to prevent limb ischemia
  - The radial and ulnar arteries are both compressed while the patient makes a tight fist to exsanguinate the palm and then slowly reopens it. When the occlusion of the ulnar artery is released, the color of the open palm is observed. Normally, the color will return to the palm within seconds; severely reduced collateral flow is present when the palm remains pale for >6–10 seconds. The predictive value of this test is poor
- *Other alternative sites include:*
  - Ulnar artery
  - Brachial artery
  - Axillary artery
  - Femoral artery
  - Dorsalis pedis and posterior tibial artery

Contd...

Contd...

*Radial artery cannulation (shown in the **Figs. 8 to 10**):*
- Over the needle technique
- Over the wire technique

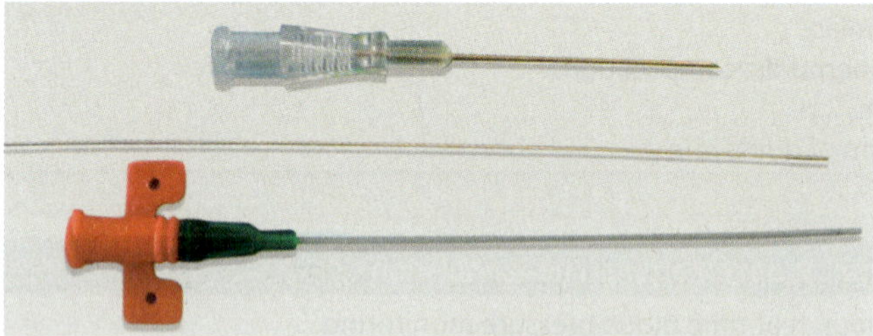

Fig. 8: Arteriofix set.

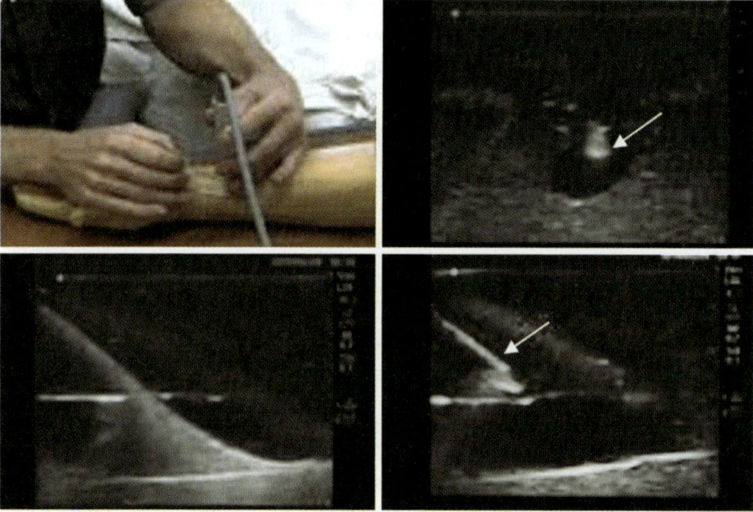

Fig. 9: Ultrasound-guided arterial line cannulation.

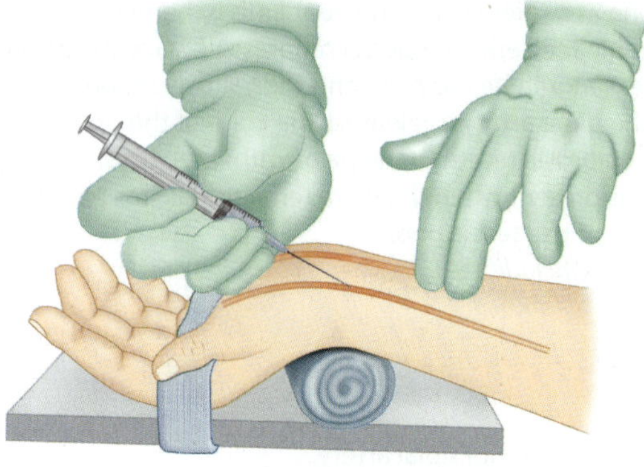

Fig. 10: Arterial line placement.

BOX 15: Arterial blood pressure tracing **(Fig. 11).**

- Invasive arterial blood pressure tracing may be underdamped or overdamped. Damping means tendency of an oscillating system to return to its resting state
- *Underdamped waveform:* Narrow and peaked tracing (higher systolic and low diastolic pressure)
- Seen with vessels having increased resistance
- Overdamped waveform (will record lower systolic and higher diastolic pressure)
- Air bubbles or blood clots
- Kinking of the catheter
- No fluid in flush bag
- Low pressure of the inflating bag
- When the tracing is underdamped or overdamped the mean arterial pressure (MAP) may still be comparable

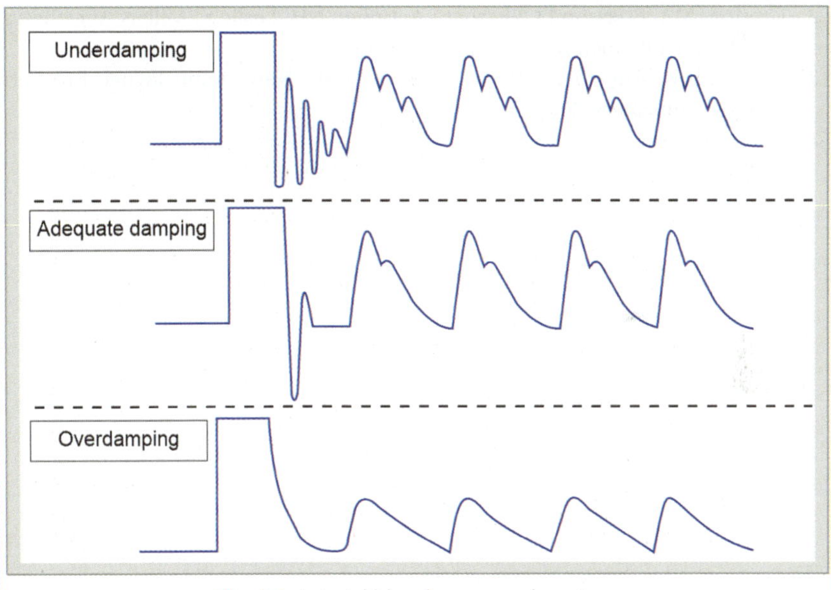

Fig. 11: Arterial blood pressure damping.

BOX 16: Square wave test.

- To test the accuracy of the arterial tracing, we use a square wave test
- The waveform will rise sharply, square off at the top when the flush is activated and the tracing returns to baseline after it is released

Now check the number of oscillations:

- It is optimally damped if there are one or two oscillations before return to tracing
- Overdamped—less than one oscillation before return to tracing
- Repeat the square test every 8–12 hours for accuracy of the tracing

BOX 17: Complications of direct arterial pressure monitoring.

- Ischemia in the cannulated limb
- Pseudoaneurysm
- Arteriovenous fistula
- Bleeding
- Embolism in the artery
- Infection
- Peripheral neuropathy
- Misinterpretation of data

SUGGESTED READING

1. Al-Shaikh B, Stacey S. Essentials of Anaesthetic Equipment, 4th edition. Philadelphia: Elsevier, Inc.; 2013.
2. Gropper MA, Eriksson LI, Fleisher LA, Cohen NH, Leslie K. Millers Anesthesia, 9th edition. Philadelphia: Elsevier, Inc.; 2019.
3. Jothinath K. Anesthesia Review, 2nd edition. New Delhi: Jaypee Brothers Medical Publishers; 2021.

CHAPTER 36

Sedation and Anesthesia in Emergency Room

Sachna P Shetty, Preeti P Doshi

BOX 1: Eligibility.

- Emergency clinicians who are trained and skilled in procedural sedation are qualified to administer sedation in the emergency room (ER) as per the American association of emergency physician
- The decision to administer sedation and the choice of specific pharmacologic agents should be tailored to each patient by the emergency clinician
- Emergency clinicians and staff should be well-versed in the medications they use and ready to handle any potential complications
- To reduce the risk of complications, appropriate drugs and dosages must be selected and administered in a properly monitored environment, with thorough patient evaluations conducted before, during, and after sedation
- Institutional and departmental guidelines for patient sedation should encompass credentialing and verification of provider competency, patient selection and preparation, informed consent, equipment and monitoring requirements, staff training and competency verification, discharge criteria, and continuous quality improvement

BOX 2: Levels of sedation and analgesia.

Procedural sedation and analgesia (PSA) are defined as "the use of anxiolytic, sedative, hypnotic, analgesic, and/or dissociative medications to reduce anxiety, pain, and/or motion. These agents facilitate amnesia or decreased awareness, ensuring patient comfort and safety during diagnostic or therapeutic procedures"

TABLE 1: Parameters of sedation levels.

Parameters	*Minimal sedation (Anxiolysis)*	*Moderate sedation and analgesia (conscious sedation)*	*Deep sedation and analgesia*	*Dissociative sedation*	*General anesthesia*
Responsiveness	Normal response to verbal	Purposeful response to verbal or tactile stimulation	Purposeful response to repeated or painful stimulation	Unarousable even with painful stimulus	Unarousable even with painful stimulus
Airway	Unaffected	No intervention required	Intervention may be required	Intervention may be required	Intervention often required
Spontaneous ventilation	Unaffected	Adequate	May be adequate	Adequate	Frequently inadequate
Cardiovascular function	Unaffected	Usually maintained	Usually maintained	Elevated	May be impaired
Monitoring	Consciousness frequently, heart rate, blood pressure (BP), respiratory rate (RR) every 15 minutes, oxygen saturation continuously, no capnography required	Consciousness, heart rate, RR, oxygen saturation continuously, BP every 5 minutes after sedation, capnography	Consciousness, heart rate, RR, oxygen saturation continuously, BP every 5 minutes after sedation, capnography required	BP at initiation, all other monitoring continuously	All monitoring continuously required

Sources: Walls RM, Hockberger RS, Gausche-Hill M. Rosen's emergency medicine: Concepts and clinical practice. Philadelphia, PA: Elsevier; 2018. Tintinalli JE, Ma OJ, Yealy DM, Meckler GD, Stapczynski JS, Cline DM, et al. Tintinalli's Emergency Medicine: A Comprehensive Study Guide, 9th edition. McGraw Hill Professional; 2019 .

BOX 3: Disposition.

- Following sedation and the procedure, patients should be observed until they return to their baseline mental status and cardiopulmonary function
- A structured assessment form should be developed according to institutional needs, following standard guidelines such as the Aldrete score **(Box 4)**
- The observation period before ending monitoring or discharging the patient depends on factors such as the amount of sedative administered, the patient's response, the duration of the procedure, and any adverse events that occurred
- Generally, patients who have regained their baseline level of consciousness are unlikely to experience further decline in consciousness. Most adverse events related to procedural sedation occur within a few minutes of administering the sedative

Caveat: Major adverse events occurring more than 5 minutes after the procedure are rare. There have been no reports of life-threatening adverse events following the discharge of ER patients who underwent procedural sedation. Patients should be advised to return if they experience respiratory issues, nausea, or repetitive vomiting

BOX 4: Aldrete score.

The Aldrete score, also known as the Aldrete recovery score, is a widely used system for assessing a patient's recovery from anesthesia.
It evaluates five criteria: Activity, respiration, circulation, consciousness, and color. Each criterion is scored from 0 to 2, with a maximum total score of 10. Here is a breakdown of the scoring system:

1. Activity:
   - *2:* Able to move all extremities on command
   - *1:* Able to move two extremities
   - *0:* Unable to move extremities
2. Respiration:
   - *2:* Able to breathe deeply and cough freely
   - *1:* Dyspnea or limited breathing
   - *0:* Apnea
3. Circulation:
   - *2:* Blood pressure within 20% of preanesthetic level
   - *1:* Blood pressure within 20–50% of preanesthetic level
   - *0:* Blood pressure greater than 50% of preanesthetic level
4. Consciousness:
   - *2:* Fully awake
   - *1:* Arousable on calling
   - *0:* Not responding
5. Color:
   - *2:* Normal
   - *1:* Pale, dusky, blotchy, jaundiced, or other abnormal color
   - *0:* Cyanotic

A score of 9 or 10 is typically required before a patient can be safely discharged from the postsedation procedure in the emergency room (ER)

BOX 5: Prerequisites.

- No fasting required
- Obtain informed consent
- Oxygen
- Airway and suction
- Monitoring equipment
- Capnography device
- Vascular access supplies
- Reversal agents
- Resuscitation medications

BOX 6: Sedation medications.

- *Propofol*
  - *Initial dose:* 0.5–1 mg/kg
  - *Onset:* 0.5 minutes
  - *Duration:* 5 minutes
  - *Repeat dose:* 0.25–0.5 mg/kg every 3 minutes
  - *Comments:*
    - Sedative and amnestic with no analgesia
    - Rapid onset and neurological recovery
    - Suitable for older adults without major comorbidities
    - Reduce dose by ≥20% (*max initial bolus:* 0.5 mg/kg) and administer slowly over 3–5 minutes
    - Respiratory depression, hypotension, and injection-site pain may occur
    - Contains egg lecithin and soybean oil
- *Etomidate*
  - *Initial dose:* 0.1–0.15 mg/kg
  - *Onset:* 5–10 seconds
  - *Duration:* 5–10 minutes
  - *Repeat dose:* 0.05 mg/kg every 3–5 minutes
  - *Comments:*
    - Sedative with no analgesia
    - Maintains hemodynamic stability, useful for patients at risk of hypotension
    - In older adults or those with kidney or liver impairment, use lower doses
    - Myoclonus, respiratory depression, injection-site pain, and nausea/vomiting may occur
- *Midazolam*
  - *Initial dose:* 0.1 mg/kg, 0.05 mg/kg in elderly over 2–3 minutes
  - *Usual individual dose:* 1–2.5 mgs, 0.5 mg in elderly, titrated to effect
  - *Maximum single dose:* 2.5 mg (1.5 mg in older adults)
  - *Onset:* 2–5 minutes
  - *Duration:* 30–60 minutes
  - *Repeat dose:* Every 2–5 minutes of 0.5–2.5 mg

Contd...

Contd...

- *Comments:*
  - Sedative and anxiolytic with no analgesia
  - Often combined with fentanyl
  - Minimal hypotension and histamine release
  - Lower doses are recommended for older adults and those with kidney or liver impairment
  - Respiratory depression may occur
- *Ketamine*
  - *Initial dose:* 1–2 mg/kg over 1 to 2 minutes
  - *Onset:* 0.5 minutes
  - Duration: 10–20 minutes
  - *Repeat dose:* 0.25–1 mg/kg every 2–5 minutes
  - *Comments:*
    - Dissociative sedative, analgesic, and amnestic
    - Minimal cardiorespiratory depression; does not inhibit protective reflexes
    - Suitable for patients at risk of hypotension or with difficult airway
    - Intramuscular administration possible with delayed onset
    - Emergence reactions common in adults
    - Nausea and vomiting may occur
    - Sympathetic stimulation, tachycardia, and hypertension may occur (rare)
    - Avoid in schizophrenia due to rigidity
- *Dexmedetomidine*
  - *Initial bolus:* 0.5–1 µg/kg over 10 minutes
  - *Infusion:* 0.2–1 µg/kg/hour
  - *Onset:* 5–10 minutes
  - *Duration:* 60–240 minutes postinfusion
  - *Repeat dose:* NA
  - *Comments:*
    - Sedative with some analgesia
    - Not amnestic
    - Suitable for patients with difficult airway or when tachycardia/hypertension is dangerous
    - It can be administered intranasally (2–3 µg/kg) for anxiolysis and sedation.
    - Lower doses are recommended for liver impairment
    - Rarely decreases respiratory drive and airway obstruction
    - Bradycardia and hypotension may occur with loading doses and rapid titration; hypertension is also observed with high-dose infusion

BOX 7: Special considerations.

- *Hypotension:* Prefer etomidate or ketamine
- *Orthopedic injuries:* Use propofol as etomidate can cause myoclonus
- *Critical illness:* Avoid etomidate; use ketamine or dexmedetomidine for respiratory complications
- *Obese, elderly, underweight, comorbid conditions, pediatric, and pregnant:* Adjust medication and dosing accordingly

BOX 8: Adult drug selection strategies.

Procedure type	*Examples*	*Recommendation*	*Alternatives*	*Comments*
Nonpainful	Radiologic imaging	Midazolam (intravenous)	Propofol (intravenous)	Midazolam has strong support and safety profile
Low pain and high anxiety	Central line placement and lumbar puncture	Midazolam (intravenous)	Propofol (intravenous) and Ketamine (intravenous)	Analgesia often achieved with local or topical agents
High pain and high anxiety	Fracture/joint reduction, abscess drainage, burn debridement, cardioversion, and chest tube placement	Midazolam + fentanyl (intravenous), propofol + fentanyl (intravenous), Ketamine (intravenous/ intramuscular)	Etomidate + fentanyl (intravenous), Propofol + ketamine (intravenous)	Significant data support the safety of fentanyl and midazolam; other choices are also supported

LOCAL ANESTHESIA

BOX 9: Local anesthesia checklist.

- Calculate the volume and check the concentration of the drug used
- Aspirate before injection
- Addition of epinephrine controls bleeding, slows systemic absorption, and can be safely used for fingers and toes unless there is digital ischemia
- *Addition of bicarbonate reduces pain:* 1 mL of 8.4% bicarbonate in 9 mL of 1% lidocaine or 29 mL of 0.25% bupivacaine
- Use small needles (25, 27, or 30G)
- Administer subcutaneously instead of intradermally
- Use a 90° angle instead of 45°
- Adverse reactions are mainly to the preservative; if present, use diphenhydramine or benzyl alcohol

BOX 10: Topical anesthetic agents.

Agent	***Active ingredients***	***Application***	***Time to effectiveness***
Intact dermis			
Eutectic mixture of local anesthetic agents (EMLA)	Lidocaine 2.5%, Prilocaine 2.5%	Apply thick layer (5-10 grams and maximum 20 grams) to area; cover with semiocclusive dressing	60 minutes
Tetracaine (amethocaine) gel (Ametop)	Tetracaine 4%	Apply 1 gram to area; cover with occlusive dressing	30 minutes
Liposome-encapsulated tetracaine	Tetracaine 5%		

Commonly used local and regional anesthesia agents and doses.

Agent	***Duration without epinephrine***	***Onset (min)***	***Max dose without/ with epinephrine (mg/kg)***	***Concentration (subdermal)***	***Concentration (regional anesthesia)***
Bupivacaine	120–240 minutes	210 minutes	3 (5)	0.500.75%	0.250.50%
Lidocaine	30–120 minutes	<1 minutes	4 (7)	0.51%	12%
Alternative if allergic				1% diphenhydramine	0.5% Benzyl alcohol with epinephrine

Sources: Tintinalli JE, Ma OJ, Yealy DM, Meckler GD, Stapczynski JS, Cline DM, et al. Tintinalli's Emergency Medicine: A Comprehensive Study Guide, 9th edition. McGraw Hill Professional; 2019.
Walls RM, Hockberger RS, Gausche-Hill M. Rosen's emergency medicine: Concepts and clinical practice. Philadelphia, PA: Elsevier; 2018.

BOX 11: Nerve blocks.

- *Definition:* Regional anesthesia technique involving infiltration of local anesthetic agents adjacent to peripheral nerves
- *Indications:*
  - Complicated lacerations
  - Abscesses
  - Fractures
  - Debridement
  - Dislocations
- *Contraindications:*
  - Active infection at the injection site
  - Use of antithrombotic drugs with coagulopathy
  - Noncompressible anatomic locations
  - Preexisting neural deficits in the block distribution area

BOX 12: Preparation.

- Obtain detailed medical history
- Prepare the patient by informing them about necessary precautions and care during recovery, and potential complications
- Establish intravenous access to manage potential toxicity
- Use a checklist to reduce medical errors
- The patient may be awake during the procedure; mild anxiolytics can be administered
- Monitor the patient during the placement of peripheral nerve blocks
- Aim to inject the anesthetic close to the nerve, avoiding intraneural injection

BOX 13: Technique.

- Use anatomical landmarks to guide the block, although ultrasound guidance improves success rates
- Ultrasound guidance reduces placement time, onset of block, required volume of local anesthetic, vascular puncture, and toxicity
- Ultrasound guidance reduces the incidence of pneumothorax and phrenic nerve paralysis
- Nerve stimulation is less preferred compared to ultrasound guidance **(Figs. 1A and B)**

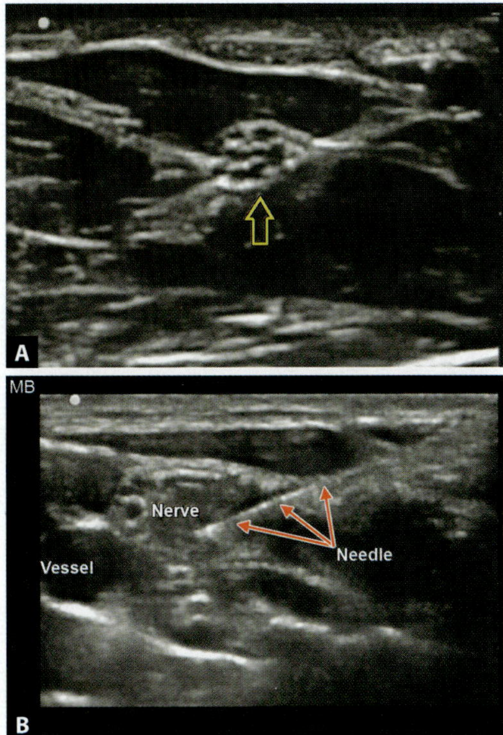

Figs. 1 and B: Ultrasound image of a nerve cross-section having white, hyperechoic, and honeycomb appearance (arrow in A).

BOX 14: Equipment for ultrasound guidance.

- High-quality portable ultrasound machine
- High-frequency probe (10–15 MHz) for superficial nerves
- Low-frequency probe (5–7 MHz) for deeper nerves

BOX 15: Technique for ultrasound-guided nerve blocks.

- Maintain aseptic precautions
- Identify the anatomical structure at the block site
- Choose the appropriate probe and cover it with a sterile plastic sheet
- Use either the inplane or out-of-plane needle insertion technique, followed by the injection of the local anesthetic around the nerves

BOX 16: Commonly used nerve blocks in roomer.

Block	***Clinical indications***	***Advantages***	***Pitfalls***
Upper extremity:			
Interscalene	Shoulder dislocation, laceration, upper arm, and deltoid humerus fracture	Good analgesia	Inconsistent block below mid humerus; avoid in patients who cannot tolerate unilateral nerve paralysis
Supraclavicular	Upper limb injury below the shoulder and abscess drainage	Broad coverage of the upper limb	Avoid in patients who cannot tolerate unilateral phrenic nerve paralysis
Infraclavicular	Elbow dislocation, forearm fracture, and wrist fractures	Lesser systemic absorption and low risk of phrenic nerve paralysis	Hyperacute needle approach
Axillary	Elbow dislocation, wrist fractures, and forearm fractures	Lesser systemic absorption and low risk of phrenic paralysis	Multiple redirections
Median	Volar lateral hand to wrist and distal phalanx of digit 13		
Ulnar	Boxer's fracture and laceration to the medial aspect of the hand		
Lower extremity:			
Fascia Iliaca	Fractures of hip, neck, and shaft of femur; abscess; laceration of anterior thigh, and hip dislocation	Higher success rate when performed above the inguinal ligament	
Femoral nerve	Femoral shaft fracture, patella fracture dislocation, proximal tibial fracture, abscess, and laceration of anterior thigh	Good vascular landmark	Risk of intravascular injection
Sciatic nerve at popliteal fossa	Leg, ankle, and foot fracture, dislocation, and spares medial malleolus in the medial leg	Spinal of the leg	Risk of compartment syndrome
Posterior tibial nerve	Laceration and foreign body to the sole of the foot and calcaneal fracture	Good vascular landmark	

BOX 17: Commonest nerve block techniques.

Fascia iliaca block:

- *Technique:* Explain the procedure to the patient and obtain consent
- Prepare the equipment, including specialized long needles and local anesthetic (30 mL of 0.25% levobupivacaine for adults ≤50 kg and 40 mL for adults >50 kg)
- Clean the skin and identify the anterior superior iliac spine and pubic tubercle
- Draw an imaginary line between these points, dividing it into thirds, with the injection site 1 cm below the junction of the lateral third and medial two-thirds
- The femoral pulse is medial to this point. Insert the needle in the sagittal plane, piercing through two distinct palpable "pops" (fascia lata and fascia iliaca)
- Aspirate to check for blood, then inject the local anesthetic slowly
- If resistance is encountered, adjust the needle
- Aspirate after every 5 mL of injection
- After the procedure, apply pressure to the injection site and monitor the patient's vital signs every 5 minutes for at least 30 minutes

Wrist block:
Technique:

- Use anatomical landmarks for nerve identification
- Insert the needle horizontally, 5–10 mm past the tendon edge, and inject after confirming negative aspiration **(Figs. 2A and B)**
- To perform a median nerve block, locate the palmaris longus tendon by having the patient flex their wrist, then insert the needle between the palmaris longus and flexor carpi radialis tendons
- For a radial nerve block, inject at the lateral aspect of the radial styloid
- For an ulnar nerve block, identify the flexor carpi ulnaris tendon by having the patient make a fist, then inject subcutaneously along the dorsal ulnar nerve branches, extending from the ulnar block insertion site to the midline of the dorsal wrist
- Insert the needle horizontally beneath the flexor carpi ulnaris tendon, 5–10 mm past the tendon edge, and inject after confirming negative aspiration

Foot block:
Technique:

- Utilize anatomical landmarks and ultrasound guidance **(Figs. 3A to D)**
- For a sural nerve block, create a subcutaneous field block extending from the Achilles tendon to the lateral malleolus
- To block the posterior tibial nerve, inject behind the posterior tibial artery
- For a deep peroneal nerve block, inject at the level of the medial malleolus, between the anterior tibial tendon and the extensor hallucis longus tendon
- For the superficial peroneal nerve, create a subcutaneous field block from the lateral malleolus to the anterior tibial tendon
- To block the saphenous nerve, create a subcutaneous field block extending from the medial malleolus to the anterior tibial tendon

Hematoma block:
Technique: Maintain aseptic conditions before injecting into the bony fracture site. Use bedside ultrasound to locate the hematoma. Confirm needle placement by aspirating blood, then inject 5–20 mL of local anesthetic into the fracture site, avoiding open wounds or fractures **(Fig. 4)**

Contd...

Contd...

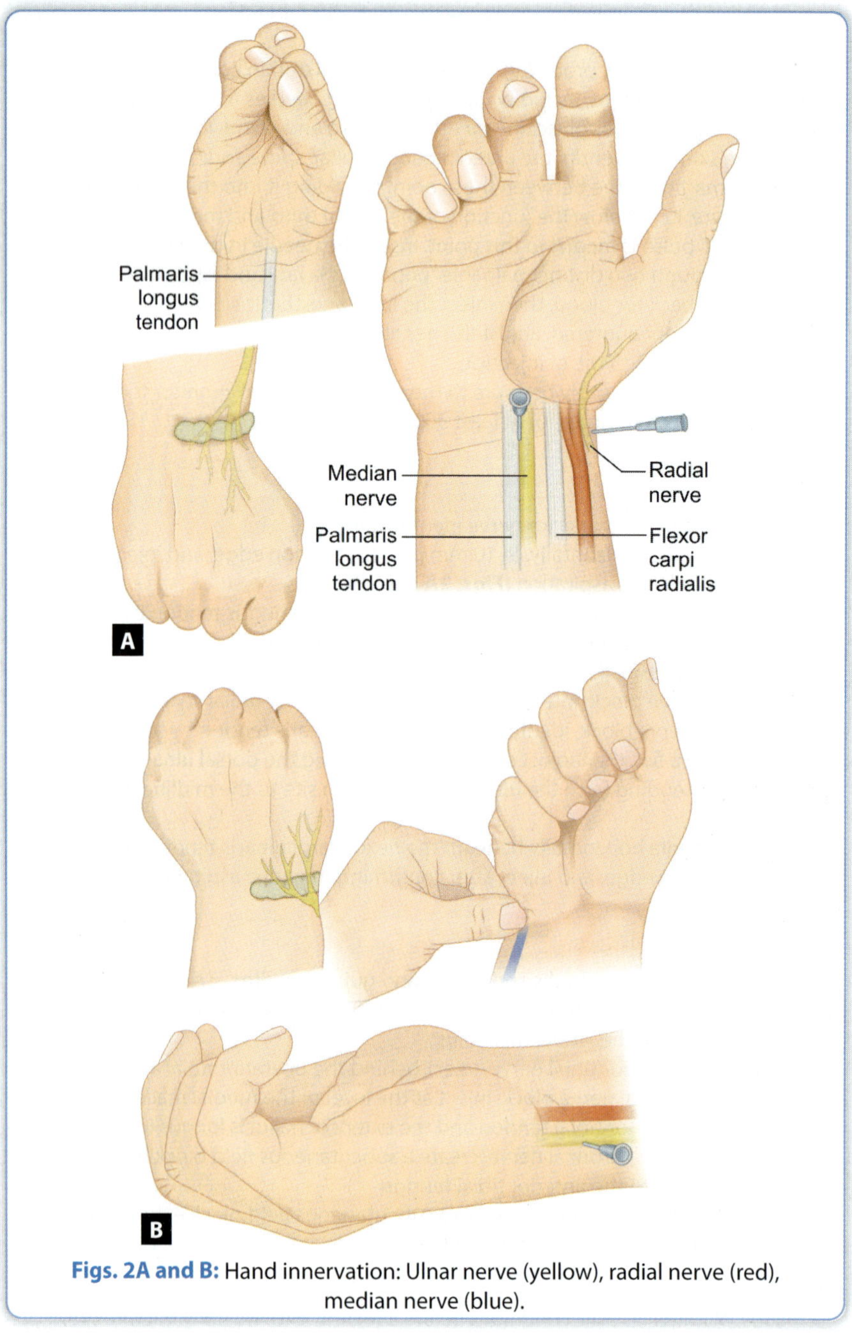

Figs. 2A and B: Hand innervation: Ulnar nerve (yellow), radial nerve (red), median nerve (blue).

Contd...

Contd...

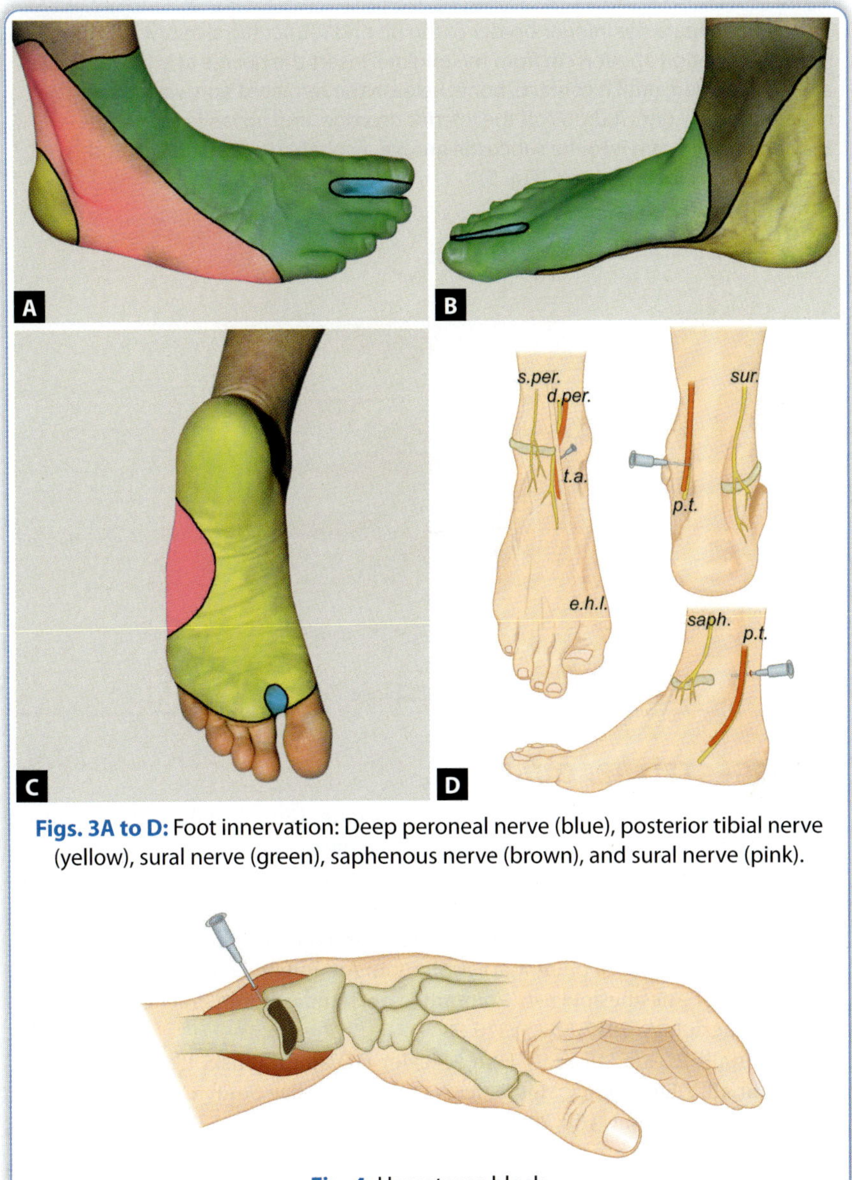

Figs. 3A to D: Foot innervation: Deep peroneal nerve (blue), posterior tibial nerve (yellow), sural nerve (green), saphenous nerve (brown), and sural nerve (pink).

Fig. 4: Hematoma block.

BOX 18: Rib block.

Technique: Palpate the inferior border of the rib and retract the skin towards the head at a location about 6 cm from the midline. Insert the needle at a 10–15° angle, aiming cephalad, until it contacts bone. Release the retracted skin, walk the needle caudally until it drops off the inferior rib edge, and advance the needle approximately 3 mm into the subcostal groove. Aspirate before injection and deposit 2–5 mL of anesthetic **(Fig. 5)**

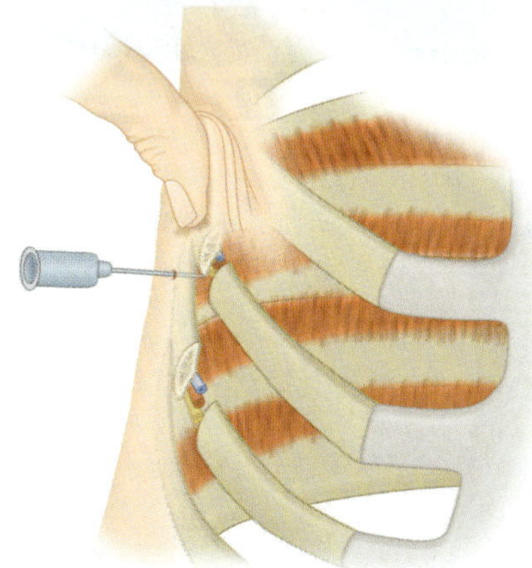

Fig 5: Rib block.

SUGGESTED READING

1. American College of Emergency Physicians. (2023). Policy Statement on Procedural Sedation in the Emergency Department. [online]. Available from https://www.acep.org/siteassets/new-pdfs/policy-statements/procedural-sedation-in-the-emergency-department.pdf [Last accessed September, 2024].
2. Practice guidelines for preoperative fasting and the use of pharmacologic agents to reduce the risk of pulmonary aspiration: An updated report by the American Society of Anesthesiologists Committee on Standards and Practice Parameters. Anesthesiology. 2017;126(3):376-93.
3. Tintinalli JE, Ma OJ, Yealy DM, Meckler GD, Stapczynski JS, David M, et al. Tintinalli's Emergency Medicine: A Comprehensive Study Guide, 9th edition. New York: McGraw Hill; 2020.

CHAPTER 37

Surgical Procedures

37.1 GENERAL PROCEDURES

Sadashiv Chaudhari, Sachna P Shetty

BOX 1: Soft tissue foreign body removal.

Materials required—surgical tray, anesthesia material, sterile drapes, ultrasonography machine

Fishhook Removal ***(Fig. 1)****:*

- *Indications:* Removal of a fishhook from nonvital structures
- *Contraindications:* Removal of hooks located near vital structures which require specialist consultation
- *Procedures:* All techniques should follow aseptic precautions and use local anesthesia or mild procedural sedation
  - *Retrograde technique:*
    - Ideal for small hooks without barbs
    - Disengage the barb by applying downward pressure on the hook's shank near the eye and remove it in the opposite direction of entry **(Figs. 2A and B)**
  - *String and Yank technique:*
    - Suitable for deep soft tissue penetration
    - Wrap a 30-silk suture firmly around the hook's bend at the point of greatest curvature
    - Apply slight traction at the skin entry point while depressing the hook's shank near the eye. Simultaneously pull the string firmly to dislodge the hook **(Fig. 3)**
  - *Needle cover technique:*
    - Effective for large hooks with a single barb
    - Advance an 18-gauge needle parallel to the hook's entrance wound until it disengages the barb. Withdraw both the hook and needle along the wound track **(Figs. 4A to C)**
  - *Advance and cut technique:*
    - Grip the hook near its bend with a needle driver
    - Push the hook along its natural trajectory until the barb passes through the skin. Clip the hook's point proximal to the barb and withdraw it along its entry path

Contd...

Contd...

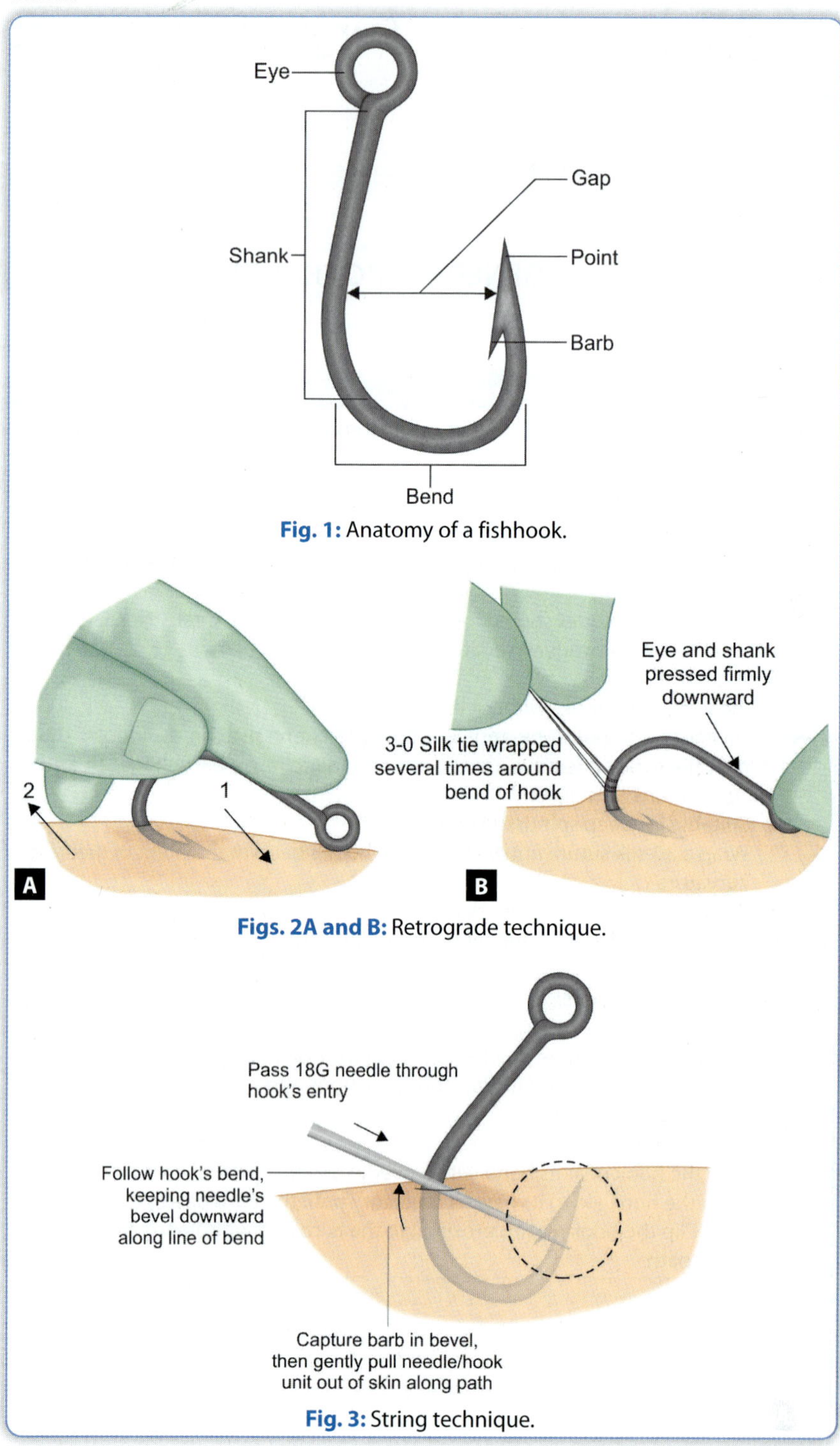

Fig. 1: Anatomy of a fishhook.

Figs. 2A and B: Retrograde technique.

Fig. 3: String technique.

Contd...

Contd...

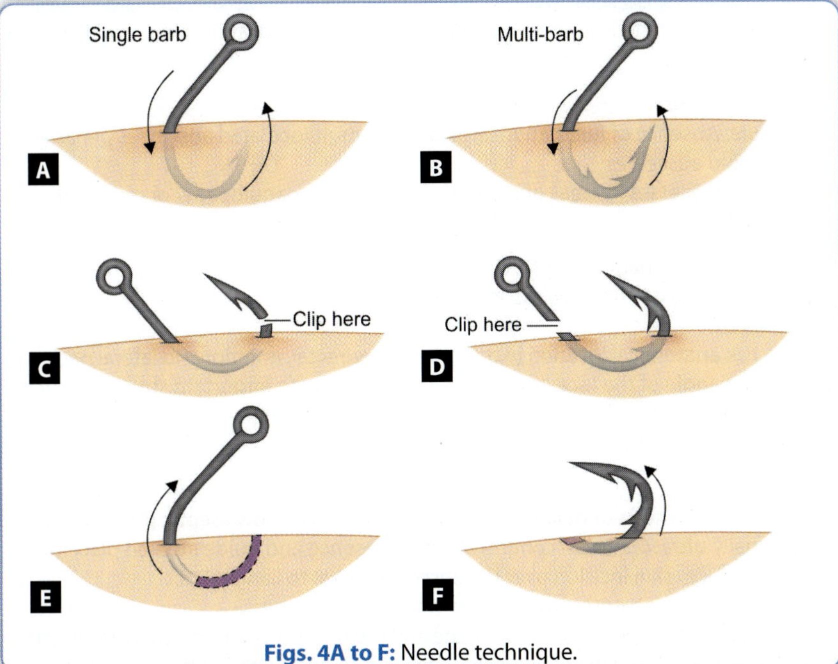

Figs. 4A to F: Needle technique.

BOX 2: Tick removal.

Procedure:
- Position the patient comfortably and follow aseptic precautions
- Grasp the tick as close to the skin surface as possible avoiding twisting or jerking to prevent mouthpart breakage
- Gently pull upward with steady even traction
- Clean the bite area postremoval and apply antibiotic ointment **(Figs. 5A and B)**

Caveat:
- Early removal is crucial to reduce the risk of Lyme disease transmission (especially after 24–48 hours of attachment)
- Monitor patients for up to 30 days for signs of tick-borne diseases
- Avoid subcutaneous lidocaine as it can irritate the tick causing regurgitation and potential disease transfer

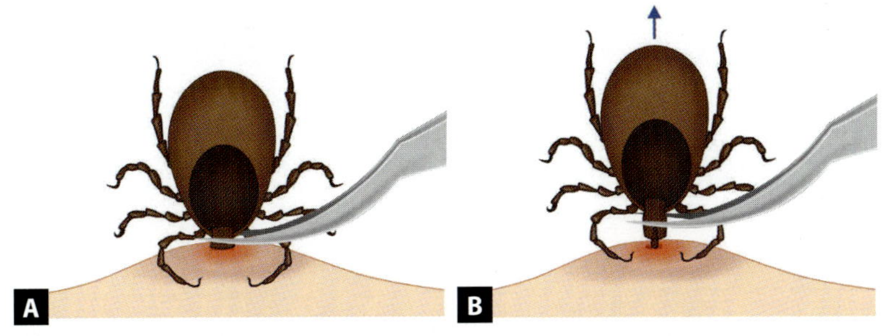

Figs. 5A and B: Tick removal.

BOX 3: Incision and drainage (I&D).

Indications: Abscesses >5 mm in diameter and accessible locations (e.g., axilla extremities trunk)

Contraindications:
- *Absolute:* Absence of fluctuation large or deep multiloculated abscesses perianal or mastoid abscesses
- *Relative:* Abscesses in areas of cosmetic importance coagulopathy or recurrent pilonidal cysts

When surgical drainage is required for the below conditions:
- Multiple abscesses (may be associated with fistulas)
- Size >5 cm
- High-risk anatomical location (e.g., perianal, perirectal, anterior and lateral neck, central triangle of the face, and breast. The proximity to important structures such as vital nerves or blood vessels should also be considered)
- Suspected mycotic or mycobacterial abscess

Procedure:
- Use local anesthesia or mild procedural sedation and follow aseptic precautions
- Optionally ultrasound can confirm abscess presence and guide incision placement
- Make a 12-cm skin incision over the abscess parallel to Langer lines
- Ensure the incision enters the abscess cavity for drainage
- Express pus after spontaneous drainage and break any loculations using a hemostat
- Pack the wound leaving a tail outside the incision and apply a dressing **(Figs. 6 and 7)**.

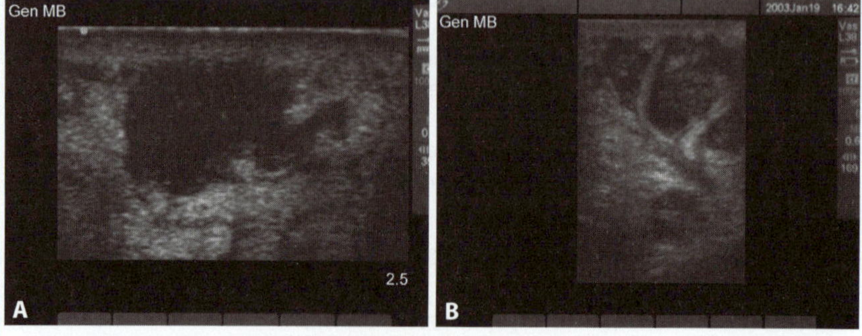

Figs. 6A and B: (A) Abscess on bedside ultrasound; (B) Multiloculated abscess.

Contd...

Contd...

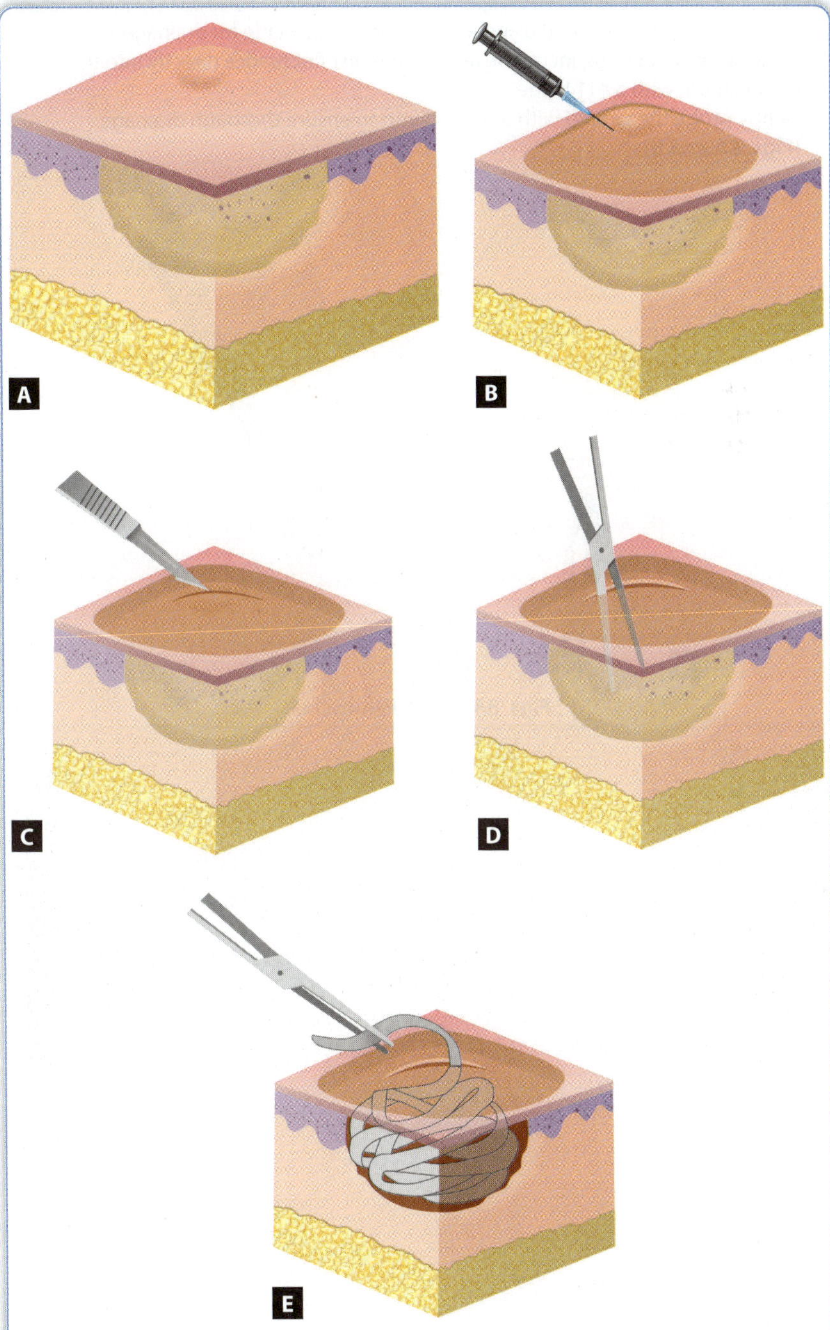

Figs. 7A to E: (A) Abscess with overlying erythema; (B) Lidocaine injection in the superficial layer; (C) Linear incision using a #11 scalpel blade; (D) Expression of purulent material and breakdown of loculations using clamps; (E) Placement of packing into the incision site (optional).

BOX 4: Paronychia.

- Elevate the eponychial fold using a flat probe or #11 blade for drainage
- In extensive infections, incise the area of greatest fluctuance directly into the eponychium with a #11 blade
- Gently probe the wound with a small clamp to ensure thorough drainage **(Figs. 8A and B)**

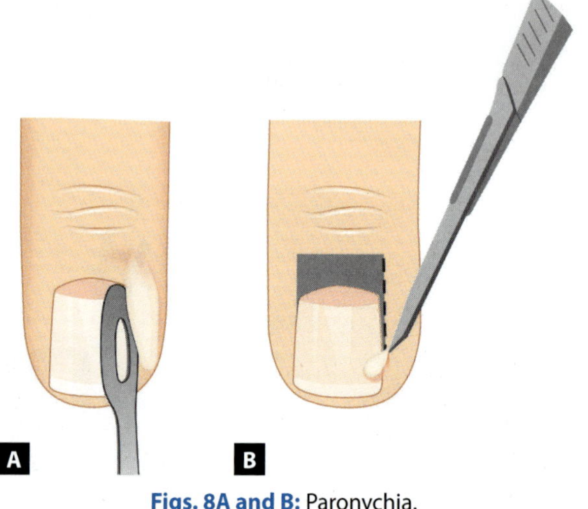

Figs. 8A and B: Paronychia.

BOX 5: Metal needle removal.

For superficial and palpable needles:
- Make an incision at one end to expose the needle
- Grasp the needle with a hemostat

For deeper needles:
- Use an ultrasound probe to locate the needle's long axis
- Make an incision closest to the skin
- Remove the needle with forceps by pulling along its long axis

Alternatively, use an industrial magnet:
- Identify the area of greatest attraction with the magnet
- Prepare and anesthetize the skin
- Make a small incision and place the magnet to attract the metallic foreign body
- Remove the needle by pulling the magnet away from the incision site
- *Caution:* Avoid using magnets in patients with pacemakers or implanted defibrillators

Long, thin foreign bodies perpendicular to the skin:
- Use forceps or hemostats if reachable to pull them straight out
- For deeper foreign bodies, enlarge the entrance wound with a skin incision
- Undermine the skin edges and apply pressure to center the foreign body before removal
- Inspect the needle and wound postremoval to ensure complete extraction **(Figs. 9A and B)**

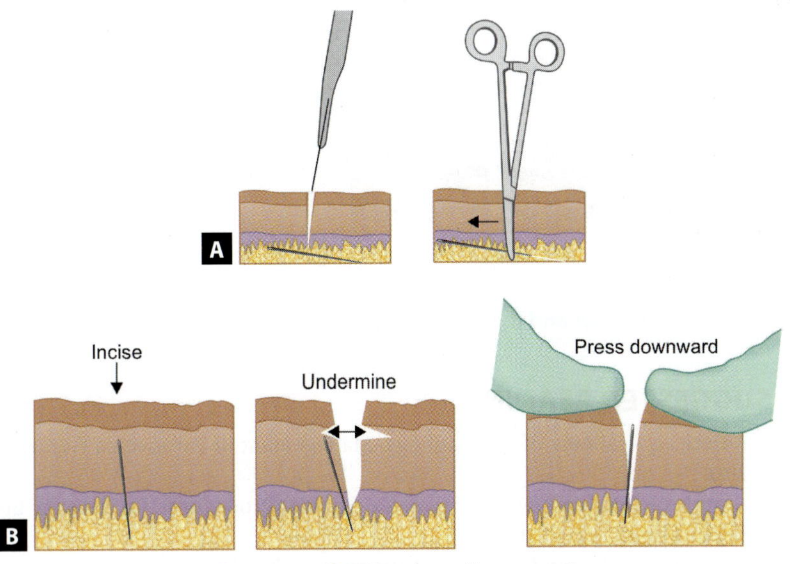

Figs. 9A and B: Metal needle removal.

BOX 6: Wood splinter or organic object removal.

Superficial splinters:
- Grasp and remove with fine-point splinter forceps
- Lift splinters parallel to the skin after incising along their long axis

Subcutaneous splinters:
- Enlarge the entrance wound with a skin incision for direct visualization and removal
- Use ultrasound to confirm the foreign body's location and axis before incising

Wood fragments:
- Create an elliptical incision around the puncture wound
- Extract the fragment within a tissue block, avoiding nerves, vessels, or tendons **(Figs. 10A and B)**

Subungual splinters:
- Remove to prevent infection, including distal phalanx osteomyelitis risk
- Use splinter forceps or a bent hypodermic needle to grasp under the nail
- Anesthetize the finger, remove a wedge of the overlying nail, or remove the entire nail for multiple foreign bodies

Cactus spines in dermis: Use forceps or remove collectively with depilatory wax, facial gel, rubber cement, or household glue

Larger spines and thorns: Remove using incision or excision techniques

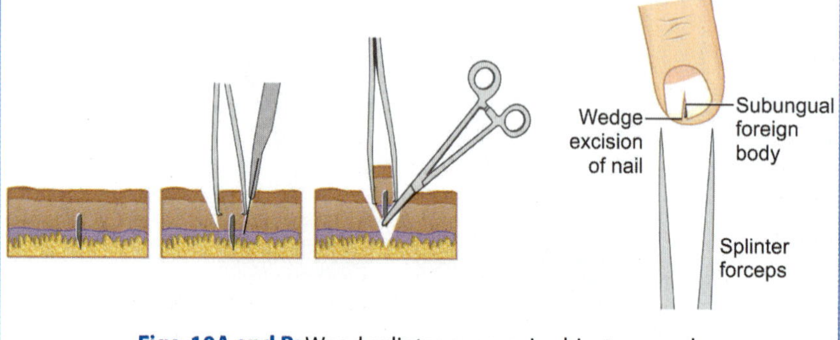

Figs. 10A and B: Wood splinter or organic object removal.

SUGGESTED READING

1. American Academy of Dermatology. Management of Paronychia Guidelines, 2020.
2. American Academy of Emergency Medicine. Procedures for Foreign Body Removal and I &D, 2020.
3. Centers for Disease Control and Prevention. Tick Removal and Prevention Guidelines, 2021.
4. Royal College of Surgeons. Management of Foreign Body Injuries, 2021.

37.2 PULMONARY PROCEDURES

Vimesh Rajput

BOX 1: Tube thoracostomy (Intercostal drain tube insertion).

Indications for thoracostomy in emergency room:
- Pneumothorax
- Tension pneumothorax
- Hemothorax
- Chest trauma with a highly unstable patient, suspected to have pneumothorax/ hemothorax with equivocal ultrasonography-focused assessment with sonography for trauma (USG-FAST)

Materials required:
- Tube thoracostomy tray (needle holder, straight artery, mosquito artery forceps, etc.)
- Implantable cardioverter-defibrillator (ICD) tube (16–32 Fr—as per the indication)
- Underwater seal bag or any collection system
- No 1 Mersilk thread—for ICD fixation
- Local anesthetic—lignocaine 2% (± adrenalin) + 0.5% bupivacaine
- Sterile gowns and drapes
- Glowes/gauze
- Povidone-Iodine or chlorhexidine-based solutions to be used

Choice of chest tube size—based on age (approximate):
- *Adults*: 16–32 Fr depending on the indication
- *Child*: 12–20 Fr
- *Infant*: 8–12 Fr
- *Neonate*: 6–10 Fr

Choice of chest tube size—based on age:
- Pneumothorax—thinner tubes like 12 or 16 Fr
- Hemothorax—broader tubes like 28 or 32 Fr

Choice of site for ICD insertion:
- Triangle of safety **(Fig. 1)** (between anterior and posterior axillary lines and imaginary perpendicular from the nipple level) corresponds to 4th or 5th intercostal space
  - Lower incision increases risk of diaphragm injury and abdominal organ injury
  - Ultrasound guidance if available should be used

*Procedure **(Fig. 2)**:*
- Try and maintain sterility even if it is a procedure in emergency room. Scrub properly and wear sterile gowns
- *Sterile skin preparation and sterile drape:* Local anesthetic infiltration in skin, subcutaneous tissue, intercostal muscle, and up to extrapleural space including the rib periosteum. Use around 5–10 mL of local solution. A trial aspiration by puncturing pleura is better to confirm the presence of air/blood
- Skin incision at appropriate site with no 11 blade. *Make sure the skin incision and the intercostal space are well aligned, in which local anesthetic agent is infiltrated*

Contd...

Contd...

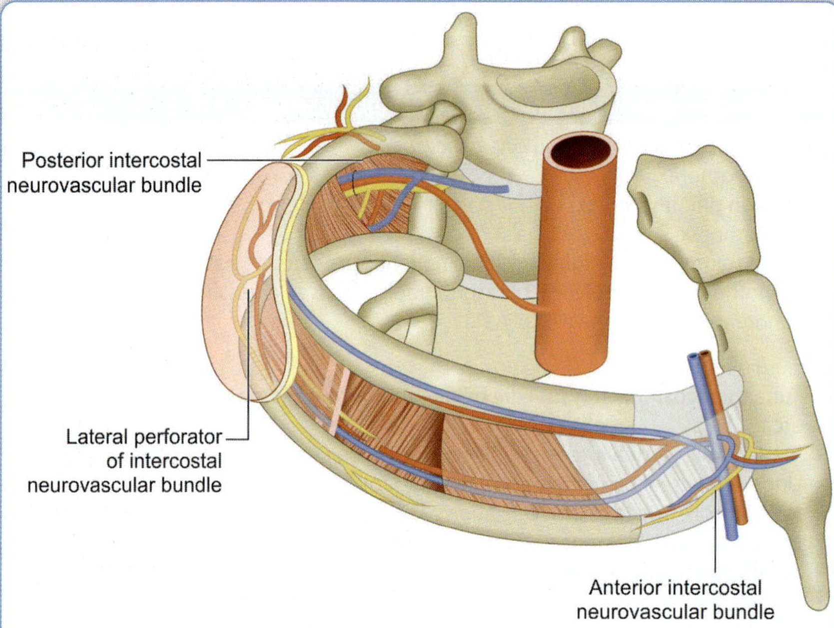

Fig. 1: Safety triangle.

- Blunt dissection with a long Kelly or a straight artery to be done. Gently hold the hemostat with the other hand close to skin to avoid uncontrolled entry into thorax
- Palpate intercostal space and mark superior margin of the inferior rib **(Fig. 2)**
- Use local infiltration liberally as per body weight
- Use Kelly over the upper margin of the rib push to enter the chest wall into the pleural cavity. Keep a guarding finger 1–2 cm away from the tip. Sudden gush of air or fluid occurs
- Make the passage bigger by opening the Kelly (artery) while still inside the pleural space
- Insert a finger in the tract to confirm there are no adhesions. This is not required in case of clear effusion/pneumothorax in a virgin chest
- Before inserting the ICDs have a gross idea of length to be inserted by measuring the TT from incision to mid-point of clavicle
- Hold the proximal end of the ICD and push through the same hole. Make sure you do not make a new tract
- Release the Kelly clamp as soon as you get the feeling of "give way" and keep pushing till the desired length is reached
- All holes of ICD should be in the chest
- Once the ICD is in the chest, fix it with an underwater seal bag or negative suction device
- A deep stitch is to be taken in such a fashion so as to avoid peritubal leak or subcutaneous emphysema with 1-0 silk
- Apply gauze below and above the ICD
- Reinforce the ICD with elastic adhesive bandage so as to prevent dislodgement
- Chest X-ray posteroanterior (PA) view should be done immediately for medicolegal purpose as well as to confirm the position of ICD

Contd...

Contd...

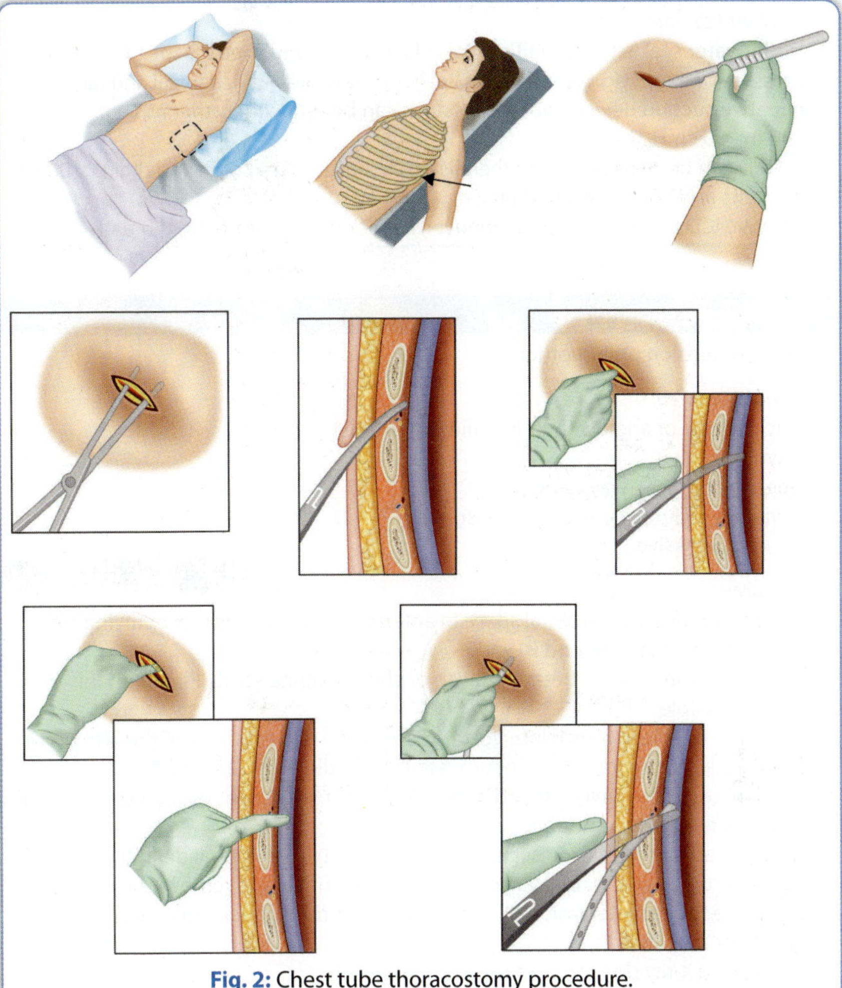

Fig. 2: Chest tube thoracostomy procedure.

Possible complications:
- *Inappropriate placement of ICD:*
  - Reposition if:
    - ICD hole in subcutaneous tissue
    - Placed too far into the chest and causes improper drainage
  - Remove and reinsert if: Placed into the abdominal cavity
- Bleeding
- Hematoma or injury to liver, spleen, heart, or lungs
- Dislodgement of ICD
- Empyema
- Persistent pneumothorax (rarely may require second ICD)
- Re-expansion pulmonary edema
- Subcutaneous emphysema

Contd...

Contd...

Important key points:
- Underwater seal acts as a uniflow valve like system and exerts 8 cmH_2O negative pressure or 6 mm Hg. Newer drains are now available—mechanical and digital negative suction devices where pressures can be reduced further as negative as –40 to –50 cmH_2O
- An ICD can be removed when there is no air leak for >24 hours and drain <100 mL in adults and <50 mL in children
- Remove ICD against Valsalva maneuver, i.e., ask the patient to hold breath

BOX 2: Needle decompression.

Indication: Tension pneumothorax

Materials required:
- Thick needle or angiocatheter (minimum of 16G)
- A syringe
- One-way or three-way valve
- Povidone-iodine or chlorhexidine solution
- Sticking adhesive

Procedure:
- Identify 4th or 5th intercostal space in anterior axillary line after identifying the affected side **(Figs. 3A and B)**
- Cleanse the area with a betadine swab or chlorhexidine scrub. Please do this as fast as possible
- Insert the needle in fourth intercostal space at the upper border of the fifth rib to avoid injury to the intercostal neurovascular bundle **(Figs. 2A and B)**
- Sudden gush of air will be heard with simultaneously patient taking normal breath and vital returning to normal
- On evacuating, the tension secures the chest cavity with ICD till definitive management. If ICD is not available, use angiocatheter and remove the needle and leave the catheter inside till definitive help arrives (if done in emergency setting or roadside)
- Get a chest X-ray done to confirm lung expansion
- Now get CT scan done to confirm or supplement the diagnosis
- Puncturing the second intercostal space in midclavicular line is obsolete

Complications:
- Failure to resolve the tension pneumothorax
- Iatrogenic pneumothorax/lung injury
- Injury to intercostal artery or nerve
- Re-expansion pulmonary edema
- Local inflammation/infections. Empyema

Important key points:
- Procedure should be done on the anterior/midaxillary line in the fourth intercostal space
- To decompress, use a 14-gauge needle for adults at least 2 inches (5 cm) long to penetrate the pleural cavity

Contd...

Contd...

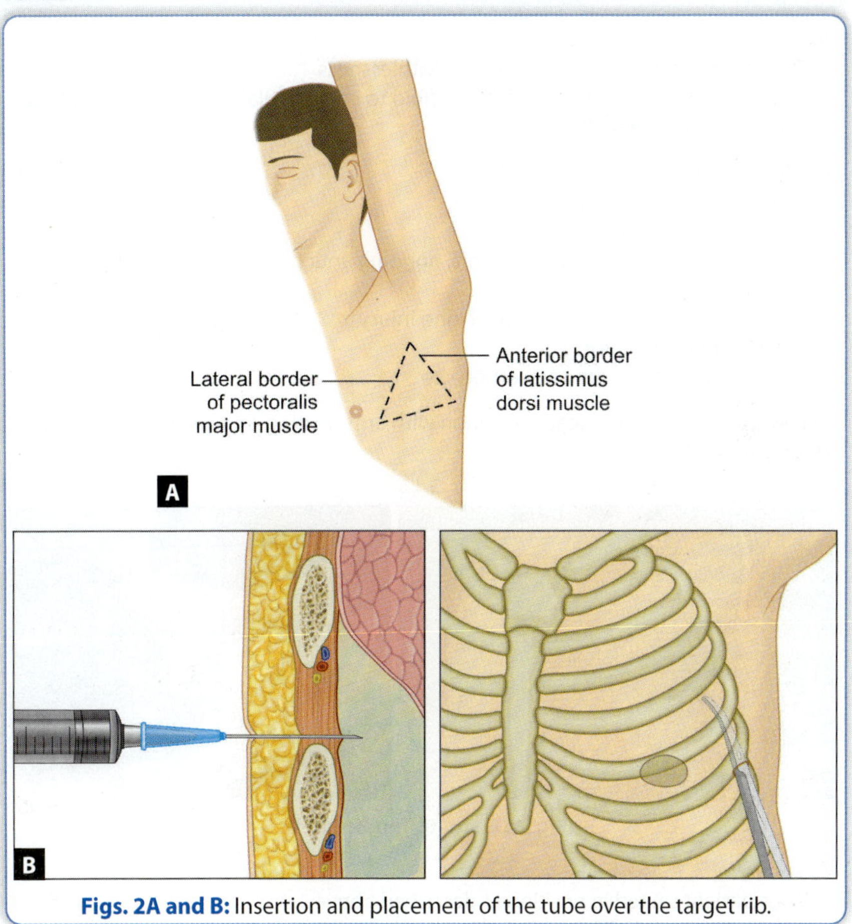

Figs. 2A and B: Insertion and placement of the tube over the target rib.

BOX 3: Thoracocentesis.

Indications:
- *Therapeutic thoracentesis:* To relieve breathlessness
- *Diagnostic thoracentesis:* To collect the fluid to come at diagnosis like tuberculosis or malignant pleural effusion

Contraindications:
- *Absolute:* None
- *Relative:*
  - Coagulopathy, thrombocytopenia, ongoing anticoagulants, or antiplatelet medications
  - Loculated effusion. Possibility of lung injury
  - Patient on ventilator
  - Local infection at site of insertion site

Patient position: Upright, seated position with arms resting on table or a Mayo trolley **(Figs. 3A and B)**

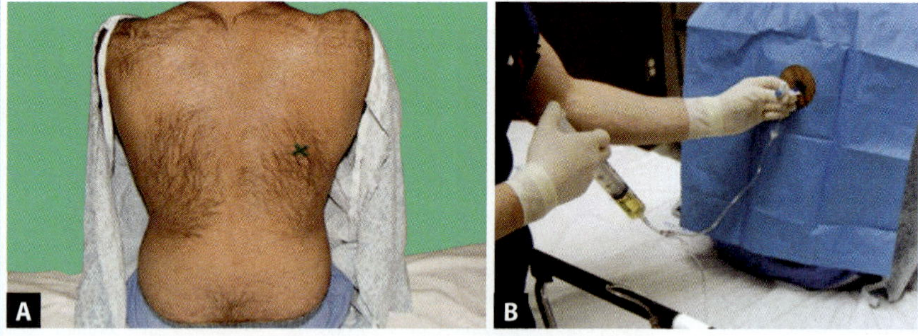

Figs. 3A and B: Thoracentesis.

Procedure:
- Place patient seated in position as described above
- Locate the pleural effusion clinically as well as on a chest X-ray. An ultrasound is the best tool to help in thoracocentesis
- Mark the site of needle insertion. Posterior axillary line or scapular line mark the 8th intercostal space **(Figs. 3A and B)**
  - Never attempt thoracentesis lower to the 8th intercostal space as injury may occur to infradiaphragmatic organs
- After painting draping and giving local anesthesia confirm clinically 8th Intercostal space or mark it with ultrasound guided. Insert the needle (16G–22G) mounted on a syringe. Keep inserting the needle with the piston of syringe pulled to create a negative suction. Once fluid start coming in syringe, stabilize the needle
- It can be a normal 18G needle or 16G angiocath. Remove not >500 mL of fluid at a time
- Carefully remove the needle avoiding excess of fluid drainage or Injury to visceral organs

Contd...

Contd...

Complications:
- Pneumothorax
- Re-expansion pulmonary edema
- Hemothorax or hematoma
- Visceral organ injury
- Air embolism
- Empyema

Considerations:
- Get trained and using ultrasound machine as much as possible
- Reexpansion pulmonary edema is a known complication of thoracentesis
- *Diagnosis:*
  - Pink frothy fluid in cough
  - Drop in saturation
  - X-ray changes
- *Treatment:*
  - Injection frusemide 40–120 mg stat provided mean arterial pressure (MAP) >70 mm Hg
  - High-flow nasal catheter O_2
  - Intubate and ventilate with 12 positive end-expiratory pressure (PEEP)

Important key points:
- Ultrasound helps in reducing the risk of complications
- Do not attempt thoracentesis inferior to the 8th intercostal space
- Avoid thoracentesis on pleural effusions <200 mL confirmed by ultrasound
- Extreme care should be exercised for thoracocentesis in a ventilated patient. Use ultrasound always in a ventilated patient

SUGGESTED READING

1. https://www.ests.org/about_ests/textbook.aspx.
2. Shields' General Thoracic Surgery.

37.3 PEDIATRIC PROCEDURES

Sachna P Shetty

BOX 1: Intraosseous access.

- *Indications:*
  - *During cardiac arrest:* If vascular access cannot be achieved after three attempts at peripheral intravenous access
  - When vascular access is unattainable in pediatric patients experiencing shock due to hemorrhage (trauma), sepsis, severe dehydration, or cardiac failure
- *Contraindications:*
  - *Absolute:* Fracture of the long bone
  - *Relative:* Previous intraosseous access attempt in the same long bone, cellulitis over the insertion site, injury to the inferior vena cava (prefer circulatory access proximal to the injury site), and osteogenesis imperfecta
- *Procedure:*
  - *Preferred site:* Proximal tibia
  - Position the patient supine with the knee flexed approximately 90°
  - Locate the tibial tuberosity, then move 2 cm distal and 2 cm medial from the tuberosity. This area is consistently flat and below the growth plate
  - Follow aseptic protocols
  - Insert the needle **(Fig. 1)** through the skin and subcutaneous tissue to the bone cortex
  - Stabilize the intraosseous device once the bone is reached
  - Apply steady, firm downward pressure with a twisting motion until the cortex is penetrated and the marrow space is reached with no resistance
  - Remove the inner trocar
  - Aspirate the marrow or infiltrate saline if there is no resistance, then connect the intravenous line **(Figs. 2 and 3)**
- *Alternative sites:*
  - Distal tibia
  - Distal femur
  - Proximal humerus

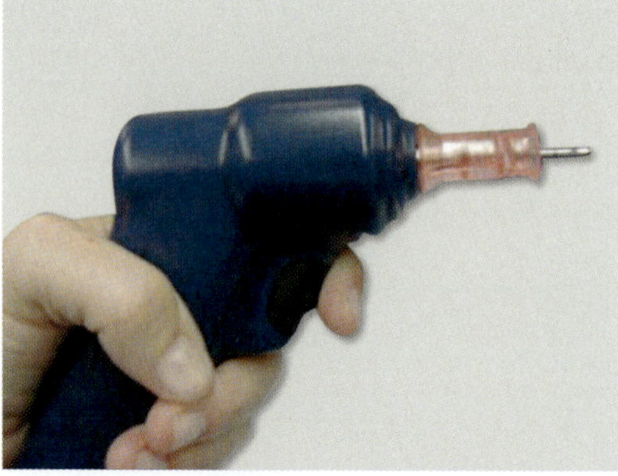

Fig. 1: Intraosseous access drilling gun.

Contd...

Contd...

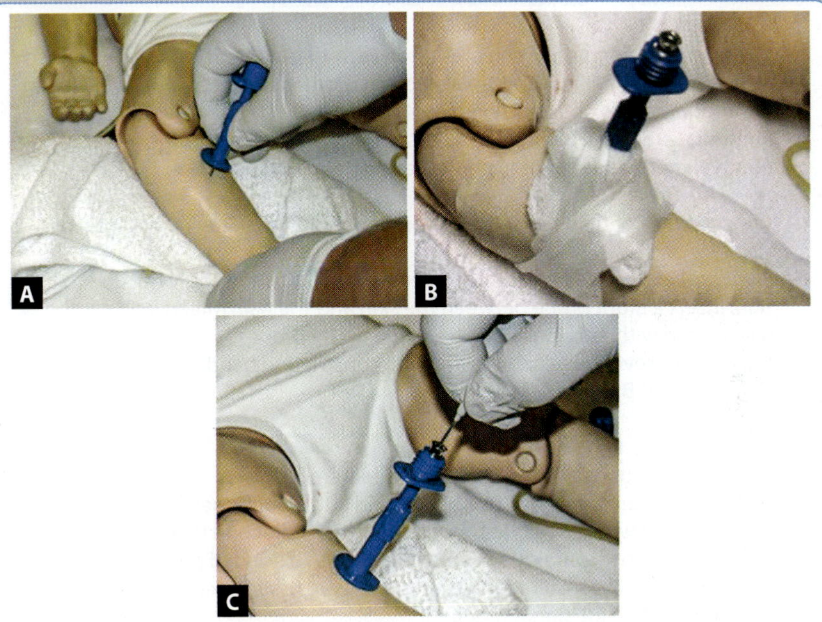

Figs. 2A to C: Procedure for the insertion of an intraosseous cannula in distal tibia.

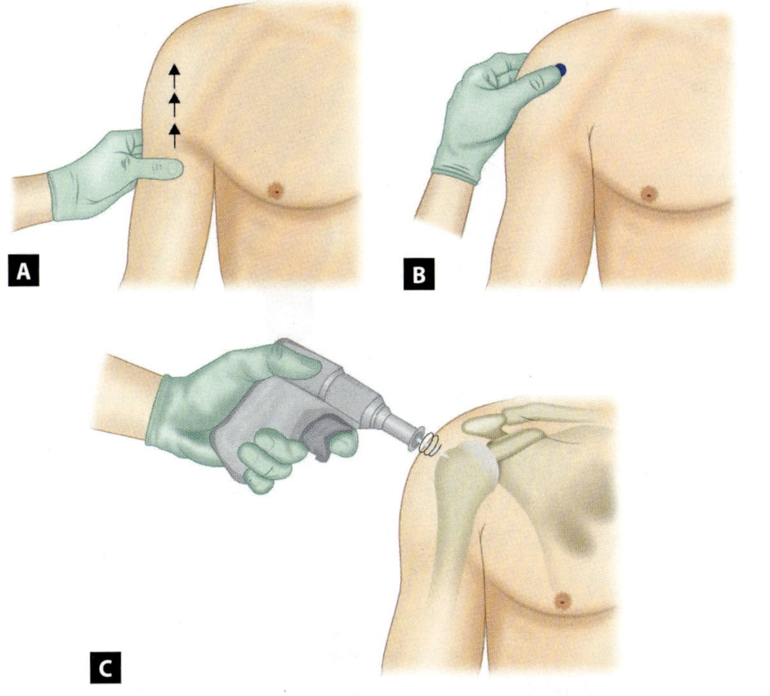

Figs. 3A to C: IO insertion into proximal humerus site.

BOX 2: Hair or thread removal.

- *Indications:*
  - Consider this diagnosis when presented with a limb that has a clearly defined circumferential, painful, and swollen distal segment next to a nonswollen and nonreddened proximal portion **(Fig. 4)**
  - Immediate removal is critical in all cases of tourniquet syndrome, with the removal method depending on the severity of the constriction
- *Removal methods:*
  - *Unwrapping:* For minimal or no edema where the offending hair or thread is visible
  - *Blunt probe cutting:* For mild-to-moderate edema, gently apply traction to the skin, insert a blunt probe between the skin and the hair/thread, and cut the hair/thread with a scalpel along the edge of the probe
  - *Incision:* For severe swelling or when the constricting band is not visible **(Figs. 5A and B)**
- *Caveats:*
  - All tourniquets must be removed
  - Identify the knot or bunched area for easier removal
  - Document neurovascular status before and after tourniquet removal
  - A 24-hour follow-up is mandatory, and return of color and blood flow may take several days if the tourniquet was in place for an extended period
  - Consider surgical consultation in cases of severe tissue edema, distorted anatomy, or if an incision is required

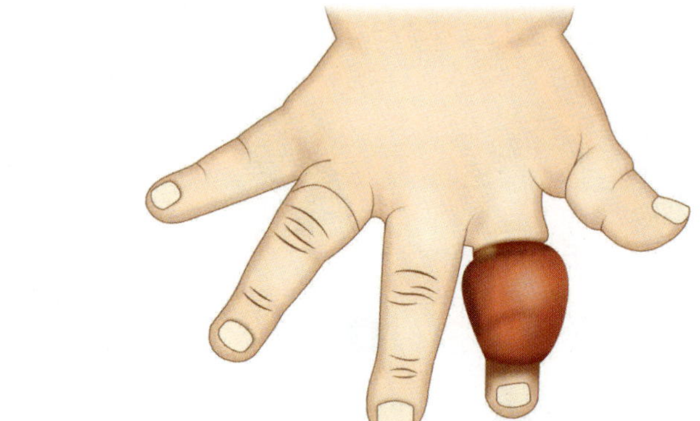

Fig. 4: Hair tourniquet.

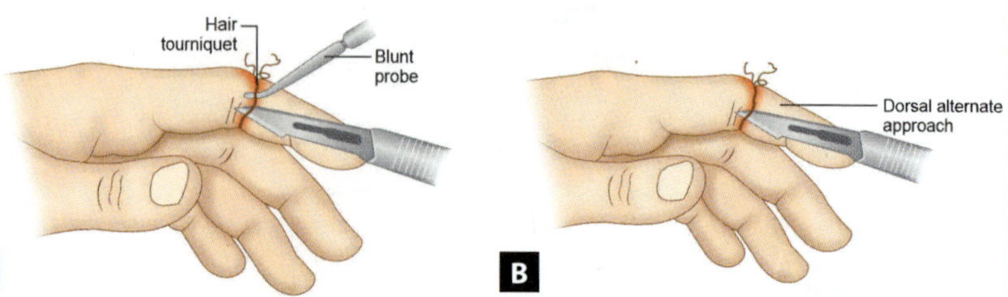

Figs. 5A and B: (A) Blunt and cut method for a tourniquet; (B) Preferable incision at 12 o'clock.

BOX 3: Penile entrapment with zipper.

- This common injury involves entrapment of the penis or scrotum in a zipper
- Interventions may include dismantling the zipper with wire cutters or surgical procedures such as circumcision
- The area should be cleansed, and local anesthesia provided
- Various methods can be used to free the zipper, including coating it with a lubricant, pulling the zipper in the opposite direction, cutting the zipper from clothing for easier handling, or cutting the sliding bar and zipper teeth
- The bottom bar of the zipper can also be cut to unzip from below

SUGGESTED READING

1. American Academy of Pediatrics. Hair Thread Tourniquet Syndrome and Other Constrictive Injuries in Children, 2022.
2. American Heart Association. Advanced Cardiovascular Life Support (ACLS) Provider Manual, 2023.
3. American Urological Association. Urological Injury Management, 2021.

37.4 FACE AND DENTAL PROCEDURES

Sachna P Shetty

BOX 1: Dislocated mandibular relocation.

Indications dislocated mandible

Procedure	• Patient should be in a sitting position with the mandible placed at the physician's comfortable position • Place the thumbs on the mandibular molars with a gauze wrapped around the thumbs to protect from patient's possible bite • Apply force in an inferior or downward direction, with the chin rotating upward and backwards **(Figs. 1A to C)**

Contraindication confirm if any displaced fracture of mandible is present as it might require surgical repair

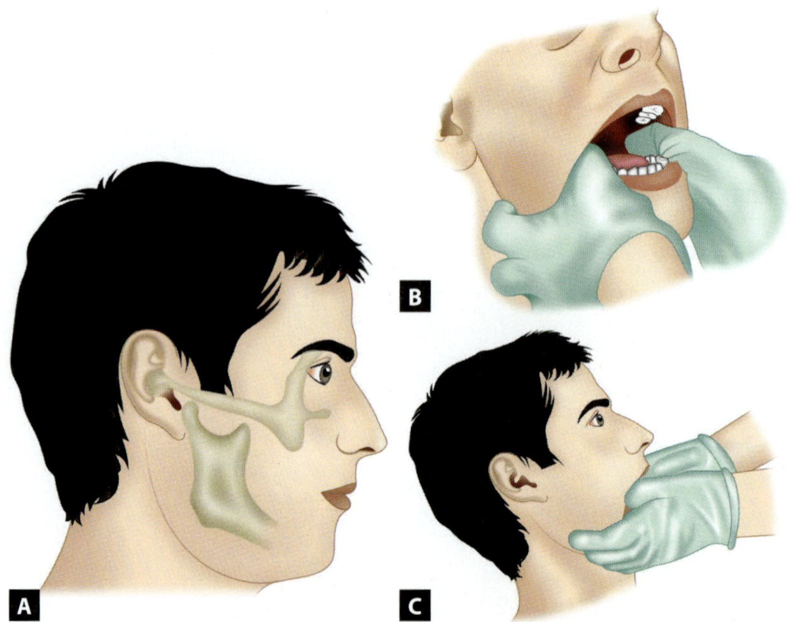

Figs. 1A to C: *Reduction in progress:* (A) In cases of mandibular dislocation, the condyle will be positioned anteriorly and superiorly to the articular eminence; (B) Place your thumbs on the mandibular molars and apply steady, downward pressure to help distract the temporomandibular (TM) joint condyles, allowing them to move back into the glenoid fossa for proper joint reduction; (C) In the lateral view, the distraction force is directed downward to move the TM joint condyle.

BOX 2: Postextraction hemorrhage control.

Indications	Recent tooth extraction site, presenting with more than indicated bleeding from the site of extraction
Contraindications	None
Procedure	• Suction the site gently, look for any clot in the extraction site and if any remove it • Look for the source of hemorrhage • Place a saline-dipped gauze at the extracted site • Instruct the patient to apply firm biting pressure, and observe for 1 hour • Frequent change of gauze might be required • If bleeding persists, an intraoral nerve block should be performed • Blocks are preferred to infiltrations as only gives temporary relief • Gently curetting of dental sockets and removal of old blood clot or granulation tissue must be done • Also look for associated arterial bleeding and if localized to soft tissue, use pressure or tie-off vessels if source identified • Fold Gel foam can also be placed on the bleeding site **(Fig. 2)** • Blood products in case of coagulopathy might be required • Follow-up with dentist
Complications	Continued bleeding due to coagulopathy or medication use or patient incompliance

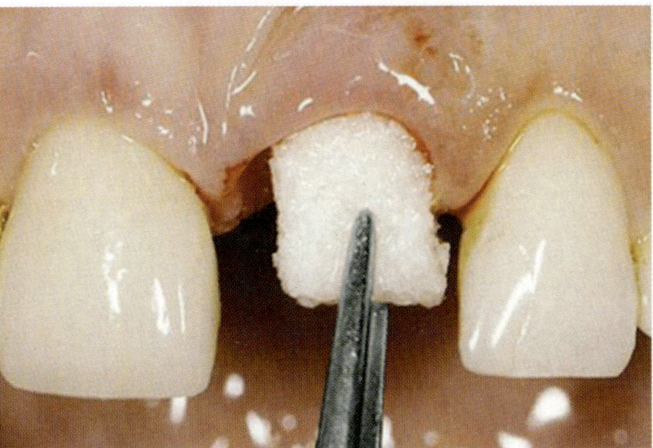

Fig. 2: Gelfoam in an extraction socket to prevent bleeding.

SUGGESTED READING

1. American College of Surgeons. Advanced Trauma Life Support: Student Course Manual. 10th ed. Chicago, IL: American College of Surgeons; 2018.
2. Killey & Kay, 1975; Fernández Sanromán, et al., 1998.
3. Malmquist, Clemens, & Wilson, 1999; Moore & Hersh, 2013.
4. Tintinalli JE, Ma OJ, Yearly DM, Meckler GD, Stapczynski JS, Cline DM. Tintinalli's Emergency Medicine: A Comprehensive Study Guide, 9th edition. New York: McGraw Hill; 2021.
5. Tintinalli JE, O. John MA, Yealy D, Meckler GD, J. Stephan Stapczynski, Cline DM, et al. Tintinalli's Emergency Medicine: A Comprehensive Study Guide, 9th edition. McGraw Hill Professional; 2019.
6. Walls RM, Hockberger RS, Gausche-Hill M. Rosen's Emergency Medicine: Concepts and Clinical Practice. Philadelphia, PA: Elsevier; 2018.

CHAPTER

38 Orthopedic Procedures

38.1 REDUCTION, SPLINTS, AND CASTS

Darius F Soonawalla

BOX 1: Splints, slabs, and casts.

- Splints, slabs, and casts are used to immobilize a limb, reducing pain and swelling
- Splints and slabs are noncircumferential accommodating swelling, and hence are safer
- Casts are circumferential, providing better immobilization, but do not permit swelling
- Slabs and casts are made from plaster of Paris or fiber cast bandages and molded onto the limb **(Fig. 1)**

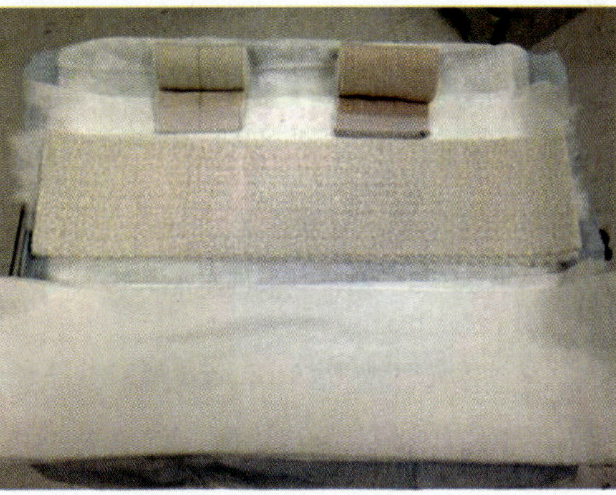

Fig. 1: Plaster of Paris and soft roll.

BOX 2: Analgesia for orthopedic procedures.

- Achieve adequate pain relief prior to attempting any reduction maneuver
- Pain relief should be tailored to the presentation and patient
- Assess safety prior to administration

Modalities used are: (mentioned in the Chapter 14)

- Hematoma block, for example, distal radius fracture
- Peripheral nerve block, for example, ring block for fingers and toes
- Intravenous (IV) agents
- Inhalation agents

BOX 3: Application of a slab.

- A stockinette may be applied on the limb first (optional)
- Cover the limb with cast padding applied in a spiral manner
- Determine the length of the slab required
- Prepare the slab using adequate layers of the plaster of Paris or fiber cast
- Dip the slab in water and gently squeeze excess water out
- An assistant holds the padded limb in the required position and the slab is placed longitudinally on the desired location
- Apply a roller bandage to fix slab in place. This molds slab to the limb
- Allow slab to harden, holding the limb immobile in the desired position **(Figs. 2A to C)**

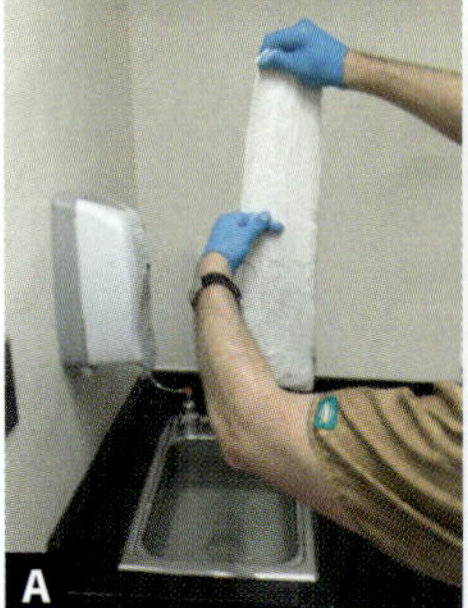

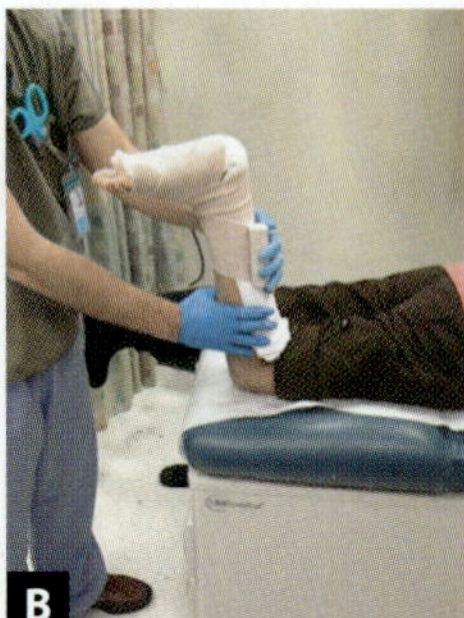

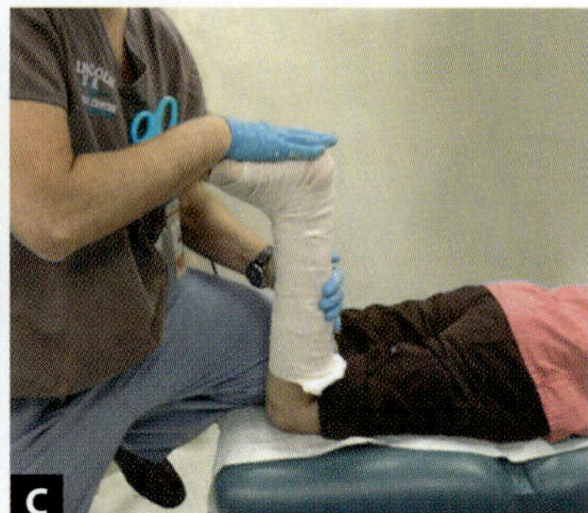

Figs. 2A to C: Application of a slab. (A) Securely hold the top of the saturated plaster with one hand using the other hand to remove excess water; (B) Use an Ace wrap to secure the slab and help contour it to the patient's extremity; and (C) Maintain the slab in a neutral anatomical position, ensuring that you avoid creating indentations with your fingertips.

BOX 4: Reduction of shoulder (glenohumeral) dislocation.

- Multiple reduction techniques are present. The traction–countertraction technique is easy and safe
- Achieve adequate analgesia or mild sedation
- Position of the patient should be supine
- Assistant provides countertraction with a bedsheet across thorax in the axilla
- With elbow bent, apply sustained traction on limb
- Reduction can be felt
- Immobilize with arm sling or shoulder immobilizer **(Figs. 3A to D)**

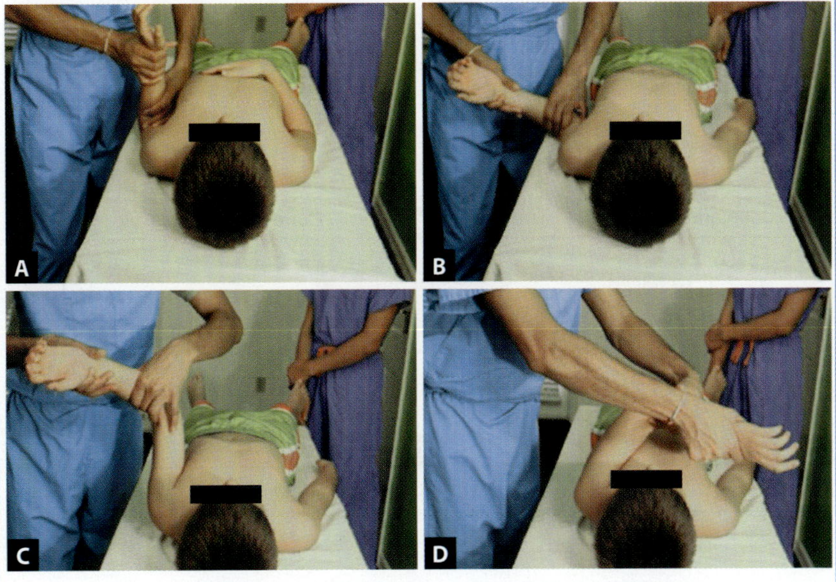

Figs. 3A to D: Reduction of shoulder (glenohumeral) dislocation.

BOX 5: Reduction of Colles' fracture.

- A Colles' fracture is a distal radius fracture with dorsal angulation
- All significantly displaced distal radius fractures should be reduced before splinting, even if surgery is planned. This helps in reducing swelling
- Give a hematoma block by entering the fracture site dorsally
- Aspirating blood confirms that the fracture site has been accessed
- About 6 cm^3 of 1% lignocaine should be injected
- Assistant supports limb just below elbow
- Apply gentle traction by holding thumb and radial three fingers
- A dorsal slab is applied from below the elbow to just proximal to the knuckles **(Figs. 4A to D)**

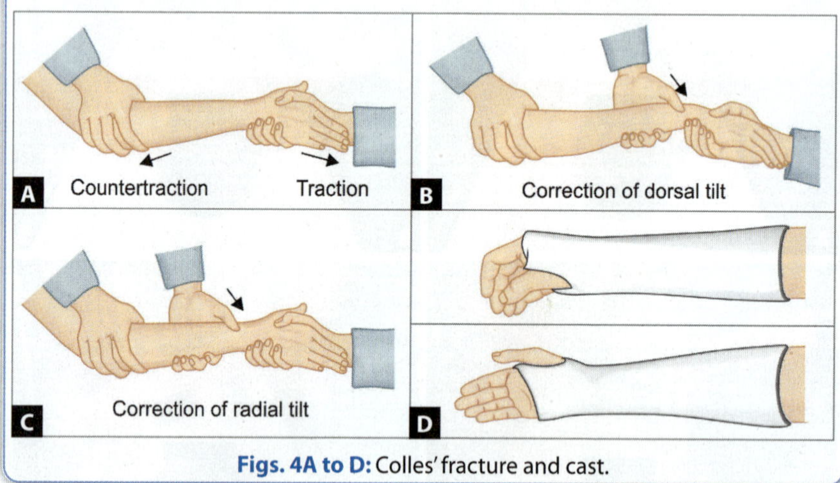

Figs. 4A to D: Colles' fracture and cast.

BOX 6: Reduction of interphalangeal joint dislocations.

- Ring block is given at the base of the finger
- Reduction is achieved by giving traction
- Immobilize with buddy strapping **(Fig. 5)**

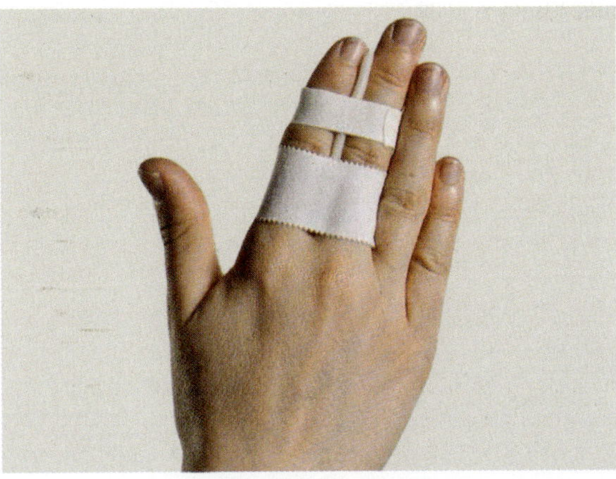

Fig. 5: Buddy strapping.

BOX 7: Commonly used splints.

Injury	***Method of immobilization***
Clavicle fracture	Figure of 8, brace with arm sling
Shoulder dislocation	Shoulder immobilizer
Proximal humerus fractures	Shoulder immobilizer
Shaft humerus fracture	U-slab with arm sling
Elbow and forearm injuries	Above elbow posterior slab with arm sling
Distal radius and wrist injuries	Below elbow slab with arm sling
Thumb injuries	Thumb spica splint
Metacarpal fractures	Short volar slab including wrist and proximal finger
Phalangeal fractures	Buddy strapping or finger cot splint
Mallet finger and distal digit injuries	Mallet finger splint
Pelvis fractures	Pelvic binder
Hip and femur fractures	Skin traction
Knee injuries	Long knee brace
Tibia fractures	Above knee posterior slab
Ankle injuries	Below knee posterior slab
Foot injuries	Short below knee posterior slab

SUGGESTED READING

1. Roberts JR. Roberts and Hedge's Clinical Procedures in Emergency Medicine and Acute Care, 7th edition. Amsterdam, Netherlands: Elsevier; 2017.
2. Walls R, Hockberger R, Gausche-Hill, Erickson TB, Wilcox SR. Rosen's Emergency Medicine: Concepts and Clinical Practice, 10th edition. Amsterdam, Netherlands: Elsevier; 2022.

CHAPTER 39

Obstetric Emergencies

Nidhi Shah Gandhi

BOX 1: Fetal heart rate (FHR).

- Fetal heartbeat is first heard sonographically at 6 weeks of gestation
- With the development of the cardiac system heart rate increases to 160 beats/min (BPM) by 10 weeks and then starts declining and is approximately 135–140 bpm by term

Principle:

- To ensure general fetal wellbeing and determine the presence of any fetal distress based on the direction and magnitude of periodic fluctuations in the heart rate
- Fetal heart rate is characterized by variability (5 BPM) over time and includes transient, accelerations of heart rate above the baseline with fetal movements and this is reassuring of fetal health
- In contrast, loss of variability and decelerations (i.e., significant slowing of heart rate well below baseline levels) is indicative of neural compromise or fetal distress

Components of FHR monitoring:

- *Baseline:*
  - <110 BPM is fetal bradycardia
  - >160 BPM is fetal tachycardia
- *Variability:*
  - Absent—0 amplitude
  - Minimal—amplitude 0–5 bpm
  - Moderate—amplitude 6–25 bpm
  - Marked—amplitude over 25 bpm
- *Accelerations:*
  - >32 weeks: Peak ≥15 bpm above baseline lasting for ≥15 seconds
  - <32 weeks: peak ≥10 bpm above baseline lasting for ≥10 seconds
- *Decelerations:*
  - Early (head compression): Uniform shape, lowest point of curve corresponds to the peak of contraction
  - Late (placental insufficiency): Uniform shape but a gradual change with the lowest point occurring after the peak of contraction
  - Variable (Cord compression): Vary in shape, duration, and intensity; no constant relation with the peak of contraction

Indications for FHR monitoring include:

- Routinely at every antenatal visit post 10–12 weeks
- High-risk pregnancies such as multiple pregnancies, preeclampsia, diabetes, growth restriction, or bleeding during pregnancy
- During labor and delivery

Contd...

Contd...

Indications for continuous fetal monitoring during Labor:

- Augmentation of labor with oxytocin
- Meconium-stained liquor
- Abnormal fetal monitoring an FHR <110 BPM or >160 BPM
- Postcontraction decelerations
- Maternal pyrexia (defined as 38.0°C once or 37.5°C on two occasions 2 hours apart)
- Unexplained fresh bleeding

Methods of FHR monitoring:

- *Auscultation monitoring:* Listening to the FHR every 15 minutes during the first stage of labor and every 5 minutes during the second stage
- *Electronic FHR monitoring:*
  - Provides continuous, real-time monitoring of FHR
  - Can be done using Doppler ultrasound or internal fetal electrocardiography (ECG)
  - External monitoring with Doppler ultrasound is preferred because it is noninvasive. If external monitoring is difficult due to poor signal quality or technical issues, invasive monitoring may be required

Procedure:

- Position the patient supine
- Palpate the maternal abdomen to locate the approximate position of the fetal heart (locate fetal back)
- Apply ultrasound gel to the maternal abdomen where fetal cardiac activity is expected
- Place the transducer probe on the gel and locate the fetal heart tones
- Once located, secure the FHR sensor to the maternal abdomen with the belt
- Position the contraction monitor sensor near the fundus to monitor uterine contractions
- Connect the FHR sensor and contraction monitor to the electronic FHR monitor to obtain FHR and uterine contraction printouts

BOX 2: Vaginal delivery.

Indications	Cervix fully dilated at 10 cm and fully effaced 1 mm with crowning of the head
Contraindications	• *Absolute:* – Indications for emergency cesarean section (C section) – Prolapsed cord – Prior C section with classic vertical incision – Placenta previa—complete/partial – Breech presentation—footling • *Relative:* – Placenta previa—marginal/low lying – Breech presentation—complete/incomplete/frank
Procedure	• Determine the fetal presentation (breech or cephalic) with Leopold's maneuvers or bedside ultrasound • If breech, follow the breech pathway • Perform a vaginal examination • Check for cord prolapse • Check effacement • Check dilation • Prepare the site • Position the mother in the extreme lithotomy position • If episiotomy required, give local anesthesia • At the time of crowning of head, give right/left mediolateral episiotomy • With good uterine contractions and maternal bearing down efforts, deliver the head in a controlled manner • Check for cord around the neck. If present, release it • Deliver the anterior shoulder with downward traction of the head • Check for shoulder dystocia. If present, follow the McRobert Rubin maneuvers • Deliver the posterior shoulder by gently pulling the trunk upward • Delayed cord clamping after milking the cord around 5 cm from the umbilicus in two places and cut • Obtain Apgar score of the baby. Initiate resuscitation if required • Keep the baby warm in the incubator • Deliver the placenta spontaneously and completely using gentle controlled traction on the clamp with one hand while placing the other hand suprapubically to push the uterus upward • If the placenta does not deliver easily, stop and wait a few minutes to allow it to come away from the uterine wall naturally and then try again • Placenta must be fully intact. If not, check for retained intrauterine placental products, and manually remove them; retained placenta may cause postpartum hemorrhage • Massage the fundus externally to prevent uterine atony, but only after all products have been removed • Repair episiotomy under all aseptic precautions or any vaginal or cervical lacerations using Vicryl rapid

BOX 3: Breech delivery.

Definition	• Breech presentation is defined as a fetus in a longitudinal lie with the buttocks or feet closest to the cervix • Incidence—34% of all deliveries at term
Types of breech presentation	• *Frank breech (50–70%):* Hips flexed, knees extended (pike position), and buttocks are the presenting part • *Complete breech (5–10%):* Hips and knees flexed (cannon ball position), buttocks +/ heels as presenting part • *Footling or incomplete (10–30%):* One or both hips extended, foot is the presenting part
Predisposing factors for breech presentation	• Prematurity • Uterine malformations • Fibroids • Polyhydramnios • Placenta previa • Fetal abnormalities such as central nervous system (CNS) malformations, neck masses, and aneuploidy • Multiple pregnancies
Types of vaginal breech deliveries	• *Spontaneous breech delivery:* No traction or manipulation is used. This generally occurs in very preterm, often previable, deliveries • *Assisted breech delivery:* It is the most common type. The infant is allowed to deliver spontaneously up to the umbilicus, post which assistance is used with the help of maneuvers to deliver the body, arms, and head • *Total breech extraction:* The fetal feet are grasped, and the entire fetus is extracted. Total breech extraction should be used only for a noncephalic second twin; it should not be used for a singleton fetus because the cervix may not be adequately dilated to allow passage of the fetal head
Indications for vaginal delivery	• Frank/complete breech presentation • >36 weeks of gestation • Estimated fetal weight between 2.5 and 3.5 kg • Flexed fetal head • Adequate maternal pelvis • No obstetric complications
Mechanism of delivery	• Engagement • Descent • Internal rotation • Lateral flexion • External rotation • Delivery of breech then body and lastly the after coming head **(Figs. 5A to D)**

Contd...

Contd...

Technique	• The fetal membranes should be left intact as long as possible to act as a dilating wedge and to prevent overt cord prolapse • Oxytocin induction and augmentation are controversial • Ensure immediate availability of pediatrician and anesthesiologist for all vaginal breech deliveries • Liberal episiotomy even in multiparas, to prevent soft tissue dystocia of the aftercoming head • Generally, follow a no touch technique unto the delivery of the umbilicus, no pull, or traction at any point • Delivery of the anterior buttock, baby's anus, and then the posterior buttock • Delivery of the trunk and lower limbs • Ensure the bank is anterior • Hold the trunk with a sterile towel to avoid the baby from slipping • Delivery of the posterior shoulder followed by the anterior shoulder • Ask the assistant to apply suprapubic pressure to maintain the head in flexed position • Delivery of the head by flexion in the order of the chin, mouth, nose, forehead, vertex, and occiput successively • *Burns–Marshall method for delivery of after coming head* allow baby to hang by its own weight, assistant applies supra pubic pressure, when the nape of the neck appears under the pubic arch, grasp the baby by the ankles with the fingers in between the two ankles and deliver the trunk by applying a steady traction in a wide arc swinging the trunk upward and forward, trunk is now depressed to deliver the vertex and occiput **(Figs. 6A to D)** • *Other methods:* Piper's forceps • *Modified Mauriceau–Smellie–Veit technique (malar flexion and shoulder traction):* Place the baby on the supinated left forearm with the hands hanging on either side • To maintain flexion of head, place the index and middle fingers of the left hand on the malar bones on either side • Place the ring and little finger of pronated right hand on the baby's right shoulder, index finger on the left shoulder, and the middle finger on the suboccipital region • Apply downward and backward traction till the nape of the neck appears below the pubic arch, now deliver the baby by following the steps as under Burns–Marshall method • *Frank breech extraction (Pinard's Maneuver)* introduces the middle and index finger up to the popliteal fossa and applies pressure and abducts the leg so that frank breech is converted to footling breech, grasp the foot at the ankle, and complete breech extraction • *Lovset's maneuver for extended arms:* Lift the baby to cause lateral flexion, rotate the trunk through 180° keeping the back anterior—delivery of posterior arm by hooking it at the elbow joint, rotate the bay in reverse direction, and deliver anterior arm similarly

BOX 4: Shoulder dystocia.

Definition	• Failure of delivery of fetal shoulders with normal traction on the fetal head • Objective criteria—head to body delivery *of >60 seconds* or the need for additional maneuvers to deliver the baby • Occurs in 0.3–3% of all vaginal deliveries
Management	*HELPERR mnemonic:* *H*—call for *Help* *E*—evaluate for *Episiotomy* *L—Legs:* Use of *McRoberts maneuver (knee to chest)* to press the thighs up against the belly so as to flatten and rotate the pelvis **(Fig. 4)** *P—Pressure:* Suprapubic pressure in an attempt to rotate and deliver the shoulder *E—Enter rotational maneuvers:* • *Rubin II rotational:* Placing two fingers on the posterior aspect of anterior shoulder and then rotating it by 30° toward the fetal chest **(Figs. 1A and B)** • *Woods corkscrew rotational:* Finger placement as per Rubin II maneuver and add two fingers on the anterior aspect of posterior shoulder and rotate the fetus 180° **(Figs. 2A and B)** • *Reverse Woods Corkscrew rotational:* The fingers are placed on the anterior aspect of anterior shoulder and posterior aspect of posterior shoulder to rotate the fetus 180° *R—Remove posterior arm: Jacquemier's maneuver* introduces the hand between the perineum and fetus, slides across the fetal chest, grasps the posterior wrist using an OK sign, and sweeps it across the fetal chest *R – Roll the patient: Gaskin all—fours maneuver (on hands and knees)* *In severe cases:* • *Intentional clavicle fracture* • *Zavanelli maneuver:* Rotate fetal head to occiput anterior position, flex the neck so chin rests on the perineum, push head gently in the vagina, and apply constant pressure to hold the head in place, another obstetrician performs C section to deliver the baby **(Figs. 3A and B)** • *Abdominal rescue under anesthesia:* Hysterotomy incision and manipulation to release the impacted shoulder followed by vaginal delivery
Complications	• Clavicle/humerus fracture • Brachial plexus injury • Hypoxia leading to ischemic encephalopathy • Intrauterine fetal death (IUFD) • Maternal trauma to the bladder, urethra, vagina, rectum, or the anal sphincter • Postpartum hemorrhage • Lateral femoral cutaneous neuropathy

Contd...

Contd...

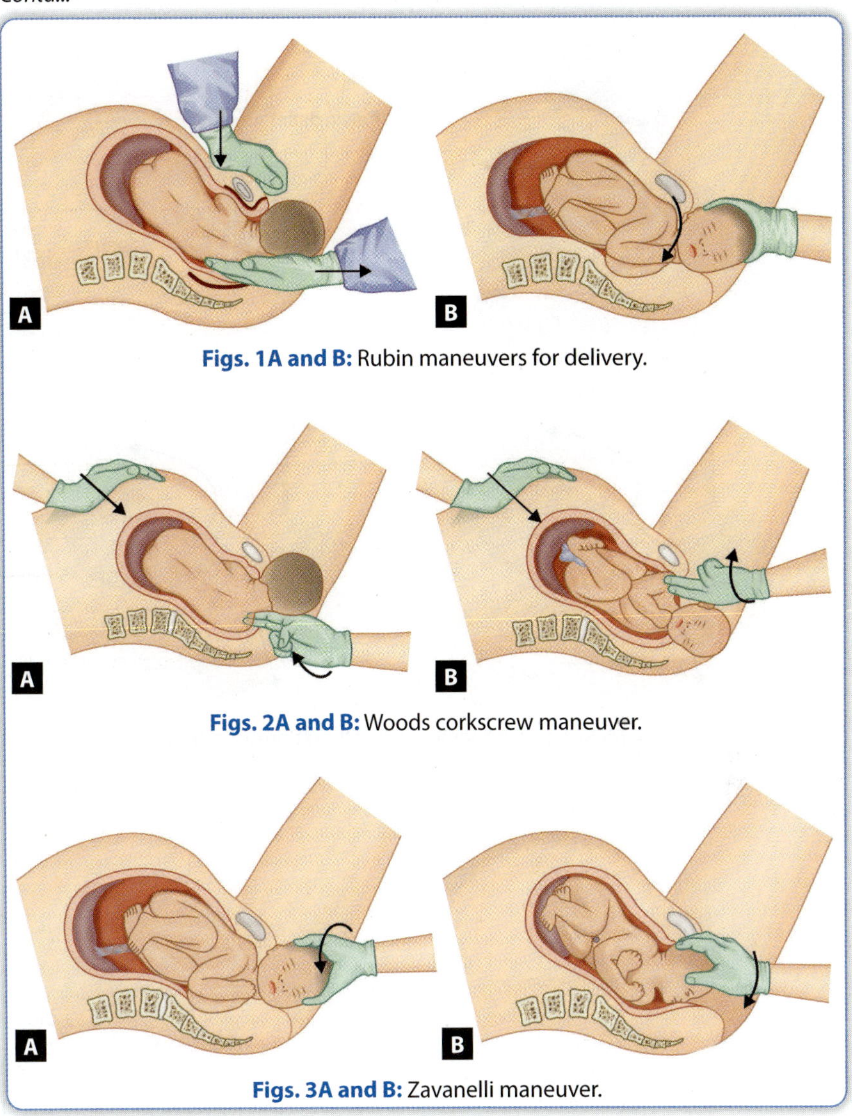

Figs. 1A and B: Rubin maneuvers for delivery.

Figs. 2A and B: Woods corkscrew maneuver.

Figs. 3A and B: Zavanelli maneuver.

Contd...

Contd...

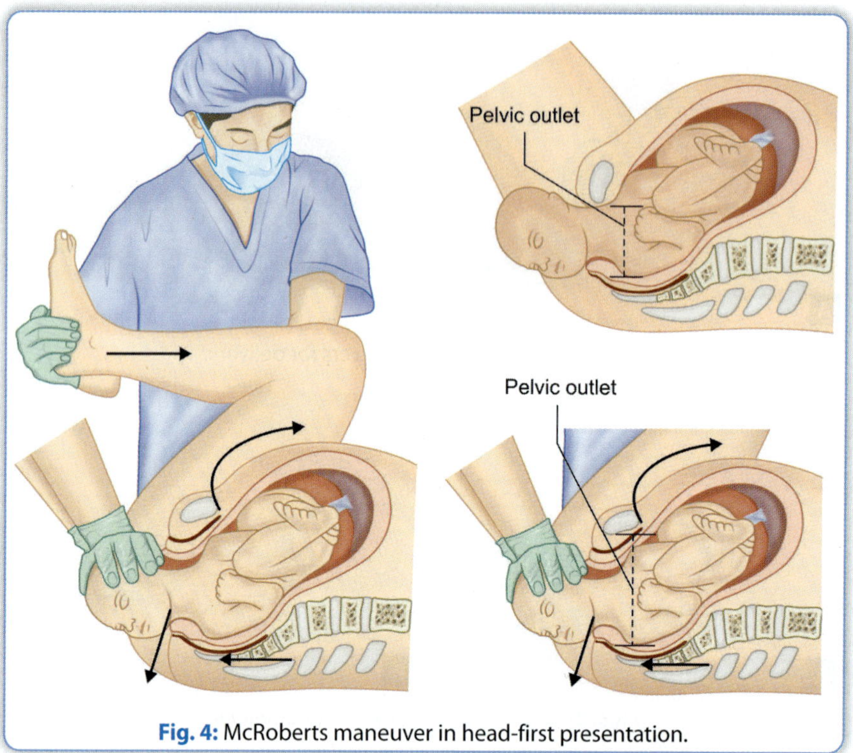

Fig. 4: McRoberts maneuver in head-first presentation.

Contd...

Contd...

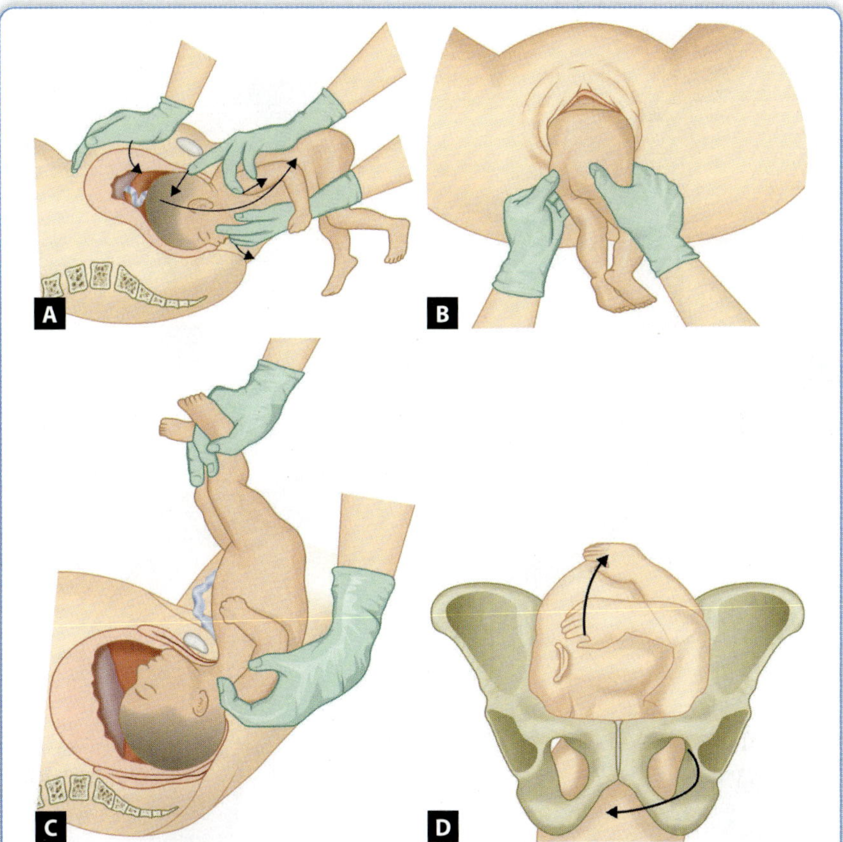

Figs. 5A to D: Techniques of delivery in various scenarios: (A) delivery of head in flexed position; (B) Correct hand placement on sacrum; (C) Correct head placement in case the abdomen is facing the anterior; and (D) Rotation toward maternal symphysis pubis to avoid nuchal arm.

Contd...

Contd...

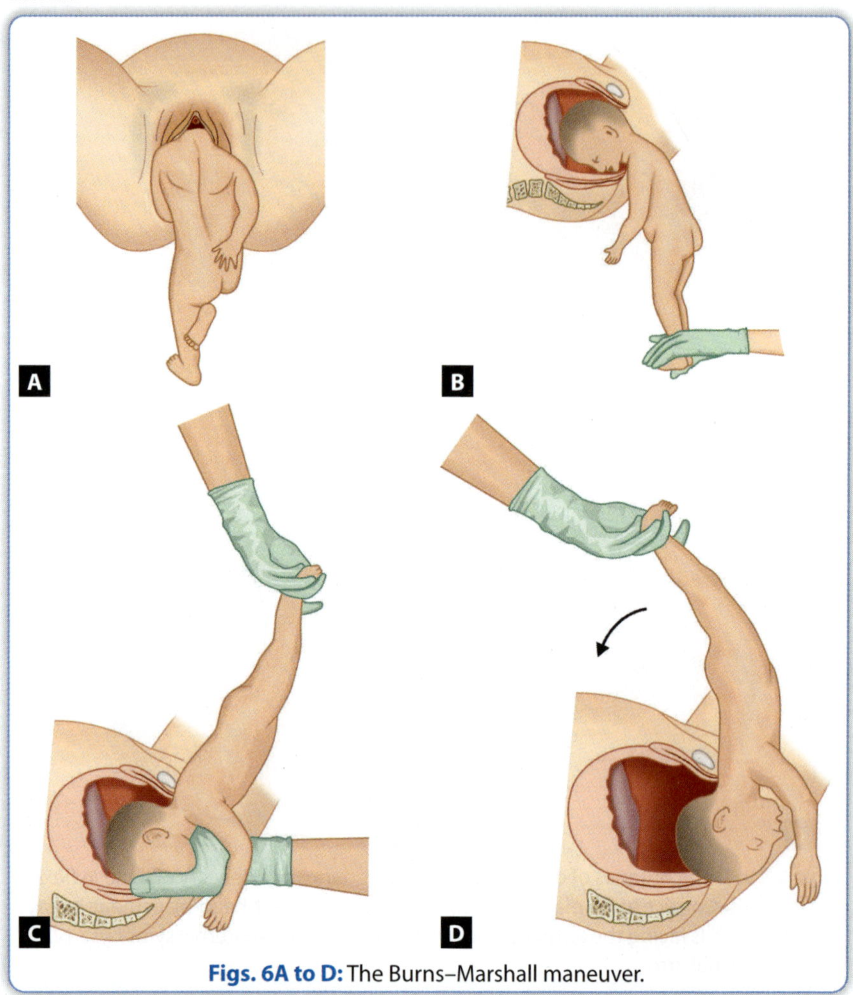

Figs. 6A to D: The Burns–Marshall maneuver.

SUGGESTED READING

1. Cunningham FG, Leveno KJ, Dashe JS, Hoffman BL, Spong CY, Casey B. Williams Obstetrics, 26e. 26th ed. Columbus, OH: McGraw-Hill Education; 2022.
2. DC Dutta, Konar H. Textbook of Obstetrics: Including Perinatology & Contraception. 9th ed. New Delhi, India: Jaypee Brothers Medical; 2021.
3. Guidelines - ACOG, RCOG, NICE and FIGO guidelines.

CHAPTER 40

Imaging

40.1 POINT-OF-CARE ULTRASOUND IN EMERGENCY ROOM

Pushkar Mahajan, Pooja P Vyas

BASICS OF ULTRASOUND

BOX 1: Probes available on the USG machine in emergency room (ER) **(Fig. 1)**.

Curvilinear	Used most commonly for abdominal scans like Point-of-care ultrasound (POCUS)/focused assessment with sonography in trauma (FAST) as it provides higher penetrance with a wider viewing window
Linear	Used to visualize superficial structures as it provides higher resolution and for Doppler examinations
Phased array	Most commonly used for performing echocardiography as it can easily fit in the intercostal spaces

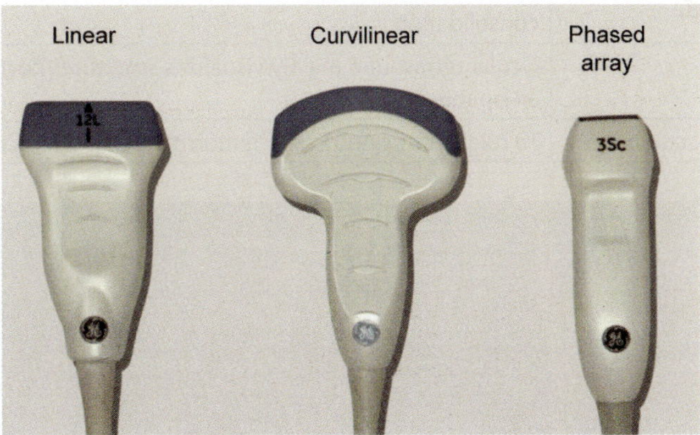

Fig. 1: Probes for the ultrasonography (USG) machine.

BOX 2: Functionality of the basic buttons on the USG machine.

B-mode	Classic greyscale 2D visualization of the tissues, default visualization technique
M-mode	Motion mode; used to objectify moving structures, thus used in echocardiography, inferior vena cava (IVC) collapsibility, and lung ultrasounds
Color mode	• It is used to visualize mobile elements in color overlay, most commonly the blood flow in vessels • By convention, red denotes flow toward the probe and blue denotes flow away from the probe
Pulsed Doppler	Spectral mode used to assess waveforms of the flowing blood seldom required in the ER

BOX 3: POCUS.

The ER physician directly performs and interprets the examination at the patient's bedside using information immediately available to come to a diagnosis and guide ongoing treatment **(Fig. 2)**.

This saves time for calling radiologists/cardiologists to do the scan and providing them with parts of the relevant history

The following are the commonly performed POCUS scans by the ER physician:

FAST	Focused assessment in trauma
RUSH	Rapid ultrasound for shock and hypotension
Thoracic ultrasound	To rule out pneumothorax/pleural and pericardial effusion/ consolidation
B-Scan	Ocular ultrasound mainly visualizes structures posterior to an opaque lens
Neonatal cranium	To rule of intraventricular hemorrhage and hydrocephalus

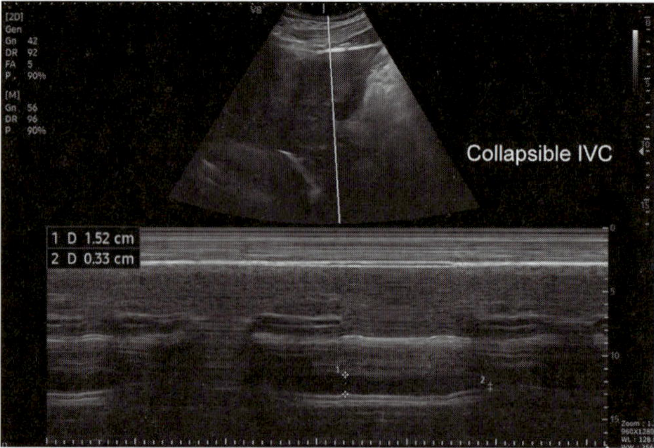

Fig. 2: Point-of-care ultrasound (POCUS).

BOX 4: FAST scan.

Patient selection	It is to be performed in all patients who have presented with blunt abdominal trauma and road traffic accidents
Purpose	It is done to rule out any intra-abdominal bleeding/hematoma that could be the cause of failed hemodynamic resuscitation of the patient
Protocol	Basic FAST scan includes four critical views, which are obtained most commonly with the curvilinear probe 1. *Right flank hepatorenal area:* – The probe is placed in the right mid-to-posterior axillary line at the level of 11th and 12th ribs – This is the Rutherford–Morison Pouch and is the most dependent part of the upper peritoneal cavity and intraperitoneal fluid and blood may collect here – Blood shows as a hypoechoic black stripe between the capsule of the liver and fatty fascia of the right kidney 2. *Left flank perisplenic area:* – The transducer is placed on the left posterior axillary line region between the 10th and 11th ribs – Fluid/blood most commonly gets collected between the diaphragm and the superior surface of the spleen 3. *Subcostal pericardium:* – The transducer is placed just to the left of the xiphisternum and angled upward under the costal margin – The pericardial examination screens for fluid between the fibrous and the visceral pericardium, and hence rules out cardiac tamponade 4. *Pelvic rectovesical or rectouterine:* – The transducer is placed midline just superior to the symphysis pubis – It helps to visualize the pouch of Douglas in females and rectovesical pouch in males, which are the most dependent areas of the lower abdomen for fluid and blood to collect
eFAST scan	This is an "Extended" FAST scan that is to be performed in patients with history of blunt thoracic trauma along with an abdominal one **(Fig. 3)**. Its protocol includes two extra thoracic views, which are commonly obtained using phased array probe: 1. Right anterior thoracic 2. Left anterior thoracic For both of these views, the probe is kept in the fourth or the fifth intercostal space in the mid-axillary line. It is mostly performed to rule out pneumothorax, thus performed on M-Mode. No Pneumothorax—sea-shore sign Pneumothorax present—barcode sign

Contd...

Contd...

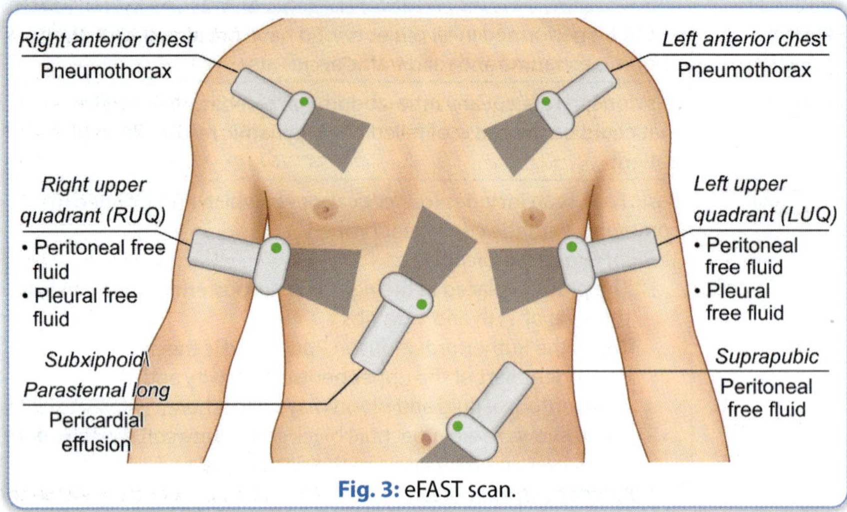

Fig. 3: eFAST scan.

BOX 5: RUSH scan.	
Patient selection	It is to be performed in all patients presenting to the ER with refractory hypotension
Purpose	It helps the ER physician to identify the cause of hypotension/shock and then take an informed decision about how to hemodynamically resuscitate the patient

USG plays an important role for the clinician to go through the following protocol:

BOX 6: Protocol.

	Organ	***Pathology***
H	Heart	• Ejection fraction (reduced) → Systolic heart failure • Ejection fraction (hyperdynamic) → Distributive or hypovolemic shock • Pericardial effusion → Tamponade • Right ventricular (RV) strain → Pulmonary embolism (PE) • Regional wall motion abnormality → Myocardial infarction • Low cardiac output → Cardiogenic, hypovolemic, or obstructive shock • High cardiac output → Distributive shock
I	IVC	• IVC collapsible → Hypovolemic or distributive shock • IVC noncollapsible → Obstructive or cardiogenic shock
M	Morrison's/eFAST	• Hemoperitoneum/Hemothorax → Hemorrhagic shock
A	Aorta	• Abdominal aortic aneurysm • Aortic dissection
P	Pulmonary	Pneumothorax

Note: Mnemonic - HIMAP

BOX 7: Thoracic ultrasound.

Patient selection	To be performed on patients presenting with breathlessness and desaturation to the ER
Purpose	To rule out pneumothorax, pleural effusion, and pulmonary edema or consolidation as a cause of the above symptoms and to begin with early targeted management
Protocol	Various intercostal spaces are to be examined using curvilinear or phased array transducer. Normal lung tissue reveals pleural sliding with respiration and A-lines due to reverberation of ultrasound waves by air in the lung tissue. **(Fig. 4B)** • *Pneumothorax:* – Findings are explained in eFAST section – Most specific USG sign for pneumothorax is the lung-point sign seen on both B-mode and M-mode at the interface of the normal and abnormal pleural space • *Pulmonary edema:* A-lines are replaced by B-lines, which appear as echogenic comet tails, not decreasing in intensity with the depth of the lung tissue and also show sliding with respiration • *Pleural effusion:* – Pleural space is seen filled up with anechoic fluid with or without mobile echoes (plankton sign) and underlying echogenic collapsed lung (jellyfish sign) **(Fig. 4A)** – Quad/sinusoid sign is seen on M-mode due to presence of mobile fluid within • *Consolidation:* A-lines are absent and the whole lung tissue can be appreciated as hypoechoic due to hepatization in the consolidation process

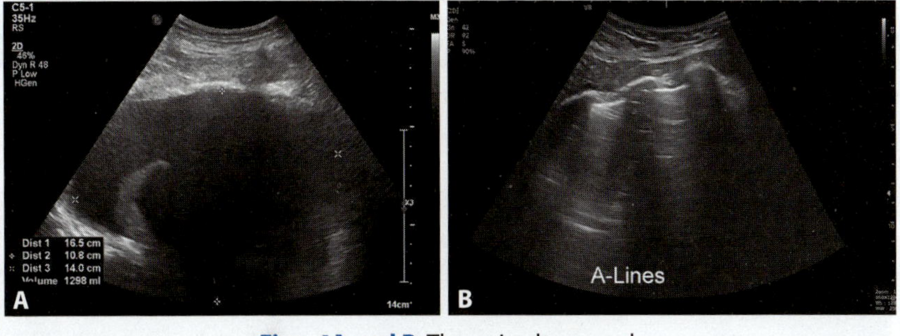

Figs. 4A and B: Thoracic ultrasound.

BOX 8: B-scan of the orbit.

Patient selection	It is to be performed in patients presenting to the ER with sudden loss of vision and are having an opaque lens (cataract) or hazy anterior chamber that limits the view by ophthalmoscopy It is contraindicated in patients with ocular trauma and postoperative patients as it increases the chances of globe rupture
Purpose	To diagnose vitreous hemorrhage and posterior wall detachment (retinal, choroidal, or hyaloid) **(Figs. 5 and 6)**
Protocol	Usually, a high-frequency linear transducer is kept on closed eyelids of the patient. Static as well as dynamic examination is performed by asking the patient to look in different gazes on a closed eyelid • *Vitreous hemorrhage:* Multiple mobile echogenic foci on dynamic examination are noted in the vitreous chamber • *Detachment:* Appears as echogenic lines seen separating from posterior wall of ocular globe. Retinal, choroidal, and hyaloid detachment can be differentiated based on the pattern of the detachment
Caution	Ocular USG can have similar findings for many different pathologies. Diagnosis should not be based on USG alone. Thorough history and ancillary imaging should be done to come to a final diagnosis

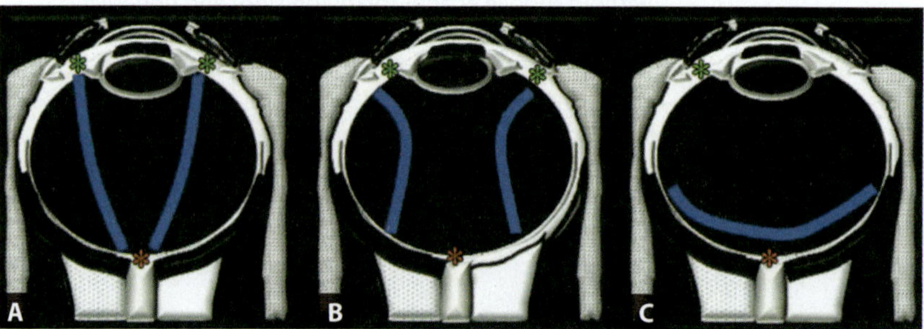

Figs. 5A to C: Posterior wall detachment. (A) retinal detachment; (B) choroidal detachment; and (C) hyaloid detachment.

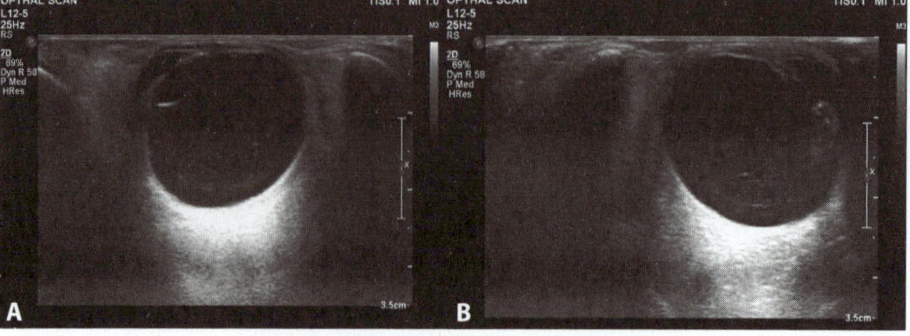

Figs. 6A and B: Vitreous hemorrhage.

SUGGESTED READING

1. Dinh V. POCUS 101. (2024). Ultrasound Machine Basics-Knobology, Probes, and Modes. [online]. Available from https://www.pocus101.com/ultrasound-machine-basics-knobology-probes-and-modes/#:~:text=The%20linear%20ultrasound%20probe%20is,then%20use%20the%20linear%20probe [Last accessed September, 2024].
2. Lorente-Ramos RM, Armán JA, Muñoz-Hernández A, García Gómez JM, de la Torre SB. US of the eye made easy: A comprehensive how-to review with ophthalmoscopic correlation. RadioGraphics. 2012;32(5):175-200.
3. Marini TJ, Rubens DJ, Zhao YT, Weis J, O'Connor TP, Novak WH, et al. Lung ultrasound: The essentials. Radiol Cardiothorac Imaging. 2021;3(2):e200564.
4. Reim P, Moore L, Minalyan A, Dinh Vi. Pocus 101. (2024). RUSH Exam Ultrasound Protocol: Step-By-Step Guide. [online] Available from https://www.pocus101.com/rush-exam-ultrasound-protocol-step-by-step-guide/ [Last accessed September, 2024].
5. Rosen CL, Wolfe RE. Ultrasound in emergency medicine. Emergency Medicine Clinics of North America. 2004;22(3):15-6.
6. Tayal V, Blaivas M, Mandavia D, Blankenship R, Boniface K, Ferre R, et al. Emergency Ultrasound Guidelines. Ann Emerg Med. 2008;53(4),550-70.
7. White S, Dinh Vi, Ahn J, Deschamps J, Genobaga S, Lang A. Pocus 101. (2024). EFast Ultrasound Exam Made Easy: Step-By-Step Guide. [online] Available from https://www.pocus101.com/efast-ultrasound-exam-made-easy-step-by-step-guide/ [Last accessed September, 2024].
8. Whitson MR, Mayo PH. Ultrasonography in the emergency department. Crit Care. 2016;20(1):227

CHAPTER 41

Ophthalmology Procedures

Tulika Goleria

BOX 1: Detailed history of the patient is important.

Vision:
- Vision of the patient should be examined at the bedside
- Patient is asked to close one eye with one hand. The patient is then made to count the fingers of the medical examiner and then distance should be gradually increased
- This procedure is then repeated for the other eye

BOX 2: Torch-light examination.

- If patient is not able to see the fingers of the medical examiner, ask them to close one eye and ask if they can see the torch light
- Project the light from different directions and ask the patient to tell from which direction the light is being projected from. This should be done in a dark room preferably
- On torch light, examine the periorbital area for swelling, tears abrasion, color or any inflammatory sign and insect bite, etc.
- Examine lids, lid margins, color conjunctival color discharge and evert lids to look for foreign bodies
- Examine conjunctiva for any congestion or hemorrhage
- Examine cornea for any impacted foreign body, tear, or any other abnormality
- Anterior chamber is also examined to see the depth
- Pupillary reaction to be checked by swinging the torch from one side to another
- Pupil size and reaction is to be documented properly, especially in road traffic accidents and if neurological cause is expected
- Eye movements are to be examined in central and in all gazes. Ask the patient to move his/her eye according to the movement of the torch by the examining doctor. Note for any restriction in movement
- This is very important in cases road traffic accidents or neurological causes

BOX 3: Tactile tonometry.

- Tactile tonometry is to examine intraocular area
- Ask patient to close the eyes
- Rest both hands on the forehead of the patient with one index finger, apply gentle pressure on globe, the supratarsal area and feel the resistance with the other finger. Both the fingers should be slightly apart
- You can roughly make out that the eye is soft tender or very hard. Very important for painful red eye patients, in ocular trauma, and acute attack of glaucoma

BOX 4: Slit lamp examination.

Procedure	• A slit lamp is used to see different structures of the eye in detail and various magnifications depending upon the type of slit lamp are available • The operator can examine the lids, lid margin, conjunctiva, conjunctival vessels, cornea anomalies, anterior chamber, and lens • Detailed examination at a higher magnification of slit lamp shows lid glands, conjunctival vessel bleeds, infections or foreign bodies of conjunctiva and cornea, inflammatory signs in anterior chamber, and in vitreous in the form of cells or flare • Removal of foreign body on slit lamp is easy and an outpatient department (OPD) procedure • Diffuse light lets us examine the blood vessels on slit lamp • Slit lamp filters are important for correct diagnosis • It has coloured filters typically built within the slit lamp, red free filter, cobalt blue, and neutral density filters • *Cobalt blue:* Used after applying fluorescein dye to evaluate for corneal abrasions and avulsions, and tear break-up time • Green filter/Red free filter: Used to increase the visibility of blood vessels • Filter is useful for the assessment of hemorrhage • Neutral density filter for corneal scar, irregularities, tear, tear debris, and foreign body • Anterior chamber examination should be done carefully to see for hyphema (Blood in case of trauma), hypopyon (pus in corneal ulcer etc), cells and flare (uveitis etc.)
Complications	• Proper sanitization is recommended to avoid spilling of infections like conjunctivitis, etc.

BOX 5: Fluoresce staining testing.

Indications and uses	• The basic principle of using fluorescein dye for corneal pathologies is that fluorescence appears green when seen with blue light or filter • Easy-to-detect small fine corneal abrasions, corneal foreign bodies, tear breakup time, and infections of the eye like corneal ulcers can be detected
Procedure	• Blue filter of the slit lamp is used to examine the eye after staining it with fluorescein strip • The slit lamp magnification and fluorescein dye that stays and stains the abrasions and their margins help us to see the finest and smallest abrasions • Fluorescein staining is used to do applanation tonometry • Seidel test is to rule out microscopic perforation of cornea or sclera in mainly post surgery cases or trauma as after staining the eye, there can be trickle of dye in the anterior chamber of eye or posterior chamber if leak is present *Caution:* Use separate strips for each eye • It should be avoided if open globe injury is expected
Complications	• Using same strip for both eyes can cause infection • Stored old fluorescein solution can cause major infections
Caveats	• Removal of contact lenses is a must before staining otherwise the lens is spoiled and whole procedure is compromised because of pooling of dye in between cornea and lens, etc. • Allergic inflammatory reaction in eye may be caused in response to dye used

BOX 6: Eye irrigation.

Indications	• Chemical (acid or alkali) injury to eye leading to burns • Removal of superficial foreign bodies or slough in the eye
Contraindications	Corneal perforation or scleral melting or perforation
Procedure	Detailed history of the patient to know the type of chemical exposure is important Explaining the patient, the procedure of irrigation and its importance and taking them into confidence is the key for a good outcome The steps involved are as follows: • Anesthetize the eye(s) with topical anesthetic drops • Completely evert the lower lid and upper lid, remove all the impacted chemical particles or slough using moist cotton buds or fine forceps • The bulbar and palpebral conjunctiva and cornea should be continuously given a wash with saline or distilled water for at least 25–30 minutes or minimum 1 liter of saline should be used • Intravenous (IV) tubing with a saline bag placed at a height ensures a smooth flow of solution and is ideal • Deep corneal injury can occur in chemical burns • With inadequate irrigation, some chemical particles may be left and may cause recurrent inflammation leading to symblepharon
Pearls and pitfalls	• Alkali burns are more harmful than acid burns, hence irrigation to be done for a longer time for alkali burns and more topical anesthetic may be used • Ophthalmological consultation is required immediately

BOX 7: Fundoscopy.

Indication	Sudden loss of vision, pain in the eye, transient vision, severe headache, history of systemic disease, trauma, and neurological symptoms *Contraindications:* Conjunctivitis and corneal ulcer
Instrument	• Direct ophthalmoscope • During fundoscopy, check the red reflex of the retina from a distance. A red glow is seen if media is clear • In case of vitreous hemorrhage or vitritis or dense cataract, the glow is absent • Patient may see black dots of various shapes, if vitreous hemorrhage is less • Check the cup disc ratio, margins of the disc, blood vessels at disc, and trace blood vessels and check for possible nicking or bleeding • Ideally, fundus examination should be done by an ophthalmologist in detail • Fundus examination is important to detect systemic disease complication in eye or to rule out intracranial pressure, etc.

SUGGESTED READING

1. Salmon JF. Kanski's Clinical Ophthalmology: A systematic Approach, 9th edition. Amsterdam, Netherlands: Elsevier; 2019.

Part 6

Interpretations/Understanding of Emergency-based Investigations

CHAPTER 42

Rapid Understanding of Arterial Blood Gases

Jamshed D Sunavala

BOX 1: Normal values of arterial blood gas (ABG).

Variables	*Normal (N)*	*Near Normal (NN)*
pH	7.40	±0.5
Partial pressure of oxygen (PaO_2)	95–100 mm Hg	>75–95 mm Hg
Arterial oxygen saturation (SaO_2)	>95%	
Partial pressure of carbon dioxide ($PaCO_2$)	40 mm Hg	±5 mm Hg
Bicarbonate (HCO_3)	24 mEq/L	±2 mEq/L
Base excess	–2 to +2	
Serum lactate	<2 mmol/L	

BOX 2: Six steps to interpret ABG.

1. **The first look:** It is done to immediately assess the underlying severity of the respiratory or metabolic derangement. The most important variable to raise the "red flag" is the pH; if the pH is <7.25, it would indicate an imminent emergency involving a critical situation encountered in intensive care unit (ICU) such as shock, organ failure, and other life-threatening cardiorespiratory and metabolic complications. Next, the ABG values need to be correlated with the clinical findings
2. **Correlate pH and $PaCO_2$** to determine the type of acid–base disorder **(Table 1)**
3. **Correlate $PaCO_2$ to HCO_3** for assessing compensation **(Box 4 and Table 2)**
4. **Mixed disorders:** Ways to suspect mixed disorders and their possible causes **(Boxes 3 and 4)**
5. **Calculate the anion gap (AG)** to know the causes of metabolic acidosis **(Boxes 5 and 6)**
6. **Analysis and causes** of metabolic alkalosis **(Box 7)**

Contd...

Contd...

TABLE 1: Groupwise, the eight possibilities of primary acid–base disorder (corrected pH vs. $PaCO_2$)

Group	*pH*	*$PaCO_2$*	*Acid–base disorders*
1	↓	↑	Respiratory acidosis
	↑	↓	Respiratory alkalosis
	↓	↓	Metabolic acidosis
	↑	↑	Metabolic alkalosis
2	N/NN	↑	Chronic respiratory acidosis or *mixed disorders:* Respiratory acidosis and metabolic alkalosis
	N/NN	↓	Chronic respiratory alkalosis or *mixed disorders:* Metabolic acidosis and respiratory alkalosis
3	↓↓	N/NN	*Mixed disorders:* Metabolic acidosis and respiratory acidosis
	↑↑	N/NN	*Mixed disorder:* Metabolic alkalosis and respiratory alkalosis

N/NN = Normal or near normal

Contd...

Contd...

TABLE 2: Primary acid–base disorders and their secondary response.

Primary acid–base disorder	***Primary disturbance***	***Secondary response***	***Magnitude of response***	***Expected response (Ex)***	***Time to complete compensation***
Metabolic acidosis	$\downarrow HCO_3$	$\Downarrow PaCO_2$	$\Delta PaCO_2 = 1.2 \times \Delta HCO_3$	Ex $PaCO_2 = 40 - [1.2 \times (24 - msHCO_3)]$	12–24 hours
Metabolic alkalosis	$\uparrow HCO_3$	$\Uparrow PaCO_2$	$\Delta PaCO_2 = 0.7 \times \Delta HCO_3$	Ex $PaCO_2 = 40 + [0.7 \times (msHCO_3 - 24)]$	12–24 hours
Acute respiratory acidosis	$\uparrow PaCO_2$	$\Uparrow HCO_3$	$\Delta HCO_3 = 0.1 \times \Delta PaCO_2$	Ex $HCO_3 = 24 + [0.1 \times (msPaCO_2 - 40)]$	<6 hours
Acute respiratory alkalosis	$\downarrow PaCO_2$	$\Downarrow HCO_3$	$\Delta HCO_3 = 0.2 \times \Delta PaCO_2$	Ex $HCO_3 = 24 + [0.2 \times (40 - msPaCO_2)]$	<6 hours
Chronic respiratory acidosis	$\uparrow PaCO_2$	$\Uparrow HCO_3$	$\Delta HCO_3 = 0.4 \times \Delta PaCO_2$	Ex $HCO_3 = 24 + [0.4 \times (msPaCO_2 - 40)]$	>5 days
Chronic respiratory alkalosis	$\downarrow PaCO_2$	$\Downarrow HCO_3$	$\Delta HCO_3 = 0.4 \times \Delta PaCO_2$	Ex $HCO_3 = 24 + [0.4 \times (40 - msPaCO_2)]$	>7 days

Δ = Change from normal value (normal values of $PaCO_2$ and HCO_3 are taken as 40 mm Hg and 24 mEq/L in the above equation)
$\downarrow\uparrow$ = Direction of primary disturbances
$\Downarrow\Uparrow$ = Direction of secondary disturbances
ms = Measured value
Ex = Expected response

BOX 3: How to suspect mixed disorders?

In metabolic acidosis (↓ HCO_3): If the level of $PaCO_2$ is undercorrected than expected for complete compensation, there is an associated respiratory acidosis. If the $PaCO_2$ is overcorrected than expected there is associated respiratory alkalosis.

In metabolic alkalosis (↑ HCO_3): If the level of $PaCO_2$ is overcorrected than the limit of expected compensation, there is an associated respiratory acidosis. If $PaCO_2$ is lower than expected then there is an associated respiratory alkalosis.

In respiratory acidosis: Here, the level of expected compensation would be a mild increase in HCO_3 in acute phase (<2 days) and a further rise if acidosis is chronic. If the rise in HCO_3 is less than expected than associated metabolic acidosis is likely, and if more than expected there is a likelihood of associated metabolic alkalosis.

In *respiratory alkalosis* similar to respiratory acidosis, there is a mild-to-moderate fall in expected level of HCO_3 depending on the acute or chronic phase of respiratory alkalosis. If the fall in HCO_3 is more than expected, then there is metabolic acidosis and if the fall is less than expected, there is associated metabolic alkalosis.

Complete compensation is N or NN pH

*For expected secondary response see **Table 2***

*Possible causes of mixed disorders are given in **Box 4***

BOX 4: Possible causes of mixed acid–base disorders in ICU setting.

Causes	***Acid–base disorders***
Septic shock Salicylate overdosage	High AG metabolic acidosis + respiratory alkalosis
Cardiorespiratory arrest	High AG metabolic acidosis + respiratory acidosis
Use of diuretics or vomiting in a patient with a chronic lung disease	Metabolic alkalosis + respiratory acidosis
Vomiting or use of diuretics in a patient with ketoacidosis or lactic acidosis	Metabolic alkalosis + high AG metabolic acidosis
Use of diuretic or vomiting in a patient of hepatic failure; pneumonia with vomiting	Metabolic alkalosis + respiratory alkalosis
Diarrhea in a patient with lactic acidosis	Hyperchloremic non-AG metabolic acidosis + high AG, and metabolic acidosis

BOX 5: Calculate the AG to know the causes of metabolic acidosis.

- $AG = (Na^+ + K^+) - (Cl^- + HCO_3)$
- Normal AG is approximately 8–12 mEq/L (upper normal = 15 mEq/L)
- AG is the difference between the serum cations and the anions as measured routinely in the laboratory, hence AG is a rough estimation of unmeasured anions

BOX 6: Causes of metabolic acidosis.

Normal AG	*High AG*
• D = *D*iarrhea • R = *R*enal – Renal tubular acidosis (RTA) – Early renal insufficiency • I = *I*atrogenic – Rapid isotonic saline infusion – Calcium chloride – Magnesium sulfate causing diarrhea – Cholestyramine causing bile acid diarrhea – Ileal conduits • P = *P*ancreatic fistula	• G = Ethylene *g*lycol ingestion • O = *O*xoproline • L = *L*actic acidosis • D = *D*-lactic acid • M = *M*ethanol • A = *A*spirin (salicylate toxicity) • R = End-stage *R*enal failure • K = *K*etoacidosis

D-Lactic acidosis occurs in patients with small bowel resection or jejunoileal bypass where large amount of carbohydrates is directly delivered to the colon, which otherwise would have been reabsorbed in the small intestine in patients with normal gut. The high load of carbohydrates delivered to the colon is metabolized into D-lactate by the colonic bacteria and it absorbed into the circulation. Hence, following high carbohydrate diet, these group of patients may succumb to metabolic acidosis with neurological abnormalities such as confusion and ataxia. D-lactate usually does not show up in the blood on normal testing as it is not sensed by the routine gas analyzer.

BOX 7: Causes of metabolic alkalosis.

Chloride responsive (urine chloride <15 mEq/L)	*Chloride resistant (urine chloride >25 mEq/L)*
H = Hypovolemia (contraction alkalosis) A = Antacids (nonabsorbable) N = Nasogastric aspiration and vomiting D = Diuretics (thiazides and loop diuretics)	C = *C*ushing syndrome R = *R*enovascular hypertension A = Primary *A*ldosteronism M = Severe hypo*m*agnesemia P = Severe *p*otassium depletion S = *S*teroids (exogenous glucocorticoids or mineralocorticoids)

The common causes of metabolic alkalosis in critically ill patients are loss of H^+ due to vomiting or gastric aspiration and intracellular shift of H^+ due to hypokalemia, administration of excessive soda bicarbonate, or contraction alkalosis.

SUGGESTED READING

1. Adrogué HJ, Madias NE. Management of life-threatening acid-base disorders. First of two parts. N Eng J Med. 1998;338(1):26-34.
2. Brend K, de Vries AP, Gans RO. Physiological approach to assessment of acid-base disturbances. N Engl J Med. 2014;371(15):1434-45.
3. Marino PL. Marino's The ICU Book, 4th edition. Philadelphia: Wolters Kluwer; 2013.
4. Rose BD, Post T, Stokes J. Clinical Physiology of Acid-Base and Electrolyte Disorders, 5th edition. New York: McGraw Hill; 2001.

CHAPTER 43

Biomarkers in Emergency Room

43.1 CARDIAC MARKERS

Sachna P Shetty

BOX 1: Introduction.

Highly-sensitive troponin I	• Commonly used quantitative cardiac marker • Detects an infarction within 3 hours, peaks in 48 hours, and stays positive for 8–10 days • Look for false positives **(Box 1)**
Troponin T	• Qualitative • Elevated in renal diseases
Creatinine kinase-MB	• Cardiac marker for infarction • Elevates in 4–8 hours and normalizes in 36 hours
N-terminal pro-B-type natriuretic peptide	• Heart failure diagnosis • Cut-off as per age

BOX 2: False-positive troponins.

- Cardiac contusion
- Cardiac procedures (surgery, ablation, pacing, and stenting)
- Acute or chronic congestive heart failure
- Aortic dissection
- Aortic valve disease
- Hypertrophic cardiomyopathy
- Arrhythmias
- Rhabdomyolysis with cardiac injury
- Pulmonary hypertension
- Pulmonary embolism
- Acute neurologic disease (e.g., stroke and subarachnoid hemorrhage)
- Myocardial infiltrative diseases (amyloid, sarcoid, hemochromatosis, and scleroderma)
- Inflammatory cardiac diseases (myocarditis, endocarditis, and pericarditis)
- Drug toxicity
- Respiratory failure
- Sepsis
- Burns
- Extreme exertion (e.g., endurance athletes)

BOX 3: Caveats.

- Patients with renal disease often have an elevated cardiac troponin T (cTnT), whereas cardiac troponin I (cTnI) elevations are less common
- For coronary artery bypass grafting (CABG), in patients with normal baseline troponin values, elevations of cardiac biomarkers above the 99th percentile upper reference limit (URL) are indicative of periprocedural myocardial necrosis

SUGGESTED READING

1. Apple FS, Jesse RL, Newby LK, Wu AH, Christenson RH, Cannon CP, et al. National Academy of Clinical Biochemistry and IFCC Committee for Standardization of Markers of Cardiac Damage Laboratory Medicine Practice Guidelines: Analytical issues for biochemical markers of acute coronary syndromes. Clin Chem. 2007;53:547-51.
2. Moon RE, Sheffield PJ. Guidelines for treatment of decompression illness. Aviat Space Environ Med. 1997;68(3):234-43.
3. Tintinalli JE, Ma OJ, Yearly DM, Meckler GD, Stapczynski JS, Cline DM. Tintinalli's Emergency Medicine: A Comprehensive Study Guide, 9th edition. New York: McGraw Hill; 2021.
4. Walls R, Hockberger R, Gaushe-Hill M, Erickson TB, Wilcox SR. Rosen's Emergency Medicine: Concepts and Clinical Practice, 10th edition. Amsterdam, Netherlands: Elsevier; 2022.

43.2 INFECTIOUS MARKERS

Sonar Narula, Jyotiprakash Panda

BOX 1: Cultures.

- *Blood culture:*
  - Blood cultures should be collected before administering the first dose of antibiotics. Cultures collected after antibiotic therapy may result in a false negative result
  - Two sets of blood cultures, i.e., two aerobic and two anaerobic/fungus bottles should be collected when possible
  - Each bottle should contain 8–10 mL of blood, as more the sample collected, better the positivity rate
  - In patients with an intravascular catheter (in place >48 hours), at least one blood culture set should be obtained from the catheter (along with simultaneous peripheral blood cultures) to assist in the diagnosis of a potential catheter-related bloodstream infection (CRBSI)
  - Overfilling the bottles should be avoided as it results in improper dilution of antibiotics and antibodies present in serum
  - Collection should be done following strict aseptic precautions. Failing which, may result in pseudobacteremia due to normal skin commensals
  - Automated blood culture systems (BACTEC™/BacTAlert™) do continuous monitoring of the culture, hence can give early information on bloodstream infections/sepsis
- *Other cultures:*
  - Urine (midstream clean-catch urine sample)/respiratory samples/surgical wounds/pus/stool or specimens from any other suspected sites of infection may be sent to the laboratory following aseptic techniques
  - Swabs/catheters tips/drain fluids are inappropriate samples and should be avoided

Interpretation/advantages:

- Culture is a highly sensitive and specific test that detects viable pathogens only. Culture positivity gives information for the identification of the pathogen as well as the antimicrobial susceptibility profile with the minimum inhibitory concentration (MIC) levels, leading to targeted and appropriate therapy
- It helps to identify the source/site of infection
- Subsequent cultures can monitor progression of infection and response to therapy
- False-negative cultures can be due to prior antibiotics given to the patient or inadequate volume collected
- False-positive results can be due to contamination during collection

BOX 2: Biomarkers.

- *C-reactive protein (CRP):*
  - CRP is an acute-phase reactant, which is elevated in inflammations due to infectious and noninfectious causes
  - CRP rises proportionally to the severity of inflammation and improves in response to appropriate antibiotic therapy if elevated due to infectious causes
  - Poor patient outcomes are associated with persistently elevated CRP levels
  - In a systematic review and meta-analysis, CRP had an estimated pooled sensitivity of 75% and a specificity of 67% for differentiating bacterial infection from noninfectious causes of inflammation
  - CRP is useful as an index of systemic inflammation but is considered less reliable than procalcitonin for bacterial infection
- *Procalcitonin (PCT):*
  - PCT is a precursor of the hormone calcitonin usually secreted by thyroid. In response to bacterial endotoxins (lipopolysaccharide) and inflammatory cytokines such as tumor necrosis factor-alpha (TNF-α) and interleukin (IL)-1β, it is secreted ectopically by neuroendocrine cells of lungs and intestine
  - It can function as a marker of inflammatory state, especially due to bacterial infections
  - PCT should not be used to guide the initiation of antimicrobial therapy in sepsis as available data suggests inadequate sensitivity and specificity for diagnosing sepsis
  - Serial PCT levels, with a cut-off of <0.5 µg/L or >80% decrease from peak levels, assist in de-escalation of antibiotics in hemodynamically stable patients
  - PCT can remain normal in the fungal infection/viral infections/early stages of bacterial infections/localized infection
  - False positive PCT can be seen in:
    - Major surgery (up to 48 hours after the surgery/trauma/burns)
    - Medullary thyroid cancer and small cell lung carcinomas
    - Chronic kidney disease (CKD)
- *Beta-d-Glucan (BDG):*
  - Invasive fungal infections are a significant cause of morbidity and mortality in patients who receive immunosuppressive therapy, such as solid organ and hematopoietic stem cell transplant (HSCT) recipients
  - BDG is an abundant fungal cell wall polysaccharide, found in most fungi and *Pneumocystis jirovecii* (PCP) with the notable exceptions of the *Cryptococcus* and the Zygomycetes (Mucor family)
  - It is most commonly used for rapid detection of invasive candidiasis, especially in critically ill immunocompromised patients, where culture positive candidemia might take up to 72 hours or may be culture negative sometimes
  - The major advantage is that BDG test can be done on serum, a readily available and easily accessible specimen, regardless of patient status
  - A meta-analysis found that the average sensitivity is 76% and the average specificity is 85%
  - Because of many potential sources of false positives (amoxicillin–clavulanate, piperacillin–tazobactam, *Pseudomonas* infections, and dialysis patients), a single positive test is of limited value
  - Serial BDG analysis from serum can significantly enhance the assays' clinical performance
  - The test has moderate sensitivity, hence a single negative test cannot exclude the diagnosis of invasive fungal infection

Contd...

Contd...

- *Aspergillus Galactomannan (GM)*:
  - GM is a polysaccharide antigen that exists primarily in the cell walls of *Aspergillus* species
  - GM may be released into the blood and other body fluids even in the early stages of *Aspergillus* invasion
  - Hence, detection of the GM level can be useful in making an early diagnosis of invasive pulmonary aspergillosis (IPA)
  - Currently, serum GM detection is considered a microbiological diagnostic criterion for *Aspergillus* infection in neutropenic patients, according to the guidelines of the European Organization for Research and Treatment of Cancer/ Mycoses Study Group (EORTC/MSG)
  - A meta-analysis of studies mainly containing immunocompromised patients reported a pooled sensitivity of 90% and a specificity of 94%
  - In nonneutropenic patients, bronchoalveolar lavage (BAL) GM can be used as an adjunctive test to radiology, histopathology, and fungal culture for diagnosis of invasive pulmonary aspergillosis (IPA)

BOX 3: Serological tests.

- *Rapid antigen/antibody detection by immunochromatography [also known as immunochromatographic test (ICT)/rapid diagnostic test (RDT)/card tests/lateral flow assays]:* Antigen/antibody detection from various specimens can help in rapid identification of the pathogen, thereby acting as point-of-care tests **(Table 1)**

TABLE 1: Samples for different assays.

Samples	***Antigen/antibody***
Blood/serum	• Malaria antigens tests [*Plasmodium* lactate dehydrogenase (pLDH), histidine-rich protein 2 (HRP2)] • Dengue (NS1 and immunoglobulin M/G (IgM/IgG) • *Leptospira* IgM • Chikungunya IgM
Cerebrospinal fluid (CSF)	• Cryptococcal antigen • Pneumococcal antigen
Urine	• Pneumococcal antigen • *Legionella* antigen

- *Enzyme-linked immunosorbent assay (ELISA):*
  - It is considered gold standard serological test for detection of antigens and antibodies of various infectious etiologies
  - It is technically more challenging and has a higher turn-around time (TAT) than ICTs

BOX 4: Polymerase chain reaction (PCR)-based tests.

- *BioFire® FilmArray® system:*
  - Useful for rapid detection of pathogens in various infectious syndromes
  - It is an automated, closed system, multiplex PCR technology used for *syndromic diagnosis of infectious diseases*
  - A BioFire® syndromic test isolates, amplifies, and detects the deoxyribonucleic acid (DNA)/ribonucleic acid (RNA) of microorganisms that cause overlapping signs and symptoms **(Table 2)**
  - It can detect pathogens in a given specimen within hours (45 minutes–2 hours) instead of days; even if the organism is difficult to grow in culture or nonviable
- *Open-system PCR tests:*
  - Open PCR-based systems can be utilized to detect the pathogens causing the sepsis directly from the blood sample, using a predefined set of primers
  - Majority of these are laboratory-developed tests and, hence are not FDA-approved. Nevertheless, they may be helpful in certain scenarios where blood cultures are either negative or a viral/fungal etiology is likely
  - Bacterial antimicrobial resistance genes can also be detected along with the identification of the pathogen

TABLE 2: Various panels available for different BioFire® tests.

Respiratory panel	Throat swab/ nasopharyngeal swab	*19 targets:* Mostly includes pathogens causing upper respiratory tract infection (URTI) and atypical pneumonia
Gastrointestinal panel	Stool	*22 targets:* Tests stool specimens for common pathogens associated with gastroenteritis
Meningitis/ encephalitis panel	CSF	*14 targets:* Identifies the most common viral, bacterial, and yeast pathogens that cause infections in the central nervous system
Pneumonia panel	Sputum/ BAL/tracheal secretions	*33 targets:* Detects pathogens causing lower respiratory tract infection (LRTI). Also provides semiquantitative results, which may help determine whether an organism is a colonizer or a pathogen

  - Blood samples (2–4 mL) collected in ethylenediaminetetraacetic acid (EDTA) tubes are preferred for PCR. Other anticoagulants have been shown to inhibit PCR
  - Cost is usually high for these tests and can be a limiting factor
  - TAT is short (24–48 hours)
  - Test may be false negative if the offending pathogen is other than the predetermined primers selected

BOX 5: Sequencing-based tests.

- Sequencing-based tests can be utilized to detect the pathogens causing sepsis directly from the blood/body-fluid samples using identification of individual genome sequences. Additionally, resistance genes can be detected as well
- Majority of these tests can detect bacteria, fungus or viruses depending on the library stored in the software, which is much wider compared to PCR-based tests
- The required blood volume for testing is 8–10 mL, which should be collected in EDTA tubes
- Due to the larger initial volume of blood specimens used for extraction of pathogen genomes, these tests have higher sensitivity compared to PCR-based tests
- Cost is usually lower as compared to PCR-based tests
- TAT is 24–36 hours

BOX 6: Basic tests.

- *Total leukocyte counts (TLC):*
  - Leukocytosis (white blood cell count >12,000/mm^3), leukopenia (white blood cell count <4,000/mm^3), and normal white blood cell count with >10% immature forms
  - When measured at presentation in the emergency room, the sensitivity and specificity of leukocytosis or leukopenia for predicting severe sepsis or septic shock versus no sepsis are estimated to be 57.1% and 78.7%, respectively
- *Platelet count:*
  - Platelets are acute phase reactants, and thrombocytosis or thrombocytopenia can be seen in patients with infection
  - Due to conditions such as disseminated intravascular coagulation (DIC), thrombocytopenia is frequently seen in patients with sepsis and septic shock
  - Thrombocytopenia is a predictor of increased mortality in patients with sepsis and is an integral component of the sequential organ failure assessment (SOFA) score
- *Serum creatinine:*
  - As a component of the SOFA score to characterize patients with sepsis, the cut-off for creatinine is <1.2 mg/dL
  - The presence of underlying chronic kidney disease (CKD) can skew the SOFA score toward increased mortality, especially when baseline SOFA is assumed to be 0
- *Serum lactate*: Lactate is considered a sensitive marker for septic shock. Patients with sepsis usually have a serum lactate >2 mmol/L
- *Serum bilirubin:* Hyperbilirubinemia at the time of admission is associated with increased mortality secondary to the development of sepsis-related acute respiratory distress syndrome
- *Urine analysis (UA):*
  - UA is considered negative for infection when nitrites, leukocyte esterase, and microscopic detection of white blood cells are absent
  - Negative UA is quite specific (92%) for the absence of urinary tract infection (UTI)
  - Sample should never be taken from the urine bag in a catheterized patient

SUGGESTED READING

1. Bennett JE, Dolin R, Blaser MJ. Mandell, Douglas, and Bennett's Principles and Practice of Infectious Diseases, 9th Edition. Amsterdam, Netherlands: Elsevier; 2019.
2. Fulton II MR, Zubair M, Taghavi S. Laboratory Evaluation of Sepsis. In: StatPearls [Internet]. Treasure Island (FL): StatPearls Publishing; 2024. Available from: https://www.ncbi.nlm.nih.gov/books/NBK594258/ [Last accessed September, 2024.

CHAPTER 44

Scoring in Emergency Room

Sachna P Shetty

BOX 1: Stroke and bleeding risk stratification.

Stroke and bleeding risk stratification with the CHA_2DS_2-VAS_c and HAS-BLED

CHA_2DS_2-VAS_c	***Score***
Congestive heart failure/left ventricle (LV) dysfunction	1
Hypertension	1
Age ≥75 years	2
Diabetes mellitus	1
Stroke/transient ischemic attack (TIA)/thromboembolism (TE)	2
Vascular disease [prior myocardial infarction (MI), peripheral artery disease (PAD) or aortic plaque]	1
Age 65–74 years	1
Sex category (i.e., female gender)	1

HAS–BLED	***Score***
Hypertension, i.e., uncontrolled blood pressure (BP)	1
Abnormal renal/liver function	1 or 2
Stroke	1
Bleeding tendency or predisposition	1
Labile international normalized ratio (INR)	1
Age (e.g., >65)	1
Drugs [e.g., concomitant aspirin or Nonsteroidal anti-inflammatory drugs (NSAIDs)] or alcohol	1

- CHA_2DS_2-VAS_c is a tool to guide stroke risk, and therefore prophylactic use of anticoagulant.
- If score is >1 for males and >2 for females, then anticoagulants are to be considered.
- Anticoagulants should be started if score is >2 for males, and >3 for females.
- HAS-BLED is a tool to guide if anticoagulant can cause bleeding when used in atrial fibrillation.
- 0–2 has low risk of bleeding and anticoagulants can be started.
- If score >3, then the chance of bleeding is increased.

BOX 2: The Acute Physiology and Chronic Health Evaluation II (APACHE II) score.

Physiological variable	***High abnormal range***						***Low abnormal range***		
	+4	***+3***	***+2***	***+1***	***0***	***+1***	***+2***	***+3***	***+4***
Rectal temperature (C)	≥41	39–40.49		38.5–38.9	36–38.4	34–35.9	32–33.9	30–31.9	≤29.9
Mean arterial pressure (mm Hg)	≥160	130–159	110–129		70–109		50–69		≤49
Heart rate (HR)	≥100	140–179	110–139		70–109		50–69	40–54	≤39
Respiratory rate	≥60	35–49		25–34	12–24	10–11	6–9		≤5
Oxygenation: • Fraction of inspired oxygen (FiO_2) ≥0.5 record first alveolar-arterial oxygen gradient (A-aDO_2) • FiO_2 ≥0.5 record partial pressure of oxygen (PaO_2)	≥500	350–499	200–349		< 200 PO_2 >70	PO_2 61–70		PO_2 56–60	PO_2 ≤55
Arterial pH	≥7.7	7.6–7.69		7.5–7.59	7.33–7.49		7.25–7.32	7.15–7.24	≤7.15
HCO_3 (mEq/L)	≥52	61–51.9		32–40.9	22–31.9		18–21.9	15–17.9	≤15

Contd...

Contd...

Physiological variable	***High abnormal range***						***Low abnormal range***		
	+4	***+3***	***+2***	***+1***	***0***	***+1***	***+2***	***+3***	***+4***
K (mEq/L)	≥7	8–6.9		6.5–5.9	3.5–5.4	3–3.4	2.5–2.9		≤2.5
Na (mEq/L)	≥100	160–179	155–159	150–154	130–149		120–129	111–119	≤110
Serum Creatinine (mqm/dL)	≥3.5	2–3.4	1.5–1.9		0.5–1.4		<0.6		
Hematocrit (%)	≥60		50–58.8	46–48.8	30–45.9		20–29.9		≤20
Total leukocyte count (TLC) (10^1/cc)	≥40		20–39.9	15–19.9	3–14.9		1–2.9		≤1
Glasgow coma scale (GCS)									

Age – Score	GCS (mentioned later)
<44 = 0	Low GCS—higher the score
45–54 = 2	
55–64 = 3	
65–74 = 5	
≥75 = 6	
Calculated on all patients newly admitted to the intensive care unit (ICU). It is an ICU mortality prediction score.	

BOX 3: CURB–65 scoring.

CURB–65 Scoring for pneumonia severity

Symptom	***Points***
Confusion	1
Urea: Blood urea nitrogen (BUN) >19 mg/dL (>mmol/L)	1
Respiratory rate ≥30 breaths/min	1
Systolic BP <90 mm Hg or diastolic BP ≤60 mm Hg	1
Age ≥65 years	1
Total	....

Score	***Disposition***
0 or 1	Outpatient care
2	Inpatient versus observation admission
≥3	Inpatient admission; consider ICU admission with score of 4 or 5

BOX 4: Scoring for pulmonary embolism/DVT.

PERC criteria rule out pulmonary embolism (PE) if no criteria present.

- Age <50?
- Pulse <100?
- Arterial oxygen saturation (SaO_2) ≥95%?
- No hemoptysis, estrogen use, surgery/trauma with hospitalization in last 4 weeks?
- No prior venous thromboembolism (VTE)?
- No unilateral leg swelling?

Modified Wells' criteria for PE

Criteria	***Points***
PE is most likely diagnosis (Dx) or suspected deep vein thrombosis (DVT)	3 each
HR >100 or prior DVT/PE	1.5 each
Immobilization/surgery in last 4 weeks	1.5
Hemoptysis or active malignancy	1 each
If ≤4: PE unlikely *If >4:* PE likely	
Clinical probability or PE	***Points***
Low	<2
Medium	2–6
High	>6

Contd...

Contd...

Wells for DVT

Criteria	***Points***
Active cancer	1
Bedridden >3 days or major surgery <12 weeks	1
Calf swelling >3 cm compared to other leg (measure 10 cm below tibial tuberosity)	1
Collateral (nonvaricose and superficial veins)	1
Entire leg swollen	1
Localized tenderness along deep venous system	1
Pitting edema confined to symptomatic leg	1
Paralysis/paresis/plaster immobilization	1
Previous DVT	1
Alternative diagnosis of DVT is more likely	–2

If point is:
0 = No risk of DVT
1–2 = Low risk, should do D-dimer testing
>3 = High risk, should undergo ultrasound (US) imaging

Geneva scoring system

Criteria	***Points***
Age >65	No: 0; Yes: +2
Previous DVT or PE	No: 0; Yes: +3
Surgery (under general anesthesia) or lower limb fracture in past month	No: 0; Yes: +2
Active malignant condition Solid or hematologic malignant condition, currently active or considered cured <1 year	No: 0; Yes: +2
Unilateral lower limb pain	No: 0; Yes: +3
Hemoptysis	No: 0; Yes: +2
Heart rate	<75: 0 75–94: +3 >= 95: +5
Pain on lower limb palpation and unilateral edema	No: 0; Yes: +4

- Preferred more in UK/USA as less subjective
- Clinical probability of PE is low if score <4, intermediate if score 5–10, and high if score >10

BOX 5: Sepsis indicator.

Criterion	*Threshold*	
	Systemic inflammatory response (SIRS)	***Quick sepsis-related organ failure assessment (qSOFA)***
Body temperature (°C)	<36 or >38	–
HR (beats/min)	>90	–
While blood cell count (103/μL) or immature forms/bands	<4 or 12 or >10%	–
Respiratory rate (breaths/min) or partial pressure of carbon dioxide (pCO_2)	>20 or <32	≥22
Systolic blood pressure (mm Hg)	–	≤100
Glasgow coma scale (altered mental status)	–	≤13

SIRS: If >2 of above, it indicates presence of infection but not necessarily sepsis.
qSOFA: It is a mortality predictor.
- >2 is high risk with poor prognosis.
- qSOFA is a superior indicator in emergency room (ER) setting for sepsis-related intervention.
- A positive SOFA score should prompt calculation of SOFA score for confirmation of sepsis.

BOX 6: HEART score indicator of cardiac event and risk stratification.

Criteria	*Points*	
History (slightly/moderately/highly suspicious)	0/1/2	
Electrocardiogram (ECG)	Normal	0
	Nonspecific	1
	Significant ST deviation	2
Age	<45	0
	45–64	1
	>65	2
Risk factors	None	0
	1–2	1
	>3 of atherosclerotic disease	2
Initial troponin	<normal limit	0
	1–3 × normal limit	1
	>3 × normal limit	2

If points:
0–3 = Patient can be discharged.
4–6 = Needs admission.
>7 = Candidates for early invasive measure.

BOX 7: Blatchford [Risk stratification criteria for upper gastrointestinal (UGI) bleed].

Risk factors at presentation	***Threshold***	***Score***
BUN (mmol/L)	6.5–7.9	2
	8.0–9.9	3
	10.0–24.9	4
	≥25.0	6
Hemoglobin for men (g/L)	120–130	1
	100–119	3
	<100	6
Hemoglobin for women (g/L)	100–120	1
	<100	6
Systolic blood pressure (mm Hg)	100–109	1
	90–99	2
	<90	3
HR (bpm)	>100	1
Melena	Present	1
Syncope	Present	2
Hepatic disease	Present	2
Cardiac failure	Present	2

Total score = 0–23

Patients with scores >0 are considered to be at risk, higher the score more the need for quicker intervention and ICU management

BOX 8: Ottawa ankle rules.

Ankle X-ray indication

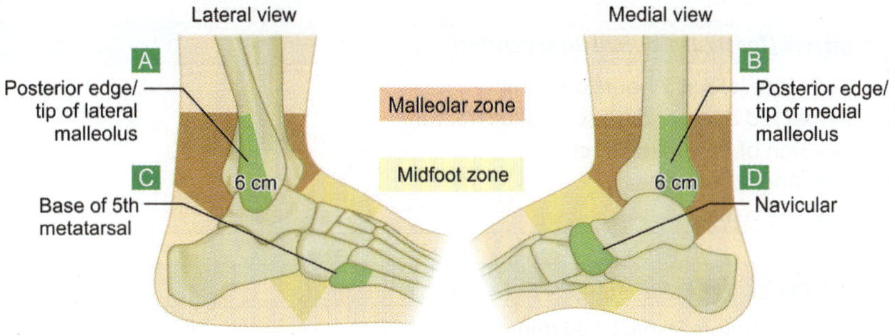

Lateral view

Medial view

A Posterior edge/ tip of lateral malleolus

B Posterior edge/ tip of medial malleolus

C Base of 5th metatarsal

D Navicular

Malleolar zone

Midfoot zone

6 cm

6 cm

An ankle radiograph should be conducted if there is pain in the malleolar region along with any of the following criteria:

- Bone tenderness at the posterior edge or tip of the lateral malleolus within the distal 6 cm **(A)**
- Bone tenderness at the posterior edge or tip of the medial malleolus within the distal 6 cm
- Inability to bear weight for at least four steps immediately after the injury and during the evaluation **(B)**

A foot radiograph series should be performed if there is pain in the midfoot region along with any of the following criteria:

- Bone tenderness at the navicular bone **(D)**
- Bone tenderness at the base of the fifth metatarsal **(C)**
- Inability to bear weight for at least four steps immediately after the injury and during the evaluation **(D)**

BOX 9: Ottawa knee rules.

Knee X-ray indications: Ottawa knee rules (acute)

- Age ≥55 years
- Isolated patella tenderness
- Tenderness at head of fibula
- Inability to flex knee 90°
- Inability to bear weight (four steps) immediately after injury and in emergency room

BOX 10: Ottawa rule for subarachnoid hemorrhage.

- Age >40 +1
- Neck pain/stiffness +1
- Witnessed level of consciousness +1
- Onset during exertion +1
- Thunderclap headache (instant peaking pain) +1
- Limited neck flexion on examination +1

If score is 0, consider ruling out SAH
But if any criterion is positive, consider workup for SAH

Exclusion criteria:
New neurological deficit, previous aneurysm, brain tumor/SAH, and chronic recurrent headache

BOX 11: Canadian computed tomography (CT) head rule.

CT head is only required in minor head injury patients with any one of these findings:

High risk (for neurological intervention)
• GCS score <15 at 2 hours after injury • Suspected open or depressed skull fracture • Any sign of basal skull fracture* • Vomiting ≥2 episodes • Age ≥65 years

Medium risk (for brain injury on CT)
• Amnesia before impact ≥30 minutes • Dangerous mechanism** *(pedestrian, occupant ejected, and fall from elevation)*

Rule not applicable if
• Nontrauma cases • GCS <13 • Age <16 years • Coumadin or bleeding disorder • Obvious open skull fracture

******Signs of basal skull fracture:* Hemotympanum, "racoon" eyes, cerebrospinal fluid (CSF) otorrhea/rhinorrhea, and Battle's sign

***Dangerous Mechanism:*

- Pedestrian struck by vehicle
- Occupant ejected from motor vehicle
- Fall from elevation ≥3 feet or 5 stairs

BOX 12: Pediatric emergency care applied research network (PECARN) head CT rule.

Younger than 2 years	*2 years or older*	
Altered mental state (AMS) or GCS <15 or Palpable skull fracture	AMS or GCS <15 or Signs of basilar skull fracture	***CT head recommended***
None	*None*	
LOC >5 seconds or Nonfrontal hematoma or Not acting normally or Severe mechanism	History of LOC or History of vomiting or Severe headache or Severe mechanism	***Observation versus CT Head***
None	*None*	
No CT required	No CT required	***Discharge***

- If GCS is low, CT is required.
- If GCS is >14 but other symptoms are present, observation is recommended for 4–6 hours to see worsening of symptoms. However, if polytrauma and strong clinical suspicion, age <3 months, and parenteral preference is there, immediate CT imaging can be done.

BOX 13: Canadian C-spine rule (assess need for C-spine imaging).

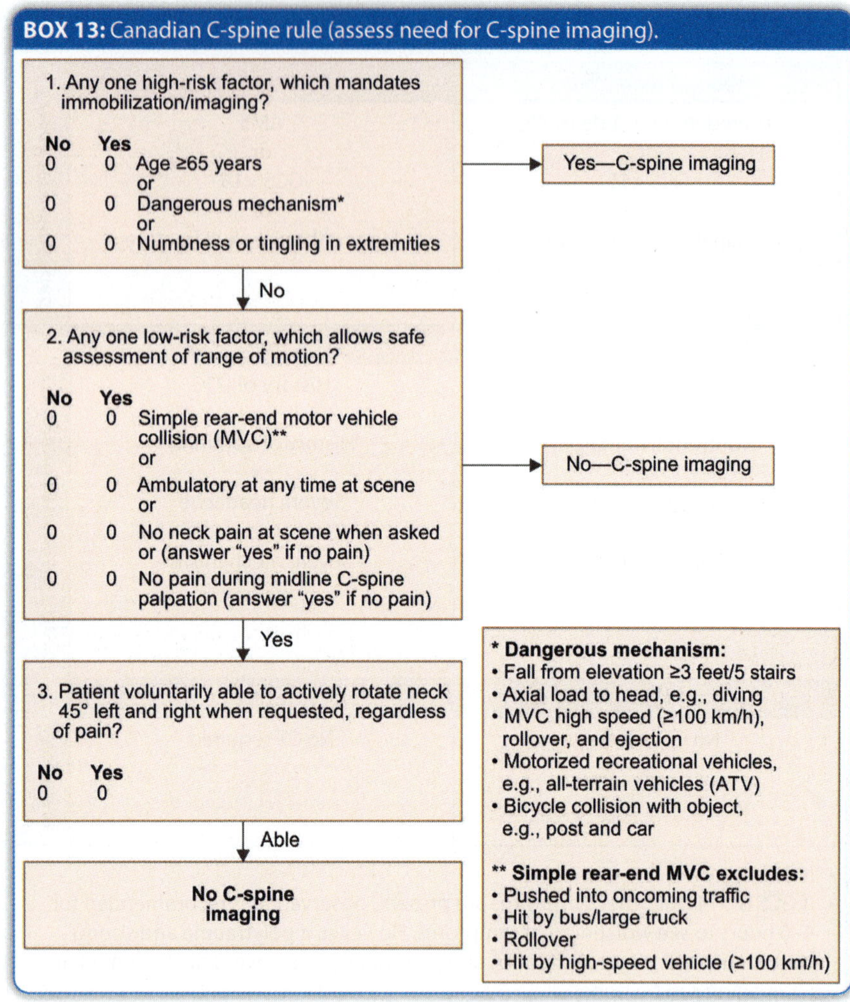

BOX 14: National emergency X-ray utilization studies (NEXUS) chest rule.

Risk factors		
Age >60 years	No 0	Yes +1
Rapid deceleration mechanism	No 0	Yes +1
• Fall from >20 feet (>6 m) • MVC >40 mph (>64 km/h)		
Chest pain	No 0	Yes +1
Intoxication	No 0	Yes +1
Altered mental status	No 0	Yes +1
Distracting painful injury	No 0	Yes +1
Tenderness to chest wall palpation	No 0	Yes +1

Result:
0 points = No thoracic imaging required
If >1 and well-appearing patient, consider only chest X-ray; if ill-appearing patient with polytrauma, consider CT imaging

BOX 15: Canadian syncope risk score.

Features		***Score***
Clinical	• Faints easily (warm/stand/emotion/pain)	–1
	• Abnormal heart [coronary artery disease (CAD)/congestive heart failure (CHF)/ cardiomyopathy (CMO)/valve replacement/ electrolyte imbalance/implantable cardioverter defibrillator (ICD)]	1
	• Increase (>180) or decrease (<90) systolic blood pressure (SBP)	2
Test	• Non-narrow QRS >130 milliseconds	1
	• Troponin elevated >99th percentile	2
	• Rotated QRS axis <-30 or >100	1
	• Increased QTc >480	2
Dx	Syncope vasovagal	–2
	Cardiac syncope	2

Risk of serious adverse events:	
–3, –2 = Very low	–1, 0 = Low
1, 2, 3 = Medium	4, 5 = High
>5 = Very high	

BOX 16: Clinical Institute Withdrawal Assessment of Alcohol Scale, Revised (CIWAr) score.

This scale objectifies severity of alcohol withdrawal by taking into consideration below symptoms:
- Nausea and vomiting
- Tremors
- Paroxysmal sweats
- Anxiety
- Agitation
- Tactile disturbances
- Auditory disturbances
- Visual disturbances
- Headache/fullness in head
- Orientation

Minimum score = 0
Maximum score = 7
- Adding each parameter, if total score exceeds 8–10, the patient might need benzodiazepine to prevent progression and control agitation.
- If score exceeds 20, patient might need ICU transfer.

BOX 17: Full outline of unresponsiveness (FOUR) score/Glasgow coma score.

FOUR score		***Glasgow coma scale***	
Eye response		*Eye opening*	
E4	Eyelids open or opened, tracking or blinking to command	E4	Spontaneous
E3	Eyelids open but not tracking	E3	To verbal command
E2	Eyelids closed but open to loud voice	E2	To pain
E1	Eyelids closed but open to pain	E1	None
E0	Eyelids remain closed with pain		
Motor response		*Verbal response*	
M4	Thumbs-up, fist or peace sign	V5	Oriented
M3	Localizing to pain	V4	Confused
M2	Flexion response to pain	V3	Inappropriate words
M1	Extension to pain	V2	Incomprehensible sounds
M0	No response to pain or generalized myoclonus status	V1	None

Contd...

Contd...

FOUR score		***Glasgow coma scale***	
Brainstem reflexes		*Motor response*	
B4	Pupil and corneal reflexes present	M6	Obeying commands
B3	One pupil wide and fixed	M5	Localizes pain
B2	Pupil or corneal reflexes absent	M4	Withdraws from pain
B1	Both pupil and corneal reflexes are absent	M3	Flexion to pain
B0	Absent pupil, corneal and cough reflex	M2	Extension to pain
		M1	None
Respiration			
R4	Not intubated, regular breathing pattern		
R3	Not intubated, Cheyne–Strokes breathing		
R2	Not intubated, irregular breathing		
R1	Breathes above ventilator rate		
R0	Breathes at ventilator rate or apnea		

BOX 18: Good outcome following attempted resuscitation (GO-FAR) score.

GO-FAR score variables	
Variable	***Score***
Neurologically intact at admission	–15
Major trauma	10
Acute stroke	8
Metastatic or hematologic cancer	7
Septicemia	7
Medical noncardiac diagnosis	7
Hepatic insufficiency	6
Admission from skilled nursing facility	6
Hypotension or hypoperfusion	5
Renal insufficiency including dialysis	4
Respiratory insufficiency	4
Pneumonia	1
Age (years)	
70–74	2
75–79	5
80–84	6
≥85	11

BOX 19: Human deficiency virus (HIV) Needle Stick Risk Assessment Stratification Protocol (RASP) score [for post exposure prophylaxis (PEP) recommendation in needle prick].

Step A	*Identify source population (choose one)*	*Score*
	Known HIV carrier: • Acute acquired immunodeficiency syndrome (AIDS) illness* • Asymptomatic	 1 10
	Unknown HIV status: • High-risk situation • Low-risk situation (other)	 100 1,000
	A value	....
Step B	*Identify inoculum type (choose one)*	
	• Fresh blood • Body fluids at risk (e.g., semen) • Dried old blood • Low-risk secretions (tears, saliva, and urine)	1 10 100 1,000
	B value	....
Step C	*Identify method of transmission (choose one)*	
	• Intravenous • Deep intramuscular • Deep transcutaneous with visible bleeding at site • Superficial transcutaneous with no visible bleeding • Mucosal contact only • Intact skin	1 10 100 200 500 1,000
	C value	....
Total score (Z) = A × B × C = ... and basic risk = 1/Z = ...		
Step D	*Estimate volume of inoculum (choose one)*	*Modifier*
	• Massive (e.g., transfusion) • Measurable (>1 mL) • Moderate (large-bore hollow needle >20 g) • Small (small-bore hollow needle <22 g) • Trace surface only (e.g., suture needle)	100 10 5 3 1
	Total risk = Basic risk × Modifier (D)	....

Total risk	***PEP recommendation***
>1/1,000	Definitely indicated
>1/10,000	Recommended but optional
>1/10,000–1/100,000	Optional but not recommended
>1/100,000	Not indicated

BOX 20: Alvarado score for appendicitis.

Symptoms and signs	***Score***
Migratory or right iliac fossa pain	1
Nausea/vomiting	1
Anorexia	1
Tenderness in right iliac fossa	2
Rebound tenderness in right iliac fossa	1
Elevated temperature	1
Laboratory tests	
Leukocytosis	2
Shift to left neutrophils	1
If score: 5–6 = Possible 7–8 = Probable >9 = Very probable	

BOX 21: Modified SAD PERSONS score.

Factor	***Points***
S = Sex (male)	1
A = Age (<19 or >45)	1
D = Depression or hopelessness	2
P = Previous suicide attempts or psychiatric care	1
E = Excessive alcohol or drug use	1
R = Rational thinking loss	2
S = Separated, divorced, and widowed	1
O = Organized or serious attempt	2
N = No social support	1
S = Stated future intent	2
If points: 6–7 = Full emergency psychiatry evaluation/treatment 9 or more = Immediate psychiatric admission	

BOX 22: Scoring for difficult airway prediction **(Fig. 1)**.

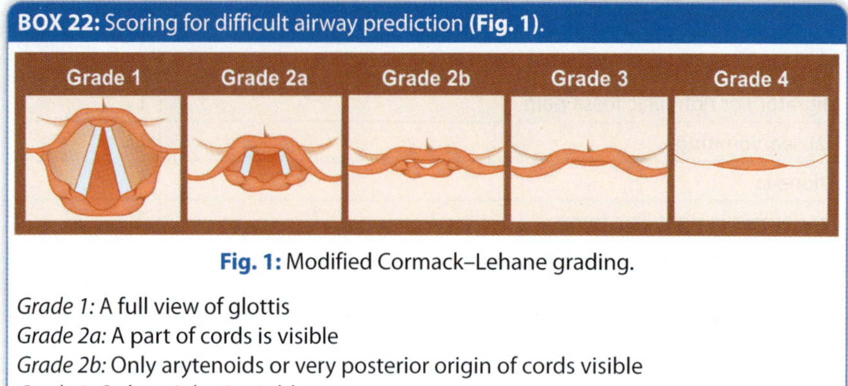

Fig. 1: Modified Cormack–Lehane grading.

Grade 1: A full view of glottis
Grade 2a: A part of cords is visible
Grade 2b: Only arytenoids or very posterior origin of cords visible
Grade 3: Only epiglottis visible
Grade 4: No glottis structure visible

SUGGESTED READING

1. Alvarado A. A practical score for the early diagnosis of acute appendicitis. Ann Emerg Med. 1986;15(5):557-64.
2. Backus BE, Six AJ, Kelder JC, Bosschaert MA, Mast EG, Mosterd A, et al. A prospective validation of the HEART score for chest pain patients at the emergency department. Int J Cardiol. 2013;168(3):2153-8.
3. Blatchford O, Murray WR, Blatchford M. A risk score to predict need for treatment for upper-gastrointestinal haemorrhage. Lancet. 2000;356(9238):1318-21.
4. Kline JA, Mitchell AM, Kabrhel C, Richman PB, Courtney DM. Clinical criteria to prevent unnecessary diagnostic testing in emergency department patients with suspected pulmonary embolism. J Thromb Haemost. 2004;2(8):1247-55.
5. Knaus WA, Draper EA, Wagner DP, Zimmerman JE. APACHE II: a severity of disease classification system. Crit Care Med. 1985;13(10):818-29.
6. Kuppermann N, Holmes JF, Dayan PS, Hoyle JD Jr, Atabaki SM, Holubkov R, et al. Identification of children at very low risk of clinically-important brain injuries after head trauma: a prospective cohort study. Lancet. 2009;374(9696): 1160-70.
7. Lim WS, van der Eerden MM, Laing R, Boersma WG, Karalus N, Town GI, et al. Defining community acquired pneumonia severity on presentation to hospital: an international derivation and validation study. Thorax. 2003;58(5):377-82.
8. Lip GY, Nieuwlaat R, Pisters R, Lane DA, Crijns HJ. Refining clinical risk stratification for predicting stroke and thromboembolism in atrial fibrillation using a novel risk factor-based approach. The Euro Heart Survey on atrial Fibrillation. Chest. 2010;137(2):263-72.
9. Mallampati SR, Gatt SP, Gugino LD, Desai SP, Waraksa B, Freiberger D, et al. A clinical sign to predict difficult tracheal intubation: a prospective study. Can Anaesth Soc J. 1985;32(4):429-34.
10. Patterson WM, Dohn HH, Bird J, Patterson GA. Evaluation of suicidal patients: The SAD PERSONS scale. Psychosomatics. 1983;24(4):343-9.

11. Rodriguez RM, Langdorf MI, Nishijima D, Baumann BM, Hendey GW, Medak AJ, et al. Derivation and validation of the Nexus Chest Decision Instrument to identify blunt trauma patients at low risk for thoracic injury. Ann Emerg Med. 2011;58(1):2938.
12. Singer M, Deutschman CS, Seymour CW, Shankar-Hari M, Annane D, Bauer M, et al. The Third International Consensus Definitions for Sepsis and Septic Shock (Sepsis-3). JAMA. 2016;315(8):801-10.
13. Stiell IG, Greenberg GH, McKnight RD, Nair RC, McDowell I, Reardon M, et al. Decision rules for the use of radiography in acute ankle injuries: refinement and prospective validation. JAMA. 1993;269(9):1127-32.
14. Stiell IG, Wells GA, Vandemheen K, C Clement, H Lesiuk, A Laupacis, et al. The Canadian CT Head Rule for patients with minor head injury. Lancet. 2001;357(9266):1391-6.
15. Stiell IG, Wells GA, Vandemheen KL, Clement CM, Lesiuk H, De Maio VJ, et al. The Canadian C-spine rule for radiography in alert and stable trauma patients. JAMA. 2001;286(15):1841-8.
16. Sullivan JT, Sykora K, Schneiderman J, Naranjo CA, Sellers EM. Assessment of alcohol withdrawal: The revised clinical institute withdrawal assessment for alcohol scale (CIWA-Ar). Br J Addict. 1989;84(11):1353-7.
17. Thiruganasambandamoorthy V, Stiell IG, Sivilotti ML, Sage NL, Yan JW, Huang P, et al. Multicenter Emergency Department Validation of the Canadian Syncope Risk Score. JAMA Intern Med. 2020;180(5):737-44.
18. Wells PS, Anderson DR, Rodger M, Ginsberg JS, Kearon C, Gent M, et al. Derivation of a simple clinical model to categorize patients probability of pulmonary embolism: increasing the models utility with the SimpliRED D-dimer. Thromb Haemost. 2000;83(3):416-20.
19. Wijdicks EF, Bamlet WR, Maramattom BV, Manno EM, McClelland RL. Validation of a new coma scale: the FOUR score. Ann Neurol. 2005;58(4):585-93.

CHAPTER 45

Archives of Images in Emergency Room

Ritu Kashikar, Jyoti Narayan

HYPERACUTE INFARCT

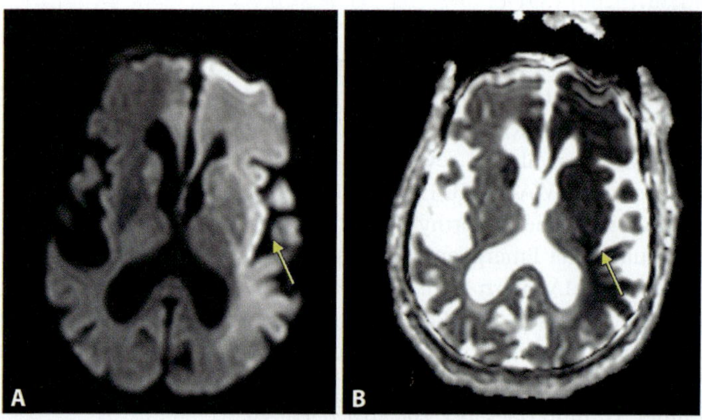

(A and B) Axial restricted diffusion in the left frontotemporoparietal lobe with corresponding drop in apparent diffusion coefficient (ADC). Large hemispheric hyperacute infarct in left frontotemporoparietal lobe. There is restricted diffusion seen with corresponding ADC drop. There is no evidence of FLAIR hyperintensity or SWI hypointensity.

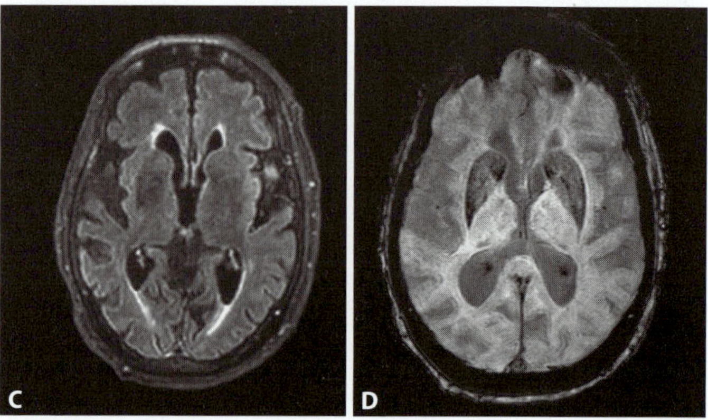

(C and D) No evidence of fluid-attenuated inversion recovery (FLAIR) hyperintensity or susceptibility weighted imaging (SWI) hypointensity within infarct in left frontotemporoparietal lobes.

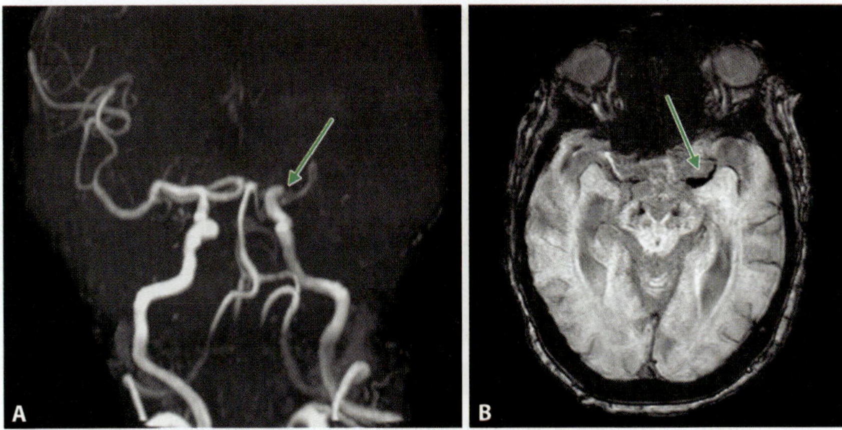

(A) There is nonvisualization of flow in left middle cerebral artery (MCA) on time of flight angiogram (arrow) and (B) There is SWI hypointense thrombus in M1 segment of left MCA (arrow).

ACUTE INFARCT-COMPUTED TOMOGRAPHY

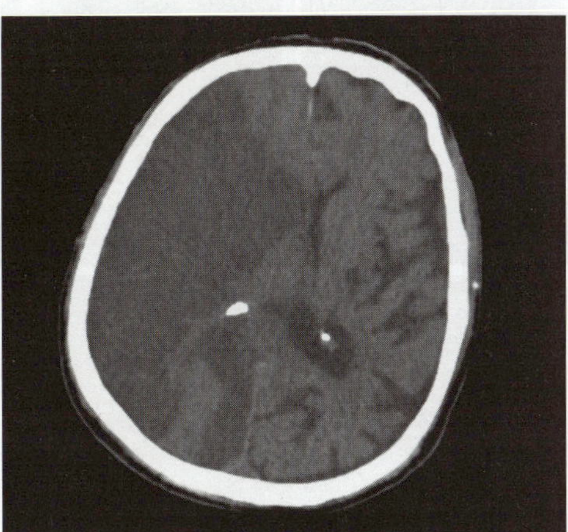

Large right hemispheric hypodense infarct in the right frontotemporoparietal occipital lobes with hypodense cerebral edema and resultant subfalcine shift to the left, and effacement of ventricles.

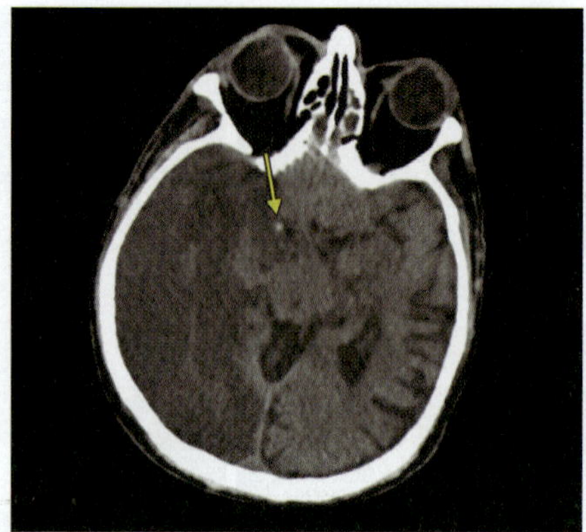

There is hyperdense MCA dot sign seen in M1 segment of right MCA.

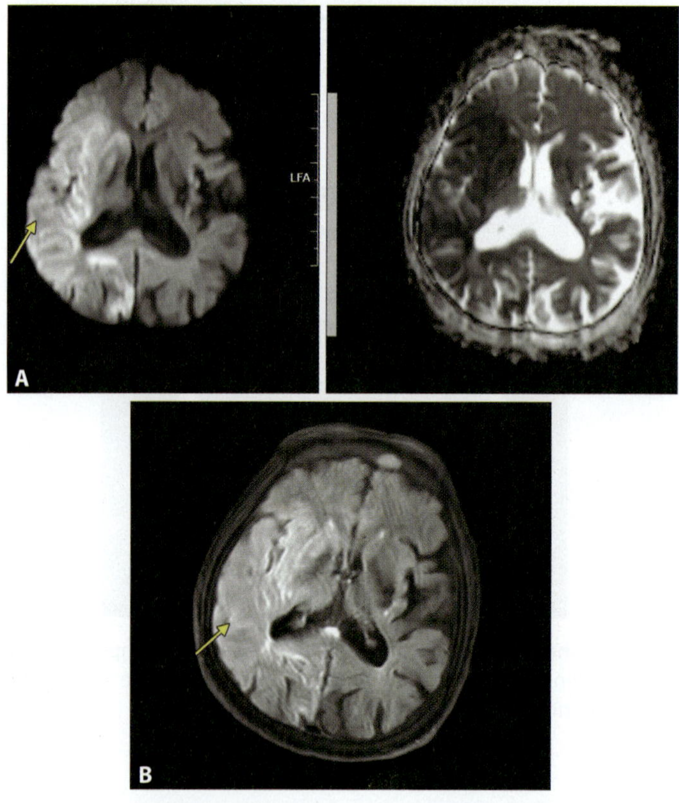

(A) Restricted diffusion (appearing hyperintense) in the right hemisphere with drop in ADC; (B) FLAIR hyperintensity also seen within the region.

INTRAPARENCHYMAL BLEED WITH INTRAVENTRICULAR EXTENSION

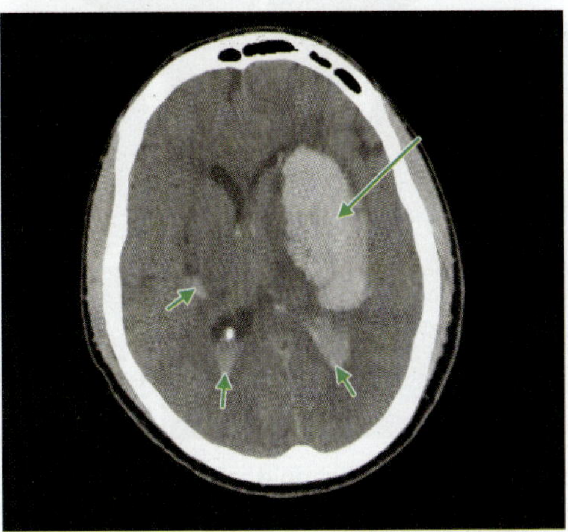

There is hyperdense intraparenchymal bleed in the left gangliocapsular region with hyperdensity extending into the occipital horns of bilateral lateral ventricles. There is another focus of hyperdensity in the right gangliocapsular region.

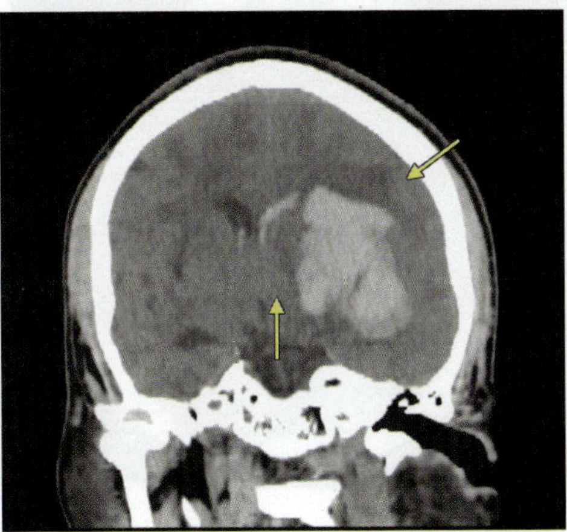

There is mass effect in the form of midline shift to the right and effacement of overlying sulci.

SUBARACHNOID HEMORRHAGE

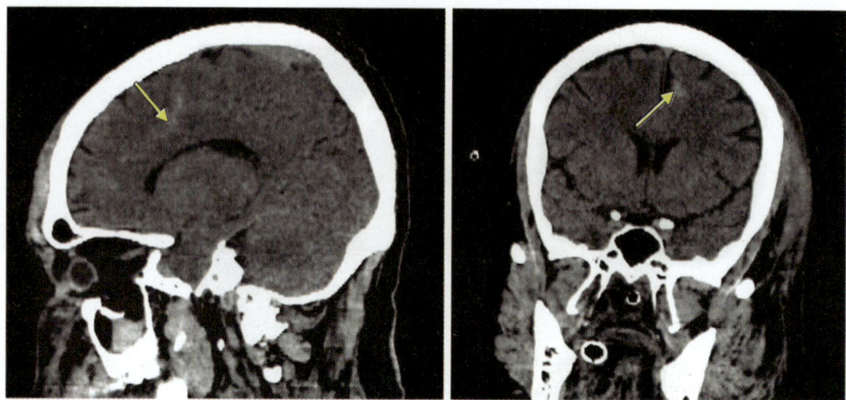

Hyperdensity is seen in the subarachnoid space in the left parafalcine region representing hemorrhage.

EXTRADURAL HEMORRHAGE

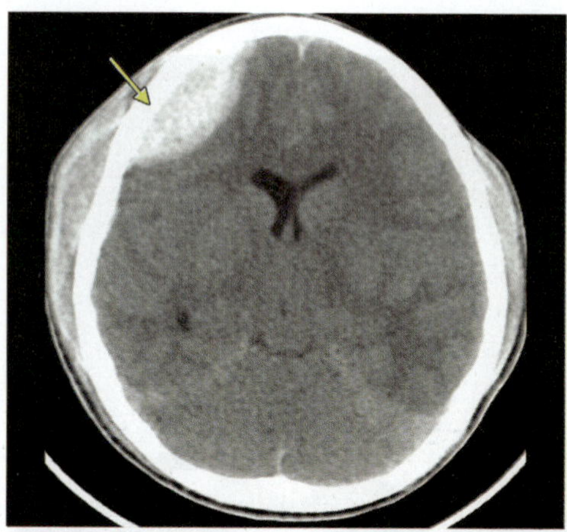

A biconvex epidural hyperdense hematoma in the right frontal region causing mild mass affect on underlying sulci and minimal subfacine shift. Hyperdense overlying subgaleal hematoma is also seen.

SUBDURAL HEMORRHAGE

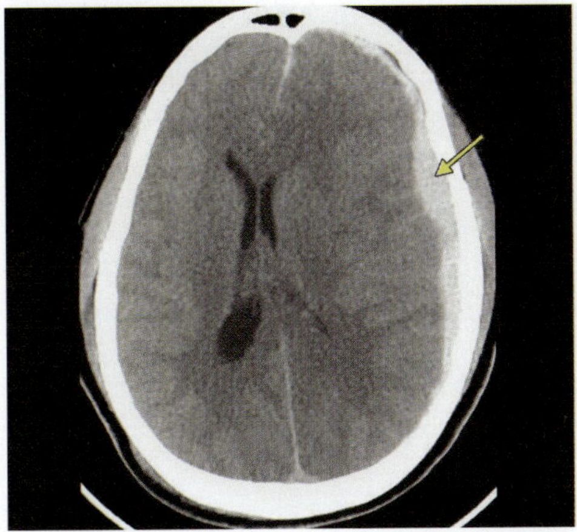

Left-sided crescent shaped subdural hyperdense hematoma, with resultant bilateral underlying sulcal effacement, edema, and midline shift.

ORBITAL FRACTURE

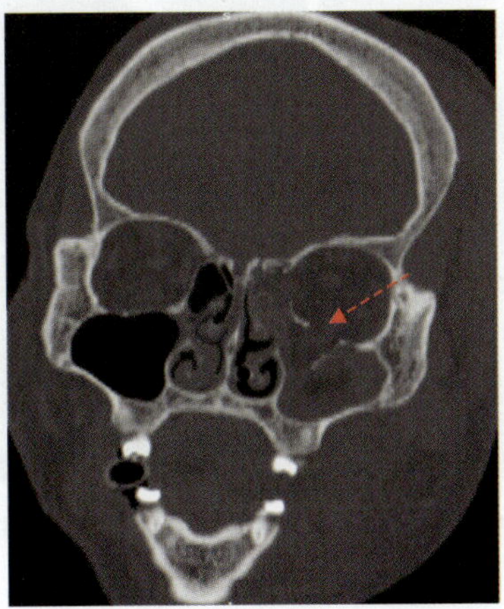

Orbital blow-out fractures occur when there is a fracture on one of the walls of orbit (inferior wall in this case) but the orbital rim remains intact. Orbital fat prolapses into the maxillary sinus and may be joined by prolapse of the inferior rectus muscle.

MULTIPLE FACIAL FRACTURES

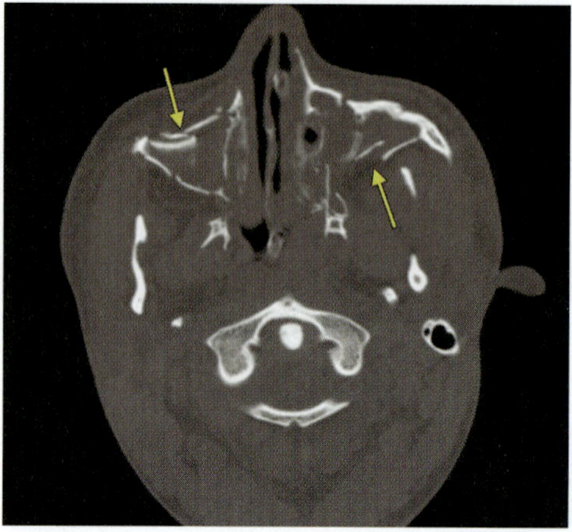

Multiple fractures involving bilateral maxillary and mandibular bones (yellow arrows) with mild displacement. There are fractures seen involving nasal septum with buckling.

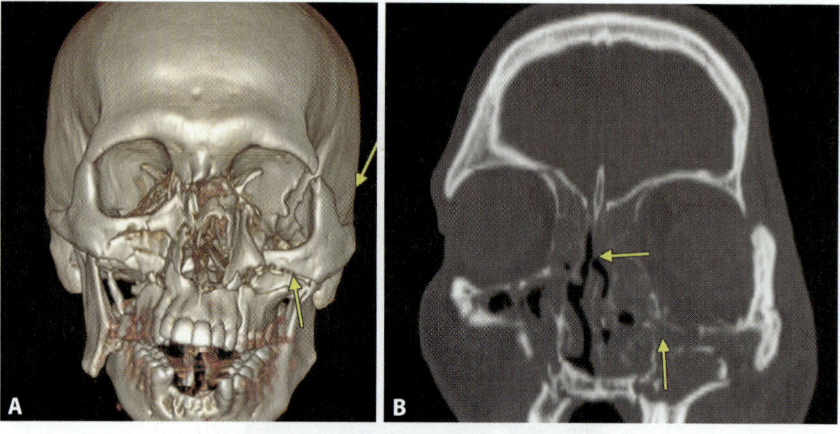

These are (A) volume-rendered images and (B) coronal reconstruction of patient with multiple facial bone fractures.

TRAUMATIC LIVER LACERATIONS

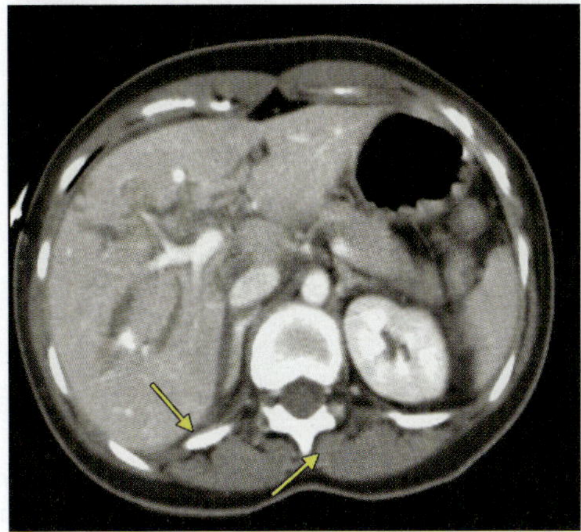

Liver lacerations appear as irregular linear/branching areas of hypodensity and hypoenhancement which is seen in both lobes of liver.

ACUTE APPENDICITIS

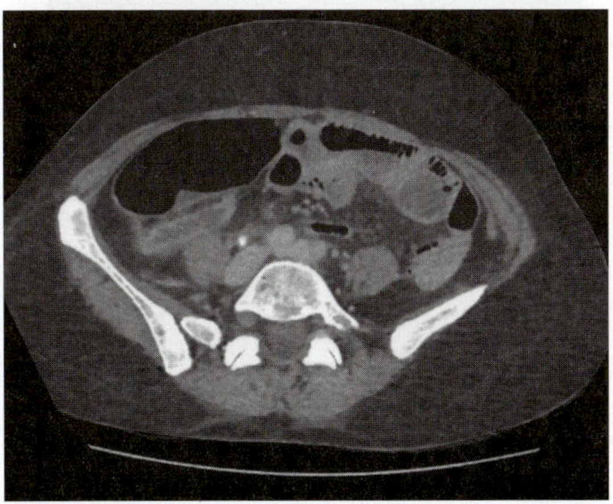

Axial postcontrast CT reveals dilated retrocecal appendix with peri appendiceal inflammation.

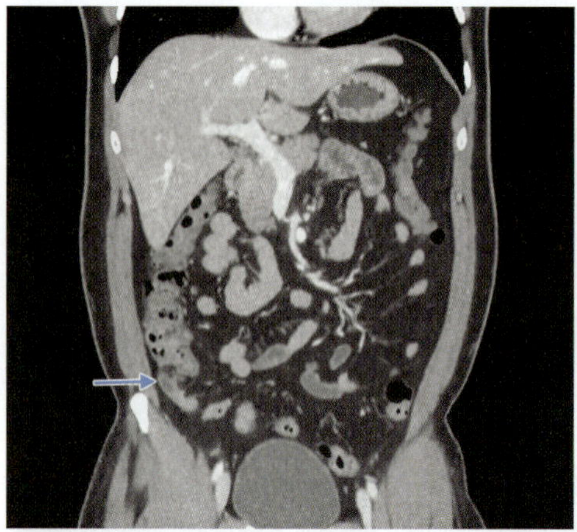

A peristaltic blind-ending tube in the right iliac fossa is the appendix (blue arrow). Increased appendiceal diameter more than 9 mm and wall thickening of more than 3 mm with enhancement and stratification with periappendiceal fluid and stranding are features of appendicitis.

PNEUMOPERITONEUM

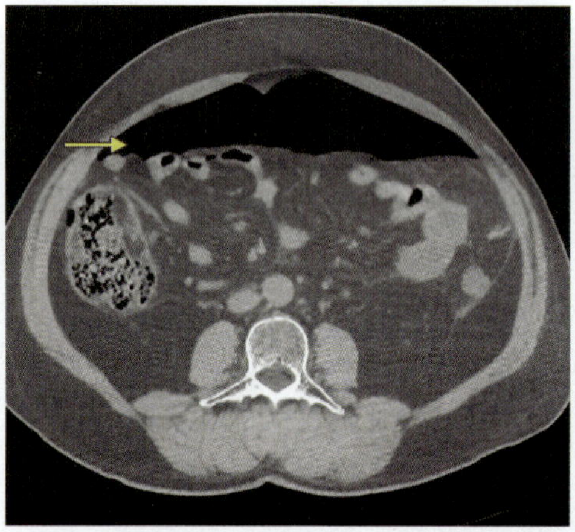

Computed tomography shows intra-abdominal air due to perforation of hollow viscera.

PULMONARY EMBOLISM

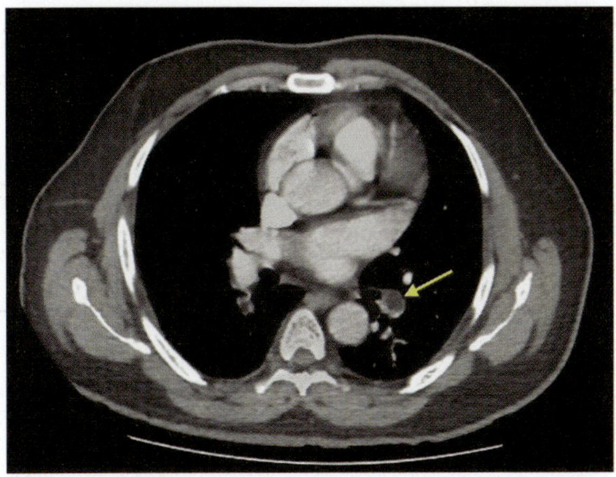

Filling defect in left descending pulmonary artery (yellow arrow) represents pulmonary thromboembolism.

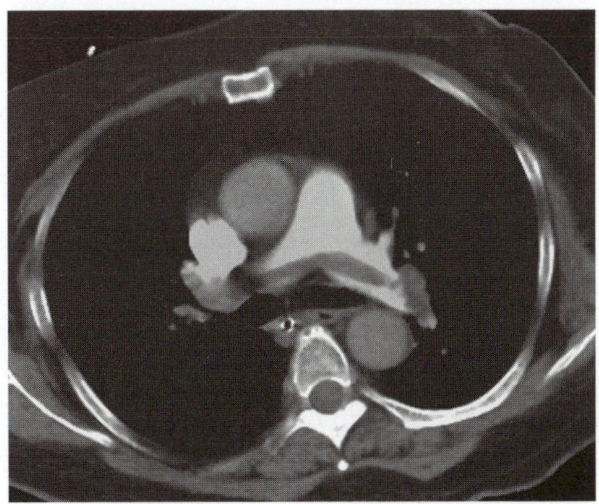

Saddle embolus—CT pulmonary angiogram (CTPA) demonstrates saddle pulmonary embolism, extending to segmental and subsegmental branches of both pulmonary artery branches.

ACUTE RESPIRATORY DISTRESS SYNDROME

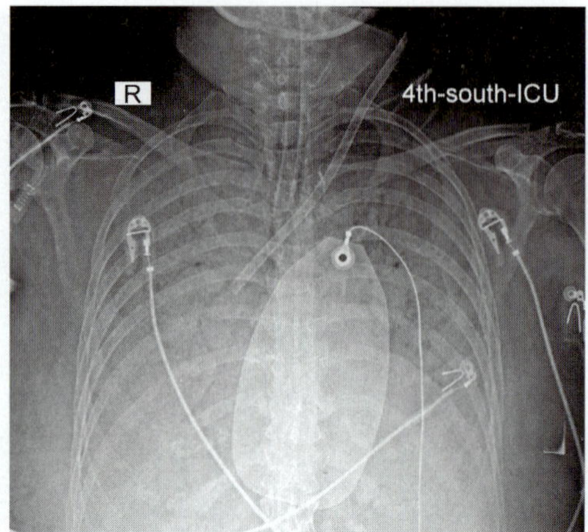

Chest radiographic findings of acute respiratory distress syndrome (ARDS) are nonspecific and resemble those of typical pulmonary edema or pulmonary hemorrhage. There are diffuse bilateral coalescent opacities.

HIATAL HERNIA

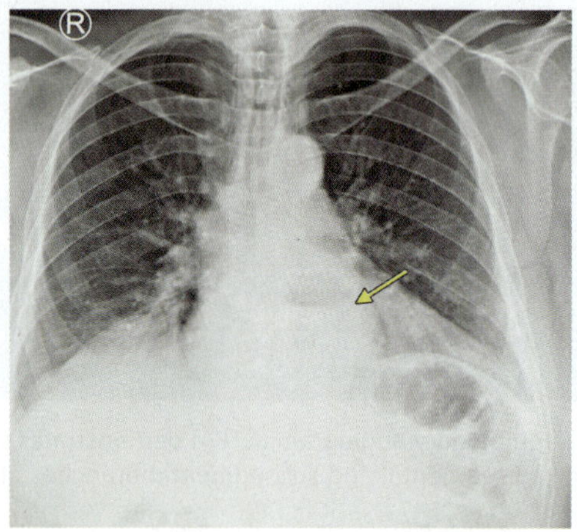

Retrocardiac opacity with gas-fluid level.

INTESTINAL OBSTRUCTION

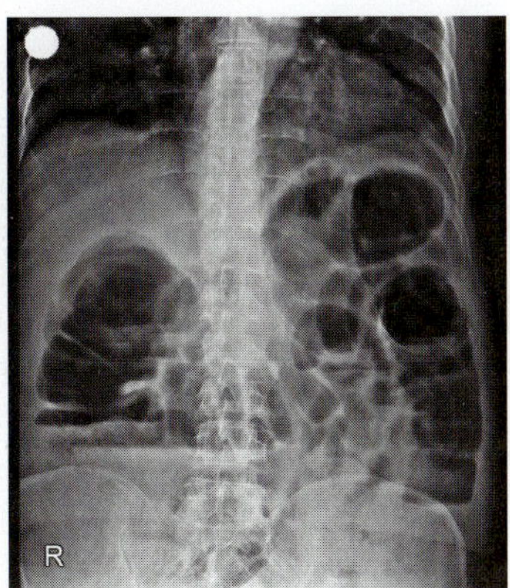

Multiple dilated loops with air-fluid level in mid abdomen.

PNEUMOTHORAX

- Visible visceral pleural edge is seen as a very thin, sharp white line
- No lung markings are seen peripheral to this line
- Peripheral space is radiolucent compared to the adjacent lung
- Lung may completely collapse

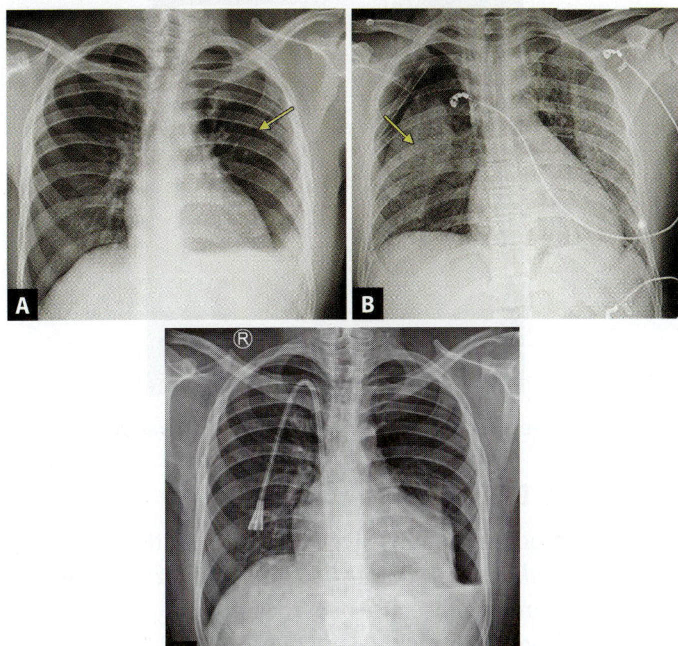

(A) Left mild-to-moderate hydropneumothorax with pleural edge (as depicted by arrows) with no distal lung markings; (B) Right moderate pneumothorax with intercostal drainage tube insertion for the same; and (C) Tension pneumothorax.

CONSOLIDATION

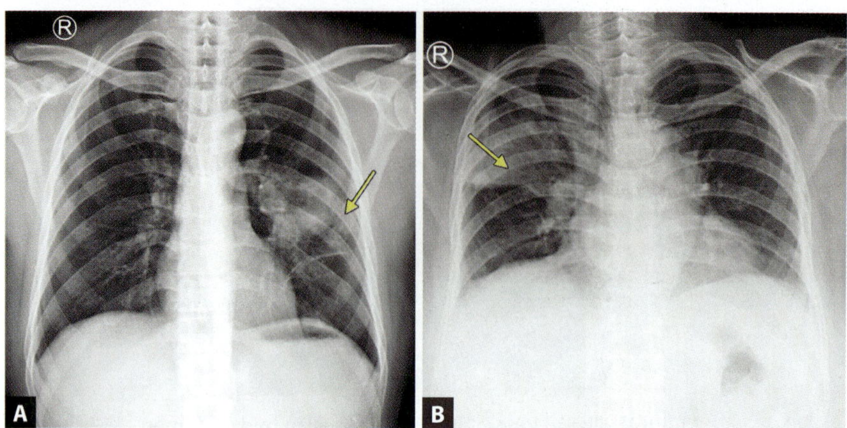

On radiographs, consolidation appears as air bronchograms with opacity which is otherwise homogeneous. (A) Left mid-zone consolidation and (B) Right upper zone consolidation.

PNEUMOPERITONEUM

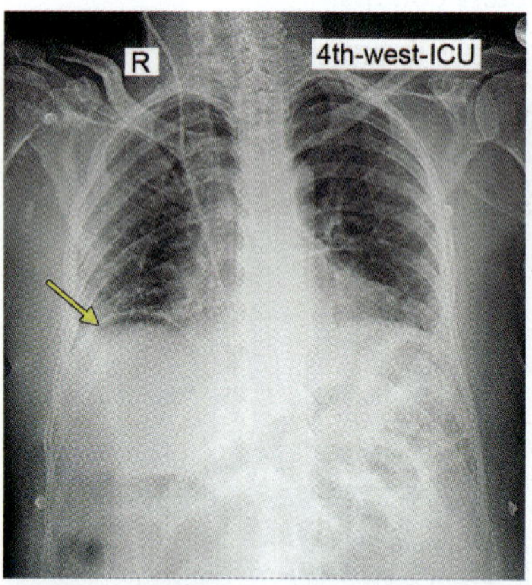

Free air seen underlying right hemidiaphragm.

PULMONARY EDEMA

- Upper lobe pulmonary venous diversion (stag's antler sign)
- *Increased cardiothoracic ratio/cardiac silhouette size:* Useful for assessing an underlying cardiogenic cause or association
- Features of pulmonary interstitial edema:
  - Peribronchial cuffing and perihilar haze
  - Septal (Kerley) lines
  - Thickening of interlobar fissures

- Features of pulmonary alveolar edema:
    - Air space opacification classically in a bat wing distribution
    - May have air bronchograms
- Pleural effusions and fluid in interlobar fissures

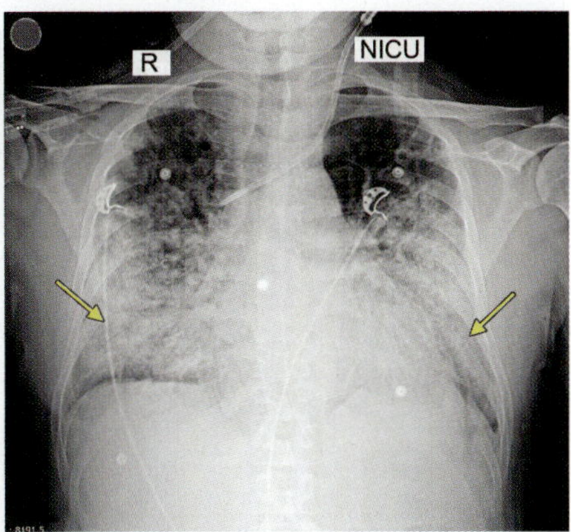

There is symmetrical area of opacity in the central region of both lungs, mild left heart enlargement with paracardiac congestion, and bilateral small pleural effusions.

PLEURAL EFFUSION IN SUPINE

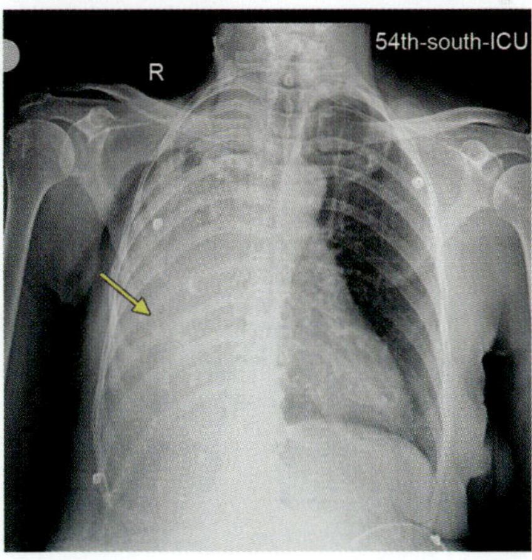

There is partial-to-gross right-sided pleural effusion.

SUBCUTANEOUS EMPHYSEMA

There are striated lucencies in the soft tissues that may outline muscle fibers. If affecting the anterior chest wall, subcutaneous emphysema can outline the pectoralis major muscle, giving rise to the ginkgo leaf sign.

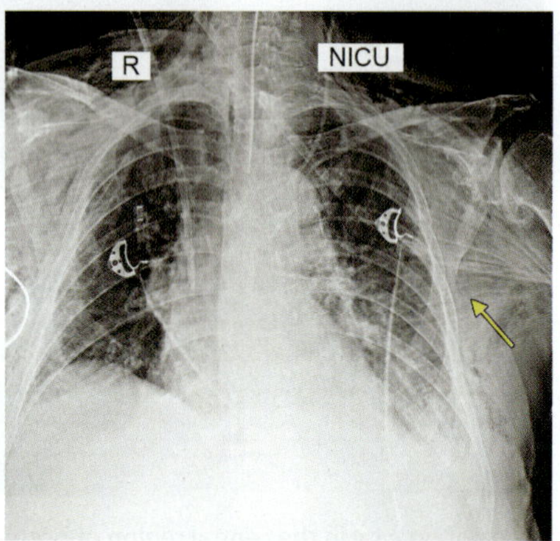

Gingko leaf sign.

CLAVICLE MIDSHAFT

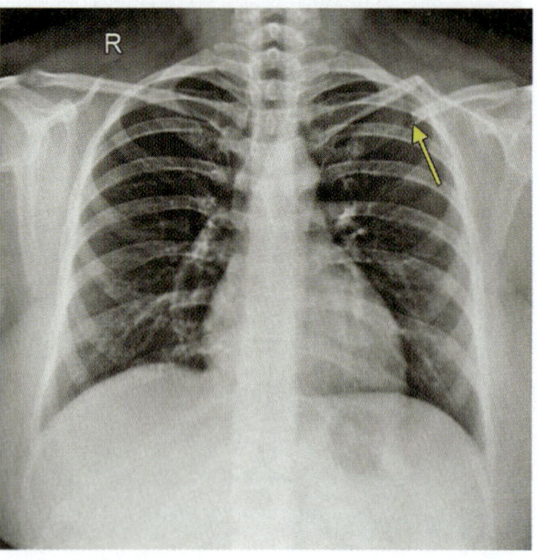

Displaced fracture of midshaft of left clavicle.

DISTAL FEMUR

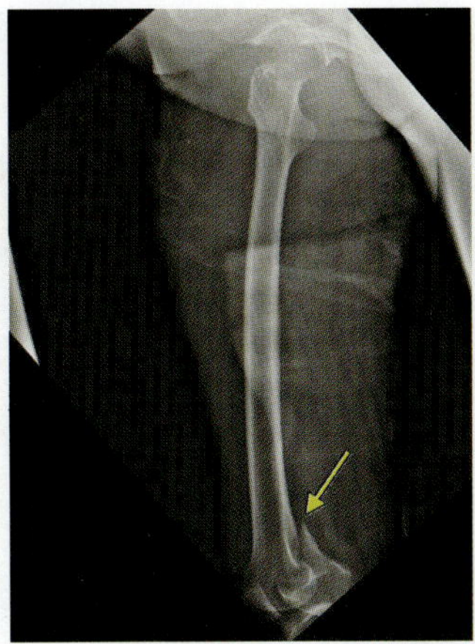

Displaced fracture of distal shaft of femur.

NECK OF FEMUR

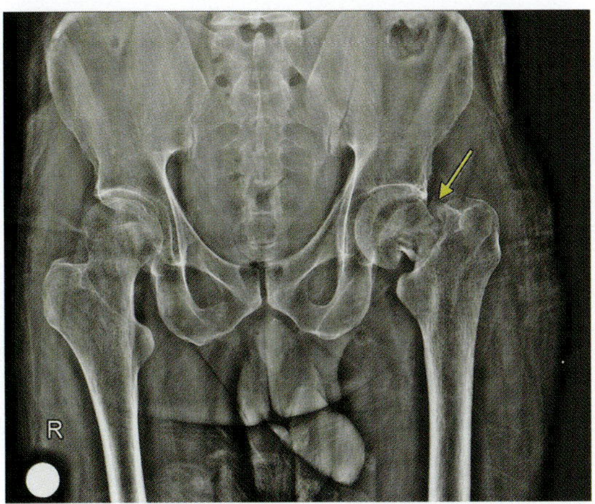

Displaced fracture of neck of left femur

NECK OF HUMERUS

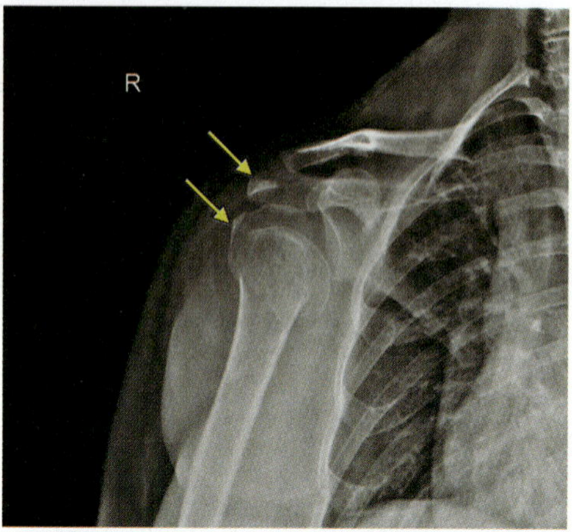

Displaced fracture of neck of right humerus with overlying soft tissue swelling.

RADIUS–ULNA

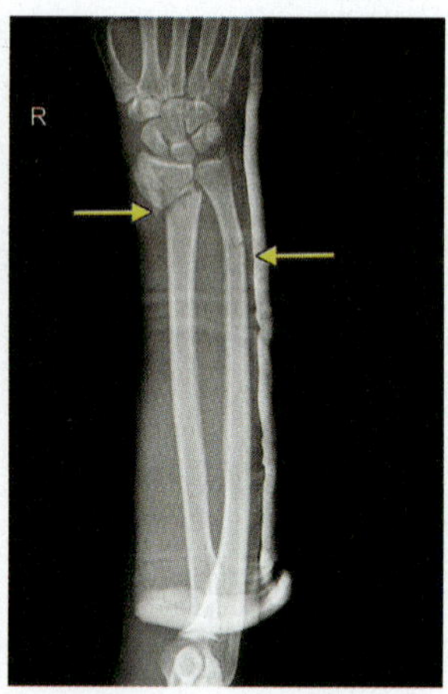

Displaced fracture of distal shaft of right radius and ulna as well as ulnar styloid process.

NORMAL IMAGES BRAIN

T1-weighted images are produced by using short repetition time (TR) and echo time (TE). The contrast and brightness of the image are predominately determined by T1 properties of tissue. Conversely, *T2-weighted images* are produced by using longer TE and TR times. In these images, the contrast and brightness are predominately determined by the T2 properties of tissue.

In general, T1- and T2-weighted images can be easily differentiated by looking the cerebrospinal fluid (CSF). CSF is dark on T1-weighted imaging and bright on T2-weighted imaging.

A third commonly used sequence is the FLAIR. The FLAIR sequence is similar to a T2-weighted image except that the TE and TR times are very long. By doing so, abnormalities remain bright but normal CSF fluid is attenuated and made dark. This sequence is very sensitive to pathology and makes the differentiation between CSF and an abnormality much easier.

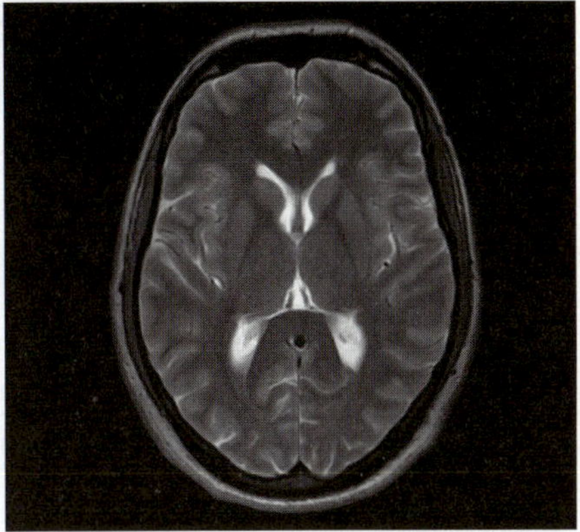

T2-weighted imaging at the level of basal ganglia. CSF and fat appear bright, gray matter appears light gray, and white matter appears dark gray.

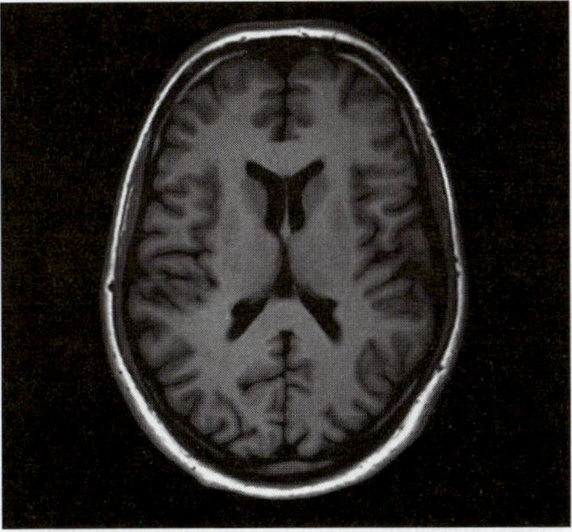

T1-weighted imaging at the level of basal ganglia. Fat appears bright, CSF appears dark, gray matter appears dark gray, and white matter appears light gray.

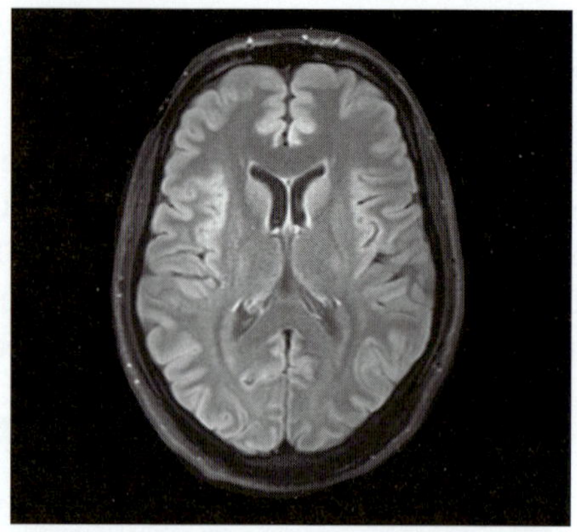

FLAIR-weighted imaging at the level of basal ganglia, CSF is suppressed, gray matter appears light gray, and white matter appears dark gray.

Tissue	***T1-weighted***	***T2-weighted***	***Flair***
CSF	Dark	Bright	Dark
White matter	Light	Dark gray	Dark gray
Cortex	Gray	Light gray	Light gray
Fat (within bone marrow	Bright	Light	Light
Inflammation (infection, demyelination)	Dark	Bright	Bright

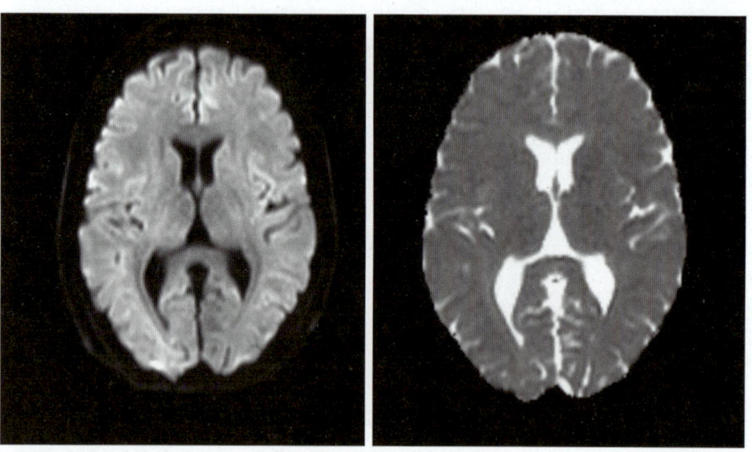

Diffusion-weighted imaging (DWI) at the level of basal ganglia with apparent diffusion coefficient (ADC).

DWI is designed to detect the movements of water protons. Water molecules diffuse relatively freely in the extracellular space; their movement is significantly restricted in the intracellular space. During ischemia, the sodium-potassium pump shuts down and sodium accumulates intracellularly. Water shifts from the extracellular to the intracellular space. As water movement becomes restricted intracellularly, this results in bright signal on DWI. Thus, DWI is a sensitive method for detecting acute stroke. ADC maps show dark signal and are derived from diffusion images.

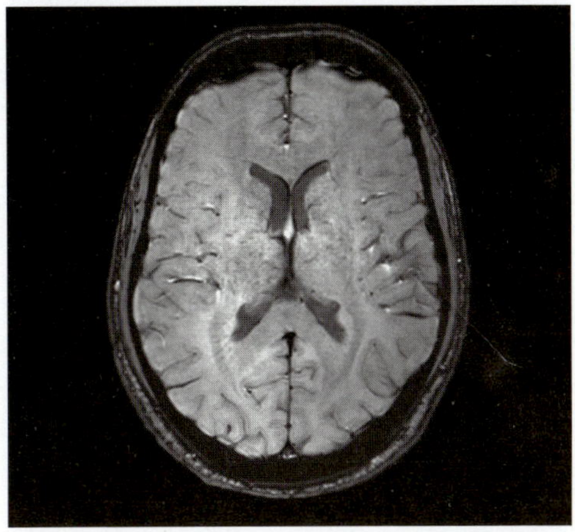

SWI at the level of basal ganglia—used to detect calfications and bleed.

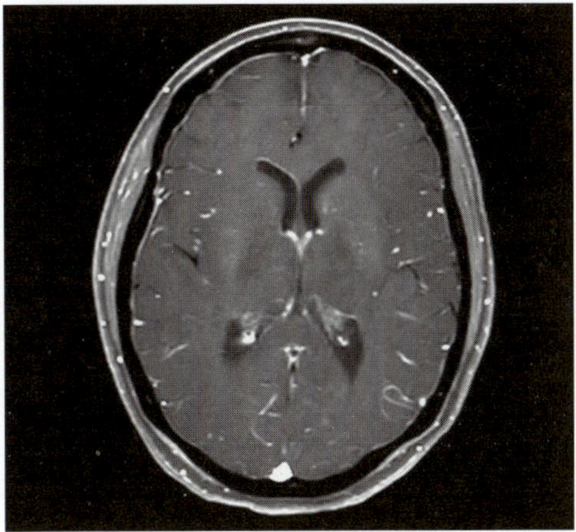

T1-weighted imaging with contrast.

When injected during the scan, Gadolinium changes signal intensities by shortening T1. Thus, Gadolinium is very bright on T1-weighted images. Gadolinium-enhanced images are especially useful in looking at vascular structures and breakdown in the blood-brain barrier

Part 7

General Approach to Emergency Room

CHAPTER 46

Triage

Sachna P Shetty

BOX 1: Introduction.

- Triage involves sorting patients based on the urgency of their need for care
- It is a critical process in every emergency room (ER) as it helps prioritize more serious cases, enabling quicker treatment for those in urgent need
- In situations where resources are limited, triage helps uphold the principle of "the greatest good for the greatest number," bringing order to otherwise chaotic circumstances and ensuring that all patients receive appropriate care

BOX 2: Method.

- Triage should be conducted within specific time frames depending on the urgency of the patient's condition: <5 minutes for those displaying emergency signs, 10–20 minutes for priority signs, and 30–120 minutes for nonurgent cases (time-frames might differ according to type of triage adapted in every institute)
- This assessment is performed by a triage nurse or another trained healthcare professional as soon as the patient arrives at the emergency unit
- Once emergency signs are identified, the emergency room (ER) physician is promptly notified, and immediate treatment is administered to stabilize the patient's condition. Early assessment and prioritization are essential for achieving favorable outcomes
- In many low-income countries, where hospitals often face high patient volumes and limited staff, triage plays a crucial role in managing patient flow and preventing deterioration by prioritizing care

BOX 3: Types.

Various triage systems are used globally, each tailored to its region. Among these, the color-coded triage system is widely used due to its simplicity. Recently, the Emergency Severity Index (ESI) has also gained traction due to its detailed set of criteria.

As outlined in the given algorithm, the ESI triage is a system used to rapidly determine the level of urgency for each patient seeking care in the ER.

- *Assessment:* Upon arrival, a nurse or healthcare provider promptly evaluates the patient's condition.

Contd...

Contd...

- The ESI triage system categorizes patients into five levels based on the urgency of their condition:
  - Level 1: Requires immediate attention (e.g., critical cases like cardiac arrest).
  - Level 2: High risk or rapidly deteriorating (e.g., severe chest pain).
  - Level 3: Needs care but not immediately life-threatening (e.g., moderate injuries).
  - Level 4: Minor issues that can wait (e.g., a sprained ankle).
  - Level 5: Nonurgent cases (e.g., a simple prescription refill).
- *Resource use:* The system also takes into account the resources a patient may require, such as tests or treatments, ensuring that those needing more intensive care receive it more quickly.

In summary, the ESI triage system enables ER staff to efficiently prioritize patients based on the severity of their condition, ensuring that the most critical cases are addressed first.

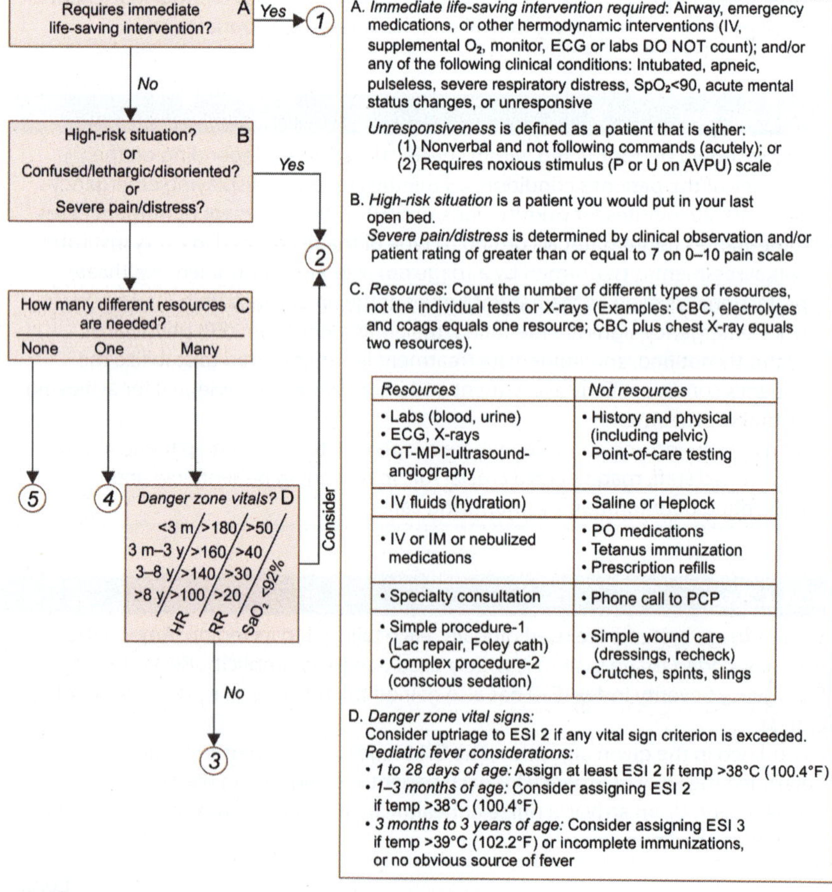

Fig. 1: Emergency severity index triage algorithm.
Source: Richard G, Williams MM. Emergency Severity Index (ESI): A Triage Tool for Emergency Departments. Emerg Med Clin N Am. 2018. https://www.escholarship.org/uc/item/6kh0x9d3

BOX 4: Color-coded triage.

This system uses colors to quickly sort patients by how urgently they need care depending on the patients' vitals and Glasgow coma scale (GCS); there can be three or four color codes **(Fig. 2)**.

	1 Red Resuscitation (0 minute)	2 Orange Urgent (15 minutes)	3 Yellow Less urgent (60 minutes)	4 Green Not urgent (180 minutes)
A	Obstructed airway Stridor	Threatened airway		
B	SpO_2 <80 RR >35 or <8	SpO_2: 80–89 RR: 31–35	SpO_2: 90–94 RR: 26–30	SpO_2: ≥95 RR: 8–25
C	HR >130 BP_{sys} <80	HR: 121–130 RR <40 BP_{sys}: 80–89	HR: 111–120 RR: 40–49	HR: 50–110
D	GCS ≤8	GCS: 9–13	GCS = 14	GCS = 15
E		Temperature >40 Temperature <32	Temperature: 38.1–40.0 Temperature: 32–34	Temperature: 34.1–38.0

Fig. 2: Commonly used color codes for triage.
Source: Gens PA, Herring MJ. The Color-Coded Triage System: Implementation and Outcomes. Ann Emerg Med. 2020. https://www.annemergmed.com/article/S0196-0644(19)31067-2/fulltext

SUGGESTED READING

1. Dhruva SM, Johnson JS. Emergency Triage: A Guide for Healthcare Professionals. Int J Emerg Med. 2019. https://www. ijem.org/articles/emergency-triage-guide
2. Gens PA, Herring MJ. The Color-Coded Triage System: Implementation and Outcomes. Ann Emerg Med. 2020. https://www.annemergmed.com/article/S0196-0644(19)31067-2/fulltext
3. Hick JL, Koenig KL. Triage in Emergency Medicine: A Comprehensive Overview. J Emerg Med. 2021. https:// www.jem-journal.com/article/S0736-4679(21)00220-7/fulltext
4. Richard G, Williams MM. Emergency Severity Index (ESI): A Triage Tool for Emergency Departments. Emerg Med Clin N Am. 2018. https://www.escholarship.org/uc/item/6kh0x9d3

CHAPTER 47

Medicolegal Queries with the Expert

Milind M Khadke

BOX 1: Who needs a medicolegal case (MLC)?

Here are some instances of MLCs. Medical officers should apply their professional judgment to recognize other potential cases that are not mentioned here:

- Assault and battery, including domestic violence and child abuse
- Accidents such as road traffic collisions and industrial mishaps
- Trauma cases with suspected foul play
- Electrical injuries
- Poisoning and alcohol intoxication
- Unexplained coma
- Chemical injuries
- Burns and scalds
- Sexual offenses
- Illegal abortions
- Suicide attempts
- Asphyxiation resulting from hanging, strangulation, drowning, suffocation, etc.
- Deaths in custody
- Fatalities occurring in the operating room
- Unnatural deaths
- Deaths due to snake bites or animal attacks
- Gunshot wounds
- Drug overdoses
- Substance abuse
- Patients arriving deceased at the accident and emergency room and those dying within 24 hours of admission without a definitive diagnosis

Source: Adapted from:

1. National Medical Council. (2016).
2. Subrahmanyam BV. Parikh's Textbook of Medical Jurisprudence, Forensic Medicine, and Toxicology: For classrooms and courtrooms. New Delhi: CBS Press; 2014.
3. Kannan K. Modi's A Textbook of Medical Jurisprudence and Toxicology, 27th edition. Gurugram, HR: LexisNexis India; 2022.

BOX 2: What materials need to be preserved as medicolegal evidence and for how long?

Medicolegal evidence should be preserved and then sent or handed over to investigating authorities for forensic examination and potential use in court. All evidence should be properly identified, sealed, and labeled. It must be stored securely and given to the investigating officer in charge of the case. Loss or destruction of evidence is a punishable offense under Section 201 of the Indian Penal Code (IPC). The evidence required to be preserved depends on the nature of the case.

- Injury cases, the following items should be preserved in sealed envelopes:
  - Clothing worn by the patient that shows evidence of injury, such as tears, bullet holes, cuts, or bloodstains
  - For multiple tears, cuts, or holes, each piece of evidence should be encircled and numbered with a matching description in the MLC report and case sheet.
  - Bullets recovered from the body should be marked with an initial or a specific mark on the bottom before preservation
  - All collected evidence should be documented in medicolegal records to establish the chain of custody for court proceedings
- In suspected poisoning cases, the following items should be preserved and forwarded for forensic examination:
  - Gastric lavage, gastric contents, vomitus, and soiled clothing
  - Blood, urine, and any other relevant body fluids depending on the ingested poison
- In cases of burns and carbon monoxide poisoning, the following items should be preserved in sealed envelopes:
  - Articles contaminated with flammable substances, such as burnt pieces of clothing or scalp hair
  - Blood (not serum) for carbon monoxide level analysis
- In sexual offense cases, the following items should be preserved in sealed envelopes:
  - Clothing worn by the patient that shows evidence of bloodstains, seminal stains, mud stains, tears, or cuts
  - Vaginal swabs, preferably from the posterior fornix, or anal swabs

Source: Adapted from National Medical Commission (2016).

BOX 3: Do medicolegal documents need to be preserved and for how long?

Indian Medical Council (Professional Conduct, Ethics and Etiquettes) Regulations 2002 prescribe a period of 3 years for preserving medical records of inpatient department (IPD) patients. However, in MLCs, the documents have to be preserved for a longer period

- Original copies of all medicolegal documents must be produced whenever requested in a court of law
- All original copies of certificates and reports issued for medicolegal purposes should be preserved until the case is finalized in court

Also, it is mandatory to take the acknowledgment from the relatives of having received a copy of medical records and preserve the receipt

BOX 4: What needs to be done with a brought-dead patient coming to emergency room (ER) in regards to issuing a death certificate?

- All brought dead patients are labeled as MLCs
- Death certificate should not be issued
- Send Police information form immediately
- Waiver of postmortem examination lies on the investigating authorities and not the doctor

BOX 5: Negligence commonly seen in ER physicians.

Inability to do the following things can amount to negligence of duties for the physician:

- Refuse to admit patient if requisite infrastructure/expertise/consultant is unavailable. Although the patient should be given first aid as required before moving the patient out
- Take requisite and timely efforts to detect the issues of patient
- Keep patient or attendant informed
- On diagnosing, take corrective steps promptly and act in accordance to medical science and medical practice. An error of judgment is acceptable but certainly not negligence
- Do not make attempts to cover or conceal the facts
- Obtain high-risk informed consent from patient/relatives
- Obtain fresh consent before any intervention, be it minor or major
- At times, risk will have to be taken but standard protocols have to be followed and there must be sound justifications for every act of omission or commission
- Delay, if any, should have a justifiable reason. Convey the reasons for delay to patient/attendant appropriately

BOX 6: Important consents for an ER physician.

Take consent only of adult/conscious/oriented patient or else the relative can give the consent.

- General consent
- Consent before any intervention, minor or major
- Consent before any surgery, minor or major
- Consent for blood transfusion
- High-risk informed consents in critically ill patients
- Any refusal/delay from the patients or attendants for any investigation or intervention should be specifically recorded in the medical records
- Consent should be signed for refusal to get admitted when the doctor has advised to admit the patient for treatment or observation
- Consent while patient/relatives want to move to another hospital

BOX 7: If patient absconds or is missing?

- If a patient is reported missing from the hospital, all efforts should first be made by the hospital to locate them. Information about the patient's absence must be communicated to the doctor, relatives, security officer, and administration. The patient or their relatives should also be contacted directly
- When all efforts to locate the patient fail, he/she will be discharged in absentia
- In case of MLCs, the Police need to be informed even if MLC intimated earlier
- In case of absconding non-MLC, same information is to be send to the Police without labeling it as MLC
- If the patient returns to the hospital after being discharged in absentia, they will be readmitted for further treatment if necessary

BOX 8: If patient sustains injury while in the hospital?

All injuries sustained in the hospital need not be reported to the Police. But all falls leading to injuries should be reported. Discretion must be exercised but in case of dilemma, it is better to inform the Police.

SUGGESTED READING

1. Bajpai M (Ed). MedLegal Year Book 2023. Mumbai: Institute of Medicine and Law; 2023.
2. Desai K. (2024). Section 201 IPC: Causing Disappearance of Evidence and Giving False Information. [online]. Available from https://www.legalserviceindia.com/legal/article-3009-section-201-ipc-causing-disappearance-of-evidence-and-giving-false-information.html [Last accessed September, 2024].
3. National Health Systems Resource Centre. (2022). Right to Health: Indian Legislations and International Documents. [online] Available from http;//qps.nhsrcindia.org/sites/default/files/2022-01/medico_legal.pdf [Last accessed September, 2024].
4. National Medical Commission. (2016). Indian Medical Council (Professional Conduct, Ethics, and Etiquette) Regulations, 2002. Guidelines on preserving medical records of IPD patients and medicolegal cases. [online]. Available from https://www.nmc.org.in/wp-content/uploads/2017/10/Ethics-Regulations-2002.pdf [Last accessed September, 2024].
5. US Department of Justice. National Institute of Justice. (2011). Crime Scene Investigation: A Guide for Law Enforcement. [online] Available from https://www.ojp.gov/pdffiles1/nij/178280.pdf [Last accessed September, 2024].
6. World Health Organization (WHO). (2014). Guidelines for medico-legal care for victims of sexual violence. [online] Available from https://iris.who.int/bitstream/handle/10665/42788/924154628X.pdf [Last accessed September, 2024].

Index

Page numbers followed by *b* refer to box, *f* refer to figure, *fc* refer to flowchart, and *t* refer to table.

A

C

D

E

G

H

I

J

K

L

Q

R

S

T

V

W

X

Z